Practical Atlas of

RETINAL DISEASE
AND THERAPY

Second Edition

Practical Atlas of
RETINAL DISEASE
AND THERAPY

Second Edition

Editor

William R. Freeman, M.D.
Professor of Ophthalmology
Department of Ophthalmology
University of California, San Diego
Shiley Eye Center
La Jolla, California

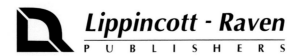

Lippincott - Raven
PUBLISHERS

Acquisitions Editor: Elizabeth Greenspan
Developmental Editor: Rebecca Irwin Diehl
Manufacturing Manager: Dennis Teston
Production Manager: Larry Bernstein
Production Editor: Erin McKenna
Cover Designer: Patti Gast
Indexer: Sandi Frank
Compositor: Maryland Composition
Printer: Phoenix Offset Ltd.

Printed in Hong Kong, P.R.C.

9 8 7 6 5 4 3 2 1

Library of Congress Cataloging-in-Publication Data
Practical atlas of retinal disease and therapy / editor, William R.
    Freeman. — 2nd ed.
        p.   cm.
    Includes bibliographical references and index.
    ISBN 0-397-51841-2
    1. Retina—Diseases—Atlases.   I. Freeman, William R.
    [DNLM: 1. Retinal Diseases—diagnosis—atlases.   2. Retinal
Diseases—therapy—atlases.   WW 17 P895 1997]
RE551.P73   1997
617.7´35—dc21
DNLM/DLC
for Library of Congress

To

My colleagues and students who have continually challenged and stimulated me.

My loving parents, Joseph and Mona, who instilled in me the desire to learn and the enjoyment of teaching.

My wife, Karen, who works to keep the balance in life and who has kept my family centered.

My children, Elana and Sam, whose love for life and each other is so radiant and who have brought more joy into my life than I could possibly have imagined. They have given me far more than I could ever give them and I am so happy to be able to be here for them.

Contents

Contributors

Gary W. Abrams, M.D.   *Professor and Chairman, Department of Ophthalmology, Kresge Eye Institute, Wayne State University, 4717 St. Antoine, Detroit, Michigan 48201*

Everett Ai, M.D.   *Director, Retina Unit, Department of Ophthalmology, California Pacific Medical Center, 1 Daniel Burnham Court, San Francisco, California 94109*

James J. Augsburger, M.D.   *Associate Clinical Professor of Ophthalmology, Oncology Unit/Retina Service, Wills Eye Hospital, 900 Walnut Street, Philadelphia, Pennsylvania 19107*

Dirk-Uwe Bartsch, M.D.   *Shiley Eye Center, University of California, San Diego, 9500 Gilman Drive, La Jolla, CA 92093–0946*

Neil M. Bressler, M.D.   *Professor of Ophthalmology, Wilmer Ophthalmological Institute, Johns Hopkins University School of Medicine and Hospital, 9th fl., 550 North Broadway, Baltimore, Maryland 21205*

Gary C. Brown, M.D.   *910 East Willow Grove Avenue, Windmore, Pennsylvania 19038*

Steve Charles, M.D.   *Clinical Professor, Department of Ophthalmology, University of Tennessee, Memphis, 6401 Popular Ave, #190, Memphis, Tennessee 38119*

Serge de Bustros, Jr., M.D.   *Director, The Retina Center, The Community Hospital, Munster, Indiana, Senior Physician, Illinois Retina Associates, The Ingalls Hospital, Harvey, Illinois, and Associate Professor of Ophthalmology, Rush Medical College, Chicago, Illinois 60602*

Eugene de Juan, Jr., M.D.   *Professor of Ophthalmology, Wilmer Eye Institute, Johns Hopkins Hospital, 600 North Wolfe Street, Maumenee 721, Baltimore, Maryland 21287*

Ann E. Elsner, PH.D.   *Associate Scientist, Schepens Eye Research Institute, Harvard Medical School, 20 Staniford St, Boston, Massachusetts 02114*

Daniel Finkelstein, M.D.   *Wilmer Eye Institute, Johns Hopkins Hospital, 600 North Wolfe Street, Baltimore, Maryland 21287*

William R. Freeman, M.D.   *Professor of Ophthalmology, Chief of Retina Service, Department of Ophthalmology, University of California, San Diego, 9415 Campus Point Drive, La Jolla, California 92093*

Alan H. Friedman, M.D.   *Clinical Professor, Department of Ophthalmology and Pathology, Mt. Sinai School of Medicine, Box 1183, New York, New York 10029*

Louis C. Glazer, M.D.   *Kresge Eye Institute, Wayne State University, 4717 St. Antoine, Detroit, MI 48201*

Dennis P. Han, M.D.   *Professor of Ophthalmology, Department of Ophthalmology, Medical College of Wisconsin, 925 N. 87th Street, Milwaukee, Wisconsin 53226*

M. Elizabeth Hartnett, M.D. *Schepens Retina Associates, 100 Charles River Plaza, Boston, MA 02114*

Alexander Irvine, M.D. *Professor of Ophthalmology, Department of Ophthalmology, University of California, San Francisco, 400 Parnassus Avenue, #750 A, San Francisco, California 94143*

Lee M. Jampol, M.D. *Louis Feinberg Professor and Chairman, Department of Ophthalmology, Northwestern University, 645 N. Michigan Ave., Chicago, Illinois 60611*

Ingrid Kreissig, M.D. *Department of Ophthalmology, University Eye Clinic, 72076 Tübingen, Germany; and Department of Ophthalmology, New York Hospital-Cornell University Medical Center, New York, NY 10016*

H. Michael Lambert, M.D. *Baylor College of Medicine, 6501 Fannin NC 200, Houston, Texas 77030*

John S. Lean, M.D. *23521 Paseo de Valencia, Suite 207, Laguna Hills, California 92653*

Hilel Lewis, M.D. *Professor and Chairman, Department of Ophthalmology, The Cleveland Clinic Foundation, 9500 Euclid Avenue, Cleveland, Ohio 44195*

Harvey A. Lincoff, M.D. *Professor of Ophthalmology, Department of Ophthalmology, Cornell University Medical College/The New York Hospital, 525 E. 68th St., New York, New York 10021*

Anat Loewenstein, M.D. *Wilmer Ophthalmological Institute, Johns Hopkins Hospital, Baltimore, MD 21287*

Kenneth G. Noble, M.D. *Associate Professor of Clinical Ophthalmology, Department of Ophthalmology, New York University Medical Center, 161 Madison Avenue, New York, New York 10016*

German Sanchez, M.D. *Asociacion Para Evitar la Ceguera en Mexico, Mexico City, Mexico.*

Paul Sternberg, Jr., M.D. *Department of Ophthalmology, Emory University, Atlanta, GA 30322*

John J. Weiter, M.D., Ph.D. *Retina Specialists of Boston, 100 Charles River Plaza, Boston, MA 02114*

Byron Wood *Charles Retina Institute, Memphis, TN 38119*

Foreword

In the four years since the publication of this practical atlas, there have been many advances in vitre-oretinal surgery and in our understanding and treatment of retinal diseases. The second edition has successfully incorporated these developments by adding four new chapters and by updating the first 18 chapters, which comprise the first edition. All chapters are illustrated and written in a style that allows the reader to quickly grasp the concepts described and to simultaneously visualize them. The succinct yet encompassing text coupled with the presentation of a wealth of excellent color illustrations make this book unique and valuable.

Stephen J. Ryan, M.D.
Professor of Ophthalmology
University of Southern California
School of Medicine

Preface to the First Edition

Retinal diseases play an increasingly important role in ophthalmology, accounting for the most common causes of blindness in the developed world. With the evolution of new diagnostic and therapeutic modalities, the ophthalmologist has become more involved in diagnostic and therapeutic decision-making for patients with retinal disease. The challenge facing the physician lies in maintaining up-to-date, practical knowledge of retinal diseases.

The *Practical Atlas of Retinal Disease and Therapy* was designed to combine the best features of traditional atlases and textbooks. Each chapter is written as a stand-alone reference that will enable the ophthalmologist to acquire a comprehensive understanding of the disease discussed. At the same time, the combination of informative yet practical material, and numerous strategically-placed color photographs, will guide the physician to a rapid diagnosis of specific disease entities and to a determination of therapeutic strategies. The reader can either concentrate on an entire chapter or browse leisurely through the text for entities of interest.

The most common retinal diseases have been grouped into 18 chapters, each written by an internationally acknowledged expert. The authors have presented the material to provide the reader with a quick but comprehensive review of the major issues. The extensive use of color photographs facilitates recognition of specific disease entities. This pragmatic atlas provides an understanding of retinal diseases, so important to the everyday practice of ophthalmology. Ophthalmologists from residents to generalists to vitreoretinal surgeons will find this book of interest.

William R. Freeman, M.D.

Preface

Retinal diseases remain the most common causes of blindness in the developed world. With the evolution of new diagnostic and therapeutic modalities, the ophthalmologist has become more involved in diagnostic and therapeutic decision-making for patients with retinal disease. In the four years since publication of the practical atlas, our understanding of many diseases has changed. New therapies have become available such as macular hole surgery and surgery for age-related macular degeneration. The challenge facing the physician lies in maintaining up-to-date, practical knowledge of retinal diseases.

The Practical Atlas of Retinal Disease and Therapy was designed to combine the best features of traditional atlases and textbooks. We recognize that the mind does not know what the eye has not seen and thus have heavily illustrated the book. Each chapter is written as a stand-alone reference that will enable the ophthalmologist to acquire a comprehensive understanding of the disease discussed. At the same time, the combination of informative yet practical material and numerous strategically-placed color photographs will guide the reader to a better understanding of retinal disease and allow more effective therapy.

Acknowledgments

For this second edition, I have once again relied on my friends and colleagues to provide for the reader a succinct atlas/text. The strength of this book lies in the authors who are all excellent educators and innovators in the field of retinal diseases. I would like to take this opportunity to thank each of them for their time and effort but most of all for their dedication to seeing our field progress.

To say that my family has been supportive of this and my other professional endeavors would be an understatement. In truth, it has been a pleasure to put this book together and to work with my colleagues and co-authors all of whom I respect and admire. My family has been my inspiration to seek out new and exciting things in life. My wife Karen has helped me raise these two gems with great dedication and care; she commands much respect for her sophisticated ways of dealing with people. My son, Samuel, who was just born at the time the first edition went to press has turned out to be an immense joy. Always happy and positive he is the epitome of the sun shining through. My daughter Elana, now seven shows us all so much love and joy that problems melt away. Y por las cosas buenas que contigo vivi.

I should also thank some of the many people who have worked with me in such a dedicated way in the area of research and teaching here at the University of California at San Diego. Dirk-Uwe Bartsch, Germaine Bergeron Lynn, David Munguia and the current fellows who have helped me with the editing of this book: Chris Macdonald, Lingyun Cheng, Caesar Avila, and Marietta Karavellas.

And to Harvey Lincoff, M.D. who has done so much and still has so much more to offer. He has been an inspiration for lifelong clinical practice, research and teaching and for other lessons in life.

Practical Atlas of Retinal Disease and Therapy, Second Edition
edited by William R. Freeman,
Lippincott–Raven Publishers, Philadelphia © 1997.

· 1 ·

Hereditary Chorioretinal Dystrophies

Kenneth G. Noble

INTRODUCTION

The hereditary chorioretinal dystrophies encompass a wide variety of disorders with many unusual, perhaps unique, fundus manifestations. As such, they provide a fascinating subject for an atlas. However, it would be a great mistake to place too much emphasis on the fundus morphology, since there may be considerable morphologic mimicking. This becomes apparent when one looks at the differential diagnosis of various appearances as illustrated in the tables included in this chapter.

A careful directed history can be very helpful in providing clues to the disease. In addition, because the majority of these disorders involve visual dysfunction (that can occur at any level of visual processing), visual function testing (psychophysical and electrophysiologic) is often critical in making the correct diagnosis.

For the purposes of this atlas, the emphasis will be on the fundus appearance. When appropriate, ancillary diagnostic tests (with examples) are included.

CLASSIFICATION

In this chapter, dystrophies are divided into two large groups. The first are the generalized dystrophies in which there is diffuse visual dysfunction, and tests of general retinal function are abnormal. The second are the localized dystrophies that usually affect the macula and posterior pole. The results of tests of generalized retinal function are normal or reflect the amount of total retina affected. Unaffected areas have normal retinal function and usually remain normal.

The extent of involvement does not always correspond to the fundus examination. In this regard, the full-field electroretinogram (ERG) is the single most important test to distinguish between these two groups. As a test of generalized retinal function, the ERG is abnormal in the generalized dystrophies and normal or nearly normal in the localized dystrophies. For each entity, the inheritance is noted as AD (autosomal dominant), AR (autosomal recessive), or XLR (X-linked recessive).

GENERALIZED DYSTROPHIES

Retinitis Pigmentosa (Rod–Cone Dystrophy) (AD, AR, and XLR)

Retinitis pigmentosa (RP) is the most common hereditary chorioretinal dystrophy and serves as the prototype for these disorders. The clinical history and fundus appearance probably represent several diseases, since it is inherited in the three Mendelian modes and is associated with numerous and varied ocular and systemic disorders (Table 1). Recent molecular genetic studies have demonstrated at least eight different chromosomes that are associated with this disorder. In addition to this genetic (nonallelic or locus) heterogeneity, there is allelic heterogeneity as exemplified by the many different mutations seen in the rhodopsin gene.

The typical history is the onset of progressive poor night vision (occasionally poor peripheral vision) in the first or second decade of life. Central visual loss is rarely the presenting symptom (except with inverse RP or cone–rod dystrophy), and visual acuity is usually preserved until the later stages.

The fundus appearance includes the classic triad of (1) attenuated arterioles, (2) bone spicule pigmentation (mostly paravenular and midperipheral), and (3) waxy pallor of the optic disc (Fig. 1). Other fundus findings can occur in the (1) macula (preretinal gliosis, pigment atrophy, and cystoid macular edema), (2) vitreous (fine pigmented cells, posterior vitreous detachment, gelatinous condensations, and veils), (3) optic nerve (optic nerve drusen), and (4) periphery (Coats-like response; choroidal atrophy, which occurs late in the course).

The XLR RP female carrier may show a fundus abnormality, either (1) patchy and focal areas of pigment alter-

K.G. Noble, M.D.: Department of Ophthalmology, New York University Medical Center, New York, New York 10016.

TABLE 1. *Pigmentary retinopathy in systemic diseases*

Metabolic disorders	Hereditary ataxias
Lipid abnormalities	Friedreich's
Bassen–Kornzweig syndrome[a]	Pierre–Marie
Refsum's disease[a]	Spastic paraplegia
Batten's syndrome	Pallidal degeneration
Haltia–Santavuori (early infancy)	External ophthalmoplegia (with or without cardiac abnormalities)
Jansky–Bielschowsky (late infancy)	Usher's syndrome
Spielmeyer–Sjögren (early childhood)	Alström's disease
Miscellaneous rare associations	Miscellaneous rare associations
Hooft's disease	Cockayne's syndrome
Letterer–Siwe disease	Charcot–Marie–Tooth syndrome
Pelizaeus–Merzbacher disease	Flynn–Aird syndrome
Mucopolysaccharide (MPS) abnormalities	Marinesco–Sjögren syndrome
MPS I-H (Hurler)	Sjögren–Larsson syndrome
MPS I-S (Scheie)	
MPS II (Hunter)	*Renal or hepatic disorders*
MPS III (Sanfilippo)	Medullary cystic disease (juvenile nephronophthisis)
Neurologic disorders	Senior–Loken syndrome
Laurence–Moon syndrome	Fanconi's syndrome
Bardet–Biedl syndrome	Alagille's syndrome
	Zellweger's (cerebrohepatorenal syndrome)

[a] Treatable disorder.

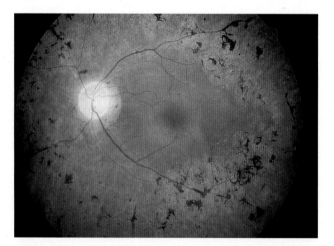

FIG. 1. The appearance of typical retinitis pigmentosa is attenuated arterioles, paravascular bone spicule pigmentation, and optic nerve pallor.

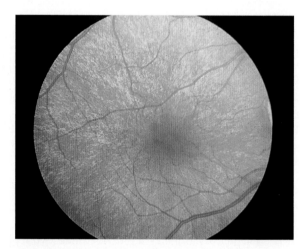

FIG. 2. X-linked retinitis pigmentosa, female carrier. The scintillating golden reflex radiates from the macula.

TABLE 2. *Golden sheen reflex*

Oguchi's disease
X-linked-recessive retinitis pigmentosa female carrier
Progressive cone dystrophies (autosomal dominant and X-linked recessive)
Stargardt's disease
Central pigmentary sheen dystrophy

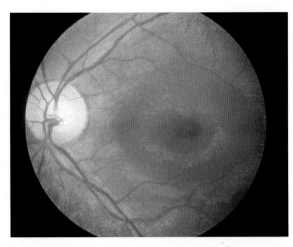

FIG. 3. Retinitis pigmentosa, inverse. Although the fundus abnormalities suggest disease localized to the posterior pole, the visual function tests confirm widespread dysfunction.

ations or (2) a scintillating golden reflex in the posterior pole (Fig. 2 and Table 2). It is important to recognize the female carrier sign because it (1) establishes the diagnosis of RP, (2) indicates the mode of inheritance, and (3) identifies women at risk for transmission of the disease.

A variant of RP has been termed inverse RP or cone–rod dystrophy because (1) the presenting symptoms are related to poor central vision, (2) the macula usually shows a fundus abnormality (Fig. 3), and (3) the ERG shows greater loss of cone-mediated than rod-mediated responses. The differential diagnosis of inverse RP includes (1) typical RP with macular degeneration, (2) progressive cone dystrophy, (3) geographic tapetoretinal dystrophies (see pseudoretinitis pigmentosa), (4) hereditary macular dystrophies, and (5) acquired macular degenerations.

A wide variety of nonocular disorders may be associated with a generalized pigmentary retinal disease that resembles RP (Table 1). The fundus appearance may be typical or atypical (Fig. 4). The two most common associations are (1) Usher's syndrome (deafness) and (2) Laurence–Moon and Bardet–Biedl syndromes (polydactyly, obesity, mental retardation, and hypogenitalism). Two less common associations are important because they are among the very few hereditary retinal dystrophies that can be treated. Abetalipoproteinemia (Bassen–Kornzweig syndrome) can be treated with intramuscular vitamin A (with a return to normal dark-adapted thresholds and an increase in the ERG response). Refsum's disease, treated with a diet low in phytanic acid, may improve the severe polyneuritis and ataxia, but probably has little effect on the associated retinal disease.

There are also some therapeutic modalities that seem effective for retinitis pigmentosa. In one study of patients with retinitis pigmentosa who met the entry criteria of age, visual field size, and ERG response, those treated with a daily regimen of oral vitamin A (retinyl palmitate) 15,000 IU had a statistically significant decrease in the rate of decline in the amplitude of the 30-Hz cone response. No other visual function study showed a statistically significant therapeutic effect. In addition, treatment for cystoid macular edema with carbonic anhydrase inhibitors seems to result in both subjective and objective visual improvement, whether the leakage occurs from the choriocapillaris through the retinal pigment epithelium (RPE) or more superficially from the perifoveal retinal capillaries. Grid laser photocoagulation has also been noted to improve or stabilize vision.

TABLE 3. *Salt-and-pepper mottling*

Syphilis
Rubella
XLR carrier RP
XLR carrier choroideremia
XLR carrier ocular albinism
Early RP
Early choroideremia
Leber's congenital amaurosis
Drug toxicity: Mellaril, Thorazine, and Clofazimine

XLR, X-linked recessive; RP, retinitis pigmentosa.

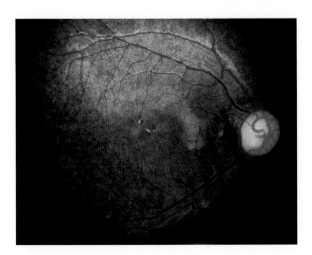

FIG. 4. Retinitis pigmentosa and systemic disease. This girl had progressive external ophthalmoplegia in association with a granular fundus and moderate reduction in the electroretinogram.

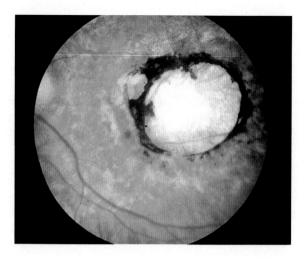

FIG. 5. Leber's congenital amaurosis with macula "coloboma." This man, like his sister, has congenital poor vision and nystagmus, an extinguished electroretinogram, and bilateral macular coloboma.

Leber's Congenital Amaurosis (AR)

Leber's congenital amaurosis probably represents a number of different diseases that share the syndrome features of (1) connatal pendular nystagmus, (2) connatal poor vision (usually profound), and (3) an absent or markedly abnormal ERG. The fundus findings are quite variable, with the most consistent finding being arteriolar narrowing. The pigment abnormalities may be very mild [salt-and-pepper mottling (Table 3)], they develop into an RP picture with pigment migration, or, in the extreme situation, there may be extensive and diffuse chorioretinal atrophy. An unusual finding is bilateral "coloboma"-like macular lesions (Fig. 5).

Pseudoretinitis Pigmentosa

Pseudo-RP is the name applied to a heterogeneous group of diseases of various etiologies (Table 4). These different diseases share only one thing in common—a fundus appearance that resembles or suggests RP. Carefully recording the patient's medical history is essential, and the ERG is often critical, since in the great majority of these diseases it will be normal or nearly normal. When the ERG is abnormal, the implicit time (measured from stimulus onset to the peak of the b wave) will usually be normal. All cases of a uniocular RP picture (Table 4) are always pseudo-RP, since RP is never truly uniocular.

The group of disorders most difficult to distinguish from RP are the geographic RPE dystrophies that have a particular and characteristic pigment distribution. The pigment may be exclusively along the retinal veins in pigmented paravenous chorioretinal atrophy (AD) (Fig. 6); in the inferior

TABLE 4. *Pseudo-retinitis pigmentosa*

Inflammations
  Syphilis
  Rubella

Drugs
  Phenothiazines
    Thioridazine (Mellaril)
    Chlorpromazine (Thorazine)
  4-Aminoquinolone
    Chloroquine
    Hydroxychloroquine
  Deferoxamine (Desferal)
  Clofazimine (Lamprene)

Resolution of retinal detachments
  Rhegmatogenous
  Nonrhegmatogenous
    Vogt–Koyanagi–Harada syndrome
    Uveal effusion
    Toxemia of pregnancy

Hereditary retinal dystrophies
  Fundus flavimaculatus
  Pigmented paravenous chorioretinal atrophy
  Geographic pigmentary dystrophies
  Female carriers
    Retinitis pigmentosa
    Choroideremia

Acquired retinal degenerations
  Peripheral reticular pigmentary degeneration
  Peripheral paving stone degeneration

Uniocular
  Trauma
    Contusion
    Intraocular metallic foreign body
    Ophthalmic artery occlusion
  Inflammation
    Chorioretinitis
    Diffuse unilateral subacute neuroretinitis
    Posterior scleritis
    Sympathetic uveitis

retina in sector RP (AD) (Fig. 7); or in a pericentral, central, or peripapillary distribution (AD and AR) (Fig. 8).

Most drugs that result in retinal toxicity are taken up by the RPE and slowly excreted. Both the daily dose and the total dose are important factors in determining the likelihood of toxicity. Progression of the retinopathy may continue following cessation. One of the more common retinotoxic drugs is thioridazine (Mellaril), which can cause numerous pigment alterations, including a salt-and-pepper mottling (Table 3), heavy pigment accumulation, a nummular area of chorioretinal atrophy, and diffuse chorioretinal atrophy (Fig. 9).

Congenital Stationary Night Blindness

Normal Fundus (AD, AR, and XLR)

As the name denotes, the history of congenital stationary night blindness is one of nonprogressive night-vision diffi-

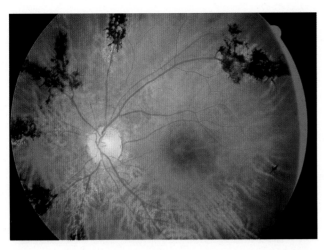

FIG. 6. Pigmented paravenous chorioretinal atrophy. Bone corpuscle pigmentation accumulates exclusively along the distribution of the veins, invariably beginning at some distance from the optic nerve. Variable degrees of chorioretinal atrophy may be present adjacent to the perivenular pigment abnormalities and surrounding the disc.

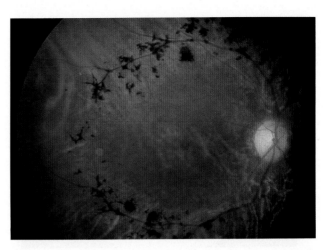

FIG. 8. Pericentral (peripapillary, annular) pigment degeneration. The pigment abnormalities emanate from the disc along the temporal vascular arcades and nasal to the disc. There is a mild pigment atrophy of the macula.

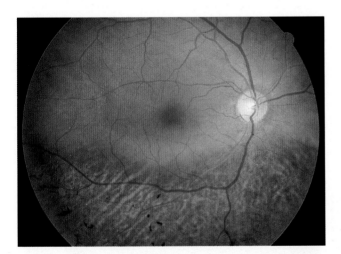

FIG. 7. Sector retinitis pigmentosa. The inferior retina is affected by a pigmentary retinopathy, whereas the superior portion is normal.

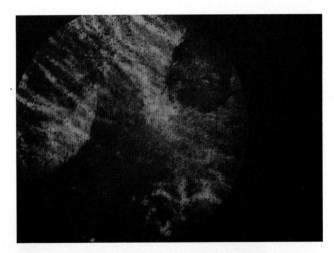

FIG. 9. Thioridazine (Mellaril) chorioretinal toxicity. Many of the pigment abnormalities seen in thioridazine chorioretinal toxicity are evident—a nummular chorioretinal atrophy, heavy pigment accumulation, and a coarse salt-and-pepper mottling.

Text continues on the following page

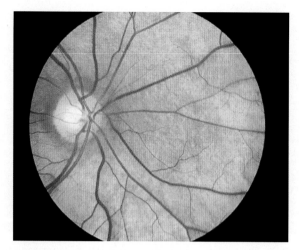

FIG. 10. Oguchi's disease. The characteristic golden metallic fundus appearance brings the retinal vessels into high relief.

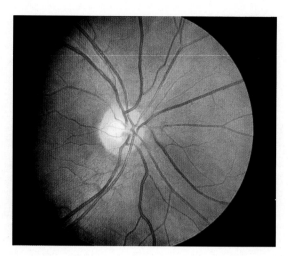

FIG. 11. Oguchi's disease (Mizuo's phenomenon). After 3 hours of dark adaptation, the abnormal retinal reflex seen in Fig. 10 has disappeared, and the fundus color appears normal.

culties beginning in early childhood. When associated with a normal fundus, visual diagnostic tests establish that there is a defect in neural transmission at either the photoreceptor or the midretinal level in each inherited type.

normal) or to visual function studies (that show a delay in neural network adaptation).

Oguchi's Disease (AR)

Oguchi's disease has a very characteristic yellowish metallic sheen (Fig. 10) (Table 2), which reverts to a normal fundus color after prolonged dark adaptation (Mizuo's phenomenon) (Fig. 11). On reexposure to light, the fundus slowly resumes this metallic yellow color. The appearance and disappearance of the abnormal fundus color are apparently unrelated to rhodopsin photopigment kinetics (that are

Fundus Albipunctatus (AR)

Fundus albipunctatus shows multiple, small, round, white dots that are monotonous in their regularity and conformity. They usually spare the macula and extend into the midperiphery (Fig. 12A). On fluorescein angiography (FA), there may be a mottling of the background choroidal fluorescence and small areas of irregular transmission, but none of the findings correspond to the observed white dots (Fig. 12B). Visual function studies demonstrate a prolonged regenera-

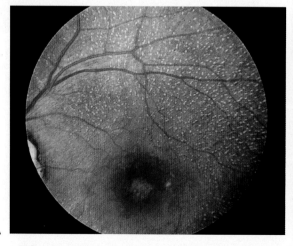

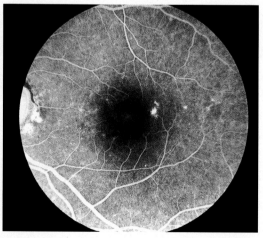

FIG. 12. Fundus albipunctatus. Small, round, white dots are seen throughout the posterior pole, sparing the macula (**A**). Fluorescein angiography shows a few areas of transmission hyperfluorescence that do not correspond to the fundus lesions (**B**).

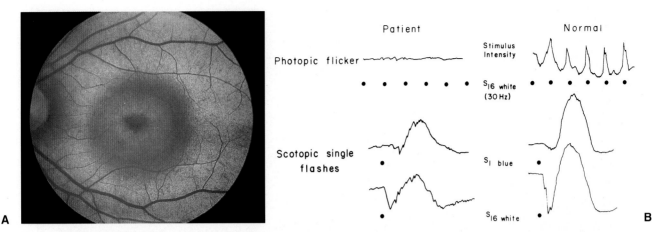

FIG. 13. Progressive cone dystrophies. This patient has two features of a progressive dystrophy: a bull's eye maculopathy and a golden reflex (**A**). However, the diagnosis is confirmed by an electroretinogram that shows an absent cone-mediated photopic flicker response and a minimally reduced rod-mediated scotopic response (**B**).

tion of cone and rod photopigments that presumably accounts for the prolonged adaptation.

Cone Dysfunction Diseases

Achromatopsia (Rod Monochromatism) (AR)

This congenital stationary disorder is characterized by (1) poor vision (20/200) and nystagmus since birth, (2) day blindness (hemeralopia) and sensitivity to light, and (3) absent color discrimination. The fundus is usually normal or may show a very mild maculopathy that is out of proportion to the visual findings. An ERG confirms the diagnosis of a diffuse cone dysfunction with an absent photopic flicker response (to a 30-Hz stimulus) and a normal scotopic response.

Progressive Cone Dystrophies (AD, AR, and XLR)

The onset of symptoms occurs in the second to fourth decades, with progressive loss of central vision and color discrimination. Nystagmus is usually not present, and hemeralopia and photosensitivity are usual additional symptoms. The fundus findings are variable, including (1) a normal appearance, (2) a nonspecific maculopathy, (3) a bull's eye maculopathy (Table 5), and (4) a golden tapetal reflex (Table 2) (Fig. 13A). Regardless of the fundus picture, the diagnosis is made by using the ERG, which shows a diffuse dysfunction of the cones with an abnormal photopic flicker follow response and a well-preserved scotopic response (Fig. 13B).

Choroidal Dystrophies

This large group of disorders is characterized by the appearance of choroidal atrophy early in the course of the dis-

ease. FA is particularly helpful, since choriocapillaris atrophy is most apparent. The putative pathogenesis is that the primary process is choroidal atrophy (an abiotrophy or dystrophy), which results in secondary RPE and photoreceptor degeneration.

Choroideremia (XLR)

The early stages of choroideremia may be confused with RP, since these patients may present with the onset of progressive night-vision and peripheral vision loss in association with diffuse pigmentary abnormalities and an extinguished ERG (Fig. 14A). However, FA demonstrates diffuse choriocapillaris atrophy (Fig. 14B), a distinctly uncommon finding in early RP. With disease progression, choroidal atrophy becomes more apparent. Beginning in the midperiphery, the atrophy spreads peripherally and centrally, with the central macula preserved until late in the course (Fig. 15).

The typical fundus appearance of the female carrier is a diffuse pigment granularity (Table 3), which is located midperipherally and is nonprogressive and unassociated with visual dysfunction. Rarely, progressive focal areas of choroidal atrophy (with abnormal visual function) can occur, and this mosaicism is explained by the Lyon hypothesis of random X-chromosome inactivation (Fig. 16).

TABLE 5. *Bull's eye maculopathy*

Age-related macular degeneration
Stargardt's disease
Progressive cone dystrophy
Chloroquine-induced toxicity
Benign concentric annular macular dystrophy
Trauma

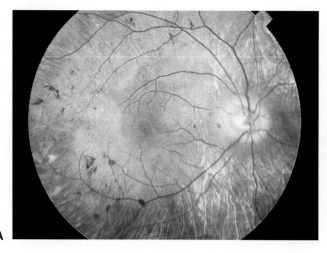
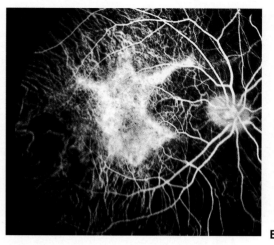

FIG. 14. Choroideremia. The posterior pole shows grayish green associated with perivenular bone spicule pigmentation not unlike that seen in retinitis pigmentosa (**A**). However, the fluorescein angiography shows diffuse choriocapillaris atrophy, sparing only the macula (**B**).

Gyrate Atrophy (AR)

This generalized choroidal dystrophy has the same symptom complex as RP and choroideremia. Unlike these other diseases, gyrate atrophy shows well-demarcated scalloped areas of choroidal atrophy with a hyperpigmented border separating normal and abnormal-appearing tissue (Fig. 17A). The lesions begin as isolated areas in the midperiphery that merge to form a garland wreath, with progression peripherally and centrally, sparing the macula until late in the disease.

FA demonstrates the sharp demarcation between normal and abnormal tissue, the former showing the normal background choroidal fluorescence and the latter showing choriocapillaris atrophy (Fig. 17B). Thus, the normal choriocapillaris background fluorescence in the early stages of gyrate atrophy is in contradistinction to the diffuse choriocapillaris atrophy in the early stages of choroideremia.

All patients with gyrate atrophy demonstrate a deficient enzyme, ornithine aminotransferase, which results in an increase in ornithine in all body fluids. In some individuals, the coenzyme vitamin B_6 (pyridoxine) stimulates activity of residual ornithine aminotransferase with a subsequent decrease in ornithine. In vitamin B_6-unresponsive patients, a low-protein diet (to restrict arginine intake) will decrease ornithine.

Generalized Choroidal Dystrophy (AD and AR)

Generalized choroidal dystrophy is usually noted in middle age in mildly symptomatic individuals who show a predominantly peripapillary or pericentral distribution of choroidal atrophy. Gradually, these areas enlarge to involve eventually the entire retina (Fig. 18A). The choroidal atrophy is vividly seen on FA (Fig. 18B).

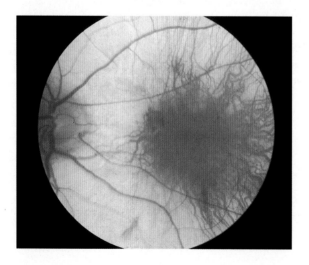

FIG. 15. Choroideremia, late stages. There is total choroidal atrophy throughout, revealing the bare white sclera. The macula is the only region with some choroid remaining.

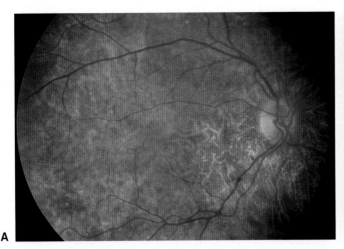
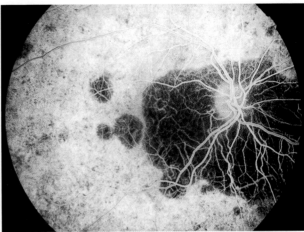

FIG. 16. Choroideremia, female carrier. This carrier has increasing visual symptoms in association with a granular salt-and-pepper fundus and peripapillary choroidal atrophy (**A**). Angiography demonstrates peripapillary and focal areas of choriocapillaris atrophy that have been increasing over time (**B**).

Crystalline Retinopathy (of Bietti) (AR)

Crystalline retinopathy is usually confined to the posterior pole, but it can progress into the periphery. The typical fundus appearance—yellow glistening intraretinal crystals in the posterior pole adjacent to areas of RPE and choroidal atrophy without crystals—confirms the diagnosis (Fig. 19A). Angiography shows transmission hyperfluorescence in the crystalline retina and choriocapillaris atrophy in the adjacent tissue (Fig. 19B).

Vitreotapetoretinal Dystrophies

The vitreotapetoretinal dystrophies are a heterogeneous group of disorders that have various vitreous abnormalities

(optically empty vitreous, fibrillar strands, vitreous veils, and sheets) in association with retinal abnormalities (retinoschisis, central and peripheral; and pigmentary dystrophy). The initial triad included juvenile retinoschisis, Goldmann–Favre disease, and Wagner's dystrophy. Additional disorders would now include Stickler's syndrome (hereditary progressive arthro-ophthalmopathy), snowflake degeneration, and AD vitreoretinochoroidopathy.

Juvenile Retinoschisis (Idiopathic Vitreous Veils) (XLR)

In this most common vitreotapetoretinal dystrophy, patients present early in life with poor vision, usually as a result of a macular schisis. The macula is elevated in a cystic appearance, with superficial linear folds radiating from the

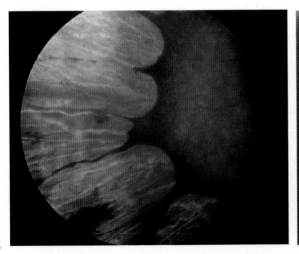
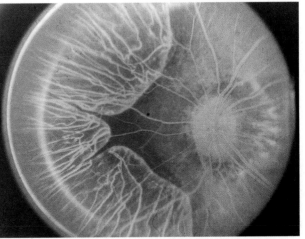

FIG. 17. Gyrate atrophy. The well-demarcated scalloped areas of choroidal atrophy are seen temporal to the macula (**A**). The sharp demarcation between the normal and abnormal choroid is confirmed on fluorescein angiography shown in the same eye, nasal to the optic disc (**B**).

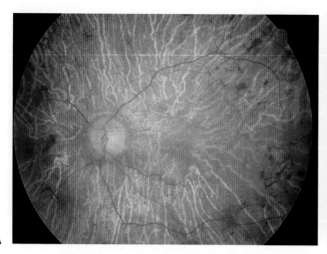
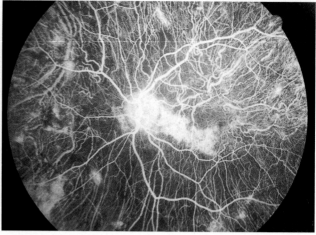

FIG. 18. Generalized choroidal dystrophy. The profound diffuse loss of choriocapillaris throughout the fundus (**A**) is best appreciated on fluorescein angiography (**B**).

fovea in a spoke-wheel fashion (Fig. 20). FA is typically normal, since the pathology is in the inner retina. In half of the patients, there is an associated peripheral schisis (of the nerve fiber layer) that is bilateral and inferotemporal, and rarely progresses to threaten central vision (Fig. 21).

When the macular schisis flattens, the resulting nonspecific maculopathy may not suggest the diagnosis (Fig. 22). This is especially true if a peripheral schisis is not present. However, the key to the diagnosis is an ERG that will always show an electronegative scotopic response (a deep negative a wave, and a b wave that does not return to the baseline) no matter what the fundus shows (Fig. 23).

Unfortunately, there are no reliable fundus findings nor visual function abnormalities that would identify female carriers.

MACULAR DYSTROPHIES

The hereditary macular dystrophies are characterized by the early onset of slowly progressive central visual loss in association with a bilateral, often symmetrical, maculopathy. The abnormal fundus picture and visual dysfunction remain confined to the macula or posterior pole. The two major differential diagnoses are acquired macular degenerations and generalized dystrophies in which the fundus abnormalities

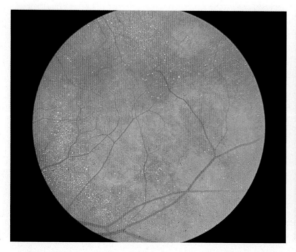
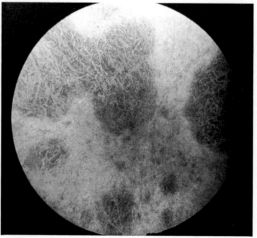

FIG. 19. Crystalline retinopathy. A comparison of the fundus (**A**) with the fluorescein angiography (**B**) demonstrates transmission hyperfluorescence in the area of the glistening yellow crystals and choriocapillaris atrophy in the adjacent areas without crystals.

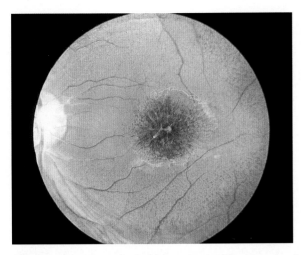

FIG. 20. Juvenile retinoschisis, macula. The macula shows linear radiating plications emanating from the fovea. There is some sheathing of the arterioles and pigment granularity of the posterior pole.

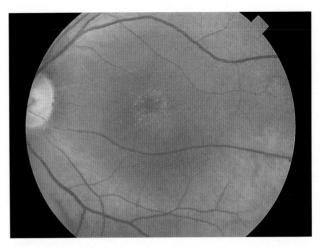

FIG. 22. Juvenile retinoschisis, flattened. The macular schisis has flattened, resulting in a few focal yellow dots.

appear confined to the macula (see inverse RP or cone–rod dystrophy).

Stargardt's Disease–Fundus Flavimaculatus (AR)

Stargardt's disease–fundus flavimaculatus is the most common hereditary macular dystrophy and serves as the prototype for these disorders. Children are symptomatic with bilateral progressive central visual loss in association with a bilateral pigmentary maculopathy, either with (Fig. 24) or without (Fig. 25A) surrounding deep yellowish-white flecks. FA may be helpful in confirming the diagnosis, since in a large majority of patients (86% in one study) there is an absence or decrease in the normal background choroidal fluorescence, with easier visualization of the retinal capillaries (the "silent" or "dark" choroid) (Fig. 25B).

Some patients have central vision preserved until later in life and present with diffuse flecks without macular degeneration (Fig. 26). These patients may ultimately develop macular degeneration.

Best's Vitelliform Macular Dystrophy (AD)

Best's vitelliform macular dystrophy is the second most common macular dystrophy and, in many ways, the most atypical. The age of onset is variable (the maculopathy has been seen shortly after birth and newly arising in the sixth decade). Vision varies considerably (from 20/20 to 20/400), fluctuates, and may improve with age. The fundus findings may be uniocular, asymmetrical, multifocal, or extramacular. Some affected individuals have normal vision and no fundus abnormalities throughout life.

The solid egg-yolk macular lesion has striking appearance

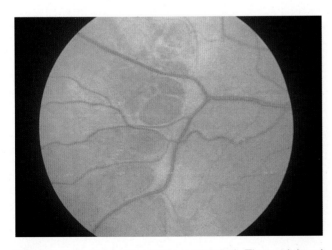

FIG. 21. Juvenile retinoschisis, peripheral. The peripheral schisis is very diaphanous and often shows superficial inner retinal holes.

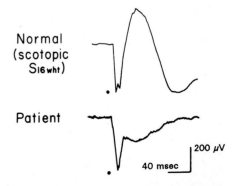

FIG. 23. Juvenile retinoschisis, electroretinogram (ERG). The key to making the diagnosis at any stage of this disease is the ERG because it will demonstrate in all patients a characteristic electronegative response (a deep a wave, and a b wave that does not return to the baseline) to a bright white flash under scotopic conditions.

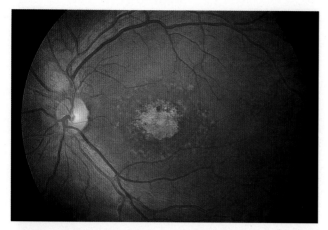

FIG. 24. Stargardt's disease–fundus flavimaculatus. The "beaten bronze" maculopathy is surrounded by parafoveal yellowish flecks.

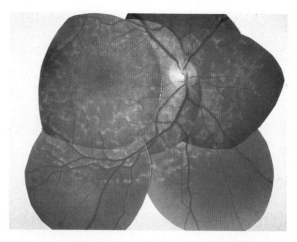

FIG. 26. Stargardt's disease–fundus flavimaculatus. Yellowish-white flecks are seen in the posterior pole, nasal to the optic disc, and beyond the temporal vascular arcades, but the macula is not affected.

(Fig. 27). However, it is not a common presentation nor is it pathognomonic (unusual morphologies of acquired macular degenerations may result in a pseudovitelliform maculopathy). When the egg yolk "ruptures," the vision declines from the previous 20/20, and the appearance has been described as a "pseudohypopion" or "scrambled egg" (Fig. 28). With resolution of the yellowish material, a nonspecific pigmentary maculopathy occurs that may be surrounded by the outline of the previous round lesion (Fig. 29). A sudden decrease in vision may be due to hemorrhage secondary to a choroidal neovascular membrane (CNVM) (Fig. 30) (Table 6).

The key to making the correct diagnosis, and establishing family members at risk, is to perform an electro-oculogram (EOG). The EOG light rise is invariably markedly abnormal in all affected individuals (the sensitivity approaches 100%), in both eyes with uniocular pathology, and in both eyes of affected individuals with a normal fundus.

Dominant Drusen of Bruch's Membrane (AD)

This disorder is usually noted fortuitously, since most individuals are asymptomatic. Therefore, the age of onset precedes the age of discovery, and the true incidence is greater than the reported incidence.

The drusen are bilateral and symmetrical, with a similar fundus morphology and topography in affected family members. They are round (unlike flecks), discrete or confluent, yellow to white, and associated with various pigment alterations. They may involve only the macula or peripapillary area, the entire posterior pole (sometimes sparing the macula), and additionally be seen in the periphery (Figs. 31 and 32).

Patients become symptomatic from degeneration of the macula caused by either yellow exudative detachments (pseudovitelliform), CNVM (Table 6), or geographic RPE and choroidal atrophy (Table 7).

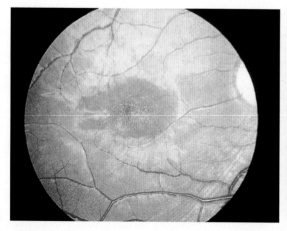

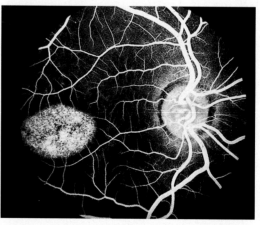

FIG. 25. Stargardt's disease–fundus flavimaculatus with a dark choroid. The pigment maculopathy is unassociated with any flecks (**A**). Fluorescein angiography shows a decrease in the background choroidal fluorescence that highlights the overlying retinal capillary circulation (**B**).

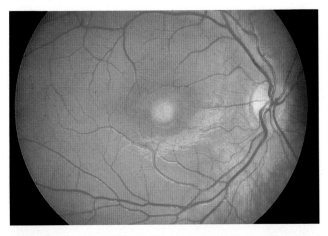

FIG. 27. Best's vitelliform macular dystrophy, egg yolk. A solid, round, yellowish lesion is present in the macula in this young boy with 20/20 vision.

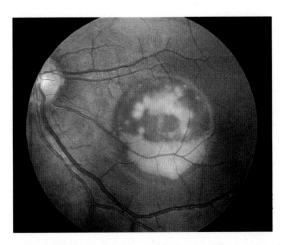

FIG. 28. Best's vitelliform macular dystrophy, pseudohypopion. The outline of the entire lesion may be seen with partial resolution of the yellowish material superiorly.

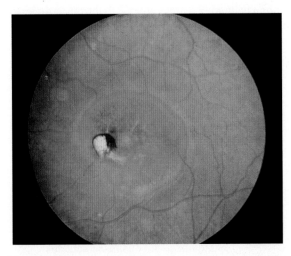

FIG. 29. Best's vitelliform macular dystrophy, atrophic stage. When the yellowish lesion has completely resolved, the atrophic changes are nonspecific. However, Best's vitelliform macular dystrophy should be suspected because of the outline of the round lesion.

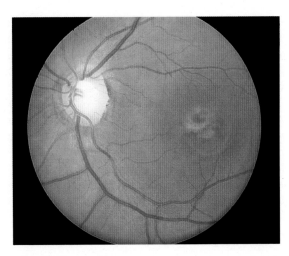

FIG. 30. Best's vitelliform macular dystrophy associated with hemorrhage. Following mild ocular trauma, this teenager noted visual loss. The subretinal hemorrhage occurred in association with a choroidal neovascular membrane.

Pigment Pattern Dystrophies (AD)

Pigment pattern dystrophies is a generic term for different dominant retinal dystrophies that share the following features: (1) variable expressivity; (2) normal or near normal vision; (3) bilateral, usually symmetrical, patterned pigment alterations (gray, black, orange, or yellow) of the macula or posterior pole; (4) normal ERG, with an occasional abnormal EOG; and (5) a benign prognosis with significant visual deterioration being unusual.

The configuration and distribution of the pigment pattern prompted the descriptive terms of butterfly dystrophy, reticular dystrophy, and macroreticular dystrophy. The pigmented pattern can be seen on funduscopy, but is graphically highlighted on FA. On occasion, sudden visual loss may result from hemorrhage due to CNVM (Table 6) (Fig. 33).

Central Areolar Choroidal Dystrophy (AD)

Central areolar choroidal dystrophy begins as a mild macular pigment granularity that progresses to a well-circumscribed area of RPE and choroidal atrophy (Fig. 34A). As

TABLE 6. *Choroidal neovascular membrane in hereditary dystrophies*

Best's vitelliform macular dystrophy
Drusen of Bruch's membrane
Hereditary hemorrhagic macular dystrophy (Sorsby's pseudoinflammatory macular dystrophy)
Fundus flavimaculatus
Pattern dystrophies of retinal pigment epithelium
Central areolar pigment epithelial dystrophy
Drusen of the optic nerve
Angioid streaks
Pathological myopia
Choroideremia

with other choroidal dystrophies, the early choroidal atrophy is appreciated by FA that demonstrates choriocapillaris atrophy (Fig. 34B). In the late stages, with further choroidal atrophy, the few remaining choroidal vessels may be seen overlying the bare sclera (Fig. 35).

There is a large differential diagnosis of central choroidal atrophy (Table 7). The diagnosis of central areolar choroidal dystrophy is confirmed by the following findings: (1) dominant inheritance; (2) bilateral, symmetrical maculopathy, confined to the posterior pole, unassociated with drusen or flecks; (3) choriocapillaris atrophy on FA; and (4) normal ERG and EOG.

Peripapillary (Pericentral) Choroidal Dystrophy (AR)

The distribution of choroidal atrophy is circumpapillary, with radiation along the temporal vascular arcades (Fig. 36). Vision is not affected until late in the course because the macula is initially spared.

Central Areolar Pigment Epithelial Dystrophy (AD)

Central areolar pigment epithelial dystrophy is either the same disorder or similar to (1) hereditary macular degeneration and aminoaciduria (dominant progressive foveal dystrophy), (2) North Carolina dystrophy and macular staphyloma (coloboma), and (3) AD central pigment epithelial and choroidal degeneration. All of these disorders have (1) variable expressivity, (2) early onset of fundus findings, (3) variable visual acuity, (4) a stable or extremely slow progression, and (5) no evidence of generalized visual dysfunction.

The fundus appearance may be mild (focal and confluent drusen and mild pigment abnormalities), moderate (CNVM, hemorrhagic maculopathy, and disciform degeneration) or marked (circumscribed area of chorioretinal atrophy—

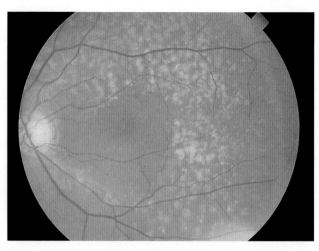

FIG. 32. Dominant drusen of Bruch's membrane. The drusen are focal and confluent, and involve the posterior and peripapillary region, but spare the macula.

staphyloma and coloboma) (Fig. 37). What is most interesting is that any type of lesion may be seen at any age, and the fundus morphology is stable and does not progress.

Hereditary Hemorrhagic Macular Dystrophy (Pseudoinflammatory Macular Dystrophy of Sorsby) (AD)

The pathogenesis of this bilateral hemorrhagic maculopathy is CNVM (Table 6), which is not associated with any other predisposing factors, such as dominant drusen, optic nerve drusen, angioid streaks, Best's vitelliform macular dystrophy, or pathologic myopia. The reparative processes suggest a postinflammatory appearance, which prompted the descriptive term "pseudoinflammatory" (Fig. 38). Whereas the initial pathology seems confined to the posterior pole, the periphery is usually subsequently involved.

TABLE 7. *Central choroidal atrophy*

Hereditary
  Primary
    Central areolar choroidal dystrophy
  Secondary
    Pigmentary dystrophies
      Retinitis pigmentosa
      X-linked recessive retinoschisis
      Favre–Goldmann syndrome
    Progressive cone dysfunction
    Macular dystrophies
      Best's vitelliform macular dystrophy
      Stargardt's—fundus flavimaculatus

Acquired
  Nonexudative macular degeneration
  Geographic, serpiginous choroidopathy
  Inflammations

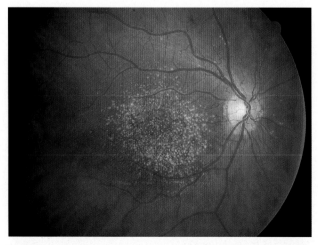

FIG. 31. Dominant drusen of Bruch's membrane. Round, yellow-white drusen are seen predominantly in the macula (a few are noted nasal to the disc) in association with mild pigmentary alterations.

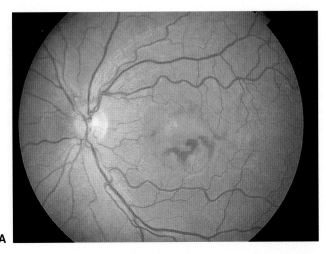
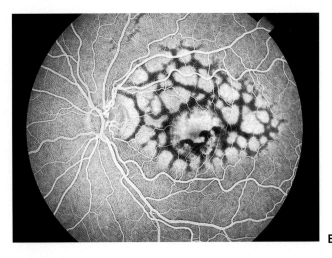

FIG. 33. Pigment pattern dystrophy. The sudden visual loss is associated with a subretinal hemorrhage in a patient with a pattern dystrophy of the posterior pole (**A**). The fluorescein angiography clearly shows the extent of the pattern (that involves a small area above the optic disc) and the association of a neovascular membrane temporal to the hemorrhage (**B**).

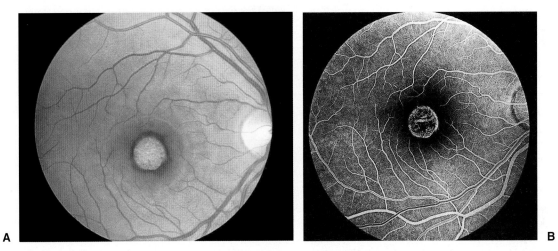

FIG. 34. Central areolar choroidal dystrophy, early. In the earlier stages, the choroidal atrophy is not as apparent on fundus examination (**A**) as it is on fluorescein angiography (**B**).

Fenestrated Sheen Macular Dystrophy (AD)

The early fundus appearance is a yellowish refractive sheen, with red fenestrations seen in the sensory retina (Fig. 39). The visual acuity is normal or near normal. One older patient showed a bull's eye maculopathy (Table 5).

MOLECULAR GENETICS

The dramatic and rapid advances in molecular genetics constitute a revolution in medicine. Nowhere has this been more profoundly felt than in the study and treatment of diseases of the eye generally and in hereditary chororetinal diseases specifically. Why is this so?

Firstly, the eye remains the only organ of the body that is available for direct visualization. This enables careful as-

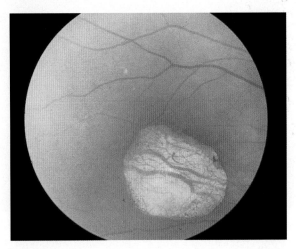

FIG. 35. Central areolar choroidal dystrophy, late. With progressive atrophy, the larger choroidal vessels are seen overlying the bare white sclera.

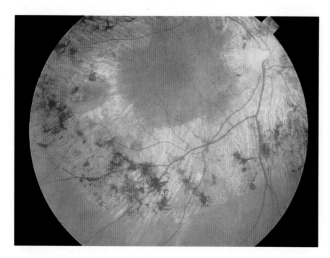

FIG. 36. Peripapillary (pericentral) choroidal dystrophy. The choroidal atrophy is well demarcated from normal tissue and surrounds the macula.

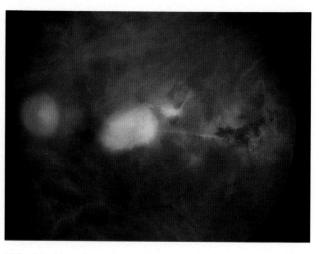

FIG. 38. Hereditary hemorrhagic macular dystrophy (pseudoinflammatory dystrophy of Sorsby). The healing stage has subretinal and intraretinal fibroproliferation in the macula and periphery that resembles some postinflammatory conditions.

sessment of the pathologic abnormalities. Secondly, a number of sophisticated tests that measure visual function, blood flow, and morphology enable a more discriminating approach to disease classification. These two features have resulted in a wide variety of large family pedigrees that have been already well studied and are ideal candidates for molecular genetic studies. Finally, an understanding of the normal visual processes (specifically phototransduction) has resulted in the identification of proteins that are potential candidates for study.

The chromosomal loci of a number of chorioretinal dystrophies have been determined by the methods of linkage analysis (and subsequently positional cloning) and by using the candidate gene approach. The chromosomal assignments for diseases mentioned in this chapter are listed in Table 8.

This listing is neither meant to be complete nor will it be in any way current because advances are too rapid for textbook publications to keep abreast. The list will inform the reader about the large number of chorioretinal dystrophies recently mapped.

The identification of a disease with a specific chromosomal locus absolutely identifies those individuals who have the disorder. In clinical terms, it confirms the correct diagnosis and avoids a mistaken diagnosis. The importance of this cannot be overemphasized. One only has to think of the role that the EOG plays in the differential diagnosis of Best's vitelliform macular dystrophy, or of ornithine levels in gyrate atrophy, to recognize how these "surrogate" genetic markers have identified affected (as well as nonaffected) individuals.

Identification of the chromosomal locus provides additional information to the family. The mode of inheritance is

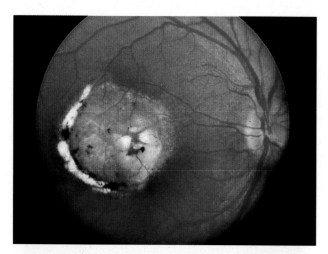

FIG. 37. Central areolar pigment epithelial dystrophy. The sharply circumscribed area of chorioretinal atrophy in the macula is the most advanced stage of central areolar pigment epithelial dystrophy (North Carolina dominant progressive foveal dystrophy). (Courtesy of Kent W. Small, M.D.).

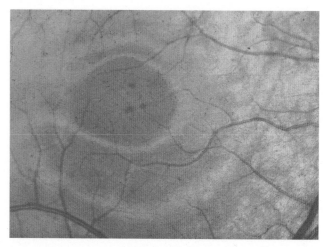

FIG. 39. Fenestrated sheen macular dystrophy. The irregular reddish lesions surrounding the fovea are in the sensory retina. (Courtesy of Frances O'Donnell, M.D.)

TABLE 8. *Chromosomal assignments of hereditary chorioretinal dystrophies*

Generalized dystrophies
 Retinitis pigmentosa
  Autosomal dominant
   3q21–q24 (rhodopsin)
   6p22.1-cen (peripherin/RDS)
   8p11–q21
   7p15.1–p13
   7q
   19q13.4
  Autosomal recessive
   3q21–q24 (rhodopsin)
   4p16.3 (rod cGMP phosphodiesterase, β-subunit)
   4p14–q13 (rod cGMP channel protein, α-subunit)
   5q31.2–34 (rod cGMP phosphodiesterase, α-subunit)
  X-linked recessive
   xp11.23
   xp21.1
   xp21.3–p21.2
  Digenic
   11p13/6p21.1-cent (ROM-1 and peripherin/RDS)
 Usher syndrome
  Type 1A
    14q32
  Type 1B
    11p13.5
  Type 1C
    11p15.2–p14
  Type 2A
    1q42-ter
 Congenital stationary night blindness
  Autosomal dominant
   3q21–q24 (rhodopsin)
   4p16.3 (rod cGMP phosphodiesterase, β-subunit)
  X-linked recessive (with myopia)
   xp11.3
 Cone–rod dystrophy
  Autosomal dominant
   18q21–q22.2
   19q13.1–q13.2
   17q
 Cone dystrophy
  Autosomal dominant
   6q25–q26
   17p
  X-linked recessive
   xq28
   qp21p11.1

Choroidal dystrophies
 Choroideremia
  xp21.1–q21.2 (Rab geranylgeranyl transferase, component A)
 Gyrate atrophy
  10q26 (ornithine aminotransferase)
Vitreoretinal dystrophies
 Juvenile retinoschisis
  xp22.1–22.2
 Stickler's syndrome
  12q13.11–q13 (collagen type II, α_1-polypeptide)
 Familial exudative vitreoretinopathy
  Autosomal dominant
   11q13.5–q22
  X-linked recessive
   xp11.4
 Neovascular inflammatory vitreoretinopathy
  11q13
 Wagner's disease/erosive vitreoretinopathy
  5q13–14

Macular dystrophies
 Stargardt's—fundus flavimaculatus
  Autosomal recessive
   1p21–p13
  Autosomal dominant
   6p21.1-cen (peripherin/RDS)
   13q24
   6q
 Best's vitelliform macular dystrophy
  11q13
  6p21.1-cent (peripherin/RDS)
 Atypical vitelliform macula dystrophy
  8q24
 Pigment pattern dystrophy
  6q21.1-cen (peripherin/RDS)
 North Carolina macular dystrophy
  6q16
 Sorsby's fundus dystrophy
  22q13.1-qter (TIMP 3)
 Dominant drusen of Bruch's membrane
  2p16–p21 (mallatia leventinese)
 Central areolar choroidal dystrophy
  6p21.1-cent (peripherin/RDS)
  17p

When known, the gene or protein is in parentheses next to the chromosome locus.

established, affected and nonaffected individuals are identified, and screening can be carried out on carriers and neonates. This information provides a firm foundation for genetic counseling.

The clinical course and prognosis of a disease depend in part on the specific mutation. An example is retinitis pigmentosa, which has been associated with allelic mutations on the rhodopsin gene that number over 70. These mutations may affect the intradiscal, intramembranous, or intracytoplasmic part of the rhodopsin molecule. Clinical investigation of families with different mutations suggests that the

severity of the disease is in part related to the location of the mutation on the rhodopsin molecule.

Once the mutation is identified, it is hoped this will be the beginning in the understanding of the mechanism of diseases. Mutations may result in an abnormal gene product, which may alter the physical structure of a molecule, affect functional activity such as an enzyme, or alter or modify cellular growth and regulation. Mutations may also result in the absence of a gene product or an accumulation of a toxic product. Molecular genetics provides a rational approach toward investigating pathogenesis. Explanations can be formulated, experiments devised, hypotheses tested—all within the framework of the known mutation and its effect.

The final step in this path is the development of a rational treatment methodology that may ultimately lead to disease cure. It should be remembered, however, that therapy for genetic diseases is not only gene therapy. Although the list is small, there are a number of diseases where pathogenesis has suggested alternative approaches, such as (1) drug therapy [vitamin A (abetalipoproteinemia) and vitamin B_6 (gyrate atrophy)], (2) diet manipulation [low-arginine diet (gyrate atrophy) and low-phytanic acid diet (Refsum's disease)], and (3) environmental adaptation (mitochondrial inherited diseases). These are all "downstream" approaches to therapy, that is, treatment of an effect that is removed from the initial event.

Further "upstream" are the attempts to replace diseased tissue with normal tissue through transplantation. Widely accepted and successful is keratoplasty for corneal dystrophies. Hopefully, RPE and photoreceptor transplantation for retinitis pigmentosa will also be a viable therapeutic alternative.

Transplantation of DNA, which is the furthest upstream approach, involves the introduction of the wild-type (normal) gene into the specifically targeted cells, resulting in the expression of the appropriate amount of the normal gene product.

The impact of molecular genetics on human disease begins with the identification of the chromosomal locus and the genetic mutation. This is the requisite for identification of disease. The "lumpers" and "splitters" of disease classification will give way to the "identifiers." Disease identification avoids the mistaken diagnosis, establishes the prognosis, and clarifies the familial inheritance pattern and family members at risk. It sets the stage for developing strategies for investigation of disease pathogenesis that ultimately, and hopefully, leads to rational treatment methods, be they upstream at the initiating events, or downstream at the final common pathways.

CONCLUSION

For over 100 years, our thinking about hereditary chorioretinal diseases has been grounded in the morphologic appearance. The proliferation of retinal atlases (first with drawings and now with gorgeous color photographs) has reinforced the concept of pattern recognition—it looks like the disease, therefore it is the disease.

The most common reason for misdiagnosis of these disorders is the reliance on the fundus appearance, and yet there is a significant amount of morphologic mimicking. Just as one example, the great majority of diseases in this chapter could, at one time or another, present as a bilateral nonspecific pigmentary maculopathy. Another example is a dominant family pedigree in which the eldest individual appeared to have central areolar choroidal dystrophy, the middle generations had the appearance of pattern dystrophy or vitelliform dystrophy, and the younger individuals appeared to have drusen or Stargardt's disease. The abnormal EOG light rise established Best's vitelliform macular dystrophy as the diagnosis.

There is no doubt that careful, directed, knowledgeable history taking is very helpful in differential diagnosis. Likewise, appropriate use of diagnostic tests can play a critical role (the use of the EOG in the noted pedigree just noted is a case in point). However, much of our way of classifying and diagnosing diseases will change in this new era of molecular medicine.

The identification of chromosomal loci and genetic mutations in various diseases is more than a new type of taxonomy. It promises to provide a basis for understanding retinal and visual processes in both health and disease. Atlases such as this one will be enhanced, not diminished, by a broader and deeper comprehension of what is illustrated.

ACKNOWLEDGMENTS

This work was supported in part by a grant from the Retinitis Pigmentosa Foundation, the Research to Prevent Blindness, and the Kirby Eye Institute.

BIBLIOGRAPHY

Carr RE, Siegel ID. *Electrodiagnostic testing of the visual system: a clinical guide.* Philadelphia: FA Davis, 1990.

Franceschetti A, Francois J, Babel J. *Chorioretinal heredodegenerations.* Springfield: Charles C Thomas, 1974.

Krill AE, ed. *Hereditary retinal and choroidal diseases.* Hagerstown, MD: Harper and Row, 1972.

Musarella MA. Gene mapping of ocular diseases. *Surv Ophthalmol* 1992;36:285–312.

Newsome DA, ed. *Retinal dystrophies and degenerations.* New York: Raven, 1987.

Renie WA, ed. *Goldberg's genetic and metabolic disease.* 2nd ed. Boston: Little, Brown, 1986.

Rosenfeld PJ, McKusick VA, Amberger JS, Dryja TP. Recent advances in the gene map of inherited eye disorders: primary hereditary diseases of the retina, choroid, and vitreous. *J Med Genet* 1994;31:903–915.

Zhang K, The-Hung EN, Crandall A, Donoso LA. Genetic and molecular studies of macular dystrophies: recent developments. *Surv Ophthalmol* 1995;40:51–61.

Practical Atlas of Retinal Disease and Therapy, Second Edition
edited by William R. Freeman,
Lippincott–Raven Publishers, Philadelphia © 1997.

· 2 ·

New Devices for Retinal Imaging and Functional Evaluation

Ann E. Elsner, Dirk-Uwe Bartsch, John J. Weiter, and M. Elizabeth Hartnett

Diagnosing and treating disease of the posterior segment are now aided by instrumentation more sophisticated than the classic ophthalmoscope, slit lamp, and fundus camera. Innovative instruments use laser scanning to view and measure the retina and choroid in ways not possible either by eye or with classic imaging methods. Infrared light is now used to visualize features unseen by other methods. Often pupil dilation is unnecessary, and light levels are comfortable. The scanning laser ophthalmoscope (SLO) features imaging combined with simultaneous presentation of stimuli for the evaluation of visual function. Several instruments enable the measurement of tissue depth and thickness. The Heidelberg retinal tomograph (HRT) and the topographic scanning system (TopSS) are instruments originally designed to measure the height of retinal features. These instruments have evolved to perform angiograms with improved discrimination from out-of-focus layers, including the Heidelberg retinal angiograph (HRA) and the AngioScan from Laser Diagnostic Technologies (LDT, San Diego, CA, U.S.A.), respectively. New interferometry techniques can provide images and thickness measurements of reflective retinal and choroidal structures as well as axial length. Sample techniques include optical coherence tomography (OCT) and laser Doppler interferometry (LDI). Estimates of blood flow are now possible not only with the SLO, but also with several devices that include new laser Doppler techniques, such as the Heidelberg retina flowmeter.

The technology driving the new devices and their clinical use has been largely the result of the international collaboration and close interaction of clinicians with optical, biomedical, and computer scientists. Successful features have often been specified by users of the instruments. Key commercial enterprises include the SLO (Rodenstock, Ottobrunn-Riemerling, Germany), the HRT and HRA (Heidelberg Engineering, Heidelberg, Germany), the TopSS and AngioScan (LDT), and OCT (Humphrey Instruments, San Leandro, CA, U.S.A.).

Many of these new techniques have moved into the clinic, providing hands-on evaluation and the impetus for further technique refinement. Clinically important features of low contrast are now reliably visualized and measured. Digitally acquiring, storing, and processing images improves comparisons across time and can prevent loss of information. Clinical research with these new quantitative techniques has already provided insights into mechanisms of several important diseases, such as retinal detachment, age-related macular degeneration (AMD), cystoid macular edema, diabetes, vein occlusion, and macular holes. Thus, our understanding of most posterior segment diseases is benefited not only by better visualization of pathology in vivo but also by quantification of the structure and function at known locations.

PRINCIPLES OF FUNDUS IMAGING WITH SCANNING LASER DEVICES

Fundus Imaging with Scanning Laser Devices

New devices can image both retinal and subretinal features with remarkable contrast. The Rodenstock SLO, the HRT, and TopSS use laser scanning to achieve high contrast, and scanning principles are also used in OCT and scanning laser Doppler flowmetry. To form an image, the fundus is illuminated with a narrow laser beam that is scanned over the surface of the retina (Fig. 1). A small fraction of this laser light leaves the eye through the pupil and is captured by a detector (Fig. 2). Thus, only one position on the fundus is illuminated at a time, and only light scattering from that position can return to the detector at a given time. Laser scanning increases the potential contrast of the image over the tradi-

A.E. Elsner, Ph.D., D.-U. Bartsch, M.D., J.J. Weiter, M.D., Ph.D., and M.E. Hartnett, M.D.: Eye Research Institute, Boston, MA 02114

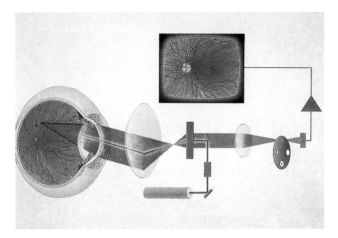

FIG. 1. The scanning laser ophthalmoscope (SLO) works by scanning a laser spot across the fundus and sampling the returning light with a selection of apertures in a plane conjugate to image plane. The live image appears on a monitor. (Courtesy of Robert Webb, Ph.D., Schepens Eye Research Institute, Boston, MA.)

tional fundus camera in which a comparatively large area is illuminated at a given time. In addition, the laser beam can be steered around cataracts and other media opacities in some cases. Another advantage over traditional fundus imaging is that lower average light levels can be used because only one location is illuminated at a given time.

The resolution depends on the imaging method, the optics of the eye, the electronics of the device, and the storage method. Most scanning instruments in the United States allow for either approximately 512 × 512 picture elements (pixels) per image, or 640 × 480 or more pixels for instruments emphasizing lateral resolution and 256 × 256 for tomographic sectioning.

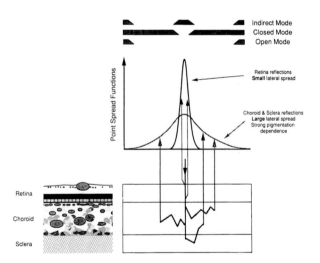

FIG. 2. Varying the sampling aperture changes the proportion of light sampled from the different layers of the fundus and from lateral positions. (Courtesy of Francois Delori, Ph.D., Schepens Eye Research Institute, Boston, MA.)

Confocal Imaging Mode

In addition to using laser scanning to illuminate the fundus, a variety of imaging modes may be used to sample the light returning from the eye (Fig. 2). In the confocal mode, a small stop is placed in the plane of the image. This stop allows the light returning directly back from the illuminated area to pass through to the detector. The stop blocks the light scattering over longer distances, either laterally or from other planes. A moderate-sized stop (direct mode) can reduce artifacts from other structures, such as the corneal reflex and vitreous opacities. A very small confocal stop emphasizes the mirrorlike aspects of the fundus, such as the foveal reflex, the roundness of blood vessels, the vitreoretinal interface, and the nerve fiber layer (Figs. 3–6).

Confocal views differ from traditional fundus photography and ophthalmoscopy. Strong reflexes with good resolution of the nerve fiber layer and other features are seen in virtually any wavelength of visible light, as well as infrared light up to 914 nm. The foveal reflex is seen in adults much older than would be typical with traditional methods. Younger eyes usually have such strong reflections from fundus structures, giving a shiny appearance to the retina, that care must be used in interpreting confocal images.

Confocal imaging allows the image information from one depth plane of the retina to be emphasized over all others because the light from other planes is blocked by a stop. In this way, it is possible to focus on a given layer of the retina. The quality of the images depends on the transparency of the layers above the plane in focus, which varies with wavelength. Many retinal opacities are highly scattering, and features beneath them cannot be imaged. Similarly, with most wavelengths of light, features cannot be seen beneath dense hemorrhages.

The principle of confocal imaging is used in several devices. The Rodenstock SLO has moderately confocal apertures, and the HRT and TopSS feature even smaller confocal

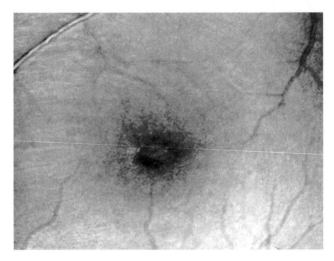

FIG. 3. Confocal SLO image of the macula in 633-nm light, normal patient.

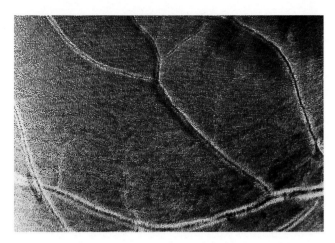

FIG. 4. The nerve fiber layer, seen as striae, imaged with a small field size with 488-nm light. (Courtesy of Joachim Nasemann, M.D., University Eye Clinic, Munich, Germany.)

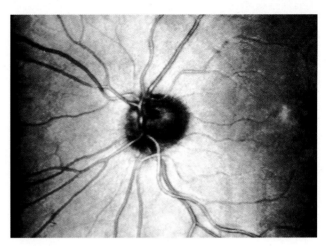

FIG. 6. SLO image, confocal and at 830 nm, same patient as in Fig. 5.

apertures. The size of the confocal aperture alone is not an indication of the depth discrimination power. The ratio between the aperture size and the focal length of the objective lens in front of the aperture is the critical parameter for comparison between instruments. These instruments are designed to image the human eye and are sold commercially and used in ophthalmic practice without needing modification. Many research versions are also in use. Several commercial and research models of scanning laser microscopes are available but are not typically meant for use in the human eye. An ophthalmoscope may be made into a microscope by increasing the magnification at the expense of reducing the field of view. Thus, detail may be gained, but it becomes more difficult to localize an area of interest or view several areas simultaneously. For example, individual blood cells within a vessel have been imaged in vivo using fluorescein angiography (FA). Magnification increase is limited by the resolution limit imposed by the optics of the human eye.

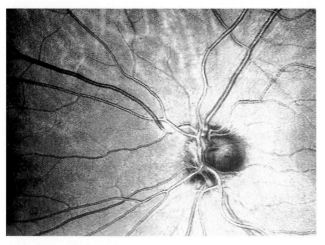

FIG. 5. SLO image, confocal and at 633 nm, of the optic disc of a normal Caucasian patient, age 28.

Typically, the smallest resolvable objects are about 10–15 μm in size.

All ophthalmic instruments that use a small stop for the returning light lose much of the potential light that is returned from the fundus. Because the potential amount of light returned through the pupil is only a few percent at best, the light intensity on the fundus must be increased to obtain an image. In addition, when the field of view is made smaller, the light falling on a given location becomes more concentrated. For some applications, so much light is needed that it is not safe for the human eye. One way around this problem has been to flash or flicker the light, as is done in fundus photography.

Indirect Mode Imaging

Anatomic structures not well seen by the traditional methods of viewing can be visualized with indirect viewing. In this mode, the light coming directly back from the eye to the detector is blocked. Light scattered over longer distances, either laterally or from other planes, can reach the detector. Indirect mode imaging is similar to viewing the fundus with a slit lamp when the lighted slit illuminates the fundus from a wide angle. When comparing indirect with confocal images, those features seen in both types of images usually have borders more indistinct in indirect mode. The contrast of features can change, depending on mode and wavelength. In 633-nm light, the healthy optic disc looks dark on a light background in confocal mode but light and indistinct on a darker background in indirect mode (Fig. 7). Blood vessels that appear dark on white in confocal mode can appear white on dark in indirect mode (Fig. 8). The appearance of features depends on not only imaging mode and wavelength but also ocular pigmentation and disease state (Figs. 9–21).

Indirect mode images can visualize features often unde-
Text continues on p 26.

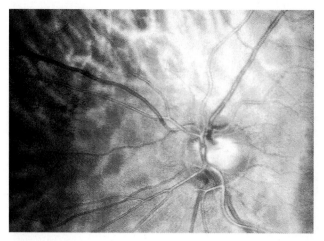

FIG. 7. SLO image, indirect and at 633 nm, same patient as in Figs. 5 and 6.

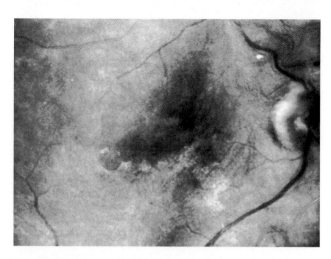

FIG. 10. SLO image in 594 nm and indirect mode of the macula of a diabetic patient following vitrectomy, showing that traction at the retinal surface prevents imaging of deeper structures.

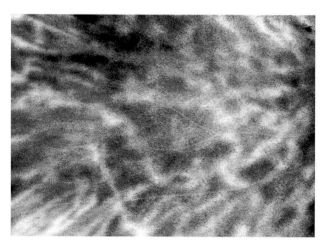

FIG. 8. SLO image, peripheral to disc, indirect and at 633 nm, same patient as in Figs. 5–7.

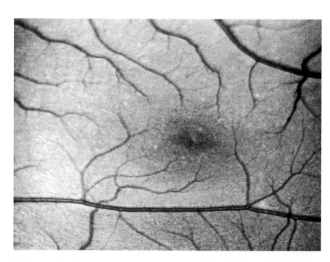

FIG. 11. SLO image of the macula of a "normal" 41-year-old patient, 543 nm and direct mode, 20° field.

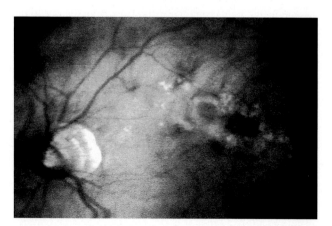

FIG. 9. SLO image of the lacquer cracks and new vessel membranes, as well as myopic disc appearance, in an undilated eye, direct mode, 830 nm. (Image by Ann Elsner and courtesy of Data Translation, Marlborough, MA; and Polaroid Corporation, Cambridge, MA.)

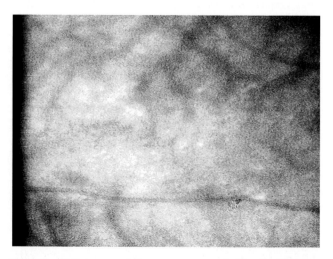

FIG. 12. SLO image of the same eye as in Fig. 11, 830 nm and indirect mode, highlighting the drusen. (From Elsner AE, et al. New views of the retina–RPE complex: quantifying subretinal pathology. In: *Noninvasive assessment of the human visual system.* Washington, DC: Optical Society of America, 1991;1:194–197, with permission.)

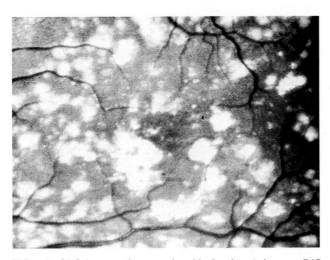

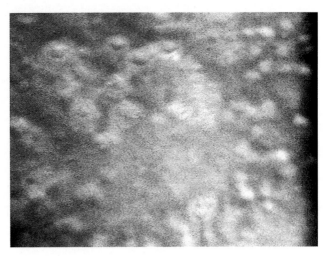

FIG. 13. SLO image of a macula with dominant drusen, 543 nm and direct mode, 20° field.

FIG. 14. SLO image of the same eye as in Fig. 13, but at 830 nm and indirect mode; the drusen are the predominant component of the image. [Image by Ann Elsner at Schwartz Electro-Optics (Concord, MA), titanium–sapphire laser, tunable from 790 to 890 nm.]

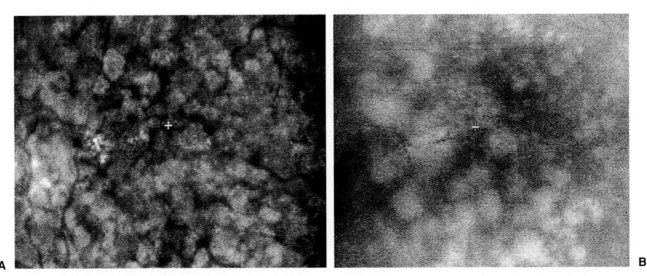

FIG. 15. SLO images of age-related macular degeneration with widespread drusen, 20° field. **A:** Confocal 790-nm image, with drusen obscuring the choroidal vessels. **B:** Indirect 633-nm image showing hyperpigmented structures beneath the drusen. [Image by Ann Elsner at Schwartz Electro-Optics (Concord, MA, U.S.A.), titanium–sapphire laser, tunable from 790 to 890 nm; courtesy of Joseph P. Walker, Glenn L. Wing, and Paul A. Raskaukas, Retina Consultants of Southwest Florida, Ft. Myers, FL.]

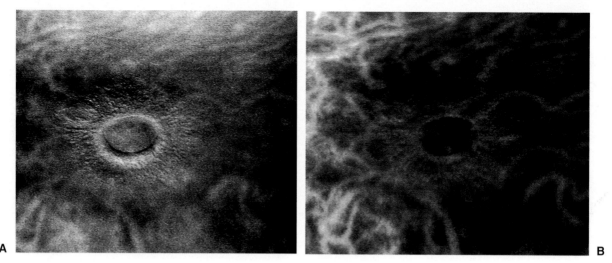

A   B

FIG. 16. SLO images of a macular hole, 20° field. **A:** Confocal, 790 nm, emphasizing superficial structures surrounding the hole. **B:** Indirect 633 nm, with improved view of the choroidal vessels in the area of the hole. (Courtesy of Joseph P. Walker, Glenn L. Wing, and Paul A. Raskaukas, Retina Consultants of Southwest Florida, Ft. Myers, FL.)

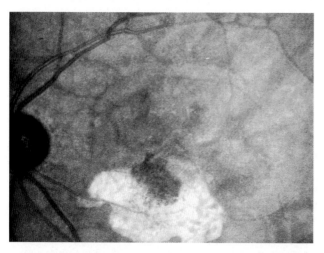

FIG. 17. SLO image of long-standing, age-related macular degeneration, 835 nm, direct mode, and large field of view. Choroidal new vessels appear darker than the surrounding fundus tissues. Laser photocoagulation produces highly backscattering scars, obscuring the view of deeper layers.

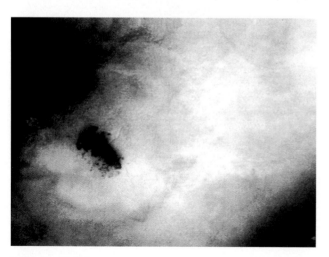

FIG. 18. SLO image of the same macula as in Fig. 17 but in indirect mode. Subretinal structures of interest are the increased thickening due to choroidal new vessels.

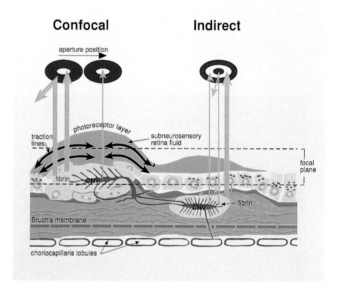

FIG. 19. An optical schematic for noninvasively detecting and localizing choroidal new vessels and exudation by using infrared imaging with an SLO. The *boldness of the arrows* indicates the amount of light from a structure. Membranes appear as thickened or elevated structures with a dark core surrounded by a brighter structure. Confocal mode visualizes those exudative components that provide contrast in the light that is backscattered: leaking new vessels, which absorb more light surrounding fundus; fibrin, which returns more light than the bright surrounding region; and feeder and draining vessels of sufficient size to have significant absorption. Fluid is visualized by the topography of the elevated retinal layers, particularly when viewed in real time during eye movements. Indirect mode allows the light that has traveled over longer distances laterally and from deeper layers to side-illuminate and retro-illuminate the borders of thickened structures, emphasizing the topography and extent of the exudation over specific components such as feeder vessels. (Adapted from Hartnett ME, Elsner AE. Characteristics of exudative age-related macular degeneration determined in vivo with confocal and indirect infrared imaging. *Ophthalmology* 1996; 103:58–71, with permission.)

24

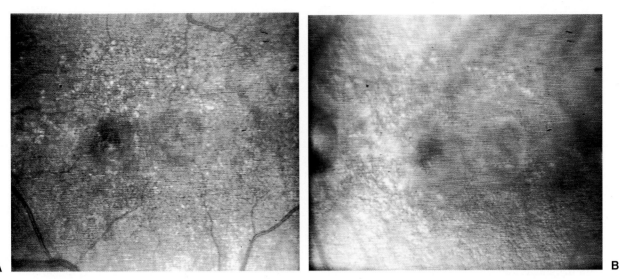

FIG. 20. SLO images of a pigment epithelial detachment temporal to a choroidal new vessel membrane, 880 nm, 40° field. **A:** Confocal image, emphasizing the darkened dome-shaped pigment epithelial detachment. **B:** Indirect mode image. Tunable near infrared wavelength by a titanium–sapphire laser. (Schwartz Electro-Optics, Concord, MA.)

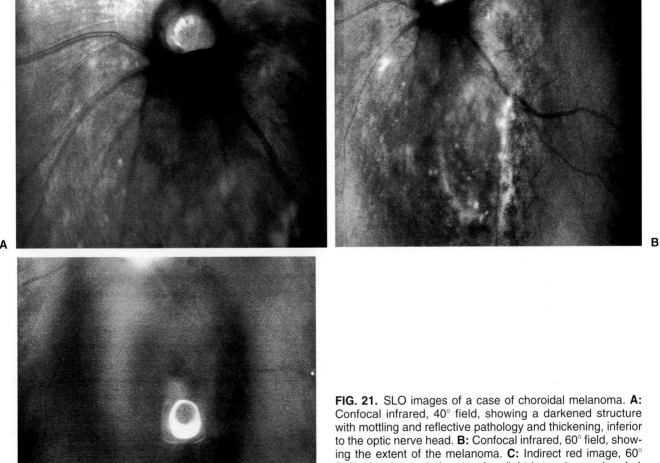

FIG. 21. SLO images of a case of choroidal melanoma. **A:** Confocal infrared, 40° field, showing a darkened structure with mottling and reflective pathology and thickening, inferior to the optic nerve head. **B:** Confocal infrared, 60° field, showing the extent of the melanoma. **C:** Indirect red image, 60° field, showing a *dark outer ring*, *light inner ring*, and a *dark center* pattern. (Courtesy of Joseph P. Walker, Glenn L. Wing, and Paul A. Raskaukas, Retina Consultants of Southwest Florida, Ft. Myers, FL.)

tectable by other methods. These features are often in deeper layers of the retina or are subretinal. For instance, choroidal blood vessels are emphasized to a greater extent at many wavelengths in indirect mode. Indirect imaging represents structures and pathology differently than merely focusing a confocal image to a different layer, because indirect imaging samples light that is scattered laterally rather than reflected back at a detector. Thus, indirect imaging often shows cysts and deposits and other thickened pathology, such as drusen, rather than the surface of blood vessels above and adjacent to them (Figs. 11–15 and 18). Although these can appear similar to craters, these are actually thickened and sometimes fluid filled. When highly backscattering tissue is present, the view of the deeper layers is poor in this region (Fig. 18). When tissue is missing, such as in a macular hole, the view of choroidal layers is improved (Fig. 16). This new method of imaging is used clinically both alone and in combination with angiography, for instance, to detect and localize choroidal new vessels (CNVs), pigment epithelial detachments (PEDs), and central serous retinopathy, as discussed below.

Monochromatic and Infrared Imaging

Most scanning instruments have only one detector, which means that the directly viewed images are monochromatic. Just as in the eye, there can be two or more detectors differentially sensitive to some physical variable (such as wavelength of light, angle of polarization, or imaging mode). Real-time color imaging has been demonstrated. Also, two images have been taken sequentially and then superimposed. Color and stereo fundus images have been produced using scanning laser imaging in this way, analogous to stereo fundus photography.

Scanning laser imaging may be performed with any wavelength of light available in gas, solid-state, or laser diodes, as long as these are powerful enough and stable. Whereas it is possible to make measurements at many wavelengths, it is impractical to do this on a routine basis, because of the amount of data in each image. The image quality depends not only on the amount of light remaining unabsorbed being high enough to form an image but also on the quality of the laser beam. Many laser diodes require extensive shaping of the laser beam to obtain good focus on the retina and subsequently a high contrast image.

There are many analogies with using filtered light for fundus photography. Laser light at 514, 543, and 594 nm emphasizes the retinal blood vessels, whereas 465- and 488-nm argon laser lines emphasize macular pigment. Hemorrhages can appear dark and of high contrast in 488- and 514-nm light but are relatively transparent to infrared light. All wavelengths of light can be used to provide a confocal image of the superficial layers, provided the ocular media are transparent (Figs. 3–6). The good contrast obtained at longer wavelengths with scanning laser devices is not found in fundus camera images because multiply scattered light reduces contrast.

Imaging with wavelengths of 780–914 nm is advantageous for viewing pathologic changes beneath the retina or blood, since infrared light is absorbed by blood and melanin to a lesser extent than is visible light. The detector in the Rodenstock SLO, the HRA, or the AngioScan is very sensitive to infrared light, whereas the photoreceptors in the eye are very insensitive. Excellent images may be obtained with light that is dim or invisible to the patient, because there is no pupil constriction. This is advantageous in imaging the eyes of children, as well as during perimetry, electrophysiology, and eye-movement testing, because infrared light does not need to interfere with the patient's response to the targets.

Recent studies by Elsner and colleagues have described the advantages of infrared imaging, not only through blood and cataract (Figs. 17–20) but also as a function of wavelength. The retina is rendered more or less transparent by varying wavelength, focus, and imaging mode. A tunable infrared laser was used to quantify the changes due to wavelength in images of drusen and subretinal deposits in AMD. At wavelengths of 790 nm or less, more superficial layers are emphasized, and choroidal vessels are not always seen. As the wavelength increases to 830 nm, the retinal vessels become less visible, but drusen more visible. As the wavelength is increased up to 890 nm, superficial features become less visible and deeper features more visible. Choroidal vessels are readily seen for wavelengths longer than about 820 nm, and these appear dark. The optic disc usually appears dark, whether in direct or indirect mode, since the surrounding retina and choroid backscatter comparatively more light.

The advantages of infrared imaging enable a wide variety of clinical uses: the noninvasive quantification of subretinal deposits in AMD and Stargardt's disease–fundus flavimaculatus, the early detection and localization of choroidal new

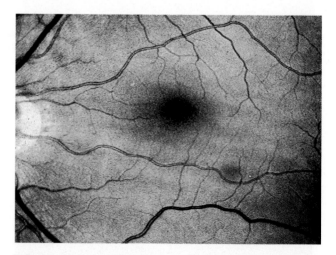

FIG. 22. SLO image of the eye of a 54-year-old normal patient following 15 minutes of dark adaptation, 594 nm, direct view. *Dark central spot* indicates a high concentration of cone photopigment. The *second dark spot* is the shadow of a vitreous floater.

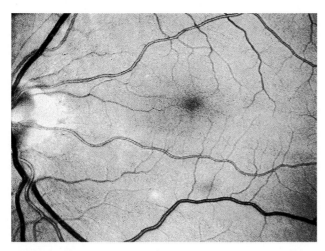

FIG. 23. The same eye as in Fig. 22, following 3 minutes of exposure to 82 μW of 594-nm light, direct view. The pigment has been bleached.

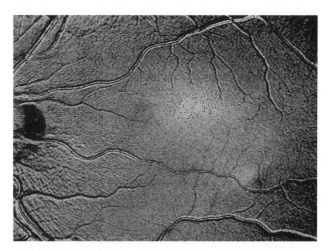

FIG. 24. Map of cone photopigment density, shown as a pseudocolor image of the log difference between the 17 and 18. In this eye, indirect mode imaging produces similar results.

vessels, and the localization of central serous retinopathy. There has been extensive correlation of FA and indocyanine green angiography (ICGA) with infrared imaging, to further the interpretation of both, often showing the extent of the pathology extending beyond the angiographic indication. Deep deposits such as drusen (Figs. 12, 14, 15, 17, and 18), as well as edema (Fig. 18), are particularly visible in infrared light with indirect mode imaging. Hartnett and Elsner have shown that many more deposits are seen, and the area covered appears greater than with traditional viewing methods. However, these remarkable views can be obtained only when the layers above the drusen are transparent. If these layers are scarred with fibrous tissue, then the large proportion of light returning from the scars washes out the contrast of the deeper layers.

The detection and localization of exudation and neoplasms are now possible via a better understanding of the interaction of red and infrared light and tissue. The normal fundus appears uniform, except for major vessels in both the retinal and the choroid, while pathologic structures in the deeper layers alter the light returning from deeper layers. Although a choroidal nevus or a plexus of normal vessels can block the path of light, these structures are rarely thicker than the surrounding ones. Thus, an optical schematic that identifies choroidal new vessels as thickened structures with a dark core surrounded by a brighter structure is clinically useful (Fig. 19). Confocal mode emphasizes the components of a choroidal new vessel membrane, such as the leaking new vessels, the surrounding fibrin, and feeder and draining vessels of sufficient size to appear dark (Fig. 20). Indirect mode emphasizes the extent of the thickened or elevated portions of exudative changes, such as new vessel membranes or PEDs. Light that is scattered multiple times across the deeper layers emphasizes the edges of thickened structures, since these are laterally or retroilluminated by scattered light (Fig.

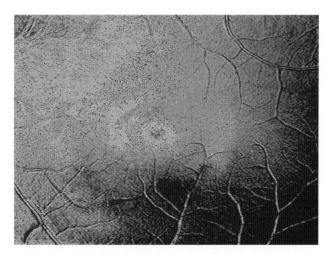

FIG. 25. Pseudocolor map of cone photopigment density in the eye of a 26-year-old patient. In young individuals and patients such as in Fig. 10, direct mode imaging can produce a high peak density but also artifacts caused by reflections of inner retinal layers.

20B). A series of images with both confocal and indirect apertures and in different focal planes is needed to represent the many pathologic components of long-standing exudative disease. The two most obvious signs of choroidal new vessel membranes are seen by comparing Figs. 17 and 18 at about one disk diameter and 3 o'clock to the pigmented region of the scar. Choroidal new vessel membranes are typically detected and localized by a dark core in confocal mode that is colocated and surrounded by elevation in the indirect mode.

A comparison in the same eye of a PED with a contiguous choroidal new vessel membrane furthers the interpretation of the views for these types of structures for confocal versus indirect imaging (Fig. 20). While choroidal new vessel membranes may be called "well defined," in comparison to • PEDs they have neither as clear-cut boundaries nor a regular, dome-shaped appearance. Both confocal and indirect modes clearly indicate the borders of the PED but to a lesser extent the topography of other thickened structures such as the vessel membrane. Both structures block light from deeper layers, proportional to their thickness and fluid content. In a sufficiently thickened or turbid structure, so little light is returned from deeper layers that imaging of deeper structures is precluded by any means, while superficial structures may even be emphasized or changed in appearance. The implications for angiography are great: these tissues may appear dark due not to nonperfusion but rather to lack of light penetration.

Neoplasms may be detected and localized early and noninvasively. SLO confocal infrared and indirect red images show a signature pattern for melanoma (Fig. 21). This is quite different from nevi, which appear flatter and of a more uniform darkness. As with other thickened pathology, the reflective and superficial pathology is emphasized in the confocal mode and topographic features in the indirect mode. The size of neoplasms, even on early detection, is often great enough to make the focal planes of the pathologic versus surrounding tissues noticeably different in confocal mode, making tomographic measurements possible. In an SLO, it is useful to use an ancillary lens to increase the field size to incorporate the entire mass in one image.

Reflectance Measurements of Pigments

Several types of ocular pigments, such as photopigment and macular pigment, can be measured with the SLO. Because the fundus is observed during measurement, one can minimize reflectance artifacts and document those that cannot be eliminated. Maps of pigment distribution are computed from the fundus images. Photopigment in rods, cones, or both together can be measured. First, the eye is dark adapted (Fig. 22). Then, it is exposed to an amount of light sufficient to bleach most of the photopigment in the normal eye (Fig. 23). A map of photopigment is obtained by taking the logarithm of each image and digitally aligning and subtracting (Fig. 24). Typically, it is not the confocal mode of imaging that is used to measure pigments in the deeper layers, because the low resolution in the axial direction, due to the optics of the human eye, allows the bright reflections from surface features to enter into these measurements (Fig. 25, using a much larger aperture than that for depth analysis).

Cone photopigment is typically greatest at the center of the fovea, where long, fragile cones are tightly packed together, and then decreases rapidly with increasing eccentricity (Fig. 26). In patients with AMD, however, the photopigment concentration is markedly less, even without evidence of exudation (Fig. 27). The photopigment loss can be remarkably well localized, even in degenerative diseases. In a patient with Stargardt's disease–fundus flavimaculatus,

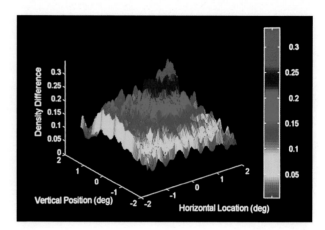

FIG. 26. Pseudocolor map of cone photopigment density in the eye of a 21-year-old normal patient. The three-dimensional map shows a high concentration of photopigment in the foveal center and a sharp decline with eccentricity.

there was a transmission defect on FA confined to the central fovea. The foveal distribution of photopigment showed a loss at this location but was normal for the surrounding tissue (Fig. 28). Photopigment mapping and other imaging techniques can also be used to study recovery from retinal detachment or other insults. Elsner and colleagues have shown that, following treatment for repair, the photopigment can require many months to reach full concentration, with recovery of visual acuity lagging. One caveat is that superficial reflections, including those caused by epiretinal membranes, following insult can increase to the extent that they obscure the view of the deeper fundus structures. The comparison of photopigment maps with visual function maps, infrared images, or angiographic images provides insights into disease mechanisms and progression.

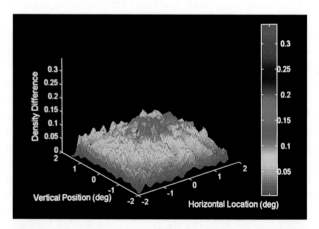

FIG. 27. Pseudocolor map of cone photopigment density in the eye of a patient with age-related macular degeneration and exudation in the fellow eye. The three-dimensional map shows a much lower concentration of photopigment in the fovea than in the eye of a young normal patient.

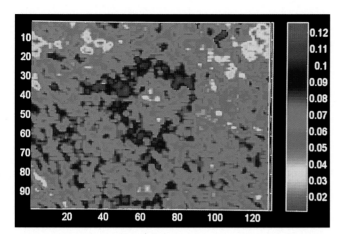

FIG. 28. En face, pseudocolor map of cone photopigment density in the eye of a patient with Stargardt's disease–fundus flavimaculatus and a central foveal defect on fluorescein angiography. There is a lack of photopigment in the central fovea at the site of the defect. The surrounding region reaches normal photopigment concentration levels, consistent with 20/40 visual acuity.

New Imaging Techniques with Charge Coupled Device Arrays

New imaging techniques are undergoing rapid development for the in vivo assessment of retina structure and physiology, all made possible by improved charge coupled device (CCD) arrays. CCD arrays are rugged, sensitive, solid state-detectors arranged in a matrix pattern that have been used in digital imaging and angiography systems, for instance, in the ICGA camera system by Topcon (Tokyo, Japan), to obtain fundus images with permissible amounts of light. The number of detector elements and their sensitivity have been increased so that images with 1024×1024 pixel resolution can now be obtained with the limited amount of light returning from the ocular fundus through the pupil of the eye. Recently, the sensitivity of CCD arrays has been improved further with intensification, cooling, and signal averaging. The spectra of extremely weak fluorophors, such as lipofuscin, have been shown by Delori and colleagues to vary with aging and pathology in AMD and Stargardt's disease–fundus flavimaculatus. Two new techniques for imaging foveal photoreceptor structure feature laser beam illumination and CCD arrays to capture images: photoreceptor alignment reflectometry and coherent imaging of the cone mosaic.

Photoreceptor alignment reflectometry measures the guidance of light by the foveal photoreceptors rapidly and objectively. Healthy photoreceptors capture light like an antenna, often aimed toward the center of the pupil. The property that the photoreceptors guide light is known as the Stiles–Crawford effect type I. For each measurement, the fovea is illuminated with a 543-nm, 5.3-log Troland laser beam, which is bright enough to bleach the photopigment. The light reflected from the fundus is captured with a CCD array in the plane of the pupil. This CCD array is sensitive over a large dynamic range so that both the weakly reflected light and the bright reflection can be measured at one time. This provides a map of how well the light is reflected back from the retina and then out of the pupil. Since the guidance for the outgoing light is assumed to be equal to the guidance of the incoming light, the image of the pupil is a map of the guidance of foveal photoreceptors. To determine how broad the guidance is, the entry position of the narrow (28 μm) illumination beam is varied. The entry position yielding the greatest reflectance indicates the main direction from which the foveal photoreceptors guide light (Fig. 29). In the healthy retina, photoreceptor guidance is maximum over a fairly narrow angle and off-axis illumination is not well guided (Fig. 30). Measurements of photoreceptor guidance have been made quite rapidly with a laser scanning version of this instrument, in contrast to the much slower psychophysical methods.

Coherent imaging of the cone mosaic provides an in vivo measure of the spacing of foveal cones in the fovea. Healthy foveal cones are so densely packed that the central ones can rarely be resolved in vivo through the optics of the human eye with incoherent light, as shown by Miller and colleagues. The elegant optical technique of Nomarski imaging described by Curcio and colleagues has provided packing density measurements for photoreceptors across the entire human macula, but only when microscope optics are used ex vivo, on retina whole mounts. Information regarding the spacing of the cone mosaic, however, can be measured in vivo by stellar speckle interferometry, a high-resolution imaging technique. A speckle pattern (Fig. 31) is obtained by illuminating the fovea with brief flashes of a narrow beam of coherent light from a 543-nm laser, while capturing images with a sensitive CCD camera. The speckle pattern indicates the spacing of the irregularities in the foveal topography (presumably in the cone mosaic). The power spectra of a series of speckle images are computed and averaged, resulting in the cone spacing from the characteristic spatial frequency for a series of retinal eccentricities. By analyzing the center versus the more eccentric portions of the foveal speckle image, the cone packing density is determined as a function of eccentricity (Fig. 32). For all normal patients, there is a clear increase in the mean cone interdistance with retinal eccentricity, with different slopes for each observer.

Rapid Data Acquisition and Video Rate Imaging

In several of these devices, the laser beam is scanned horizontally and vertically, and the timing is designed to synchronize with a wide range of video and computer equipment. The image of the fundus is viewed in real time on a monitor, typically with a frame rate of 25 or 30 times per second (Hz) in commercial devices. The field rate is 50 or 60 Hz. This allows the patient's eye and head movements to provide the perception of depth to optic disc and retinal

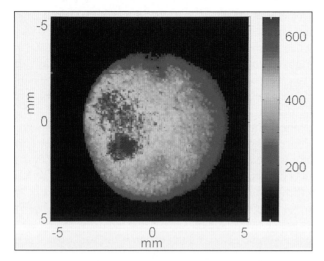

FIG. 29. Pseudocolor map of light guided by the foveal photoreceptors in the eye of a normal subject, determined from light reflecting from the retina and captured in the plane of his pupil. The light illuminates the fovea perpendicular to the axis of the photoreceptors. (Courtesy of Stephen Burns, Ph.D., Schepens Eye Research Institute, Boston, MA.)

pathology. Floaters and vitreous opacities are readily visualized. The venous pulse at the optic disc is readily seen. Blood flow through the capillaries and major vessels can be seen on FA, and eye movements can be quantified. Imaging with SLOs enables a better perception of depth in images. This is partly due to the larger stereopsis that is possible with these instruments. Since the illumination pupil can be as small as 1 mm, a larger angle of separation between illumination points can be achieved.

Images presented continuously enable the observer to obtain an average perception of several images to compare successive views in a natural way. The HRT and the TopSS store the data digitally in an image buffer, which improves the perceived resolution of individual nerve fiber bundles, the lamina cribrosa, and other structures. This improvement in perceived resolution is due to image processing by the human observer. Single images of low contrast or small structures never equal the quality of the live video.

Video recording has several practical advantages. Images recorded on videocassette recorder are readily replayed for consulting physicians, the patient, and family members. It is unnecessary to develop film to make a diagnosis. Video recording also allows rapid screening and replay, particularly of uncooperative patients. Displaying the images on a large monitor is an easy way to magnify the images; the actual resolution is not improved, but important details are more readily seen this way.

For rates of image acquisition less than video rates, sequences of images can yield the perception of depth of lesions, such as displayed on the TopSS, HRT and HRA, as well as the sequence of blood flow. This enables many physiologic parameters to be quantified, such as blood flow, photopigment bleaching and regeneration, and eye position.

Fluorescein and Indocyanine Green Angiography

Understanding the retinal and choroidal circulation is the goal of new angiographic techniques. Good contrast (Figs. 33 and 34), high data rates during the transit, and the ability

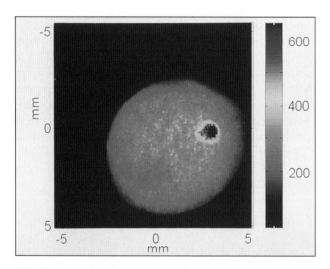

FIG. 30. Pseudocolor map showing the lack of guiding of light when light illuminates a normal fovea from the edge of the pupil, marked by the bright reflex on the left side of the pupil. Since the light enters at a wide angle from the axis of the photoreceptors, the returning light is uniformly distributed across the pupil (that is, unguided by the photoreceptors). (Courtesy of Stephen Burns, Ph.D., Schepens Eye Research Institute, Boston, MA.)

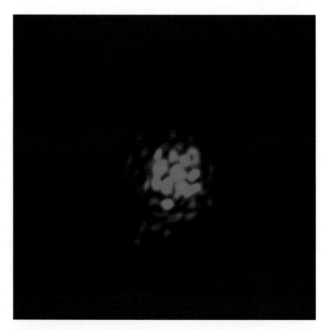

FIG. 31. Typical speckle image of the normal fundus at 0.5° retinal eccentricity, resulting from a brief exposure to 543-nm laser light. The speckle pattern is correlated with the structure of the cone mosaic. (Courtesy of Susana Marcos, Spanish National Center for Scientific Research, Madrid, Spain.)

to observe blood flow are the main advantages of using the Rodenstock SLO, the HRA, or the AngioScan. The success of the angiogram can be improved by monitoring eye position and focus during the test. It is unnecessary to delay treatment while film is being developed. Digital angiography with scanning laser devices is performed in a similar manner to that with a video or CCD camera, except that images can be acquired at a much higher rate. Both can have rates higher than film photography (which is about 1/second). Newer research instruments include confocal apertures and a choice of barrier filters.

In FA, the main dye technique for imaging the retinal circulation, the illumination light with an SLO is typically 100–160 μW of 488-nm argon laser light, which is well tolerated and within safety limits, although longer wavelengths have been used. ICGA aimed primarily at imaging the choroidal circulation is a much newer technique. A much longer wavelength (780–810 nm) and a higher-power light (1–2 mW/cm^2 at the retina) is used than for FA. The light is barely visible, is not uncomfortable, and is within the safety limits for the time used. In angiography techniques, light returning from the retina is filtered so that mainly light of any wavelength longer than the illumination wavelength is measured, similar to photographic and video camera methods.

Both FA and ICGA methods should always be preceded by and compared with reflectance control images, which are often of outstanding contrast with scanning laser devices. Red-free images are taken at a light level much less than that used for angiography, in the commercial Rodenstock SLO at

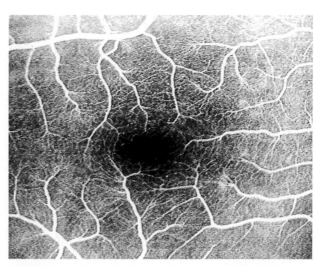

FIG. 33. SLO fluorescein angiogram of the macula of a normal patient. Foveal capillaries are seen at the field size with greater magnification (20° field size).

488 nm (argon blue) (for example, see Figs. 4 and 35), although 514 nm (argon green) is also possible. Infrared images, discussed above, emphasize different features, depending on the wavelength and mode of imaging used. For autofluorescence and angiographic images, a filter is placed in the path of the light returning from the retina. Fluorescence images must be distinguished from pseudofluorescence, which is the leakage of backscattered light through the filter. One appropriate control used by Elsner and colleagues is the comparison of contrast of features in the red-free or infrared image to the same loci in the autofluores-

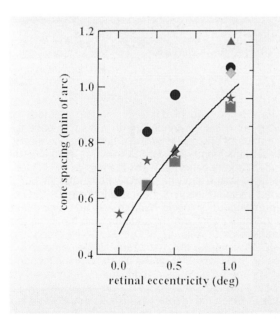

FIG. 32. Cone spacing at different foveal eccentricities, obtained in vivo by means of stellar speckle interferometry, as shown in Fig. 31. Different normal patients are represented by *different symbols*. The *solid line* represents a fit of the histologic data obtained by Curcio et al., averaging over subjects and retinal regions. (Courtesy of Susana Marcos, Spanish National Center for Scientific Research, Madrid, Spain.)

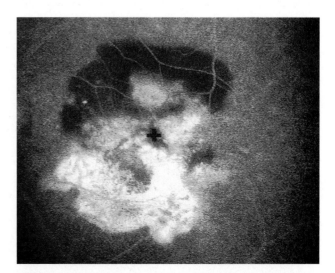

FIG. 34. SLO fluorescein angiogram, late phase, of the same case as in Figs. 17 and 18. The *black cross* is a fixation target produced by turning off the 488-nm laser at these locations. This angiogram precedes those 835-nm images by 2 weeks. Fluorescein and infrared images, however, from the same sessions produced the same findings: the 835-nm light images through the hemorrhage.

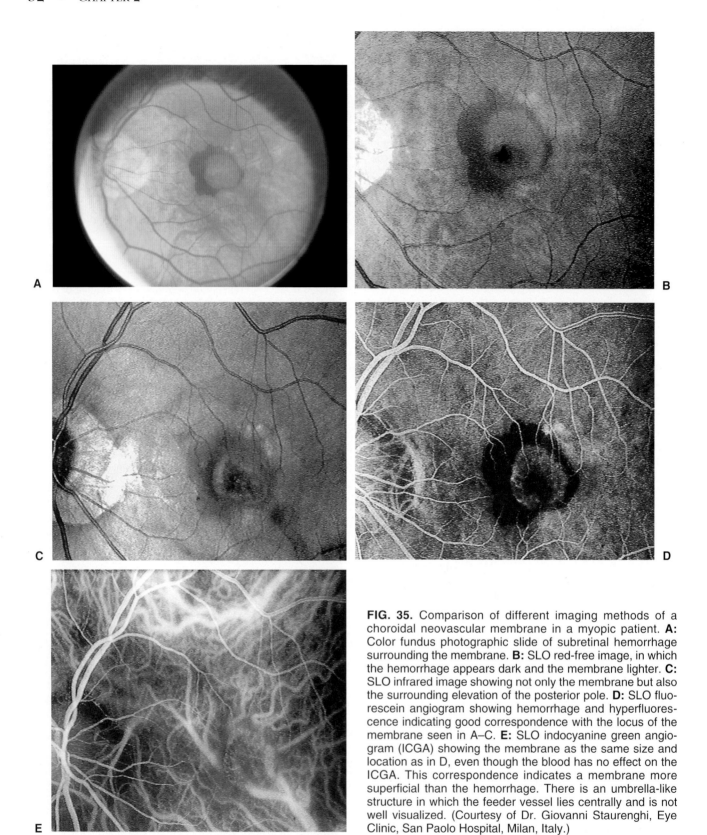

FIG. 35. Comparison of different imaging methods of a choroidal neovascular membrane in a myopic patient. **A:** Color fundus photographic slide of subretinal hemorrhage surrounding the membrane. **B:** SLO red-free image, in which the hemorrhage appears dark and the membrane lighter. **C:** SLO infrared image showing not only the membrane but also the surrounding elevation of the posterior pole. **D:** SLO fluorescein angiogram showing hemorrhage and hyperfluorescence indicating good correspondence with the locus of the membrane seen in A–C. **E:** SLO indocyanine green angiogram (ICGA) showing the membrane as the same size and location as in D, even though the blood has no effect on the ICGA. This correspondence indicates a membrane more superficial than the hemorrhage. There is an umbrella-like structure in which the feeder vessel lies centrally and is not well visualized. (Courtesy of Dr. Giovanni Staurenghi, Eye Clinic, San Paolo Hospital, Milan, Italy.)

cence image to be distinguished from pseudofluorescence. The contrast must be greater with the filter than in the red-free image or infrared image (with no filter). Autofluorescence for short wavelengths is readily found. Autofluores-

cence for pathology is difficult to determine for infrared wavelengths; pathologic structures can be 1000 times brighter than the surrounding tissues, and filter leakage is inevitable.

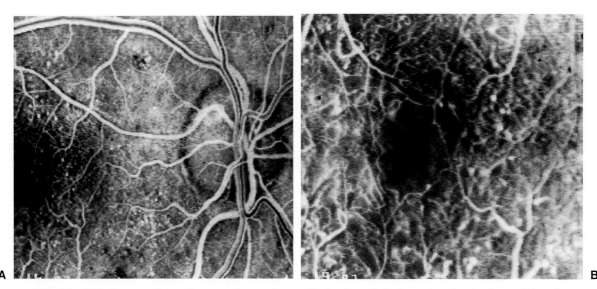

FIG. 36. SLO fluorescein angiogram of macular capillaries in a diabetic patient for the large (**A**) and small (**B**) fields of view. (Courtesy of Sebastian Wolf, M.D., Ph.D., Eye Clinic, Aachen, Germany.)

We have developed several techniques to superimpose the graphics of the SLO during the angiogram to determine a fixation point (Fig. 34) or measure the sensitivity to targets near the area of proposed laser photocoagulation. In this manner, treatment can be guided by the expected loss of useful vision.

Different features of the retinal and choroidal circulations are emphasized by the choice of several parameters: field of view (Figs. 33, 34, and 36), type of dye (Figs. 35, 37, and 38), concentration of dye, technique of administering dye, plane of focus, dilation of pupil, amount of light, wavelength of light, amplification of video signal, mode of imaging, and speed of image acquisition, as well as digital versus analogue (usually videotape) format of data storage. Simultaneous FA and ICGA have been performed using two detectors by Bischoff and colleagues or using a single detector with the il-

lumination for FA versus ICGA alternating line by line, that is, interlaced lines of video (HRA, Fig. 38). While this allows image registration with minimal postprocessing, the caveat remains that there is only one focusing mechanism. The main advantage of simultaneous FA and ICGA is that it provides an easier, quicker way for physician to visualize neovascular membranes, since both types of angiograms are taken at the same time and field size, allowing better comparison. A potential disadvantage is that a compromise must be made for individual variations in focal planes for the two tests, because of different elevations of the pathology of the retinal and choroidal circulations, and individual differences in the focal power of the eye for short versus long wavelength light (that is, axial and lateral chromatic aberrations). One possible solution is axial scanning during acquisition, which is available in an automated process on the HRA. Si-

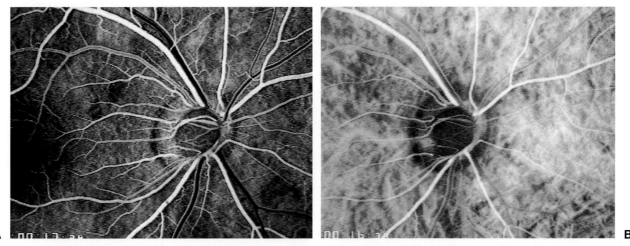

FIG. 37. SLO fluorescein angiogram (**A**) compared with SLO indocyanine green angiogram (**B**), in which the choroidal vessels are much more pronounced. (Courtesy of Sebastian Wolf, M.D., Ph.D., Eye Clinic, Aachen, Germany.)

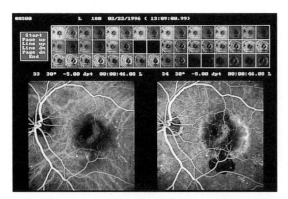

FIG. 38. Simultaneous fluorescein and indocyanine green angiography with the Heidelberg retinal angiograph showing subretinal neovascularization in age-related macular degeneration. (Courtesy of D.-U. Bartsch, M.D., and William R. Freeman, M.D., Shiley Eye Center, University of California–San Diego, La Jolla, CA.)

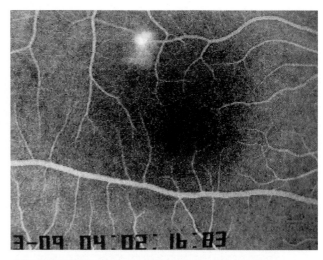

FIG. 40. SLO fluorescein angiogram demonstrating leakage from central serous retinopathy, 2 minutes and 16 seconds after injection. (Courtesy of Joachim Nasemann, M.D., University Eye Clinic, Munich, Germany.)

multaneous images in different axial positions are recorded. The reviewer can choose useful image pairs.

The standard clinical dose of sodium fluorescein (5 ml of 10% sodium fluorescein), injected in the typical manner into a patient who is well dilated, gives excellent angiographic results (Figs. 33 and 34). The resolution of small features can be superior to that of clinical photographic angiography in the same individuals. High-contrast images of features as small as foveal capillaries can obtained for several minutes after injection (Fig. 33). Areas of suspected leakage can be confirmed, with good contrast in both early and late phases of the angiogram (Figs. 33–45). Subtle leakage is readily seen (Figs. 36, 39, and 40). Because excellent results are also obtained with smaller doses of fluorescein, followed by a flush of saline, both eyes of the same patient can be studied in a single visit. Pupil dilation is not always necessary to obtain a good image of the major retinal vessels (Fig. 45). Because there is good contrast, we find that oral administration

of fluorescein produces excellent results of phases after the transit.

The main differences between ICGA and sodium fluorescein angiography (SFA) and are the better binding of ICG to blood proteins, the excitation and fluorescence at longer wavelength, and the much lower fluorescence (only 4% of the fluorescence of SF). One advantage is that the feeder and draining vessel complex may be identified on ICGA without masking (Figs. 46 and 47) from large amounts of dye leakage from either CNVs, retinal anastomoses, or retinal pigment epithelial cells, making the early-phase ICGA information crucial, as discussed by Wolf and colleagues. The contrast must be sufficient for even small feeder vessels, however, and this is provided by scanning laser techniques (Figs. 48–51) and proper focusing on the layers of interest (Fig. 51). Photocoagulation of the region of only the feeder

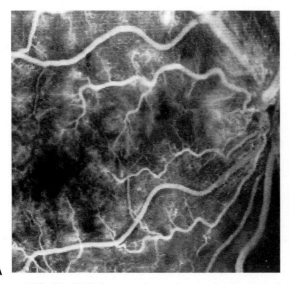

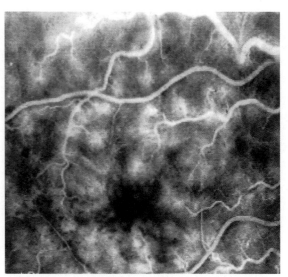

FIG. 39. SLO fluorescein angiogram for the large field (**A**) and small field (**B**) sizes of an eye with a macular edema. (Courtesy of Sebastian Wolf, M.D., Ph.D., Eye Clinic, Aachen, Germany.)

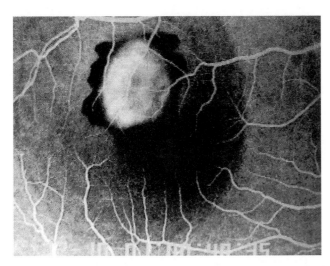

FIG. 41. SLO fluorescein angiogram of idiopathic subretinal neovascularization. (Courtesy of Joachim Nasemann, M.D., University Eye Clinic, Munich, Germany.)

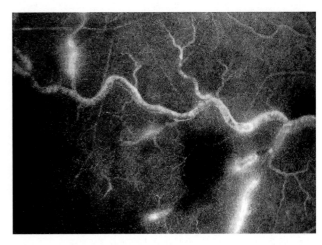

FIG. 42. SLO fluorescein angiogram of vascular staining in the eye of a patient with a severe vaso-occlusive periphlebitis. (Courtesy of Joachim Nasemann, M.D., University Eye Clinic, Munich, Germany.)

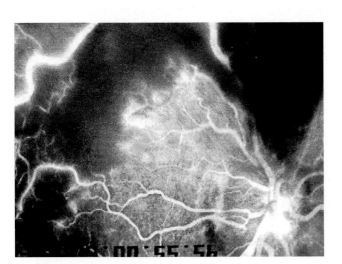

FIG. 43. SLO fluorescein angiogram of severe ischemic hemicentral retinal vein occlusion showing areas of capillary nonperfusion. (Courtesy of Joachim Nasemann, M.D., University Eye Clinic, Munich, Germany.)

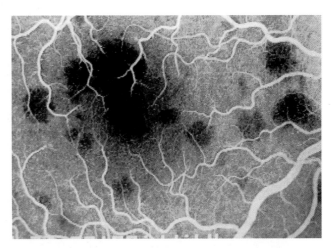

FIG. 44. SLO fluorescein angiogram of deep retinal hemorrhages in optic disc vasculitis with periphlebitis. Inflammatory signs are not seen in the early phase. (Courtesy of Joachim Nasemann, M.D., University Eye Clinic, Munich, Germany.)

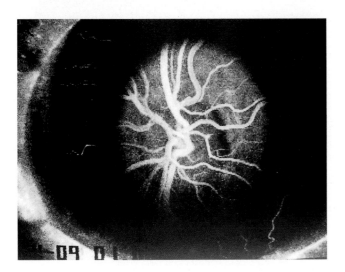

FIG. 45. Early iris phase of a simultaneous retina iris fluorescein angiogram in a 44-year-old normal woman. Blood flow through the anterior segment is measured by comparing the arrival time of fluorescein dye with the retinal vessels and the iris vessels. To image the blood vessels of the iris and the optic disc simultaneously, a 20-diopter planoconvex lens with a central perforation is placed between the SLO and the patient's eye. The peripheral part of the image is the iris, but the central part is the optic disc. (Courtesy of Joachim Nasemann, M.D., University Eye Clinic, Munich, Germany.)

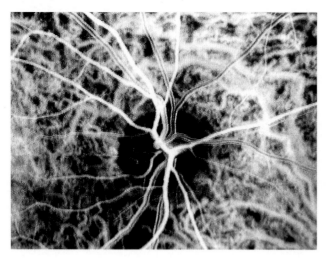

FIG. 46. SLO indocyanine green angiogram of a normal eye, emphasizing choroidal vessels. (Courtesy of Andreas Scheider, M.D., University Eye Clinic, Munich, Germany.)

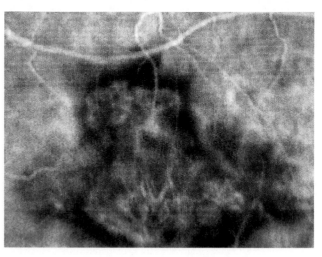

FIG. 47. SLO indocyanine green angiogram of subretinal neovascular membranes. (Courtesy of Andreas Scheider, M.D., University Eye Clinic, Munich, Germany.)

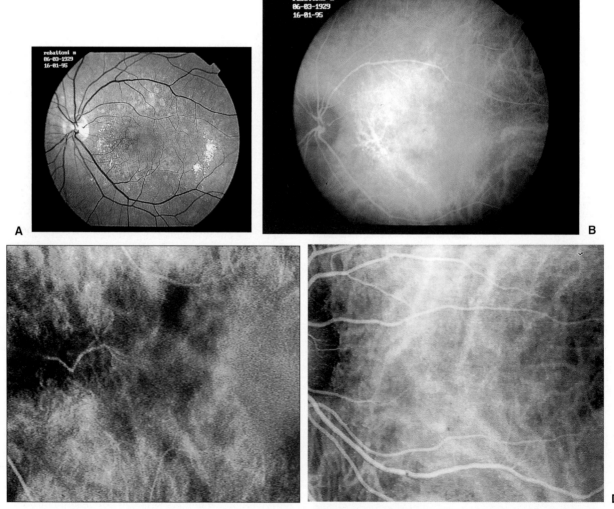

FIG. 48. Comparison of indocyanine green angiography (ICGA) with a Topcon digital fundus camera system versus angiography with an SLO system. **A:** Red-free fundus slide of a case of retinal pigment epithelial detachment (temporal) with choroidal neovascular membrane, concomitant with age-related macular degeneration. **B:** Early phase of the ICGA with a Topcon system. **C:** Early phase of the SLO ICGA, clearly showing a feeder vessel that crosses the fovea, of a choroidal neovascular membrane. **D:** Midphase ICGA with an SLO, showing that the extensive choroidal fluorescence in this phase obscures the feeder vessel. (Courtesy of Dr. Giovanni Staurenghi, Eye Clinic, San Paolo Hospital, Milan; and Dr. Ferdinando Bottoni, Eye Clinic, San Gerardo dei Tintori Hospital, Monza, Italy.)

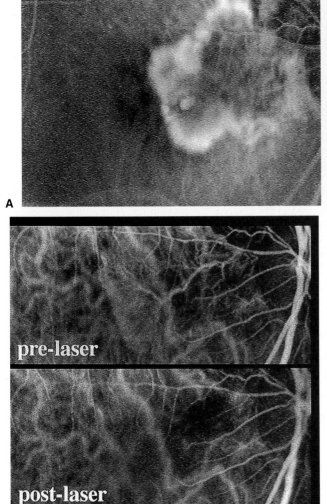

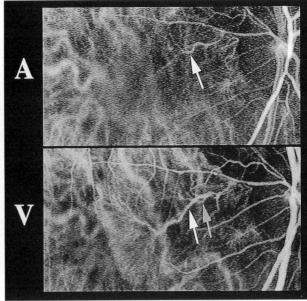

FIG. 49. SLO angiographic study of the eye of a patient with age-related macular degeneration, showing the effect of treatment of the feeder vessel of a choroidal new vessel membrane. **A:** Fluorescein angiogram (before treatment), showing extensive hyperfluorescence at the border of the membrane leakage. There is also a well-demarcated cyst in the foveal area. **B:** Indocyanine green angiogram (ICGA), early phase, in which *arrows* indicate the feeder vessel (A) and the draining vessel (V). **C:** Comparison of ICGAs before treatment (A) and after treatment (B), showing that the vessel is closed. (Courtesy of Dr. Giovanni Staurenghi, Eye Clinic, San Paolo Hospital, Milan, Italy.)

vessel, without ablating the entire CNV, may become an option for preserving good vision (49).

For the late phase, good visualization of leakage of ICG is possible at later phases than with SF, for which diffusion of dye through tissue lowers the contrast. Typical late-phase images in ICGA are taken at around 20–45 minutes (Figs. 50 and 52). Imaging with SLOs typically offers better contrast and brighter images in the late phase than with conventional fundus cameras. The advantages, particularly for ICGA, are due to the same factors that make infrared imaging possible. Only one region is illuminated, so long-range scatter and fluorescence are minimized and contrast is maximized. SLOs have a small illumination area and large light collection area in the plane of the pupil so that fluorescence is captured effi-

ciently. The point detectors in SLOs are more efficient in comparison to area detectors in fundus cameras. The disadvantage of the scanning principle is the occurrence of motion artifacts within the brief scanning time within an image: fragmented or misleading images of good contrast can occur instead of blurred images.

The confocal aperture in combination with the ICGA allows a depth discrimination between retinal and choroidal layers even in angiograms (Figs. 51 and 53). It was noted that it is easier to discriminate against retinal layers, since light from deeper choroidal layers is scattered in superficial retinal layers and thus detected even if the focal plane is within the retinal layers. Confocal ICGA enables visualization of tumor vessel patterns in patients with ocular melanoma (Fig.

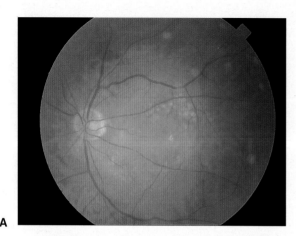

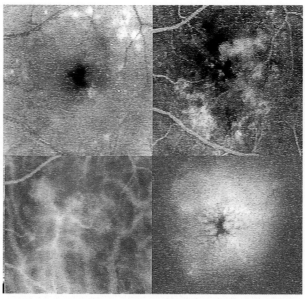

A **B**

FIG. 50. Comparison of different imaging methods used in the eye of a patient with occult new vessel membrane, which is well visualized only on indocyanine green angiography (ICGA). **A:** Color fundus slide showing an ill-defined membrane complex. **B:** SLO red-free (*top left*), SLO fluorescein angiogram (*top right*), SLO ICGA early phase (*bottom left*), and SLO ICGA late phase (*bottom right*). (Courtesy of Dr. Giovanni Staurenghi, Eye Clinic, San Paolo Hospital, Milan, Italy.)

53). Previous studies have shown that certain vessel patterns and appearances in histologically examined tumors lead to a significantly better prognosis of tumor malignancy. ICGA with confocal SLOs appears to enable in vivo imaging of these patterns.

The choroidal circulation is particularly important in several diseases, such as age-related maculopathy or choroidal melanoma, because the new vessels originate from the choroid (see, for example, Figs. 47–54). With ICGA, CNVs can be identified that are sometimes difficult to visualize with FA (50). In inflammatory disease, the choroidal circulation may show much more leakage than in many other diseases (Fig. 55). This, taken together with improved visualization through hemorrhage or in darkly pigmented fundi, indicates that ICGA may be the technique of choice in some diseases. ICGA may provide a complementary technique, and the comparison between both types of angiography, as well as infrared imaging, may provide new information regarding pathophysiology (Figs. 48–50) (see also Chapter 9 by N.M. Bressler).

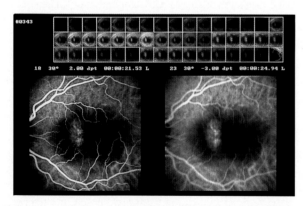

FIG. 51. Confocal indocyanine green angiogram taken with the Heidelberg retinal angiograph. The two images were taken at the same phase of the angiogram in different confocal layers. The **left image** was focused onto retinal layers, allowing clear identification of retinal vessels. The **right photograph** is focused onto deeper choroidal layers, and the retinal vasculature is almost invisible. (Courtesy of D.-U. Bartsch, M.D., and William R. Freeman, M.D., Shiley Eye Center, University of California–San Diego, La Jolla, CA.)

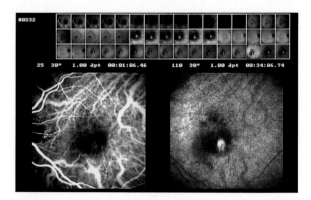

FIG. 52. Confocal indocyanine green angiogram of subretinal neovascularization in the early phase (**left**) and the late phase (**right**), with the Heidelberg retinal angiograph. The extent of the membrane can be appreciated in the early phase. The late-phase angiogram confirms leakage. Note the excellent visibility of retinal vessels as dark vessels against a dimly fluorescent background consistent with staining of the choriocapillaris.

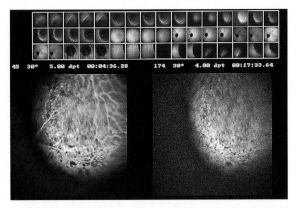

FIG. 53. Confocal indocyanine green angiogram of a choroidal melanoma with the Heidelberg retinal angiograph. Imaging with this instrument enables visualization of vessel structures within the tumor better than with fluorescein angiography. (Courtesy of D.-U. Bartsch, M.D., and William R. Freeman, M.D., Shiley Eye Center, University of California–San Diego, La Jolla, CA.)

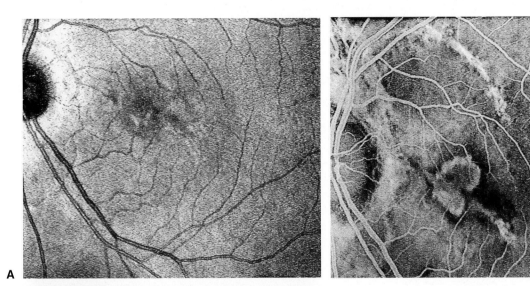

A

B

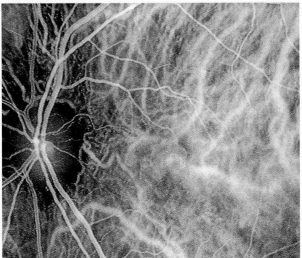

C

FIG. 54. Comparison of SLO infrared imaging, fluorescein angiography, and indocyanine green angiography (ICGA) in the visualization of choroidal new vessels in angioid streaks. **A:** Infrared image showing the membrane as a circular, inhomogeneous region that appears elevated. Within this region, the membrane is centrally located and growing from the main angioid streak. **B:** Fluorescein angiogram with the linear hyperfluorescence indicating the cracks. The membrane is demarcated by circular hyperfluorescence. **C:** ICGA clearly showing the membrane but not the cracks. (Courtesy of Dr. Giovanni Staurenghi, Eye Clinic, San Paolo Hospital, Milan, Italy.)

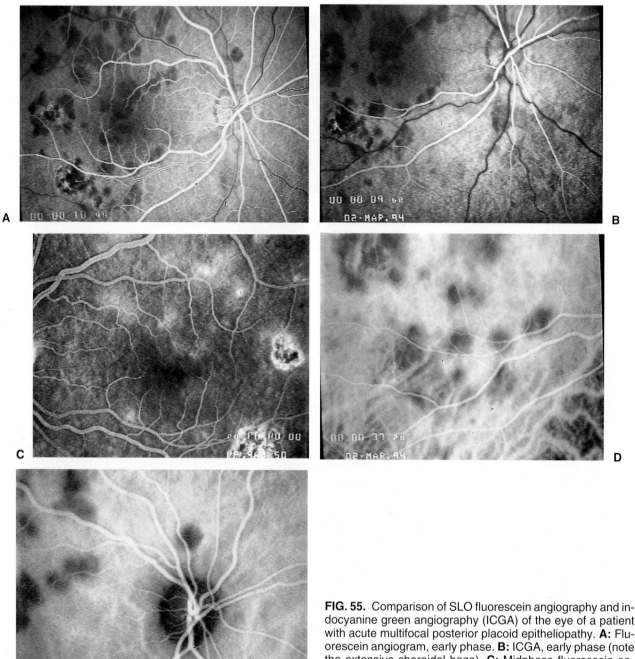

FIG. 55. Comparison of SLO fluorescein angiography and indocyanine green angiography (ICGA) of the eye of a patient with acute multifocal posterior placoid epitheliopathy. **A:** Fluorescein angiogram, early phase. **B:** ICGA, early phase (note the extensive choroidal haze). **C:** Midphase fluorescein angiogram. **D,E:** Midphase ICGA showing the macula and the optic nerve head, respectively.

As with any type of imaging, resolution is gained at the expense of field of view. In the Rodenstock instrument, a commercially available SLO, each resolution element is a 10- or 20-mm spot for the small and large fields of view, respectively. With the small field of view, the inner capillary loop surrounding the foveal avascular zone and individual capillaries may be readily resolved (Figs. 33 and 56–58). These are easily seen on videotape because the visual system integrates over several frames to identify each capillary clearly. The perifoveal capillaries are readily seen in normal subjects for several minutes after injection of fluorescein dye.

There is good contrast in the angiograms and monochromatic images, particularly notable for subtle features, which opens up many new diagnostic possibilities, such as the early detection and quantitative measurement of cystoid macular edema. The cystic formations in macular edema are well visualized by the early phase of FA (Figs. 59–61). This suggests that the origin of cystoid macular edema depends more on choroidal circulatory defects than retinal defects, as suggested by Arend and colleagues.

When the larger field of view is used to see the disc and the area within the vessel arcades, resolution is decreased.

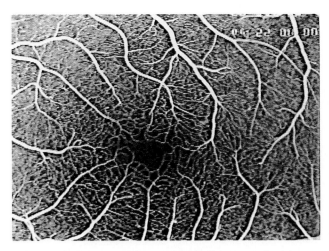

FIG. 56. SLO fluorescein angiogram of the eye of a 31-year-old normal patient, 20° field, showing the foveal avascular zone and several intercapillary loops. (Courtesy of Oliver Arend, M.D., Eye Clinic, Aachen, Germany.)

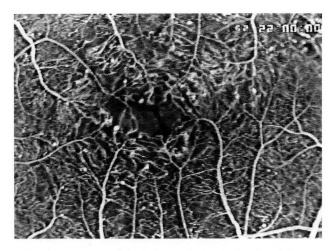

FIG. 59. SLO fluorescein angiogram, as in Fig. 57, of the eye of a 33-year-old diabetic patient with cystoid macular edema, showing clearly visualized cysts. The retinal capillary changes are less pronounced than in the age-matched patient without cystoid macular edema in Fig. 58. (Courtesy of Oliver Arend, M.D., Eye Clinic, Aachen, Germany.)

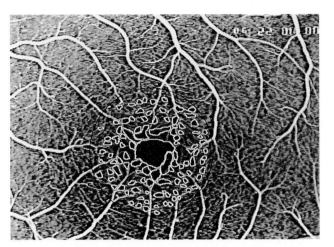

FIG. 57. Objective quantification of macular capillary density from the angiogram in Fig. 56. Perifoveal intercapillary areas within a 5° circle (*black*), centered on the foveal avascular zone, are marked by using digital image processing. (Courtesy of Oliver Arend, M.D., Eye Clinic, Aachen, Germany. After Arend et al., 1991.)

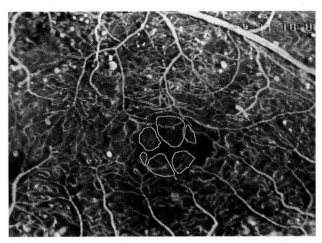

FIG. 60. Objective quantification of the area of cystic formations from the angiogram in Fig. 59. The outer diameters of cysts within a 2.5° circle (*black*), centered on the foveal avascular zone, are marked by using digital image processing. (Courtesy of Oliver Arend, M.D., Eye Clinic, Aachen, Germany. After Arend et al., 1995, with permission.)

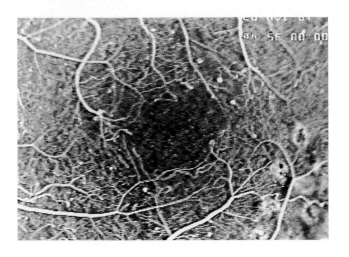

FIG. 58. SLO fluorescein angiogram, as in Fig. 57, of the eye of a 33-year-old diabetic patient. The foveal avascular zone is nearly triple the size of that in a normal patient, and there is strikingly decreased capillary density. (Courtesy of Oliver Arend, M.D., Eye Clinic, Aachen, Germany. After Arend et al., 1994.)

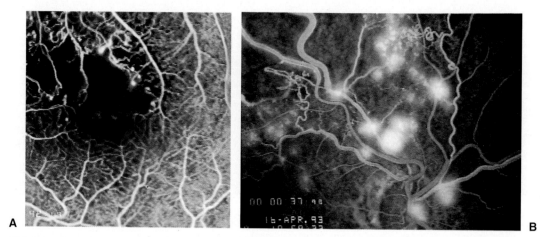

FIG. 61. SLO fluorescein angiogram showing branch retinal vein occlusion concomitant with ischemia and cysts. **A:** Macula. The cysts are clearly visualized as hyperfluorescence during the early portion of the angiogram. **B:** Peripheral region showing dilated vessels and extensive leakage. (Courtesy of Andreas Remky, M.D., Eye Clinic, Aachen, Germany.)

Most individual capillaries cannot be seen with this field of view, but retinal pigment epithelial defects and areas of leakage that are clinically important often can be seen because of the good contrast. One strategy is to begin the angiogram with the large field to identify potential defects and then switch to the higher resolution (Figs. 36 and 39) to examine these defects. The foveal avascular zone may be much larger in diabetics, presumably because of capillary dropout, implying ischemia (Fig. 58).

In branch retinal vein occlusion, the treatment regimen depends in part on the presense of ischemia. FA with the SLO enables rapid but exact determination of the status of ischemic macular disease. If ischemia is present (Fig. 61),

then photocoagulation treatment is contraindicated. If the retina does not appear to be ischemic, then treatment is advised.

Subtle features can be detected and localized by infrared imaging as well as FA. For instance, central serous choroidopathy (Fig. 62) has been shown to be detected by infrared imaging (Fig. 63). The extent of the thickened, fluid-filled portion of the lesion is highly correlated with the extent as determined by FA, as shown by Remky and colleagues. Thus, determination of the progression or regression, and potential photocoagulation treatment, may be assisted by infrared imaging, which is noninvasive, rapid, and can be performed through poor media.

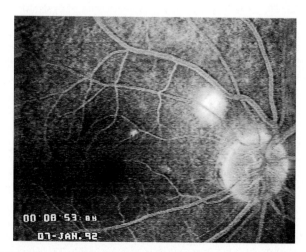

FIG. 62. SLO fluorescein angiogram of a patient with central serous retinopathy, showing the focal region of hyperfluorescence. (Courtesy of Andreas Remky, M.D., Eye Clinic, Aachen, Germany.)

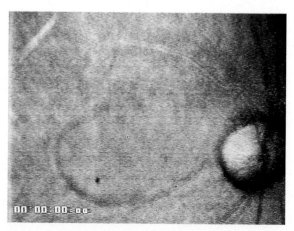

FIG. 63. SLO infrared image of the eye in Fig. 62, showing a large thickened area in the macula. (Courtesy of Andreas Remky, M.D., Eye Clinic, Aachen, Germany.)

BLOOD FLOW

Video rate recording of FA documents the transit time of dye from arteries to veins when a bolus of dye is clearly visible. The larger field of view, which shows simultaneously the major retinal vessels and the macula, is useful to measure arteriovenous passage time, that is, the time for the dye bolus to pass from a given artery to the corresponding vein so that the major arteries and veins can be seen, as well as the macula. Blood flow by this measure decreases in diseases such as diabetes. The blood flow in capillaries and small vessels can also be measured, quantifying the flow rates of either the bolus of dye or a portion of the blood column with both stained and less-stained blood components (Fig. 42). With the greater resolution available at the smaller field size, nonperfusion of vessels is seen immediately (Fig. 36). Blood flow through perimacular capillaries can decrease and size of the foveal avascular zone can increase in diabetes (Figs. 58 and 59).

The characteristics of the perceived blood flow depend on the size of the vessel, and measurements that are difficult in normal subjects become possible in patients with retinal circulatory disorders. When the arteriovenous passage time is measured, the stained dye bolus is measured against the background of the as-yet unstained blood. For flow through vessels, it is typical to wait until the entire vessel column has had stained blood passing through it and then to image the portions of the blood that stain versus those that do not stain. The latter stand out at video rates as dark, moving spots, flowing along between stained or partially stained elements. Measurements of blood flow differ, depending on whether the flowing blood components are in the center of a vessel or near the edge, which has greatly reduced flow. This can be due to the nature of laminar blood flow.

Blood Flow Measurement with Laser Doppler Velocimetry

Blood flow through a selected retinal vessel may also be measured with several methods using the Doppler shift principle, such as laser Doppler velocimetry or laser Doppler flowmetry (LDF) or scanning laser Doppler flowmetry (SLDF). For laser Doppler velocimetry, a blood vessel of interest, which must be 40 μm or more in diameter, is selected with the aid of an imaging device. In contrast to the methods just described, the image of the eye does not provide the data. Instead, a safe amount of laser light illuminates a cross section of a vessel and is then scattered back to a detector by both moving particles in the blood and the vessel walls. The frequency of the light is shifted according to the velocity of the moving blood particles. The velocity varies with the position of particles within the vessel, with the center particles

achieving a maximum velocity (Fig. 64). The vessel walls provide a reference measurement. The frequency shift is too small to be detected as a change in wavelength, but the interference of the shifted frequency light and the reference light reflected from stationary objects (vessel walls) will cause a measurable intensity oscillation that enables the calculation of a power spectrum and particle velocity by using a fast Fourier transform. Volumetric retinal blood flow is calculated from the cross-sectional area of the vessel and the mean blood velocity.

There are several variations on this technique, as well as advances in equipment. Infrared light may be used to illuminate the blood vessel. This is particularly important because there is a complex response to light by the blood flow in the retina and choroid, and there is potential for the light from the measuring device to influence the results. Blood flow can follow the frequency of a flickering light. With this new infrared technique, visible light is an experimental variable.

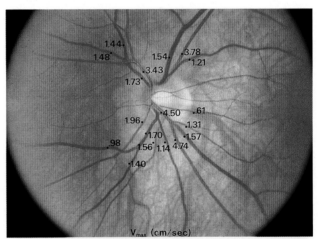

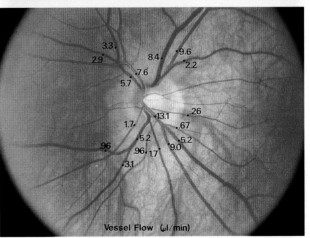

FIG. 64. Center-line maximal velocity V_{max} (**A**) and blood flow (**B**) in several retinal vessels, measured with laser Doppler velocimetry. (Courtesy of Charles Riva, D.Sc., Scheie Eye Institute, Philadelphia, PA.)

Scanning Laser Flowmetry

By combining LDF with scanning laser technology, SLDF can be used to obtain two-dimensional images of particle motion in the posterior pole of the eye. An example of such an image is presented in Figs. 65 and 66. Because of the Doppler effect, an intensity oscillation can be measured. The oscillation frequency is proportional to the red blood cell velocity. The temporal variation of the reflected light is measured, Fourier transformed, and parameterized, yielding three parameters: *volume* (number of blood cells), *flow* (number of blood cells times their velocity), and *mean velocity* (division of flow by volume). Several research groups have conducted preliminary experiments showing a high degree of linearity for the velocity measurements. More investigations of this method are needed for measuring the background velocity at zero flow (zero offset).

Depth Transfer Function Evaluation

Depth measurements of structures in the eye are obtained with confocal scanning laser tomographs by evaluating the change of reflected laser light intensity through the retina. The confocal imaging mode of an SLO is used to acquire a stack of typically 32 images of a structure, focused over a series of depth planes. Laser light is reflected at each retinal boundary that involves a change in refractive index between the two adjacent retinal layers. Each interface is imaged in the overall depth transfer function as a curve with a Gaussian profile. The half-width of this Gaussian profile is governed by the optics of the imaging system and the optics of the eye. Provided that the individual Gaussian profiles are separated far enough, it is possible to discriminate between them.

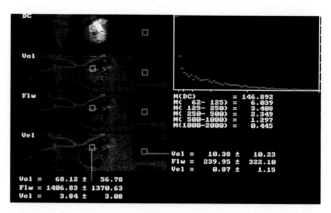

FIG. 66. Scanning laser Doppler flowmetry image of an optic nerve head. The scanning area was focused on the level of the lamina cribosa at the bottom of the cup. The **top photograph** shows the corresponding fundus view. The **second, third, and fourth images** show a map proportional to red blood cell volume, flow, and mean velocity, respectively. (Courtesy of D.-U. Bartsch, M.D., and William R. Freeman, M.D., Shiley Eye Center, University of California–San Diego, La Jolla, CA.)

Thus, the center line of each profile can be extracted from the composite depth transfer function, and the axial position of the retinal boundary can be calculated (Figs. 67–70).

In the case of the commercial instruments—the HRT and the TopSS—it was found that Gaussian profiles of depth have a half-width of 300–450 μm. The half-width is wavelength dependent, and since the TopSS uses 790 nm compared with 633 nm, it is expected to have a somewhat larger half-width. Both use light of long wavelength, thereby avoiding many of the problems associated with hemorrhage or media opacities at shorter wavelengths. Thus, the anterior and posterior surfaces of large retinal cysts can be visualized (Figs. 71 and 72). Future improvements to the optical resolution of the confocal scanning laser tomograph are designed to enable the detection of the anterior and posterior surfaces of the retina and thus the thickness. Preliminary work on the improvement of resolution is being performed at several institutions.

Retinal Tomography

Two commercially available instruments—the HRT and the TopSS—use the depth transfer function evaluation to create a three-dimensional map of the retinal surface. By detecting the center line of the depth transfer function, they can reproducibly measure the location of the retinal surface. A variety of patient studies have been performed with these instruments. Most applications have centered around imaging of the optic nerve head in glaucoma, and confocal scanning laser tomographs have been found to be useful in the follow-up of glaucoma patients. Researchers have found that retinal tomography offers a robust indicator of the degree of glaucomatous optic nerve damage. These instruments have es-

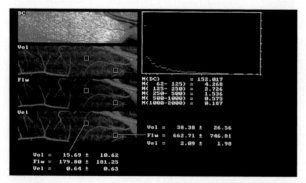

FIG. 65. Scanning laser Doppler flowmetry image of an optic nerve head. The scanning area was focused on the retinal surface surrounding the cup. **Top photograph** shows the corresponding fundus view. The **second image** shows a map proportional to the total number of moving red blood cells at the measurement location (volume). The **third image** shows a map proportional to the total number of red blood cells times their velocity (flow). The division of the second and third parameters yields the **fourth image** proportional to the mean velocity of the red blood cells. (Courtesy of D.-U. Bartsch, M.D., and William R. Freeman, M.D., Shiley Eye Center, University of California–San Diego, La Jolla, CA.)

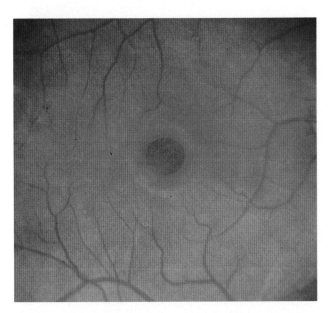

FIG. 67. Color fundus slide of the right eye of a 67-year-old woman with a full-thickness macular hole. Retinal examination revealed a cuff of subretinal fluid surrounding the hole. (Courtesy of D.-U. Bartsch, M.D., and William R. Freeman, M.D., Shiley Eye Center, University of California–San Diego, La Jolla, CA.)

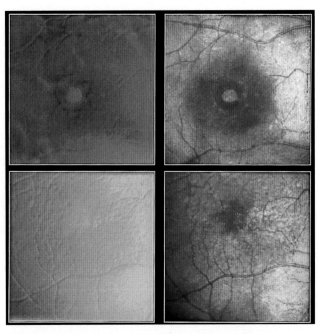

FIG. 69. Color-coded height images taken by tomography of an eye with epiretinal membrane before and after surgical removal as in Fig. 68. Note that the retinal wrinkles have all but disappeared after surgery. (Courtesy of D.-U. Bartsch, M.D., and William R. Freeman, M.D., Shiley Eye Center, University of California–San Diego, La Jolla, CA.)

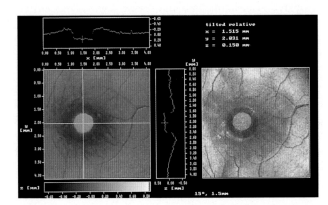

FIG. 68. Color-coded height image generated with a confocal scanning laser (Heidelberg retinal) tomograph (*left side*). *Lighter colors* represent lower elevations. The *right side* of the graph shows a vertical and horizontal cut through the macular hole at the location of the *white cross* in the fundus view. (Courtesy of D.-U. Bartsch, M.D., and William R. Freeman, M.D., Shiley Eye Center, University of California–San Diego, La Jolla, CA.)

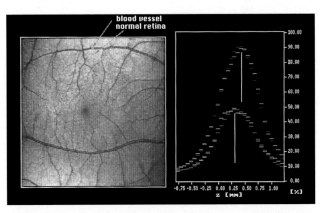

FIG. 70. Depth transfer function in the eye of a normal subject. The *blue line* was taken at the apex of a retinal blood vessel, while the *black line* was taken on the retina without large vessels. It can be seen that light from deeper retinal layers beyond the internal limiting membrane is detected by confocal instruments. (Courtesy of D.-U. Bartsch, M.D., and William R. Freeman, M.D., Shiley Eye Center, University of California–San Diego, La Jolla, CA.)

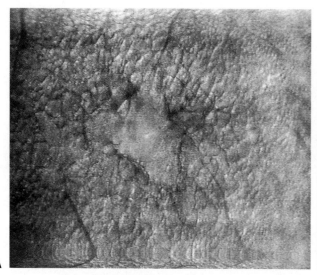 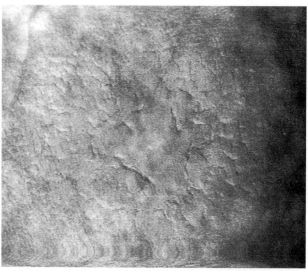

FIG. 71. SLO image showing cystoid macular edema caused by uveitis, 850 nm, 20° field. The entire macula is covered by cysts. A large, central cyst is covered by smaller, multiple cysts. **A:** Direct mode, emphasizing superficial structures. **B:** Indirect mode. The borders of the cyst are well visualized, especially in the big cyst in the center. Tunable near infrared wavelength by a Chr–lithium–SaF laser (Schwartz Electro-Optics, Concord, MA). (Courtesy of Andreas Remky, M.D., Schepens Eye Research Institute, Boston, MA.)

tablished themselves as an adjunct to other photographic methods. Other areas of retinal imaging that employ scanning laser tomographs include visualization of macular hole formation (Fig. 65), cyst formation, epiretinal membranes (Fig. 69), and exudation associated with AMD. Bartsch and colleagues have reported the ability to measure the change in surface topography following vitrectomy. Retinal tomogra-

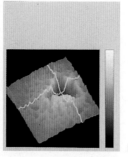

FIG. 72. Topographic scanning system (TopSS) images of the same eye as in Fig. 71, 790 nm, 10° field. **A:** The average of 32 images that differ in the plane of focus. The cysts are visualized as depressed areas. The scale on the *left side* of the image represents the height values of the vertical axis of the crosshair in the image. The scale on *top* of the image represents the height values on the horizontal axis. Notice the depth of the large cyst in the center. **B:** Color-coded height map generated with a confocal scanning laser tomograph (TopSS) (*left side*) of the same eye. *Darker colors* represent lower elevations. The height map provides a three-dimensional representation of all of the cysts. (Courtesy of Eva Beausencourt, M.D., Schepens Eye Research Institute, Boston, MA.)

phy enabled measurements of surgical success before vision improved following the surgical trauma.

The HRT and the TopSS use long-wavelength light, in contrast to early instruments, so that deeper structures are readily imaged. The HRT or the TopSS may be used to quantify cysts (Figs. 71 and 72) and exudative AMD (Figs. 73 and 74). The findings from infrared imaging with the SLO can be compared, validating that thickened regions on indirect mode represent elevations. Infrared imaging with the SLO shows that cystic structures can be much more widespread than may be appreciated by clinical means (Fig. 72). The borders of the cysts often are touching.

CNV data may be interpreted in light of the data from cysts in which there is also fluid accumulation. Bartsch and colleagues have shown that cysts are imaged as depressed structures. The fluid within a PED is imaged is a similar manner as a depressed structure (Fig. 74). This indicates that the major backscattering source is below the retinal surface, presumably at the deeper fluid–tissue boundary.

Scanning Laser Polarimetry

Some research efforts in glaucoma focus on the measurement of changes in the nerve fiber layer thickness. A modified SLO [nerve fiber analyzer (NFA)] from LDT creates a thickness-equivalent map based on the retardation of polarized light. The instrument records 20 image pairs with crossed analyzer axis with different incident direction of polarization of the illuminating laser light. A cornea polarization compensator was designed to cancel the retardation caused by the cornea. Using Fourier ellipsometry, it is then

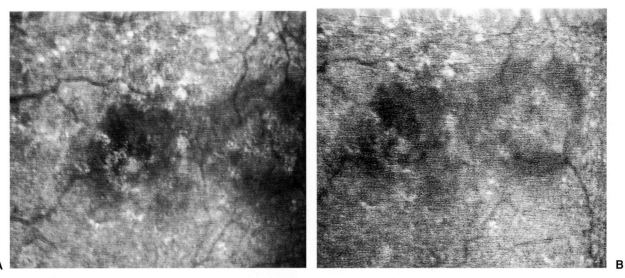

FIG. 73. SLO images of a pigment epithelial detachment temporal to a choroidal new vessel membrane, 880 nm, 40° field. **A:** Confocal image, emphasizing the darkened dome-shaped pigment epithelial detachment. **B:** Indirect mode image. Tunable near infrared wavelength by a titanium–sapphire laser. (Schwartz Electro-Optics, Concord, MA.)

possible to calculate the retardation caused by the birefringent nerve fiber layer. An example of the recorded retardation map is shown in Fig. 75. The instrument is still being evaluated and tested to determine accuracy and specificity. The first reports have been encouraging, even though some researchers observed a dependence of measured retardation on light reflectance. This caused artifacts when imaging bright structures such as the sclera at the center of the optic nerve head and in laser scars.

Interferometry Techniques

Interferometry techniques are based on two beams of light interacting to produce interference fringes. Interferometry has long been used in a subjective manner, with the patient resolving the finest possible fringes or targets, to estimate potential visual acuity through cloudy media. In contrast, new interferometry techniques provide objective information about ocular tissues in an axial direction. Two or more beams of light illuminate the eye, the more mirrorlike ocular structures return the light in the direction of a detector, and interference fringes are created by the light beams. The detector senses not merely the amount of light at a given time, as in scanning laser measurements and angiography, but the pattern of interference. The distance between the groups of interference fringes and the amplitudes of the fringes can be used to measure intraocular distances.

Interferometry in an axial dimension is used in ways similar to ultrasound but has several advantages, since light rather than sound is used. The theoretical resolution for retinal and choroidal structures is finer for interferometry be-

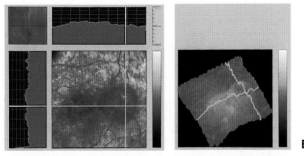

FIG. 74. Topographic scanning system (TopSS) images, 790 nm, 15° field, of a pigment epithelial detachment on the temporal side of the macular and a choroidal new vessel on the nasal side. The area with the pigment epithelial detachment is elevated with a depressed center. **A:** As in Fig. 72A. **B:** As in Fig. 72B.

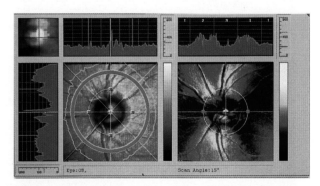

FIG. 75. Scanning laser polarimetry of a normal optic nerve head. The image is color coded. Color is proportional to the calculated nerve fiber layer thickness. *Black–red–yellow–white* is the color scale for the increasing nerve fiber layer thickness.

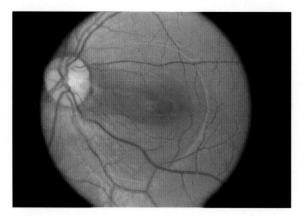

FIG. 76. Color fundus photograph of an eye with an optic nerve head pit on the temporal side, which is more likely to correspond to macular schisis, and a serous detachment of the neurosensory retina.

cause the wavelength of light is much smaller than that for sound and also because there is much better penetration. Furthermore, as with other optical techniques, there is no probe touching the eye. The strength of the interference signals depends on, among other things, the strength of the illumination beam after it passes through the tissues and the difference in indices of refraction. The index of refraction changes must occur within a small distance for effective backscattering, which leads to interference fringes. In general, structures that are strongly backscattering are potentially well visualized with both confocal imaging with scanning laser devices and by interferometry. Structures that cause multiple

scattering, backscattering at a more oblique angle, or backscattering over a longer distance produce a weaker interferometry signal but are potentially imaged by indirect mode imaging in scanning laser devices, as well as other scattered light methods. Recent ocular interferometry techniques feature a fine resolution made possible by new light sources, such as superluminescent diodes in the near infrared, that feature high spatial coherence and low temporal coherence. As in all interferometry techniques, however, the distance between or thickness of ocular tissues depends on their index of refraction, which is unknown for many structures in the eye, particularly pathologic ones.

Optical Coherence Tomography

OCT combines interferometry (in the axial direction) with scanning in a lateral direction to provide a cross-sectional image of vitreal, retinal, and choroidal tissues. Measurements of the thickness of retinal structures can be computed as long as the index of refraction can be estimated. Fujimoto, Swanson, and colleagues used an image alignment program to register the axial information of adjacent scans so that layers are continuous despite eye movements. In contrast, Fercher and colleagues have a dual-beam interferometry method that uses one set of beams to compensate for eye movements so that additional image alignment of the scans in unnecessary.

Macular holes, which may benefit from surgery, are differentiated from cysts or other abnormalities by using the ex-

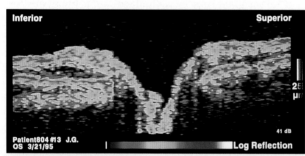

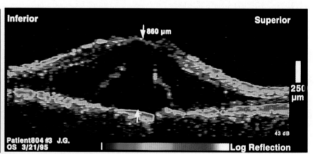

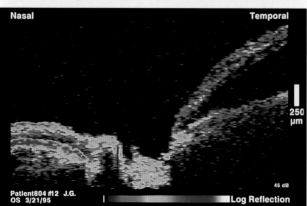

FIG. 77. Pseudocolor images from optical coherence tomography of the eye in Fig. 76 with the optic nerve head pit. Highly reflective or backscattering structures are represented as *bright, warm colors*. A gradual or minimal changing in refractive index or other factor causing low interference is represented by *dark, cool colors*. **A:** Vertical scan centered on the optic nerve head pit (bright, depressed region) and including the peripapillary retina. **B:** Horizontal scan centered on the pit (bright, depressed region). The retinal layers temporal to the pit are low in reflectivity and displaced by nonreflective spaces, interpreted as fluid-filled schisis regions. **C:** Vertical scan through the macular cyst region. The potential diagnosis of a macular hole is ruled out by the continuity of the retinal layers, albeit the uppermost layer is thin and a cool color. Dark regions bordered by *blue* are interpreted as schisis cavities filled with fluid. (Courtesy of Jay S. Duker, M.D., New England Medical Center, Boston, MA.)

cellent axial resolution of the coherence methods, for example, as described by Hee and colleagues. The goal is to determine whether all of the retinal layers are present and contiguous as well as which fluid cavities are connected, as in the case of an optic nerve head pit (Fig. 76). A commercial OCT instrument from Humphrey Instruments, based on the Fujimoto instrument, is used in combination with a slit lamp to provide a pseudocolor image (Fig. 77) and is also described by Krivoy and colleagues. The strength of the interference signal is color coded. Strong signals are represented by warmer colors (for example, red) and weak interference by cooler colors (for instance, blue) or darker colors. Thus, a continuous layer of tissue that differs strongly in the index of refraction from a closely adjacent structure should appear as a continuous band of a warmer color. If the gradient of the index of refraction changes only gradually or minimally, such as in turbid fluid, then a darker color is shown.

Laser Doppler Interferometry

LDI employs interferometry with a detector that moves, causing a Doppler shift. Fercher, Hitzenberger, and their colleagues have applied LDI to the measurement of axial length, analogous to the ultrasound A-scan measurements, even through moderately cataractous lenses. Schmid and colleagues have achieved an accuracy of $+/-20$ μm. LDI employs the dual-beam (or Michaelson) interferometer of Fercher and of Hitzenberger and colleagues so that eye movements may be compensated for (Fig. 78). Since there is no probe touching the eye in these measurements, there is no artifact from depth of the probe placement. In cases of severe corneal irregularities, however, it can be difficult to obtain

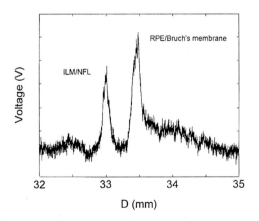

FIG. 78. Uniaxial reflectance profile 5° inferior to the fovea of the human fundus, obtained with laser Doppler interferometry (LDI). Average of thirteen consecutive scans. Peaks likely correspond to reflections from the inner limiting membrane (ILM)/nerve fiber layer (NFL) and retinal pigment epithelium (RPE)/Bruch's membrane. The x-axis indicates the optical distance (D) from the cornea, and the y-axis the intensity of the interference fringes converted to a voltage. (Courtesy of G.F. Schmid, G.I. Papastergiou, C.E. Riva, R.A. Stone, and A.M. Laties, Department of Ophthalmology and Scheie Eye Institute, University of Pennsylvania, Philadelphia, PA.)

enough direct backscatter to make a measurement. The result is a weak, rather than an erroneous, signal.

Digital Image Processing

All of the previously described techniques depend on digital processing for quantitative results. The cost in both time and money, as well as the incompatibility with the almost exclusive use of a 35-mm-slide format in most institutions and practices, cause many of these techniques to be accepted slowly. It is highly desirable to record images and data directly to digital media so that no information is lost in the transfer from analogue media such as tape or film. Then, there can be repeated later reproduction of results without loss of image quality as well as the addition of digital archival and processing systems. With the use of standardized file format, image data can be transmitted rapidly via the Internet or in offices with local area networks. In some techniques (such as blood flow from FA, tomography, and pigment density from reflectometry), digital image processing is possible without previous analogue storage of the data. Recent developments in computer-imaging products have made possible the recording of sufficient images or data at high rates to digital media quickly and inexpensively.

Visual Stimuli for Functional Assessment

There are several advantages of visual function testing with the SLO. First, the stimuli are visible on the retina during the test. The stimuli are placed as precisely as eye movements allow, either on pathologic or normal tissue. Second, several types of functional assessment may be performed: fixation assessment, pursuit eye movements, perimetry, pattern and focal electroretinography, visual evoked potentials, dark adaptation, and so on (Figs. 79–81). Full-color movies have even been shown to examine eye-movement patterns in patients with neurologic deficits. Third, the retinal function of many patients with ocular media opacities may be assessed when testing with conventional means is difficult.

Some instruments provide an infrared background to image the eye and a visible wavelength for the stimuli. The stimuli may be monochromatic or a mixture of wavelengths, determined by which lasers are used; even white targets are being used. Newer blue-on-yellow techniques to isolate the short-wavelength-sensitive cone pathway response have been implemented by Remky, Elsner, and their colleagues. An argon line (458 nm) and a Helium Neon laser (594 nm) provide excellent results, minimizing the artifact of media opacities in older subjects by careful alignment of the entrance pupil. Because the light is scanned, there is no speckle. The field of view is more uniform in brightness than the view on most television monitors, with the exception of visible *raster lines* (the small horizontal lines caused by scanning the light source line by line). These are visible when television monitors are viewed closely.

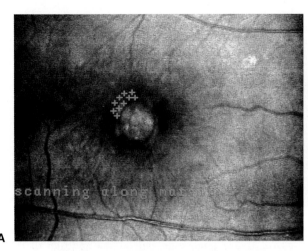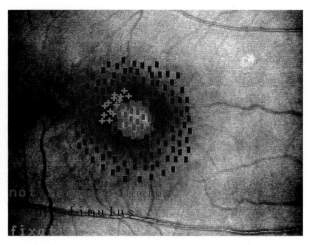

A   B

FIG. 79. Perimetry in a macular hole displayed in 780-nm light of an SLO, showing positions of fixation (**A**). **B:** Relative and absolute scotomas compared with a macular hole. (Courtesy of F. Acosta, M.D., Eye Research Institute, Boston, MA.)

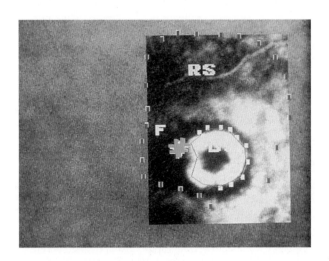

FIG. 80. Subretinal new vessels as shown in fluorescein angiogram, with the fixation (F), the dense scotoma (*red line*), and the area of relative scotoma (RS) plotted on the live video image of an SLO. (Courtesy of X. Reynaud, M.D., Eye Research Institute, Boston, MA.)

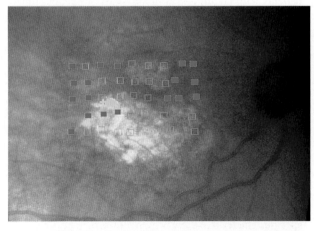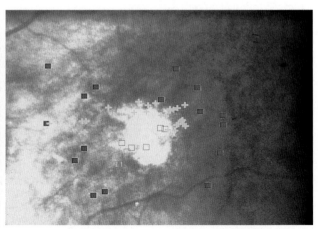

A   B

FIG. 81. Comparison of the sensitivity and fixation maps for an eye with age-related macular degeneration, following photocoagulation for choroidal new vessels. The *solid symbols* are areas where the stimulus was seen, and the *open symbols* correspond to areas with a dense scotoma. **A:** An eye with good fixation. **B:** A eye with poor fixation. (Courtesy of Sebastian Wolf, M.D., Ph.D., Eye Clinic, Aachen, Germany; and Ann E. Elsner, Ph.D., Schepens Eye Research Institute, Harvard University, Boston, MA.)

The light level can be set for virtually any clinical test. Several SLOs use white and a variety of colors for visual function tests. For cone perimetry with monochromatic stimuli or 594 or 633 nm, a full range of light levels have been investigated, from the dim stimuli that are typically used in bowl perimetry to backgrounds and stimuli bright enough to bleach most of the cone photopigment. Performance is not as accurate at very high light levels as at those levels used in modern bowl perimeters. Thus, the light levels used in bowl perimeters [1.7 log Td] are dim enough to be very comfortable but bright enough to lead to good performance in many subjects. However, this dim stimulus is not bright enough to pass through certain types of pathologic tissue to reach functioning cones. One example is the neovascular net and hemorrhage associated with AMD. For determination of scotoma size in similar cases, it is much better to use a brighter background and target (for example, 3.7 log Td).

The choice of tests available is limited by the temporal and spatial resolution, as is true in other video systems. Unlike phosphors in a cathode ray tube monitor, however, there are no phosphors to persist, and each spot is illuminated for only a few nanoseconds. The rate at which this spot can be modulated in brightness is determined by the computer video system used. Most video systems in the United States have one complete image each 33 ms: a 30-Hz frame rate and a 60-Hz field rate. Some computer systems permit 71 Hz. However, flicker rates and flash repetition rates are commonly limited to stimuli that are integer multiples of 33 ms. Square-wave flicker of the same pixels is 15 Hz maximum.

The size of target, gratings, checks, or lines must be a multiple of about 1.8 minutes of arc for each element. The finest resolution square-wave grating is 15–20 cycles per degree. This is more than adequate for assessing acuity outside the fovea, as well as the acuity in young children and patients

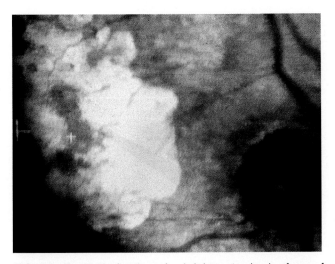

FIG. 82. Eccentric fixation of a bright cross in dry form of age-related macular degeneration. The *small cross* (added to image) indicates the preferred retinal location in other situations. (Courtesy of R. Schuchard, Ph.D., Wilmer Eye Institute, Baltimore, MD.)

with low vision, but not for assessing foveal acuity at high contrast in patients with good retinal function. Clearly, Snellen acuity targets for 20/20 (1.0) visual acuity cannot be presented accurately unless there is additional minimization of the stimuli on the retina. For perimetry, it is unnecessary to have a smaller target because microsaccadic eye movements in a person with excellent fixation are larger than 1.8 minutes of arc. It is usually useful to use larger targets of low contrast.

The rate of image acquisition determines the quality of the eye-movement assessment. The rate is suitable for characterizing several types of slow eye movements: pursuit, fixation, and components of the vestibulo-ocular reflex. Retinal versus target position as the result of voluntary, involuntary, or vestibularly driven saccades is assessed very accurately both horizontally and vertically (Fig. 82). We have demonstrated that an SLO in combination with a commercial eye-movement tracker can provide the basis for image and retinal stabilization. This would provide more accurate perimetry as well as benefit functional testing of children and adults with poor fixation. However, only a field rate greater than the usual 50 or 60 Hz would allow the measurement of certain parameters of fast eye movements, such as acceleration and peak velocity.

Sunness and colleagues have developed a technique to correct for eye movements during macular perimetry using the SLO, and have used this extensively in testing patients with geographic atrophy, a form of advanced AMD in which scotomas develop in the central field but often spare the foveal center itself until late in the course of the disease (Fig. 83). The examiner identifies two retinal landmarks, such as vessel bifurcations, and plans a set of retinal sites to be tested. The computer randomizes the order of stimulus presentation. This method differs from other fundus perimetry in that the examiner positions a cursor over the retinal landmark prior to the presentation of each stimulus. The computer corrects the stimulus position to be presented for any change in landmark position. The final results are displayed on a digitized retinal image in their correct retinal locations (Fig. 84).

PITFALLS

Media opacities are no longer the severe limitation that they were for older imaging devices, but there are still problems. Measurements around vitreous floaters and some cataracts are possible in instruments with narrow input beams.

It is difficult to perform measurements with any optical technique when insufficient light returns to the photodetector. For instance, ICGA has been clinically useful with a 1-mm pupil, but the image quality is reduced. Dense optical filters are produced when biological material either absorbs or strongly scatters light. Examples are the blood in a dense hemorrhage, clumped pigment, and cell and flare, and the

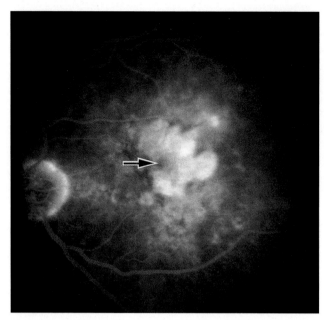

FIG. 83. Photographic fluorescein angiogram of an eye with geographic atrophy.

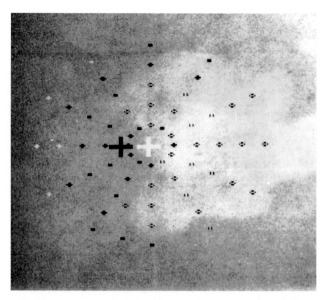

FIG. 84. Results from landmark-driven fundus perimetry, using the SLO in the eye in Fig. 83. The *white cross* is the fixation cross seen by the subject, whereas the *black cross* merely indicates the computer input to the instrument and is not seen by the subject. The results from the different target positions are coded in either *black or white*, according to which will be more visible on the fundus image. The *solid symbols* are areas where the stimulus was seen, and the *open symbols* correspond to areas with a dense scotoma. (Courtesy of Janet Sunness, M.D., Wilmer Eye Institute, Baltimore, MD.)

fluid in a large PED. An image obtained may provide information not provided by fundus photography or clinical examination but may be nonetheless nonquantitative or even misleading. For example, on FA, a PED has early, uniform, and progressive filling. The view of the deeper fundus layers, the potential site of fluid source, is often obscured during late phase. On ICGA, a thick PED has a dark, uniform appearance, which is due to the scatter of light by fluid (Fig. 85). The view of the deeper layers is again blocked during the late phase. This dark region has been mistaken for nonperfusion, and therefore ischemia, as well as a melanoma. Instead, the correct interpretation is that the health of the underlying tissues is unknown. Treatment therefore should be determined by the potential for vision and the effectiveness of treatment of the source of the fluid. A typical source of the fluid is thought to be leakage from choroidal new ves-

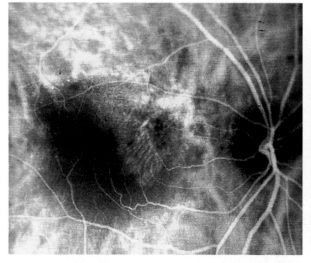

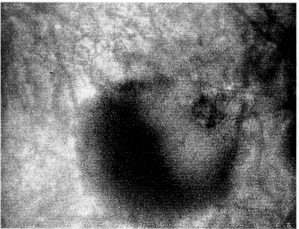

A

B

FIG. 85. SLO indocyanine green angiogram (ICGA) of a pigment epithelial detachment associated with age-related macular degeneration: early phase (**A**) and late phase (**B**). There is not a uniform filling of ICG into the fluid space but rather a clear visualization of the new vessels at the edge and superficial to most of the fluid. The failure of the light to penetrate the pigment epithelial detachment leads to a lack of conclusion regarding the extent of the vessels.

sels, which are readily identified as notching into the raised, fluid-filled area. However, difficulty remains in determining the extent of the vessels into the PED due to the blockage of light by the fluid.

Similarly, light may not be adequately reflected, because of a loss of reflectance in the retinal pigment epithelium and choroid. Quantitative light–tissue interactions in advanced disease are only beginning to be studied. Furthermore, imaging is difficult in a fundus with a highly backscattering structure, such as a fibrous scar, adjacent to an absorbing structure, such as a hemorrhage. Because of a lack of dynamic range, one image cannot represent both loci accurately. Detector systems or CCD arrays with much larger dynamic ranges, however, such as those used in the new photoreceptor techniques, are not yet in widespread use.

Interpretation of the results is sometimes made more difficult by invoking the automatic or technologically advanced features of new devices as well as by image processing. Although the Rodenstock SLO features an automatic video gain setting, it is particularly important not to use this during angiography. The HRA and AngioScan do not have an automatic video gain. Automatic gain varies the video gain in an unknown manner, often decreasing the contrast during the transit, and results in poor early-phase information. Further, it becomes difficult to distinguish between dye leakage over time as opposed to transmission defects in the successive frames. Similarly, if the images are processed to increase the contrast of only selected features or frames, then an erroneous impression of continuing dye leakage can result. Such techniques can give the erroneous impression of ICG dye leakage into PEDs or active CNVs.

Great caution has to be exercised when using digital image manipulation techniques such as digital image subtraction or contrast enhancement. Digital manipulation cannot increase the amount of data in a given image. Most methods will actually cause a data loss (image subtraction, and brightness and contrast adjustment). In addition, digital image manipulation typically increases background noise and in some cases leads to misleading artifacts. Some of these technologies may enable better visualization if the image is recorded too darkly. The operator has to ensure that the original image was recorded with the best possible dynamic range of light intensity. Otherwise, background noise is amplified to a level where image information is obscured.

Images may not be properly interpreted if the reviewer is unaware of the special properties of confocal imaging, which records images of one axial location: the plane of focus. If an object with a significant axial size is imaged, each confocal section image will show only a portion of the object. Out-of-focus regions appear dark, and these dark regions may be misinterpreted as hypofluorescent whereas the in-focus regions are interpreted as huperfluorescent (Fig. 86).

The clinical and experimental uses of these new techniques are beginning to drive technology in new directions, which in turn allows new noninvasive measurements in human eye disease that address questions of natural history, di-

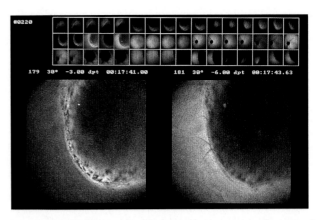

FIG. 86. Heidelberg retinal indocyanine green angiogram of a choroidal melanoma. The confocal imaging mode allows light collection from only one plane. The image can be misinterpreted if the reviewer is unaware of the sectional imaging mode. The reviewer may interpret the image as hyperfluorescent in the plane of focus compared with other retinal layers.

agnosis, and prognosis. Future developments in the imaging field will include finer video resolution, improvements in optical resolution, and more integration of computer technology into retinal imaging devices. These developments will further improve our ability to measure a variety of retinal parameters in ways that are currently not possible.

ACKNOWLEDGMENTS

This work was supported by the National Institutes of Health, National Eye Institute (grant EYO7624), the Perkin Fund, and the Chartrand Foundation (A.E.E.), and by the Whitaker Foundation and Stern Foundation grants (D.-U.B.).

BIBLIOGRAPHY

Acosta F, Lashkari K, Reynaud X, Jalkh AE, van de Velde F, Chedid N. Characterization of functional changes in macular holes and cysts. *Ophthalmology* 1991;98:1820–1823.

Arend O, Wolf S, Jung F, et al. Retinal microcirculation in patients with diabetes mellitus: dynamic and morphologic analysis of perifoveal capillary network. *Br J Ophthalmol* 1991;75:514–518.

Arend O, Wolf S, Remky A, et al. Perifoveal microcirculation with non-insulin dependent diabetes mellitus. *Graefes Arch Clin Exp Ophthalmol* 1994;232:225–231.

Arend O, Remky A, Elsner AE, Bertram B, Reim M, Wolf S. Quantification of cystoid changes in diabetic maculopathy. *Invest Ophthalmol Vis Sci* 1995;36:608–613.

Arend O, Remky A, Elsner AE, Wolf S, Reim M. Indocyanine green angiography in traumatic choroidal rupture: clinico-angiography case reports. *German J Ophthalmol* 1995;4:257–263.

Arend O, Remky A, Harris A, Bertram B, Reim M, Wolf S. Macular microcirculation in cystoid maculopathy of diabetic patients. *Br J Ophthalmol* 1995;79:628–632.

Arend O, Wolf S, Harris A, Reim A. The relationship of macular microcirculation to visual acuity in diabetic patients. *Arch Ophthalmol* 1995;75:610–614.

Bartsch D-U, Freeman WR. Laser–tissue interaction and artifacts in confocal scanning laser ophthalmoscopy and tomography. *Neurosci Biobehav Rev* 1993;17:459–467.

Bartsch D-U, Freeman WR. Axial intensity distribution analysis of the human retina with a confocal scanning laser tomograph. *Exp Eye Res* 1994;58:161–173.

Bartsch D-U, Intaglietta M, Bille JF, Dreher AW, Gharib M, Freeman WR. Confocal laser tomographic analysis of the retina in eyes with macular hole formation and other focal macular diseases. *Am J Ophthalmol* 1989;108:277–287.

Bartsch D-U, Bille JF, Dreher AW, Intaglietta M, Gharib M, Freeman WR. Analysis of the human macula by confocal laser tomography. In: Nasemann JE, Burk ROW, eds. *Laser scanning ophthalmoscopy and tomography*. Munich: Quintessenz, 1990:215–223.

Bartsch D-U, Weinreb RN, Zinser G, Freeman WR. Confocal scanning infrared laser ophthalmoscopy for indocyanine green angiography: preliminary results. *Am J Ophthalmol* 1995;20:642–651.

Bertram B, Wolf S, Fiehofer S, Schulte K, Arend O, Reim M. Retinal circulation times in diabetes mellitus type I. *Br J Ophthalmol* 1991; 75:462–465.

Bertram B, Wolf S, Schulte K, et al. Retinal blood flow in diabetic children and adolescents. *Graefes Arch Clin Exp Ophthalmol* 1991;229:336–340.

Bischoff PM, Niederberger JH, Torok B, Speiser P. Simultaneous indocyanine green and fluorescein angiography. *Retina* 1995;15:91–99.

Burns SA, Elsner AE. Color-matching at high illuminances: photopigment optical density and pupil entry. *J Opt Soc Am [A]* 1993;10:221–230.

Burns SA, Kreitz M, Elsner AE. Apparatus Note: A computer controlled, two color, laser-based optical stimulator for vision research. *Appl Opt* 1991;30:2063–2065.

Burns SA, Wu S, Delori F, Elsner AE. Direct measurement of human cone photoreceptor alignment. *J Opt Soc Am [A]* 1995;12:2329–2338.

Chen JF, Elsner AE, Burns SA, et al. The effect of eye shape on retinal responses. *Clin Vision Sci* 1992;7:521–530.

Chi QM, Tomita G, Inazumi K, Hayakawa T, Ido T, Kitazawa Y. Evaluation of the effect of aging on the retinal nerve fiber layer thickness using scanning laser polarimetry. *J Glaucoma* 1995;4:406–413.

Curcio CA, Sloan KR, Kaline RE, Hendrickson AE. Human photoreceptor topography. *J Comp Neurol* 1992;292:497–523.

Delori FC. Spectrophotometer for noninvasive measurement of intrinsic fluorescence and reflectance of the ocular fundus. *Appl Opt* 1994;33: 7439–7452.

Delori FC, Dorey CK, Staurenghi G, Arend O, Goger DG, Weiter JJ. In vivo fluorescence of the ocular fundus exhibits retinal pigment epithelium lipofuscin characteristics. *Invest Ophthalmol Vis Sci* 1995;36: 718–729.

Delori FC, Staurenghi G, Arend O, Dorey CK, Goger DG, Weiter JJ. In-vivo measurements of lipofuscin in patients with Stargardt's disease. *Invest Ophthalmol Vis Sci* 1995;36:2327–2331.

Dreher AW, Bailey ED. Retinal nerve fiber thickness measurements by scanning laser polarimetry. In: *Vision science and its applications*. Washington, DC: Optical Society of America, 1994:122–125 (*Technical digest; vol 2*).

Drexler W, Hitzenberger CK, Sattmann H, Fercher AF. Measurement of the thickness of fundus layers by partial coherence tomography. *Opt Eng* 1995;34:701–709.

Elsner AE. Scanning laser ophthalmoscopy, tomography, and visual function evaluation. *Clin Vision Sci* 1992;7:v–viii.

Elsner AE, ed. *Scanning laser ophthalmoscopy, tomography, and microscopy*. New York: Plenum, 1997 [*in press*].

Elsner AE, Burns SA, Delori FC, Webb RH. Quantitative reflectometry with the SLO. In: Nasemann JE, Burk ROW, eds. *Laser scanning ophthalmoscopy and tomography*. Munich: Quintessenz, 1990:109–121.

Elsner AE, Burns SA, Kreitz MR, Weiter JJ. New views of the retina–RPE complex: quantifying subretinal pathology. In: *Noninvasive assessment of the human visual system*. Washington, DC: Optical Society of America, 1991;1:150–153.

Elsner AE, Burns SA, Hughes GW, Webb RH. Reflectometry with a scanning laser ophthalmoscope. *Appl Opt* 1992;31:3697–3710.

Elsner AE, Burns SA, Weiter JJ. Retinal densitometry in retinal tears and detachments. *Clin Vision Sci* 1992;7:489–500.

Elsner AE, Burns SA, Webb RH. Mapping cone pigment optical density in humans. *J Opt Soc Am* 1993;10:52–58.

Elsner AE, Staurenghi G, Weiter JJ, Buzney SM, Wolf S, Wald KJ. Infrared imaging in age related macular degeneration: retinal pigment epithelial detachments. In: *Noninvasive assessment of the visual system*. Washington, DC: Optical Society of America, 1993:282–235 (*Technical digest; vol 3*).

Elsner AE, Hartnett ME, Weiter JJ, Buzney SM, Burns SA. Advantages of infrared imaging in detecting choroidal new vessels. In: *Vision science and its applications*. Washington, DC: Optical Society of America, 1995:192–195 (*Technical digest; vol 1*).

Elsner AE, Burns SA, Weiter JJ, Delori FC. Infra-red imaging of subretinal structures. *Vision Res* 1996;36:191–205.

Fercher AF, Hitzenberger CK, Drexler W, Kamp G, Sattmann H. In vivo optical coherence tomography. *Am J Ophthalmol* 1993;116:113–114.

Freeman WR, Bartsch D-U. New ophthalmic lasers for the evaluation and treatment of retinal disease. *Aust NZ J Ophthalmol* 1993;21:139–146.

Gorrand J-M, Delori FC. A reflectometric technique for assessing photoreceptor alignment. *Vision Res* 1995;35:999–1010.

Hartnett EM, Elsner AE. Characteristics of exudative age-related macular degeneration determined in vivo with confocal direct and indirect infrared imaging. *Ophthalmology* 1996;103:58–71.

Hee MR, Puliafito CA, Wong C, et al. Optical coherence tomography of central serous retinopathy. *Am J Ophthalmol* 1995;120:65–74.

Hee MR, Puliafito CA, Wong C, et al. Optical coherence tomography of macular holes. *Ophthalmology* 1995;102:748–756.

Hitzenberger CK. Optical measurement of the axial length of the eye by laser Doppler interferometry. *Invest Ophthalmol Vis Sci* 1991;32: 616–624.

Huang D, Swanson EA, Lin CP, et al. Opt Coherence Tomogr *Sci* 1991;254:1178–1181.

Krivoy D, Gentile R, Liebmann JM, Stegman Z, Walsh JB, Ritch R. Imaging congenital optic disc pits and associated maculopathy using optical coherence tomography. *Arch Ophthalmol* 1996;114:165–170.

Marcos S, Navarro R, Artal P. Coherent imaging of the cone mosaic in the living human eye. *J Opt Soc Am* 1996;13:897–905.

Miller D, Williams DR, Morris GM, Liang J. Images of the cone mosaic in the living human eye. *Vision Res* 1996;36:1067–1079.

Nasemann JE, Burk ROW, eds. *Scanning laser ophthalmoscopy and tomography*. Munich: Quintessenz, 1990.

Remky A, Arend O, Elsner AE, Toonen F, Wolf S, Reim M. Digital imaging of central serous retinopathy using infrared illumination. *German J Ophthalmol* 1995;4:203–206.

Riva CE, Petrig BL, Grunwald JE. Retinal blood flow. In: Shepherd AP, Oberg PA, eds. *Laser–Doppler blood flowmetry*. Boston: Kluwer Academic, 1990:349–383.

Scheider A, Kaboth A, Neuhauser L. Detection of subretinal neovascular membranes with indocyanine green and an infrared scanning laser ophthalmoscope. *Am J Ophthalmol* 1992;113:45–51.

Schmid GF, Petrig BL, Riva CE, Shin KH, Mendel MJ, Laties AM. Measurement of intraocular distances in humans and chicks with a precision of better than +/−20 micrometers by laser Doppler interferometry. *Appl Opt* 1997;35:3358–3361.

Schuchard RA, Fletcher DC. Preferred retinal locus: a review with applications in low vision rehabilitation. *Ophthalmol Clin North Am* 1994;7:243–256.

Staurenghi G, Aschero M, La Capria A, Gonella P, Orzalesi N. Visualization of neovascular membranes with infrared light without dye injection by means of a scanning laser ophthalmoscope. *Arch Ophthalmol* 1996; 114:365.

Sunness JS, Bressler NM, Maguire MG. Scanning laser ophthalmoscope analysis of the pattern of visual loss in age-related geographic atrophy of the macula. *Am J Ophthalmol* 1995;119:143–151.

Sunness JS, Schuchard RA, Shen M, Robin GS, Dagnelie G, Haselwood D. Landmark-driven fundus perimetry using the scanning laser ophthalmoscope (SLO). *Invest Ophthalmol Vis Sci* 1995;36:1863–1874.

Toonen F, Remky A, Janssen V, Wolf S, Reim M. Microperimetry in patients with central serous retinopathy. *German J Ophthalmol* 1995;4: 311–314.

Wald KJ, Elsner AE, Wolf S, Staurenghi G, Weiter JJ. Indocyanine green videoangiography for the imaging of choroidal neovascularization associated with macular degeneration. *Int Clin Ophthalmol* 1994;34:11–325.

Weinreb RN, Shakiba S, Zangwill L. Scanning laser polarimetry to measure the nerve fiber layer of normal and glaucomatous eyes. *Am J Ophthalmol* 1995;119:627–636.

Wolf S, Toonen H, Arend O, et al. Zur Quantifizierung der retinalen Kapillardurchblutung mit Hilfe des Scanning-Laser-Ophthalmoskops. *Biomed Tech (Berlin)* 1990;35:131–134.

Wolf S, Arend O, Toonen H, Bertram B, Jung F, Reim M. Retinal capillary blood flow measurement with a scanning laser ophthalmoscope: preliminary results. *Ophthalmology* 1991;98:996–1000.

Wolf S, Arend O, Toonen H, Bertram B, Reim M. Measurement of retinal micro- and macrocirculation in patients with diabetes mellitus with scanning laser ophthalmoscopy. *Clin Vision Sci* 1992;7:461–469.

Wolf S, Wald KJ, Kuckelkorn R, Remky A, Arend O, Reim M. Detection of persistent choroidal neovascularization using indocyanine green choroidal angiography. *Retina* 1993;13:81–82.

Wolf S, Wald K, Elsner AE, Staurenghi G. Indocyanine green choroidal videoangiography: a comparison of imaging analysis with the scanning laser ophthalmoscope and the fundus camera. *Retina* 1993;13:266–269.

Wolf S, Arend O, Bertram B, et al. Hemodilution therapy in central retinal vein occlusion: one-year result of a prospective randomized study. *Graefes Arch Clin Exp Ophthalmol* 1994;232:33–39.

Wolf S, Remky A, Elsner AE, Arend O, Reim M. Indocyanine green video angiography in patients with retinal pigment epithelial detachments. *German J Ophthalmol* 1994;3:224–227.

Wolf S, Wald KJ, Remky A, Arend O, Reim M. Evolving peripapillary choroidal neovascular membrane demonstrated by indocyanine green choroidal angiography. *Retina* 1994;14:465–467.

Zwick H, Gagliano DA, Ruiz S, Stuck BE. Utilization of scanning laser ophthalmoscopy in laser induced bilateral human retinal nerve fiber layer damage. *SPIE* 1995;2393:189–193.

Practical Atlas of Retinal Disease and Therapy, Second Edition
edited by William R. Freeman,
Lippincott–Raven Publishers, Philadelphia © 1997.

· 3 ·

Uveitis Affecting the Retina and Posterior Segment

Alan H. Friedman

INTRODUCTION AND CLASSIFICATION

It is quite useful to subdivide the lesions occurring in the fundus into four general categories. One can classify lesions in the fundus in association with retinal necrosis; the prototype of such lesions is toxoplasmosis. Viral lesions that cause acute retinal necrosis syndrome or viral-associated lesions are often herpesviruses. The second class of fundus diseases are those associated with nodular lesions. The prototype of nodular fundus disease is sarcoid. The differential diagnosis of multinodular lesions is metastasis or benign choroidal tumors such as hemangioma. The third class of disease of the fundus is multifocal choroiditis. Sarcoidosis, syphilis, tuberculosis, acute multifocal placoid pigment epitheliopathy, sympathetic ophthalmia, and other conditions are associated with multifocality. The fourth category of posterior uveitis to be discussed in this series includes lesions commonly associated with vasculitis, such as Eales's disease, Behçet's disease, and multiple sclerosis.

Toxoplasmosis

Toxoplasmosis is one of the most common causes of uveitis in the world. In some areas, nearly 50% of all uveitis is associated with toxoplasmosis. In our own series of 1,000 cases of uveitis, toxoplasmosis probably accounts for about 10%. The causative organism is the parasite *Toxoplasma gondii*, which is an obligate intracellular parasite that is a normal habitant of the intestinal epithelium of felines. The cat sheds the oocysts in feces. The oocysts are picked up by sheep, cattle, and pigs. People are infected by eating raw meat or through intraplacental transfer. Rodents and birds are a reservoir. Either small domestic cats or larger felines that are kept in zoos are generally infected with the parasite.

About 95% of human ocular toxoplasmosis is probably congenital, and 5% is acquired. The disease is normally seen in healthy adults, usually in their teens, 20s, or early 30s. The disease is manifested by recurrences; eventually, the condition may burn itself out. Patients in their 40s or older may have no further recurrences, although even patients in their 80s may develop recurrences. Most patients are healthy and immunologically intact. However, the disease is seen in immunosuppressed individuals. In a study that we performed, 15 cases of ocular toxoplasmosis occurred in acquired immunodeficiency syndrome (AIDS) patients. The disease had a strikingly different presentation in that it was seen in both eyes and was observed in multiple foci and often associated with central nervous system (CNS) involvement. For this reason, AIDS patients with ocular toxoplasmosis must undergo computed tomography (CT) or magnetic resonance imaging (MRI) of the brain. The prevalence of ocular toxoplasmosis interestingly is about 1 in 10,000 births in the United States, whereas it occurs in about 1 in 1,000 births in France. It is even more common in Brazil.

The clinical diagnosis of ocular toxoplasmosis may be supported by serologic tests such as enzyme-linked immunosorbent assay (ELISA) or by indirect hemagglutination inhibition titers. ELISA for immunoglobulin G demonstrates past infection and supports the diagnosis of ocular toxoplasmosis. Figure 1 shows an infected retinal pigment epithelial cell that looks absolutely normal. Figure 2 shows the prototypical involvement of a scar with reactivation adjacent to it. Figure 3 shows lesions in 40-year-old woman who had three previous episodes of active toxoplasmosis and who developed a new lesion adjacent to the fovea. One can see the lesion adjacent to fixation. As time progresses, one can see how the most recent lesions are being incorporated into the two previous lesions. Eventually, the recent lesion subsides, and the appearance is of one large scar adjacent to the previous scar. By 3 months after onset, normal vision has returned. A curious feature appearing in Fig. 3E, which was taken several months later, is new tortuosity of vessels adja-

A.H. Friedman, M.D.: Department of Ophthalmology, Mount Sinai School of Medicine, New York, NY 10029-6574

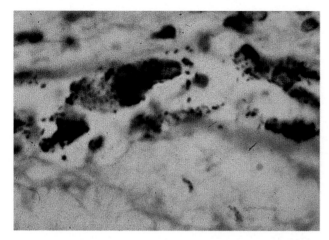

FIG. 1. Photomicrograph of retinal pigment epithelium showing intact toxoplasmosis cysts within epithelial cells.

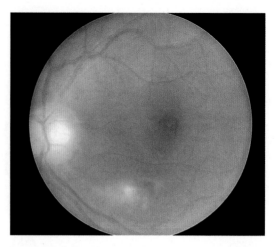

FIG. 2. Fundus showing a healed, scarred toxoplasmosis area with an active lesion just nasal to it.

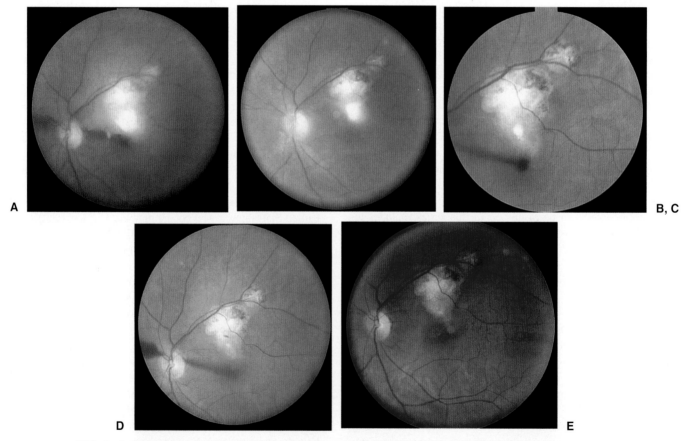

FIG. 3. A–E: Progress of toxoplasmosis. The most recent episode, the third definite area of activation, is just adjacent to the fovea. As the lesion ages, one can see lesions 2 and 3 coalescing until there is a large scar. In the later photograph, one can see tortuosity of retinal vessels, indicating superficial preretinal fibrogliosis. Vision returned to 20/20. (Photos taken at monthly intervals.)

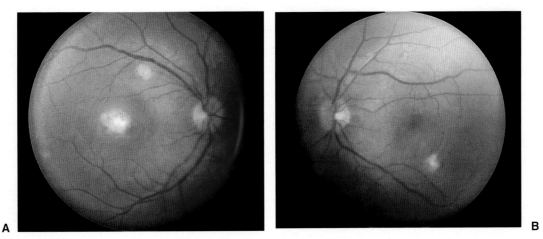

FIG. 4. A,B: An AIDS patient with bilateral ocular disease. The toxoplasmosis was not associated with a preexisting scarred area. In the right eye (A), there were multifocal lesions.

cent to the fovea demonstrating an area of preretinal fibrogliosis. In AIDS patients, CNS involvement with toxoplasmosis may also be present and may be life threatening. Figure 4 shows two separate foci in the same eye and bilateral lesions. Additionally, large areas of retinal necrosis encompassing an entire quadrant may be seen. Multiple active lesions may be seen in AIDS patients. The MRI showed three separate lesions in the brain that were ring shaped and showed enhancement in the outer part of the ring.

Treatment of patients with ocular toxoplasmosis may consist of quadruple therapy consisting of Pyrimethamine (loading dose of 75 mg followed by 25 mg/day). Pyrimethamine may be administered with folinic acid 5 mg three times per week. Clindamycin (300 mg) may be administered four times daily. Triple sulfa (a 1-g loading dose followed by 0.5 g four times daily) and prednisone (40–60 mg/day, depending on the patient's weight) can both be used. Patients are usually treated for 3 weeks and tapering the medication is

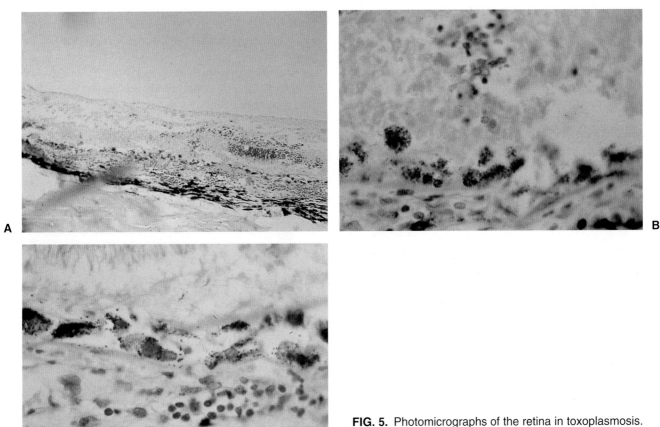

FIG. 5. Photomicrographs of the retina in toxoplasmosis. Note the large areas of retinal necrosis (**A**) and the presence of organisms in the retina (**B**) and retinal pigment epithelium (**C**).

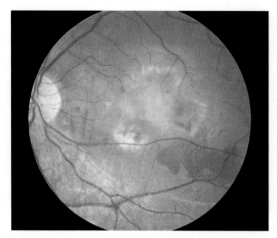

FIG. 6. Focus of subretinal neovascularization that occurred in a child. There is a disciform response with subretinal hemorrhage.

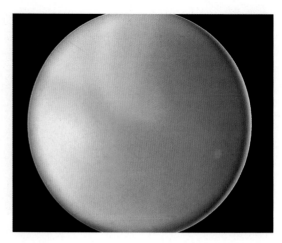

FIG. 8. Total exudative retinal detachment secondary to toxoplasmosis.

then considered, depending on the therapeutic response. Alternatively, Bactrim DS 500 mg twice daily by mouth may be used in place of pyrimethamine or clindamycin.

A number of complications are associated with ocular toxoplasmosis. The first is massive necrosis (Fig. 5), which is usually seen in immunosuppressed patients and is often associated with CNS toxoplasmosis. The areas of retinal pigment epithelium and retina are equally involved. Here, the patient shows extensive necrosis in the superior nasal quadrant. Figure 5A displays large areas of retinal necrosis. Organisms are seen (Fig. 5B,C) in the retinal pigment epithelial cell in the overlying retina; no special stains are required. Another complication of ocular toxoplasmosis is choroidal or subretinal neovascularization (Figs. 6 and 7), which generally occurs in teenagers, and the subretinal neovascular membrane is usually adjacent to an inactive choroidal scar. Figures 6 and 7 show the scar and the area of subretinal neovascularization superior and temporal to the scar in an 8-year-old girl. In the involved area, one can see the area of ex-

udative retinal detachment and hemorrhage. The angiogram quite nicely delineates the focus of subretinal neovascularization. As the study progresses, one can see the large amount of leakage into the macula. This eventually developed into a full-blown disciform macular scar; a choroidal–retinal vascular anastomosis developed during the process. In the late phase, the vascular arcades were drawn into the central area of the large scar.

Another associated problem in ocular toxoplasmosis is chorioretinal vascular anastomosis. Preretinal fibrogliosis is also common. Total retinal detachment may also occur because of toxoplasmosis. Figure 8 shows a documented case of ocular toxoplasmosis 10 years before reactivation. The disease was quiescent for 10 years, and a large focus of reactivation developed with exudative detachment. A branch artery occlusion (Fig. 9) may occur at the site of retinal

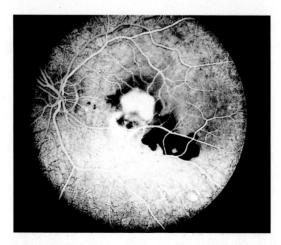

FIG. 7. Fluorescein angiogram shows subretinal neovascularization from toxoplasmosis.

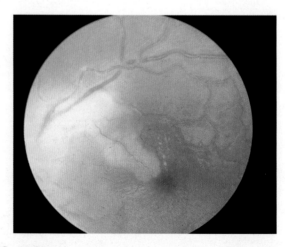

FIG. 9. Branch retinal artery occlusion secondary to toxoplasmosis. Note the beading on the retinal arteriole and the superficial retinal edema in the arteriole leading to the macula area. There is a large area of retinal necrosis just superior and temporal to the optic nerve.

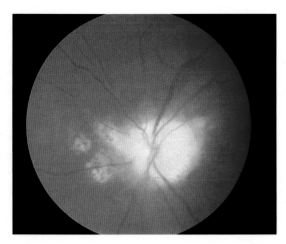

FIG. 10. Optic neuritis secondary to toxoplasmosis. A lesion is at the nasal border of the optic nerve, with two additional lesions in the retina away from the nerve.

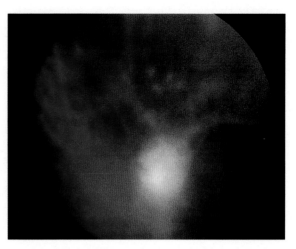

FIG. 12. A peripheral lesion of *Toxocara canis*.

necrosis. One can see areas of necrosis and arteritis. Superficial retinal edema extends into the macular area with a macular scar. The angiogram will show an area of nonperfusion in the necrotic area. Foci of retinal arteritis may also be seen in toxoplasmosis, quite similar to what one might see in Behçet's disease. Figure 10 shows lesions in a young woman who first developed optic neuritis at the age of 7. This was thought to have been related to demyelinating disease, although a few years later a second episode occurred outside the optic nerve. Toxoplasmosis titers at the time were positive. Because the lesion was on the nasal side of the disc, it was not treated. She subsequently developed additional foci of inflammation, none of which were treated (see also Chapter 5 by E. Ai).

Toxocara

Toxocariasis is a common disorder that is caused by ascarids (roundworms). It is a cosmopolitan disease, and stud-

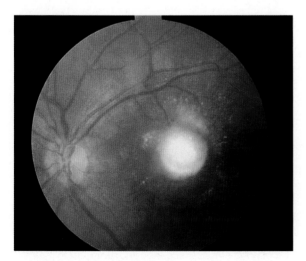

FIG. 11. Macular granuloma of *Toxocara canis*.

ies in New York State show that 73% of puppies are affected. They usually carry the parasite for the first year of life. The infection is acquired in utero by transplacental migration of larvae, and nearly all puppies possess mature egg-laying worms by 3 months after birth. Growth of the ova are inhibited in adult dogs. Human infection is accidental and is due to pica, ingestion of ova on the coat of infected pets, or licking the face of infected puppies. Two syndromes can be associated with *Toxocara canis*. In visceral larval migrans, first-stage and second-stage larvae in the gut emerge from the outer shell, penetrate the gut mucosa, enter the portal circulation, and travel in the intestinal lymphatics. The larvae enlarge in the liver and may travel to the lungs, brain, eyes, and skin. Visceral larval migrans is usually manifested by fever, hepatosplenomegaly, leukocytosis, and eosinophilia. The course of visceral larval migrans usually is benign. The second syndrome is ocular larva migrans. In this disorder, the larvae enter the eye via the ophthalmic artery or via the retinal or uveal circulation. This is usually a unilateral event. Three syndromes are seen. The first two consist of a posterior granuloma (Fig. 11) and a peripheral granuloma (Fig. 12) perhaps involving the pars plana. Either of these two can develop into the third form, endophthalmitis, which is often associated with the destruction of the larvae. This is manifested as granulomatous inflammation. The area of necrosis is usually associated with a central zone of necrosis and eosinophilia and the presence of the larvae. To date, *Toxocara canis* is the exclusive organism that one associates with dogs and puppies, whereas the *Toxocara cati* (associated with felines) has not been demonstrated in humans. The diagnosis is usually confirmed by means of ELISA serology performed on undiluted serum.

The treatment of ocular toxocariasis remains an enigma. Corticosteroids may be helpful. Surgery may be contemplated if a focal lesion is present in the pars plana. Figure 11 shows the typical posterior pole granuloma. A white lesion is associated with an overlying clear vitreous. In this particular patient, an ELISA performed at the Centers for Disease

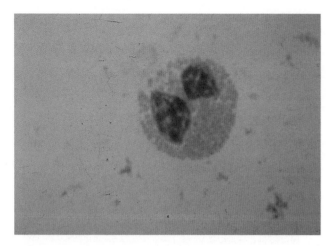

FIG. 13. An eosinophil that was aspirated from the vitreous of a patient with *Toxocara*.

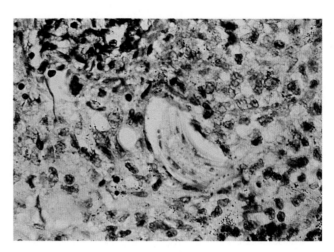

FIG. 14. The *Toxocara* parasite within the chorioretinal granuloma.

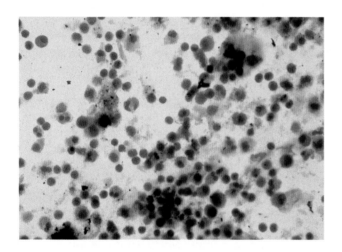

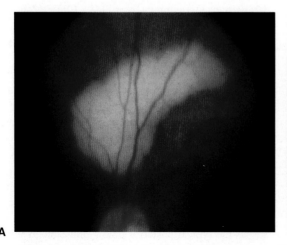

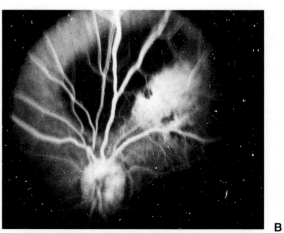

FIG. 15. In the adjacent area of Fig. 14, numerous eosinophils in the retinal tissue.

FIG. 16. A,B: Fundus showing exudation along with the *Clonorchis sinensis* superior and temporal to the disc. Fluorescein angiogram (**B**) demonstrates the presence of the parasite much better.

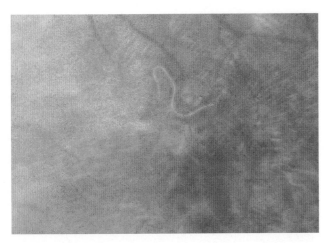

FIG. 17. The presence of a roundworm in the subretinal space, leading to diffuse unilateral subacute neuroretinitis.

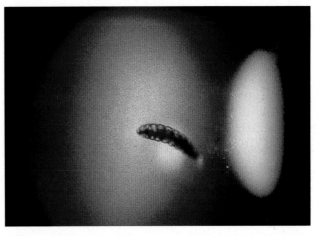

FIG. 19. Fly larva in the vitreous cavity (in the same patient as in Fig. 18). (Courtesy of Gordon Klintworth, Duke University, Durham, NC.)

Control showed a positive titer of 1:128. In some patients, it can be helpful to aspirate aqueous or vitreous and look for eosinophils (Fig. 13). Figure 12 shows a more peripheral granuloma in a patient. Serial sections, taken from the blind eye of a child, through the area of the posterior pole demonstrated the larvae in the midst of the granulomatous inflammation (Fig. 14). In another area, a larva is associated with a fair number of eosinophils (Fig. 15).

One must approach the treatment of patients with suspected toxocariasis with some trepidation. A parasitologist treated one patient with mebendazole, which killed the larva, but a quiet process in the pars plana was converted into a florid endophthalmitis following destruction of the organism.

Other Parasitic Infections

Other parasitic infections can be seen in the posterior segment. Figure 16 shows the fundus of a 42-year-old man from Asia who had emigrated to the United States and who complained of a scotoma superior to the disc in the left eye. There was a large area of retinal exudation, but between the area of exudation and the disc was a bottle-shaped organism pointing toward the disc that was better seen on the fluorescein angiogram (Fig. 16B). The organism was the Chinese liver fluke. The patient refused any treatment because his central vision was quite normal. Figure 17 shows a patient with a roundworm lying between the retina and pigment epithelium. This type of worm is responsible for diffuse unilateral subacute neuroretinitis described by Don Gass. Organisms migrating into this area and within the subretinal space destroy retinal pigment epithelial cells and photoreceptors alike.

Figure 18 shows the typical snail tracks of a fly larva migrating through the subpigment epithelial space. These tracks crisscross back and forth. The fly larva was found in the vitreous (Fig. 19). It was removed by vitrectomy. Many of the fly larvae, particularly those associated with cattle,

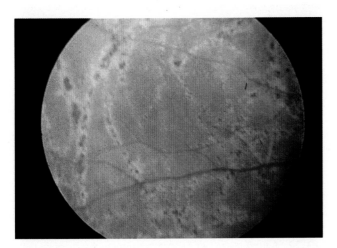

FIG. 18. Small tracks caused by fly larva in fundus. (Courtesy of Gordon Klintworth, Duke University, Durham, NC.)

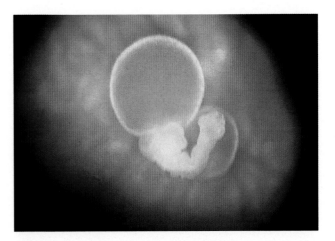

FIG. 20. Two cysts of *Cysticercus cellulosae* in the vitreous. The anterior macula has evaginated, and scolex is quite prominent.

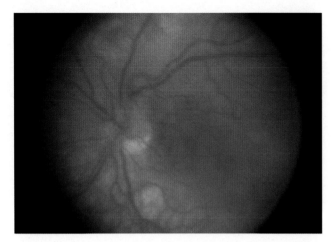

FIG. 21. Fundus of the same patient as in Fig. 20, following vitrectomy.

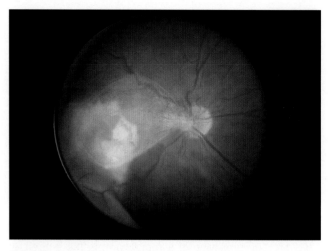

FIG. 23. A cysticercus in the subretinal space involving the macular area.

sheep, or horses, spend a portion of their life cycle in a warm-blooded animal. Sometimes the brain or the eye is inadvertently the warm environment in which the animal spends a portion of its life cycle.

Cysticercus cellulosae is the larval form of *Taenia solium*, the pork tapeworm. Cysticercus is in a cyst form during one phase of its development. Figure 20 shows two cysts of cysticercus in the vitreous of a young child from Guatemala who came to the emergency room with a seizure. When the scolex evaginates, one can see the scolex with its suckers and hooklets on the rostellum. The two cysts were removed via vitrectomy (Fig. 21). In Fig. 22, the scolex can be seen with a double row of hooklets and at least three of its four suckers. Cysticerci can also be observed in a subretinal location (Fig. 23). The most comprehensive ophthalmic review on cysticercosis in humans was written by Von Graefe in the late 19th century. He described 170 cases. The disease is less common in Western countries; however, in Third World countries, the disease still remains a serious problem.

ENDOGENOUS BACTERIAL INFECTIONS

Numerous cases of tuberculosis involvement of the retina and choroid have been described. Figure 24 shows a large tubercle in the choroid that developed during the course of miliary tuberculosis. Tubercles are large foci of necrotizing, granulomatous inflammation associated with exudation. Macular stars (Fig. 24) may be seen in association with these inflammatory masses. In another patient, vasculitis has been a component with foci of retinal necrosis. In eyes that have been enucleated as a result of tuberculosis, there is caseous necrosis in the choroid with an overlying retinal detachment (Fig. 25). In the areas of caseous necrosis are acid-fast bacteria (Fig. 26). One patient with AIDS was seen who had a choroidal lesion (possibly due to *Mycobacterium avium*) adjacent to the disc. The lesion did not respond to antituberculous therapy and enlarged slightly over the short course of follow-up. The patient died, but was not autopsied.

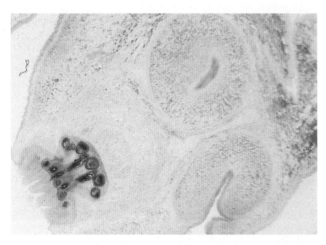

FIG. 22. A light micrograph of the cysticercus scolex showing the double row of hooklets and three of four suckers.

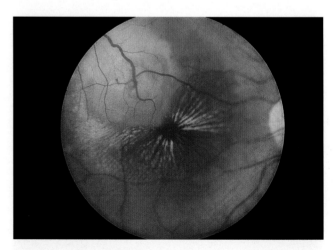

FIG. 24. A tubercle superior and temporal to the macula, with a portion of a macular star in a patient with miliary tuberculosis.

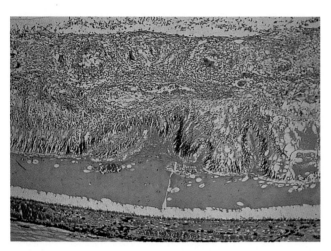

FIG. 25. An area of exudative detachment in a patient with tuberculosis of the eye.

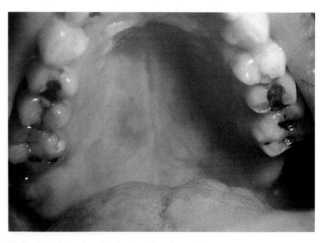

FIG. 27. A lesion in the hard palate of a patient with syphilis.

In association with bacterial endocarditis, endogenous infectious fundal lesions can develop that at first can be small and white in the retina and appear similar to those seen in endogenous fungal infections. These are associated with small hemorrhages. Eventually, these lesions may become full-blown abscesses with exudative detachments of the retina.

Syphilis is another bacterial disease that is still quite common, particularly in the population at high risk for developing AIDS. Sexually promiscuous people continue to run a high risk for the disease. Numerous patients have been seen with secondary syphilis; the spirochete *Treponema pallidum* is the causative agent. There are two general forms of the disease: the congenital form with the typically salt-and-pepper fundus and the acquired form (usually in the secondary stage) with a uveitis manifested as either an iritis, iridocyclitis, chorioretinitis, vitritis, or optic neuritis. Diagnosis is dependent on serologic testing with a Venereal Disease Research Laboratory or fluorescent treponema antibody absorption test. Syphilis remains one disease for which penicillin treatment has been quite effective. The primary phase

of the disease occurs at the site of inoculation, with development of a chancre in about 3 weeks. Lymphadenopathy in the area is quite common, and the lesions can be seen on the genitalia, rectum, mouth, and lips. The primary phase lasts about 3–12 weeks, and the organism can be demonstrated on dark-field examination; serology is positive. In Fig. 27, there is a lesion in the apex of the mouth, and biopsy demonstrated the presence of treponemas with silver stains (Fig. 28). Figure 29 shows the anterior segment in a patient who, in the course of his secondary syphilis, had anterior uveitis. One can see a ring of pigmentation on the anterior lens capsule where posterior synechiae were broken. Note also the haziness caused by the amount of vitritis present. Ultrasound in this patient showed an exudative retinal detachment. For all unexplained chronic or recurrent, unilateral, or bilateral cases of anterior uveitis, one must perform a serologic test for syphilis. Figure 30 shows the development of subretinal neovascularization in association with multifocal chorditis. An area of hemorrhage is visible within the macular lesion. Figure 31 shows luetic, optic neuritis. In the late phase of

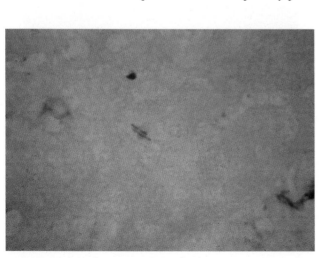

FIG. 26. In the same patient as in Fig. 25, acid-fast bacilli were in the area of necrosis.

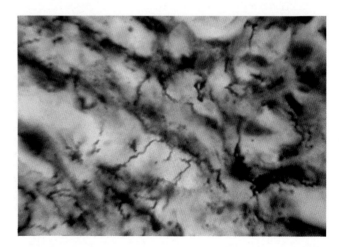

FIG. 28. A biopsy specimen with silver stain demonstrating spirochetes.

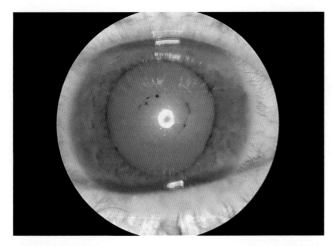

FIG. 29. The anterior segment in a patient with syphilis who has iridocyclitis. Note the pigment ring on the anterior lens capsule.

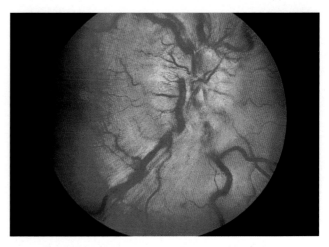

FIG. 31. Optic neuritis in a patient with syphilis.

BEHÇET'S DISEASE

syphilis, focal areas of retinal pigment epithelial hyperplasia may occur (Fig. 32). This particular patient had gone blind from syphilis and developed secondary glaucoma. The eye was enucleated and on gross examination the areas of retinal pigment epithelial hyperplasia were present. On microscopic examination, note the invasion of the choroid by retinal pigment epithelial cells as well as retina pigment epithelium present in the overlying atrophic retina (Fig. 33A,B). There are foci of retinal pigment epithelial cells within the choroid, as demonstrated by the trichrome stain (the red delineates glia, whereas the blue delineates the fibrous components of the choroid) (Fig. 33C). There are also large foci of gliosis within the choroid, indicating retinal pigment epithelium. Proliferation of the retinal pigment epithelium along with glial hyperplasia into the choroid is one of the classic findings of ocular syphilis.

Behçet's disease is an uncommon disorder in the eastern part of the United States. Approximately 75% of patients are males, usually between the ages of 20 and 40 years, and nearly all of them are from the Eastern Mediterranean basin (being of either Egyptian, Lebanese, Greek, Turkish, or Italian background). The patients manifest lesions in the mouth, with ulcers on the tongue, lips (Fig. 34), hard palate, and/or genitalia. It is occasionally associated with polyarthritis of large and small joints. The ocular involvement is manifested by recurrent episodes of iridocyclitis that may be quite severe and produce a hypopyon—devastating necrotizing retinal vasculitis with retinal vascular occlusions manifested by attenuation and nonperfusion in areas with retinal hemorrhages, retinal infarcts (Figs. 35 and 36), optic nerve ischemia, and edema (Fig. 37). Vitreous hemorrhages may be seen as well. Of the major symptoms, oral ulcers are seen at

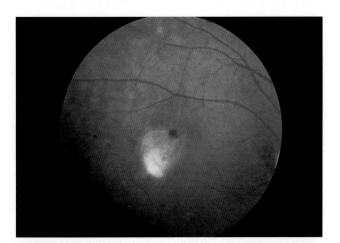

FIG. 30. An area of subretinal neovascularization hemorrhage at the border and evidence of multifocal choroiditis as a result of syphilis.

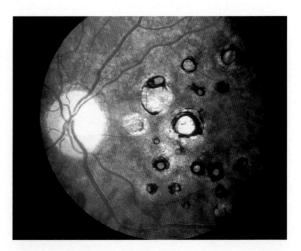

FIG. 32. Multifocal choroiditis with atrophic areas, with pigment hypertrophy at the borders, in a patient with syphilis. (Courtesy of Maurice Luntz, Mount Sinai School of Medicine, New York, NY.)

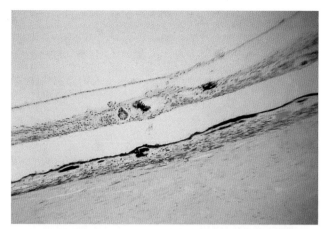

A

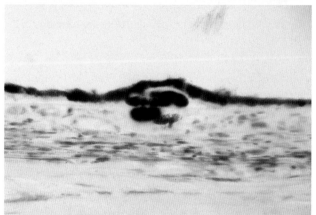

B

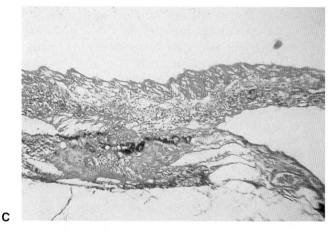

C

FIG. 33. **A:** Evidence of retinal pigment epithelial invasion of the choroid, as well as pigment migration into the retina in syphilis. **B:** Evidence of retinal pigment epithelial hyperplasia within the choroid in syphilis. **C:** Trichrome stain shows glial proliferation (*red*) within choroid.

some time or other in over 90% of patients, skin lesions are seen in over 80% of patients, ocular lesions are seen in about 80% of patients, and genital lesions are seen in about 80% of patients. At the site where blood is drawn, patients may develop a small focal necrotizing lesion. The condition is treated with prednisone and other immunosuppressive agents, such as chlorambucil or cyclosporine. Treatment must often continue for a number of years. I have seen pa-

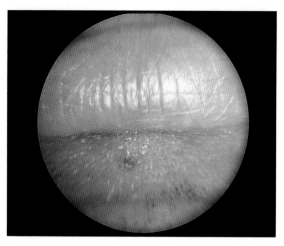

FIG. 34. The lip of a patient with Behçet's disease showing ulceration.

tients develop reactivation 1 year after discontinuance of treatment. In some patients, continuation of treatment for at least 5 years has been undertaken as a result of reactivations every time the medication is tapered. Anteriorly, hypopyon

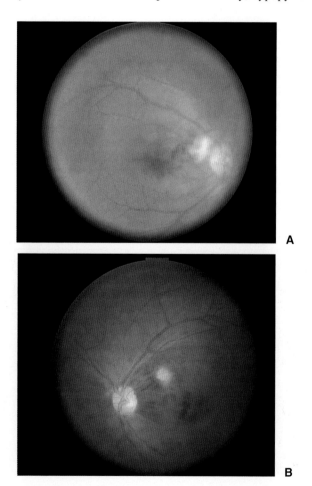

A

B

FIG. 35. **A,B:** The right and left eyes of a patient with Behçet's disease. Note the white areas of retinal necrosis with associated retinal hemorrhage. There is evidence of arteritis as well.

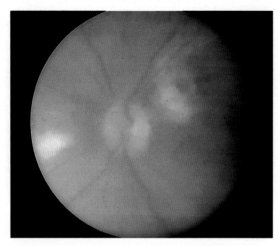

FIG. 36. Several lesions of necrosis with significant overlying vitreous haze in a patient with Behçet's disease.

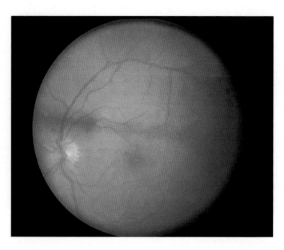

FIG. 38. A patient with pars planitis. Note the haziness of the vitreous.

and severe iridocyclitis occur with a significant fibrinous exudation into the anterior chamber. In this particular patient, an ulceration on the lip (Fig. 34) and an ulceration of the hard palate were seen. Figure 35 shows areas of retinal necrosis, with associated hemorrhage and, in the opposite eye, hemorrhages and areas of necrosis. Note the lack of highlights in the posterior pole. The highlights are seen outside of the posterior pole. This patient had significant disease, and the vision had been reduced as a result of multiple infarcts. Another area of infarction occurs superiorly nasal to the disc, and here again there is significant overlying vitreous reaction (Fig. 36).

INTERMEDIATE UVEITIS

Intermediate uveitis consists of a number of conditions, among them classic pars planitis, sarcoidosis, toxocariasis,

multiple sclerosis, and toxoplasmosis. The most common is classic pars planitis, which is of unknown etiology and usually occurs in two groups of people: one group peaks around the age of 5–10 years, whereas the second group peaks in their late teens and early 20s. Males and females are equally involved, and the disease lasts for 5–10 years. Of a large group of patients followed for 10 years, approximately 80% had a visual acuity of 20/40 or better. Patients usually complain of floaters and blurred vision, and the ocular signs are those of conjunctival hyperemia or a quiet eye (in younger individuals). A mild iridocyclitis may be associated with cells in the vitreous that appear as individual cells, snowballs, or debris (Fig. 38). Posterior synechiae rarely form. Inferiorly, there is a "snowbank" of pars plana (Fig. 39). There may also be an associated patchy peripheral vasculitis and, later on, peripapillary retinal edema or cystoid macula edema (Fig. 40). The snowbank, after many years, may ac-

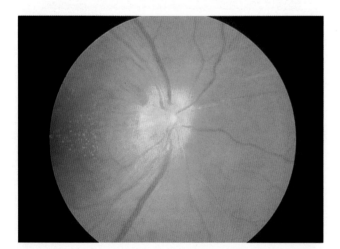

FIG. 37. The disc in a patient with Behçet's disease. Note the elevation and hyperemia of the disc with hemorrhages on the disc in the retina within an associated vasculitis temporal to the disc.

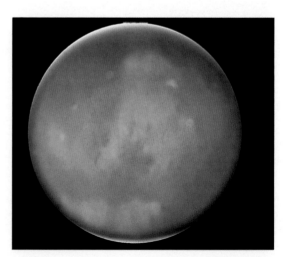

FIG. 39. In the same patient as in Fig. 38, note the exudation on the pars plana inferiorly with associated hemorrhage in the retina and aggregation of inflammatory cells in the vitreous.

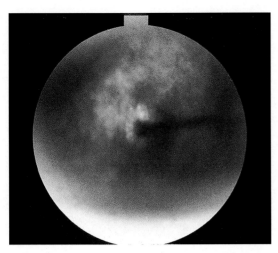

FIG. 40. A patient with pars planitis who had cystoid macular edema as demonstrated by intravenous fluorescein angiography.

tually vascularize and lead to recurrent vitreous hemorrhages.

In Fig. 39 is the trailing edge of a snowbank, with exudation in the periphery associated with vitreous hemorrhages and small aggregates in the vitreous inferiorly. However, cystoid macular edema is a serious problem and, on angiography, the typical flower-petal arrangement of the edema in the outer plexiform layer of the retina can be readily delineated (Fig. 40). Figure 41 shows one eye obtained at autopsy, with nongranulomatous inflammation in the stroma as well as in the epithelial layers of the ciliary body. The epithelial layer of the nonpigmented ciliary epithelium is quite edematous, and there is a fibroglial membrane on the anterior surface. Inflammatory cells have accumulated in the overlying vitreous. A high-power view shows these to be almost exclusively monocular cells. The usual complications seen in addition to cystoid macular edema and pars plana neovascu-

larization with vitreous hemorrhage are posterior subcapsular cataract and secondary glaucoma.

Retinal detachment is rare. Treatment of classic pars planitis can often be difficult. The usual course is to wait until the visual acuity has dropped below 20/40; then, the vitreous component causes significant symptoms, or cystoid macular edema develops. In these instances, treatment with either topical or periocular corticosteroids might be helpful. Monthly injections are usually given of posteriorly placed methylprednisolone (Depo-Medrol) (80 mg). If this does not work, a short course of oral prednisone may be effective. Methazolamide (Neptazane) (50 mg twice daily) may be effective in some patients for the macular edema. Cryotherapy is useful in treating any neovascular component of the pars plana. A short course of immunosuppressive therapy, such as a combination of prednisone and cyclosporine, may be helpful to patients with intractable cystoid macular edema.

SARCOIDOSIS

Sarcoidosis is a common disease in the eastern part of the United States, particularly in the New York City area. It accounts for 15% of all uveitis that we see, compared with 2%–4% of uveitis in other areas of the country. Women account for over 80% of our patients, with a predilection for young black women in their 20s and 30s. A second group consists of elderly white women in their 50s and 60s. Sarcoidosis is a systemic disease. Between 25% and 50% of patients with sarcoidosis will develop ocular manifestations. The disease lasts less than 2 years in most patients. Only 13% of patients have the disease for more than 7 years, and 7% of patients develop a chronic form of the disease. The lungs, particularly the parenchyma, are involved in over 80% of patients, whereas the lymph nodes draining the lungs involve about 75% of patients. On the average, approximately 40% of patients have ocular involvement, whereas about

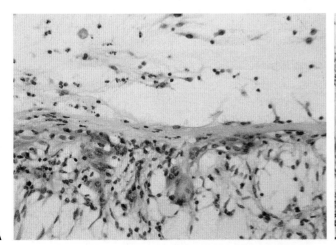

A

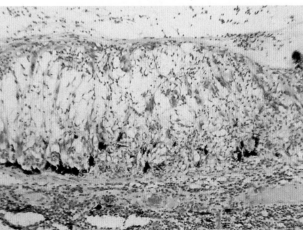

B

FIG. 41. A,B: Photomicrographs of the autopsy eye of a patient who had pars planitis. Note the edema of the nonpigmented epithelium of the ciliary body with a preretinal fibroglial membrane with a nongranulomatous inflammation in the ciliary body, as well as in the overlying vitreous.

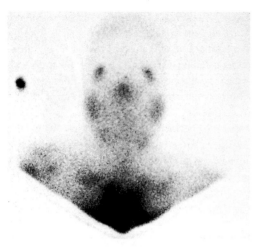

FIG. 42. A gallium scan of the upper body of a patient with sarcoid. Note the positive areas in the orbit, nasopharynx, and parotid gland. The chest is also enhanced.

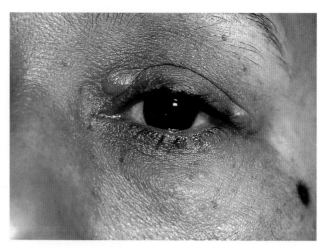

FIG. 44. A typical sarcoid eyelid lesion with a waxy nodule along the lid margin.

30% will have skin involvement. Further down the list are liver, spleen, CNS, and gastrointestinal tract involvement. Useful laboratory tests are the chest x-ray, serum lysozyme, and serum angiotensin-converting enzyme, as well as the gallium scan of the orbits, sinuses, lungs, liver, and spleen.

In our sarcoidosis clinic, the Siltzbach–Kveim test is standard. An antigen is prepared from the spleen of patients with sarcoidosis. The tested area is then biopsied in 6 weeks. Other areas that can be biopsied are conjunctiva (only when nodules are seen) and the lacrimal gland. Figure 42 shows a positive gallium scan with lung, lacrimal gland, and parotid gland uptake. Nearly 70% of patients will have some form of lacrimal gland problem usually manifested by dry eye, al-

though a number of patients show enlargement of the lacrimal gland. In these patients, biopsy is useful. Of the 40% of patients who developed uveal tract problems, 35% have pure anterior disease, 10% have pure posterior disease, and 55% have a combination of anterior and posterior segment diseases. In the eyelid, two different types of lesions may be seen. The first type, lupus pernio, is an inflammatory nodular lesion that is rather widespread (Fig. 43). In the second type, small nodules with minimum coloration occur 1 or 2 mm back from the lid margin (Fig. 44). When biopsied, the lesions show granulomatous inflammation in the dermis (Fig. 45).

In the conjunctiva, diffuse nodular involvement can be seen (Fig. 46). The conjunctiva on biopsy shows foci of epithelioid cells in the substantia propria. The anterior uveitis is typically "granulomatous" and is manifested by large nodules in the inferior angle, as well as by keratic precipitates of the mutton fat type on the corneal endothelium. Vasculariza-

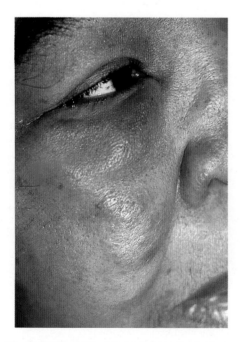

FIG. 43. Sarcoid of the skin as evidenced by lupus pernio.

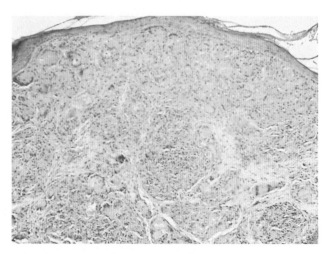

FIG. 45. A biopsy of one such sarcoid lesion showing granulomatous inflammation in the dermis.

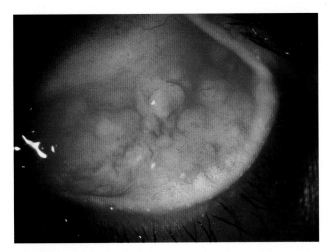

FIG. 46. A nodular infiltration in the conjunctiva in a patient with sarcoidosis.

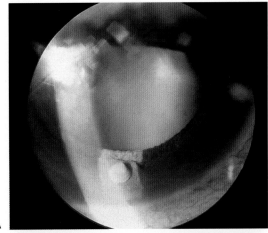

A

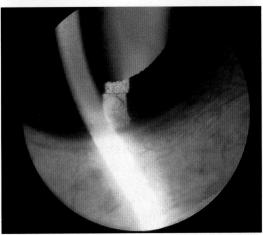

B

FIG. 48. A,B: A nodule on the iris surface (Busacca nodule); following treatment with topical corticosteroids, the lesion "melts away."

tion of these nodules is also seen in tuberculosis, but only indicates the long-standing nature of the processes. Large nodules in the angle may also be seen (Fig. 47). Following corticosteroid treatment, the nodules clear, thus leaving a grayish lucent area at the limbus, with broad peripheral ante-

rior synechiae. Patients may develop rather widespread posterior synechiae as well (Fig. 48).

Over a period of several weeks, the nodules shrink and eventually disappear, leaving no trace. In those eyes that respond poorly to treatment, one sees rather extensive granu-

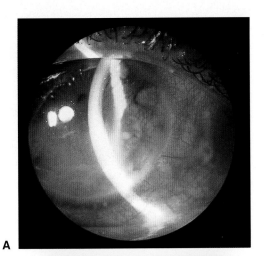

A

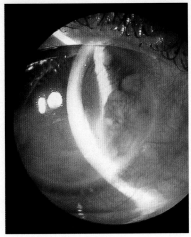

B

FIG. 47. A,B: Serial images of large nodules in the iridocorneal angles of a sarcoid patient.

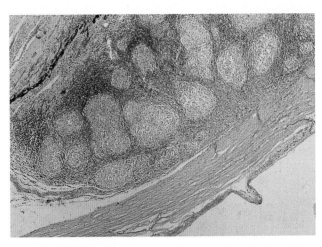

FIG. 49. Granulomatous inflammation in the ciliary body in a case of sarcoidosis.

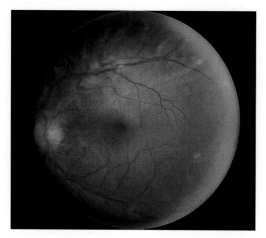

FIG. 50. Sarcoidosis with periphlebitis.

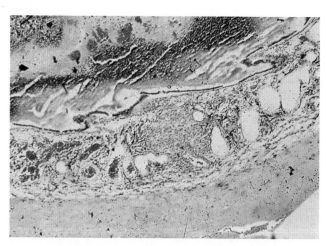

FIG. 53. Photomicrograph showing severe anterior and posterior segment sarcoidosis. In the choroid, one can see the focal granuloma. The overlying retina shows hemorrhage in the outer plexiform layer.

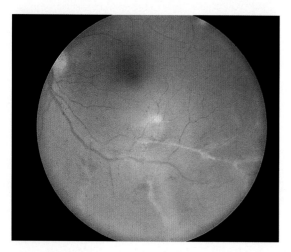

FIG. 51. Sarcoidosis with evidence of arteritis and hemorrhage in the retina.

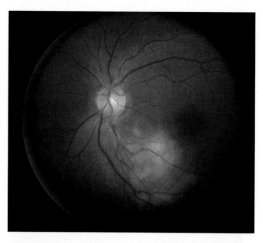

FIG. 54. Sarcoidosis, with granuloma in the choroid.

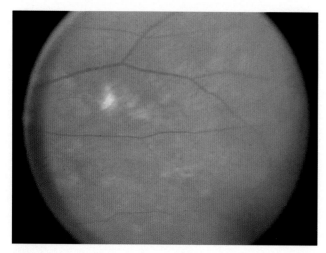

FIG. 52. Sarcoidosis and multifocal choroiditis. Note the small yellowish nodules in the fundus.

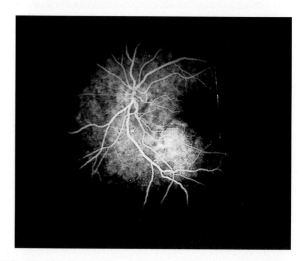

FIG. 55. Intravenous fluorescein angiogram of the same sarcoid lesion as in Fig. 54. Note staining in the late stages.

the course of corticosteroid treatment, one can see partial or complete resolution. The microscopic counterpart of a large choroidal nodule is seen here as a focus of rather significant granulomatous inflammation in the choroid (Fig. 56). The patient had bodywide sarcoid. In the eye, this was manifested by diffuse chorioretinal depigmentation and degeneration, with constriction of the visual field and an abnormality in the electroretinogram (Fig. 57). Figure 58A shows one of the more dramatic cases of optic nerve head sarcoid. This particular case was followed over a series of months, and the nodules are seen emanating from the optic nerve with surrounding inflammation in the choroid containing areas of exudation (Fig. 58). Nodules are larger as time goes on.

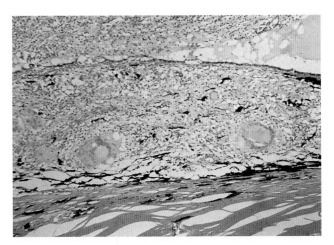

FIG. 56. A focus of granulomatous sarcoid inflammation in the choroid and subretinal space.

lomatous inflammation overwhelming the anterior segment (Fig. 49). Another problem is neovascularization of the anterior segment, with occlusion by broad peripheral anterior synechiae associated with rubeosis iridis. Posteriorly, a variety of problems in the fundus are seen, such as vascularization nodules, strings of pearls or beading in the vitreous, and nodules in the choroid or, rarely, in the retina. These nodules in the choroid may be small or large. "Candle-wax drippings" or perivasculitis is quite common. Focal hemorrhages along retinal vessels and neovascularization have also been seen. Optic neuritis and orbital pseudotumor are also common findings. Multiple foci of vascular cuffing of retinal veins are common (Fig. 50).

In the retina, arteries are similarly involved (Fig. 51). Figures 52 and 53 show nodules in the choroid. Histopathologically, we were able to locate areas of granulomatous inflammation in the choroid. The overlying retina shows hemorrhages in the outer plexiform layer (Fig. 53). Large nodules near the disc can be seen (Figs. 54 and 55). During

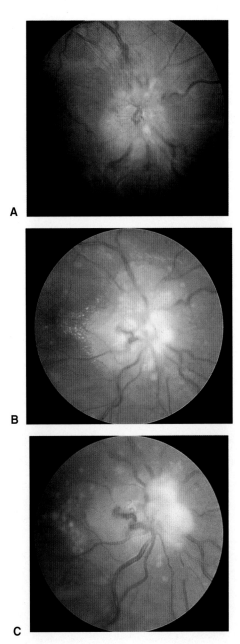

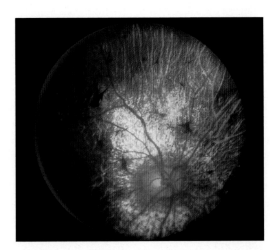

FIG. 57. A patient who had widespread sarcoid throughout his body, and diffuse retinal and retinal pigment epithelial and choroidal atrophy. His electroretinogram was extinguished, and he had severe visual field changes.

FIG. 58. A: Evolution of optic nerve sarcoid. Note the presence of nodules in the adjacent retina and on the surface of the optic nerve. Note also the opticociliary shunt vessel on the optic disc (B,C).

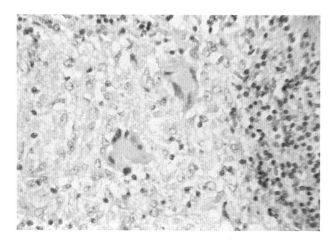

FIG. 59. Biopsy specimen of the optic nerve of a sarcoid patient showing granulomatous inflammation.

(Note the optic ciliary shunt vessel in Fig. 58C.) Biopsy revealed granulomatous inflammation in the optic nerve and its sheaths (Fig. 59). The optic nerve on CT scan shows incredible thickening right up to the optic canal (Fig. 60). In this particular patient with bilateral optic nerve involvement due to sarcoid, treatment with cyclosporine and prednisone returned vision from finger counting to 20/50 in each eye (Fig. 61). Note how the color of the optic nerves has returned. A peripapillary edema residue gives the peripapillary ring a yellow–white hue. In many patients, there is obvious enlargement of the lacrimal glands. Focal granulomata in the gland can be seen with trichrome stain.

SYMPATHETIC OPHTHALMIA

Sympathetic ophthalmia (SO) is a cosmopolitan disease. It is rare, with probably fewer than 50 cases per year reported in the United States. Historically, in 1890, 5% of perforating injuries were associated with the development of SO. As late

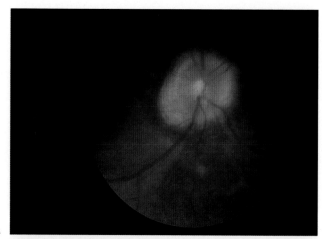
A

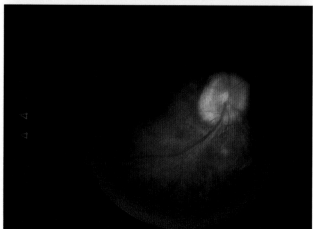
B

FIG. 61. A,B: Involvement of the optic nerve with sarcoidosis. Treatment with prednisone and cyclosporin A reduced optic neuritis dramatically. The nerve showed peripapillary edema residues. Vision returned to 20/40 from finger counting.

as 1975, fewer than 0.1% of perforating injuries developed because of SO. During the period from 1975 to 1980, 0.2% of enucleated eyes received in 26 ocular pathology laboratories across the country showed SO, whereas 1% of eyes received by the Armed Forces Institute of Pathology showed SO. Curiously, during the 1967 Israeli–Arab war, no cases of SO were reported although 10% of all casualties were eye injuries. SO is an incurable disease. Once acquired, patients usually do not spontaneously go into remission from the disease. Rather, they may go on to a lifelong association with uveitis. Regarding etiology, two types of injuries are associated with SO: the first includes blunt-to-perforating trauma, with an incidence of 0.44%; and the second includes cases following intraocular surgery, such as vitrectomy, filtering surgery, and cataract extraction, and accounts for an incidence of 0.06%. Onset occurs in approximately 17% of cases within 1 month, 50% within 3 months, 65% within 6 months, and 90% within the first year. Reportedly, cases have occurred years or perhaps decades following the injury. Eight percent of cases in the literature occurred after enucleation of

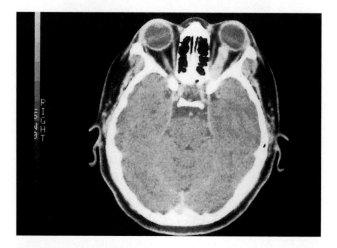

FIG. 60. Computed tomographic scan of the optic nerve. Note the intense thickening.

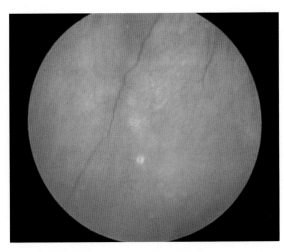

FIG. 62. A Dalen–Fuchs nodule in a patient with sympathetic ophthalmia.

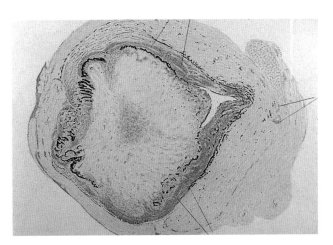

FIG. 64. A drawing depicting panuveal inflammation in sympathetic ophthalmia. (From Fuchs *Atlas of Pathology*, circa 1900.)

the exciting eye. Signs of SO are diminished visual acuity in about 60% of patients, conjunctival hyperemia in 50% of patients, keratic precipitates in 30% aqueous cells and flare in 50% posterior synechiae in 15% of patients, cells in Berger's space in 10%, vitreous cells in 25%, and macular or peripapillary edema in 20% of cases. In the sympathizing eye, the earliest symptom is blurred vision occurring in 60% of patients and photophobia in 30% of patients. Blurred vision may be due to a decreased amplitude of accommodation. This is an early sign of cyclitis. In the periphery of eyes with SO, one can see Dalen–Fuchs nodules (Fig. 62). The retinal pigment epithelium overlying the Dalen–Fuchs nodules is attenuated, and inflammatory cells are at the level of Bruch's membrane (Fig. 63). Depigmentation of the choroid and retinal pigment epithelium especially in the posterior pole can produce devastating visual sequelae. Pathologically, one finds diffuse granulomatous uveal inflammation with epithe-

lioid cells, lymphocytes, multinucleated giant cells, eosinophils, and a few plasma cells (Figs. 64–68). Generally, but not universally, there is a sparing of the choriocapillaris (Fig. 66).

Epithelioid cells contain phagocytosed uveal pigment (Fig. 67). Dalen–Fuchs nodules are seen that are collections of lymphocytes beneath the retinal pigment epithelium and anterior to Bruch's membrane. The granulomatous inflammation may extend into the scleral canal. Macular edema, with fluid accumulating in the outer plexiform layer as well as serous detachment of the sensory retina in the posterior pole, can be occur (Fig. 69). Historically, 25% of cases have been associated with an element of phacoanaphylactic endophthalmitis. In the injured eye, one may see uveal prolapse, with a track of the wound at the limbus (Fig. 65). There is extensive inflammation, and Fig. 66 is an artist's drawing of panuveal inflammation from Fuchs' *Atlas of*

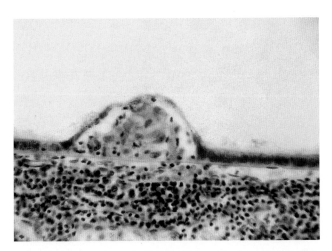

FIG. 63. Photomicrograph of a Dalen–Fuchs nodule. Note the thinning of the overlying retinal pigment epithelium with cellular infiltration between Bruch's membrane and the overlying pigment epithelium.

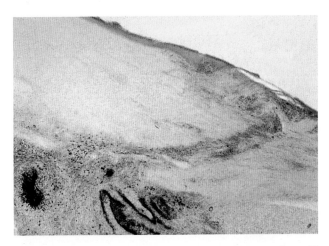

FIG. 65. Photomicrograph showing a limbal laceration with incarceration of the iris in a patient with sympathetic ophthalmia.

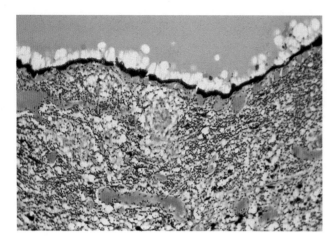

FIG. 66. Granulomatous inflammation in the choroid of a patient with sympathetic ophthalmia. Note the sparing of the choriocapillaris and the exudate in the subretinal space.

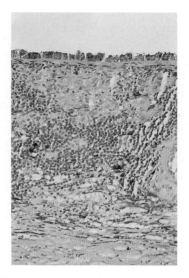

FIG. 68. Photomicrograph of granulomatous inflammation showing eosinophils in sympathetic ophthalmia.

Pathology, written at the turn of the century (Fig. 66); the pinkish areas represent epithelioid cells, whereas the dark zones are lymphocytic infiltration that has given rise to a "marbleized" appearance. Eosinophils may be readily seen among the lymphocytes (Fig. 68). Immunopathologic studies have shown that the lymphocytes predominantly within the Dalen–Fuchs nodules are T suppressor cells and cytotoxic T cells. Lymphokines, such as interleukin 2 and γ-interferon, and major histocompatibility complex class II antigens can also be demonstrated. Immunofluorescent stains demonstrate T lymphocytes in Dalen–Fuchs nodules.

Treatment of SO is proportional to the amount and location of the intraocular inflammation. Severe cases must be treated with oral prednisone, adding cyclosporine and azathiaprine as necessary. The latter two drugs are particularly suited to treatment of SO in children.

VOGT–KOYANAGI–HARADA SYNDROME

Vogt–Koyanagi–Harada syndrome, which was actually described by Jonathan Hutchinson in 1892, is usually associated with a prodrome of headache, stiff neck, pain, fever, nausea, and meningeal signs. If a spinal tap is performed at that time, lymphocytosis can be demonstrated in the cerebrospinal fluid. The prodrome lasts approximately 1–2 weeks and is followed by the ophthalmic phase manifested by multiple areas of retinal pigment epithelial leakage of fluorescein angiography, retinal edema, exudative retinal detachment, and papilledema. The ophthalmic phase is followed by the convalescent phase, which is associated after 1

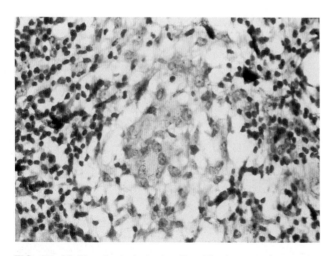

FIG. 67. Multinucleated giant cells with pigment phagocytosis in sympathetic ophthalmia.

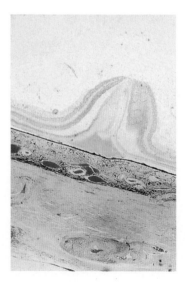

FIG. 69. Serous detachment of the sensory retina. Note also the inflammation around the emissary, in this case, of sympathetic ophthalmia.

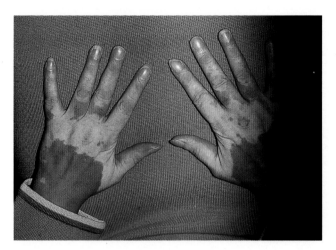

FIG. 70. The hands of a patient with Vogt–Koyanagi–Harada syndrome. Note the symmetric nature of the vitiligo.

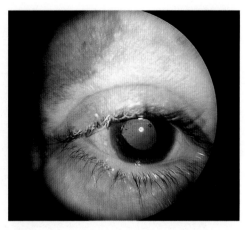

FIG. 72. Vitiligo, poliosis of the eyelashes, and vitiligo of the limbus. The patient's status is post cataract extraction with insertion of posterior chamber intraocular lens.

month with perilimbal vitiligo and after several months with generalized vitiligo, alopecia, poliosis, and sensorineural hearing loss. In the United States, the disease occurs commonly among blacks with Native American ancestry; Native American peoples, Hispanics, Eskimos, and Asiatic Americans are also involved. Immunologic studies have shown the presence of retinal S antigen or at least antibodies to retinal S antigen in patients with Vogt–Koyanagi–Harada syndrome. Patients with the full-blown syndrome may require a hearing aid because of sensorineural hearing loss, a wig because of alopecia, and makeup to cover the areas of vitiligo. Perilimbal vitiligo is the most constant sign and is seen in over 90% of patients, whereas sensorineural hearing loss, skin vitiligo, poliosis, and alopecia are seen in only about 25%–40% of patients. Patients can have significant symmetric vitiligo of the skin of the hands (Fig. 70). This is quite typical in Vogt–Koyanagi–Harada syndrome in that the same areas of each side of the body are involved. In diseases

like thyrotoxicosis and diabetes mellitus, similarly the vitiligo is symmetric whereas, in conditions like leprosy and syphilis, vitiligo is quite haphazard. Perilimbal vitiligo (Fig. 71) is common, as is perilimbal vitiligo combined with poliosis of the upper-lid eyelashes. In many patients, the uveitis may be under control, but vitiligo of the skin progresses even with prednisone therapy (Fig. 72). Figure 73 shows a fundus photograph of exudative detachment of the posterior pole. (Note that the retina is thrown up into folds.) There is marked hyperemia of the optic nerve, and fluorescein angiography shows multiple areas of retinal pigment epithelium leakage (Fig. 74A) indicative of multifocal chorditis. A later phase of the angiogram shows the near confluence of the multifocal areas, along with leakage from the optic nerve (Fig. 74B).

In the convalescent phase, focal areas of retinal pigment epithelial hyperplasia developed (Fig. 75). (Note also the depigmentation of the intervening choroid, referred to as the sunset glow sign.) In some patients, when the exudative de-

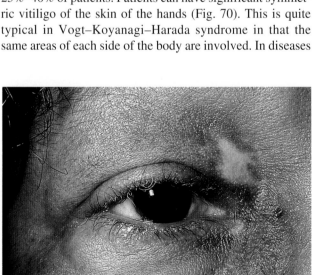

FIG. 71. Perilimbal and skin vitiligo in Vogt–Koyanagi–Harada syndrome.

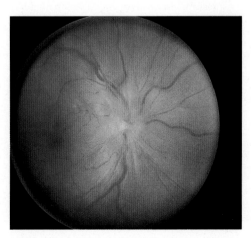

FIG. 73. An exudative detachment of the posterior pole in Vogt–Koyanagi–Harada syndrome.

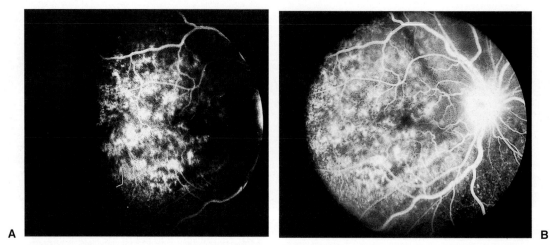

FIG. 74. Early (**A**) and slightly later (**B**) angiograms of a posterior pole. Note the areas of multifocal choroiditis with focal leakage in Vogt–Koyanagi–Harada syndrome.

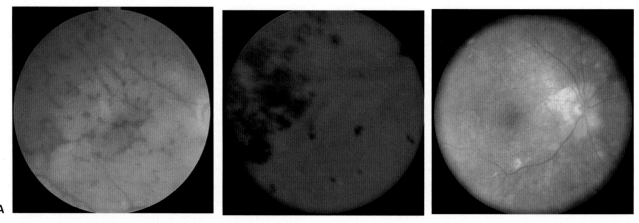

FIG. 75. A–C: Various areas of retinal pigment epithelial hyperplasia following resolution of the exudative detachment in Vogt–Koyanagi–Harada syndrome. Areas between the foci of retinal pigment epithelial hyperplasia showed vitiligo of the choroid, giving rise to the sunset glow sign.

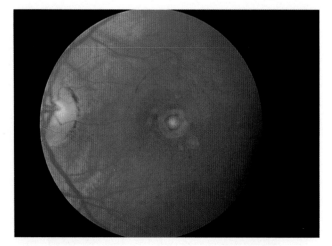

FIG. 76. Macular fibrosis following resolution of the exudative detachment.

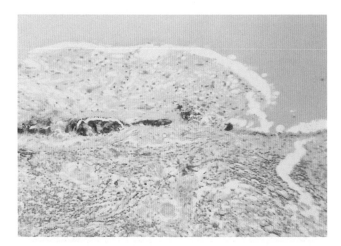

FIG. 77. Granulomatous inflammation in the eye in Vogt–Koyanagi–Harada syndrome. Note that the granulomatous inflammation extends through the choriocapillaris into the subretinal space. Note also the exudative response.

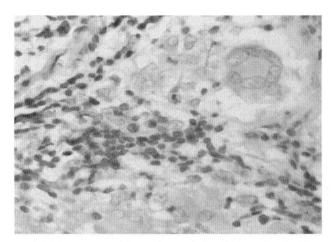

FIG. 78. Multinucleated giant cells and epithelioid cells in Vogt–Koyanagi–Harada syndrome.

tachment clears, macular fibrosis causes irretrievable central visual loss (Fig. 76). In this particular patient, vision had returned to 20/30, but she developed an exudative detachment several years afterward due to the ingrowth of subretinal neovascularization. She was treated with high-dose corticosteroids and her vision improved.

Histopathologically, granulomatous inflammation is present in the choroid, with extension through the choriocapillaris and pigment epithelium into the subretinal space, with an overlying serous retinal detachment (Fig. 77). High-power microscopy shows foci of multinucleated giant cells, epithelioid cells, and lymphocytes (Fig. 78). Vitiligo is an interesting component of Vogt–Koyanagi–Harada syndrome. Numerous etiologies have been proposed for the cause: an immune hypothesis suggests a circulating immune factor, an activated T cell, or perhaps an antibody; a neural hypothesis suggests that the neural innovation of the melanocyte is affected; lastly, a hypothesis suggests an autodestruct mechanism in the limbal melanocytes. None of these three mechanisms have been proven to date. In a patient with vitiligo of

the skin, poliosis of the eyelashes, and limbal vitiligo, a cataract was operated on and a sample of limbal tissue was obtained at the time of cataract surgery. DOPA stains as well as Fontana–Masson stains for melanin were both negative, indicating the loss of melanocytes. The disease is treated with a high dose of corticosteroids, often in association with cyclosporine if the corticosteroids are not effective. A number of patients can be treated with perhaps 5 mg/kg of cyclosporine per day, along with a lower dosage of prednisone. Corticosteroids are usually continued for the rest of the patient's life.

LEUKEMIC INFILTRATION

Leukemia may be associated with some form of ocular involvement in over 50% of cases. Cotton-wool spots with attendant hemorrhages are quite common. However, less common are actual leukemic infiltrations of the retina (Figs. 79 and 80). Retinal metastases, as in this case of bronchogenic carcinoma metastatic to the retina, often produce a difficult diagnostic picture (Figs. 81 and 82). Myelinated nerve fibers

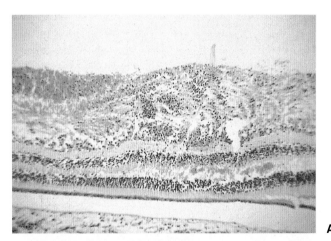

A

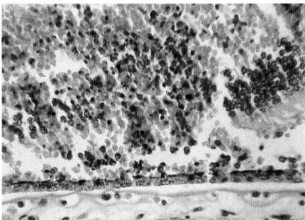

B

FIG. 80. A,B: The same patient as in Fig. 79. Note the leukemic infiltration in the retina and subretinal space. Hemorrhage appeared after the photograph was taken.

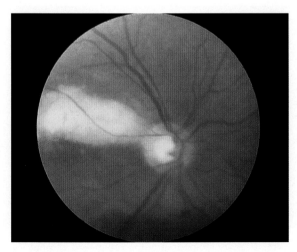

FIG. 79. Leukemic infiltration in the retina.

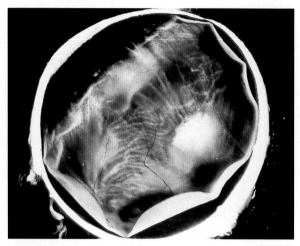

FIG. 81. Retinal metastasis. (Courtesy of Don Nicholson, Bascom Palmer Eye Institute, Miami, FL.)

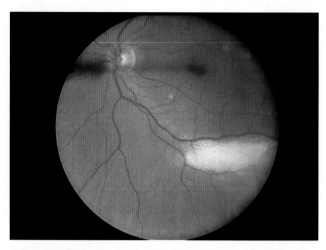

FIG. 83. Myelinated nerve fibers in the retina. Note the feathered appearance distally and a hint of myelination in the area between the disc and large area.

may be mistaken for a pathologic condition in some rare instances. The white color, the level of retinal involvement, and the feathery peripheral border should be quite apparent (Fig. 83).

PRIMARY INTRAOCULAR OCULAR LYMPHOMA

One particular syndrome that should be kept in mind—particularly in patients aged 50 and older who have either unexplained vitritis or multifocal lesions in the retina or subpigment retinal pigment epithelium—is primary intraocular lymphoma, which is known to most ophthalmologists as reticulum cell sarcoma. Although rare, many cases have been reported. Although this disease, which is certainly underdiagnosed because the necessary test—vitreous aspiration/vitrectomy—is not done, is most commonly seen in those aged 50 and older, we have seen patients as young as 25 years of age. The cell that produces the lymphoma most often is the lymphocyte. In total, 85% of cases are B lym-

phocyte derived, and 15% of cases are T lymphocyte derived. The condition is usually bilateral in about 80% of patients, and about 20% of patients have concomitant CNS involvement. A CT scan or preferably MRI with gadolinium is absolutely necessary. The condition is manifested by vitreous cellular involvement or with multifocal intraretinal or subretinal pigment epithelial infiltrates. These infiltrates, which are usually white or may be associated with hemorrhage (Fig. 84), are small and discrete at first and then eventually become confluent. Sometimes the lesions, when first seen, are rather nodular at the level of the pigment epithelium with overlying mottling of retinal pigment epithelial cells. The lesions, as noted here, in this particular instance are multiple and small. They may be single, as noted in the particular patient whose condition was thought to have been a lesion of toxoplasmosis but it did not respond to antitoxoplasmosis therapy and became larger after 4 weeks of quadruple therapy (Fig. 85). When the patient developed bilateral vitreal infiltrations, a vitreous biopsy was done.

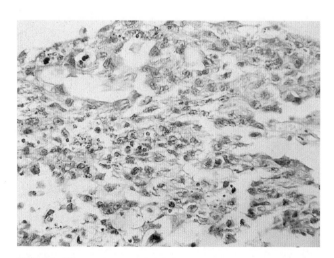

FIG. 82. Photomicrograph of the same lesion as in Fig. 81, showing metastatic bronchogenic carcinoma in the retina.

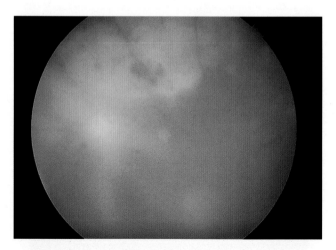

FIG. 84. Primary lymphoma of the retina and vitreous. Note the overlying vitreous haze.

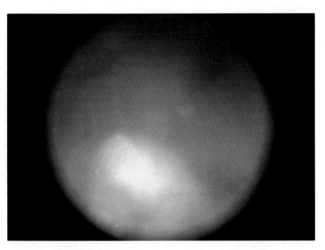

FIG. 85. A solitary focus of lymphoma inferior and temporal to the disc. Note the overlying vitreous haze.

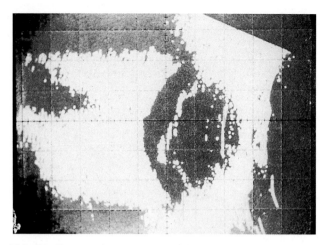

FIG. 87. B-scan ultrasonogram of the same patient as in Fig. 86. Note the thickening of the detached posterior vitreous face.

Some patients developed such a large cellular aggregation that when a posterior vitreous detachment developed, a collection of cells formed on the detached posterior vitreous face (Fig. 86). This was well documented on B-scan ultrasound (Fig. 87). Presented here is the ultrasound of that case of lymphoma, and a rather large subretinal pigment epithelial nodule in another patient with lymphoma (Fig. 88). (Note the speckling of the pigment epithelium overlying it.) Fluorescein angiography shows that the lesion fluoresces during the course of the angiogram (Fig. 89). Figure 90 shows a case where discrete lesions are apparent throughout the posterior pole (Fig. 90A), whereas the other eye has confluent lesions (Fig. 90B). This particular case looks not unlike that seen in the acute retinal necrosis syndrome (Fig. 84). The CT scan shows a large nodule in the temporal lobe (Fig. 91). Rare cases may have a vasculitic presentation.

It is the vitreous biopsy that must be performed and depended on for diagnosis. The material that is removed (usu-

ally 0.5 ml) can either be spun down (in a Cytospin centrifuge) or filtered (through a Millipore filter). The cells are large, with large nuclei and scant cytoplasm; bizarre forms may be present with mitotic figures (Fig. 92A). The nucleus may be seen bulging through the nuclear membrane into the cytoplasm (Fig. 92B). Treatment entails combination radiotherapy, usually 2,000 rad of therapy to the eye and brain, along with high-dose intravenous cytosine arabinoside. As seen in Fig. 93, there can be complete resolution of the disease. In the days before chemotherapy was added to the regimen, radiotherapy was often not enough to cure the disease. In this particular patient who had a T-cell lymphoma, lesion enlargement can be seen. In this patient, treated with radiotherapy alone, the disease recurred 1 year later and then systematized, producing lesions along the large intestinal tract (as seen by the abdominal CT). At autopsy in a patient who died following radiotherapy and core vitrectomy, "exudation" at the level of the pars plana can be seen. Histopathol-

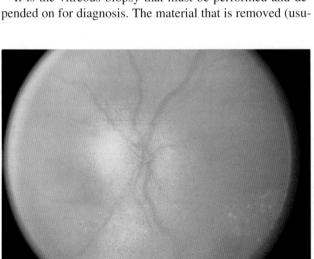

FIG. 86. Note the dense infiltration of the vitreous, with collection of lymphoma cells on the posterior surface of the vitreous face (*right*).

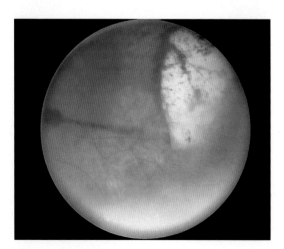

FIG. 88. A large subpigment epithelial nodule. Note the mottling of the overlying pigment.

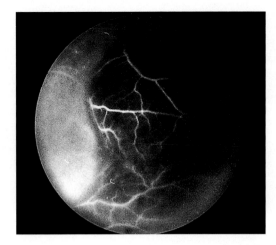

FIG. 89. Lesion stains on fluorescein angiography.

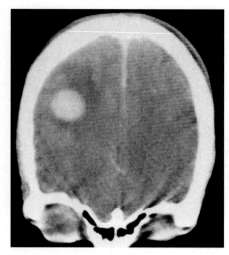

FIG. 91. Computed tomographic scan showing a large nodule in the temporal lobe.

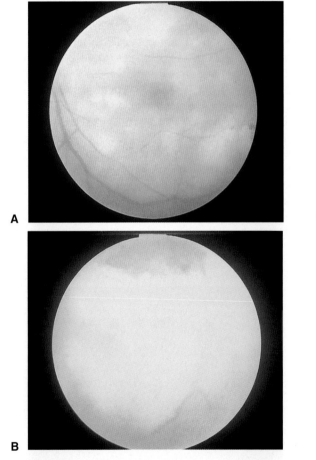

FIG. 90. Right (**A**) and left (**B**) eyes of the same patient as in Fig. 89. Note the multiple white intraretinal and subretinal lymphoma lesions. They have coalesced in B.

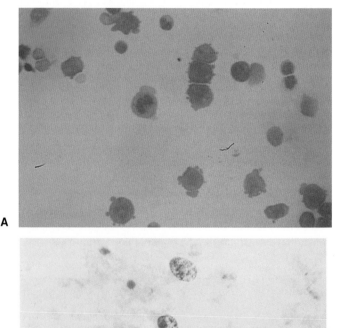

FIG. 92. Vitreous aspirates that were subjected to Cytospin. **A:** Note the large bizarre-looking cell with large nuclei, some with mitotic figures and distinct pleomorphism. **B:** A distortion of the nucleus projects into the cytoplasm in this case of ocular lymphoma.

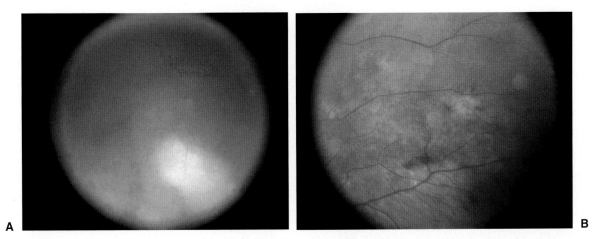

FIG. 93. A patient with ocular lymphoma before (**A**) and after (**B**) radiotherapy and chemotherapy. The lesion resolves completely.

ogy revealed the effect of the core vitrectomy, with residual cells in the cortex of the vitreous and high-power view showing the cells were malignant lymphoma (Fig. 94).

OTHER UNUSUAL CAUSES OF VITREOUS CELLS

Vitreous cells may be present in patients with retinitis pigmentosa. This is not an inflammatory disease, and the vitreal cellular presence does not mandate treatment with anti-inflammatory agents.

A group of patients who are in their 50s and 60s develop cells in the vitreous. These may or may not be associated with multifocal choroidal lesions (Figs. 95 and 96). They may be associated with Whipple's disease, and it may be necessary to biopsy the vitreous if the visual acuity is affected even in the absence of systemic disease because an ocular form of Whipple's disease has been well described by Schepens and colleagues. In these patients, vitreous aspira-

tion may be necessary with careful examination of the cells in the aspirate sediment (Fig. 97). They should be stained with periodic acid–Schiff (PAS), and PAS-positive granules should be looked for (Fig. 98). Patients with Whipple's disease (Fig. 99) will respond nicely to a course of combined antibiotic and corticosteroid therapy.

Some elderly patients, for no apparent reason, develop a mild cellular response in the vitreous without significant loss of vision, and no treatment is necessary.

FUNGAL LESIONS

Endogenous fungal endophthalmitis has been regularly reported in certain groups of patients, particularly intravenous drug abusers, immunosuppressed patients (those with AIDS, burns, lymphoma, leukemia, or cancer, or those on chemotherapy), and patients on hyperalimentation. The most common organisms are the *Candida* species, followed

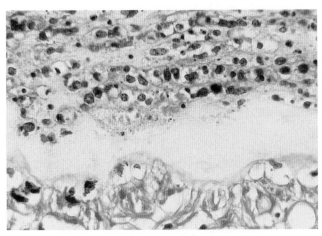

FIG. 94. High-power photomicrograph of the pars plana showing malignant cells in the vitreous.

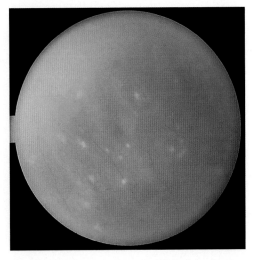

FIG. 95. Multifocal lesions in Whipple's disease.

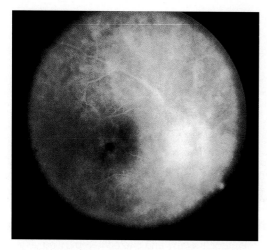

FIG. 96. The lesions light up. There is cystoid macular edema, retinal vasculitis, optic nerve edema, and leakage of dye.

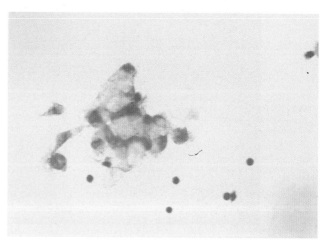

FIG. 98. Periodic acid–Schiff (PAS) stain showing PAS-positive inclusions in the cells in the vitreous in Whipple's disease.

by the *Aspergillus* species and *Cryptococcus neoformans*. The early lesion is seen as a solitary intraretinal white lesion (Fig. 100); later, multiple lesions may develop and can contain a hemorrhagic component. These lesions can coalesce and then burgeon into full-blown endophthalmitis. Histopathologic examination shows areas of retinal necrosis (Fig. 101) replete with fungi (Fig. 102). Treatment is with intravitreal and intravenous antifungal agents.

The (presumed) ocular histoplasmosis syndrome is another fungal disease and is a common disorder found in the Ohio, Missouri, and Mississippi River valleys. It particularly involves inhabitants of Ohio, Indiana, and western Maryland. Similar patients have been described in Great Britain and Germany. Following an initial exposure to *Histoplasma capsulatum*, patients develop an acute respiratory illness with fever, malaise, and lymphadenopathy. Ocular disease, although never associated with anterior segment inflammation or vitreous cellular infiltration, is manifested by the following: (1) numerous small to medium-sized punched-out atrophic spots ("histospots") numbering from 1 to 30 or more in the fundus, involving the choroid and retinal pigment epithelium and with a slight propensity for the superior temporal quadrant (Fig. 103); (2) a peripapillary pigment ring with pigment at the border (Figs. 104 and 105); (3) a macular scar that may be associated with episodes of exudation (Fig. 106) and may occur with subretinal neovascularization (Fig. 107) (occurring 20 or so years after initial exposure to *H. capsulatum*). This leads to disciform-type macular response with hemorrhage (Fig. 105), exudation, and scarring. Treatment of the macular component with

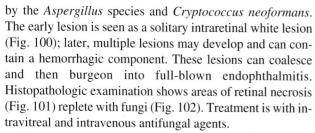

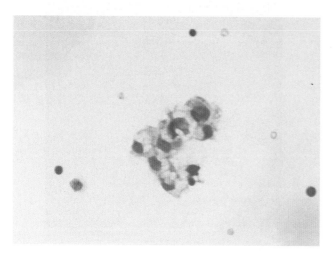

FIG. 97. Macrophages in the vitreous aspirate in Whipple's disease.

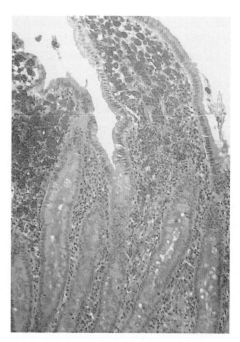

FIG. 99. Jejunal biopsy specimen from a patient with Whipple's disease showing PAS-positive occlusion in the villi.

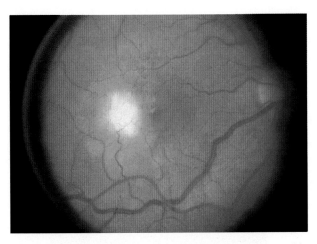

FIG. 100. A patient who is an intravenous drug abuser with a necrotizing retinitis of *Candida albicans* etiology. There is a white lesion in the retina.

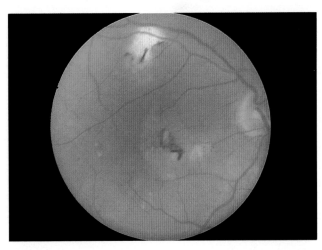

FIG. 103. A patient with (presumed) ocular histoplasmosis syndrome with histospots superior and temporal to the disc and in the macula.

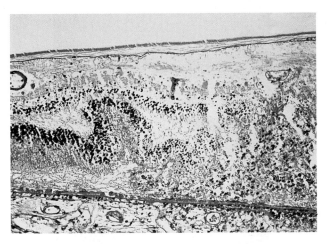

FIG. 101. Photomicrograph showing extensive retinal necrosis.

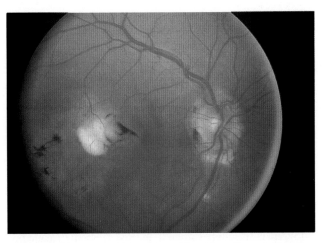

FIG. 104. Numerous histospots with peripapillary and macu-

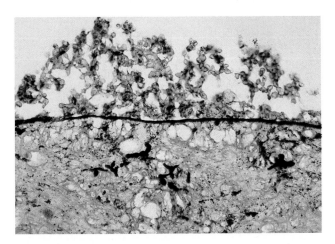

FIG. 102. A silver stain (Gomori methenamine silver) showing *Candida* organisms in the retina.

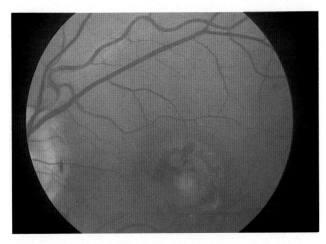

FIG. 105. A peripapillary lesion along with evidence of subretinal neovascularization with hemorrhage and leakage.

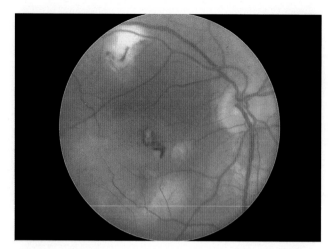

FIG. 106. The same patient as in Fig. 103, but with retinal exudation.

high-dose corticosteroids, argon (green), or krypton laser photocoagulation is helpful, depending on the proximity of neovascularization next to the foveola.

PNEUMOCYSTIS CARINII CHOROIDITIS

A new ocular inflammatory/infectious syndrome developed in AIDS patients due to infection by *Pneumocystis carinii*. The condition has been observed predominantly in patients undergoing prophylactic therapy following *P. carinii* pneumonia. Patients develop multifocal cream-colored lesions within the choroid (Fig. 108). Visual acuity is nearly always preserved. Intravenous fluorescein angiography is diagnostic (Fig. 108) in that the pattern of the angiogram is strikingly similar to the involvement in acute posterior multifocal placoid pigment epitheliopathy. The lesions are dark early in the study but stain during the later phases.

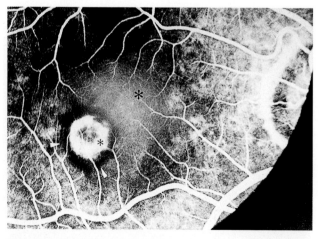

FIG. 107. A patient with (presumed) ocular histoplasmosis syndrome with a peripapillary lesion and subretinal neovascularization with leakage around the area (*).

Histopathologic study of postmortem eye has unequivocally found organisms in the choroid. Treatment with systemic antipneumocystis medications like pentamidine or Bactrim is effective in eradicating the organism.

COMMON PITFALLS

In treating patients with retinal necrosis with steroids alone, serious complications could ensue, particularly in patients with toxoplasmosis. Extensive retinal necrosis with

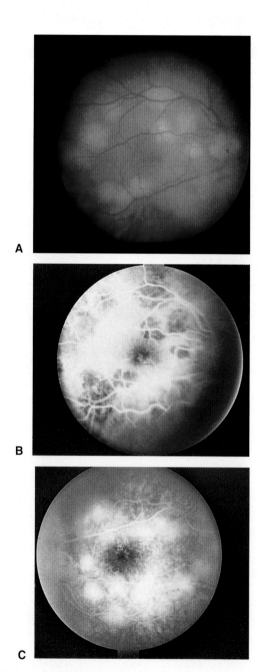

FIG. 108. A–C: Multifocal cream-colored lesions with the choroid. The intravenous fluorescein angiography pattern is similar to the involvement in acute posterior multifocal placoid pigment epitheliopathy

detachment can occur. Lesions have been treated with prednisone alone because of a failure to diagnose toxoplasmosis. The necrotizing lesion can extend and develop a large exudative detachment that can not be repaired surgically, and the patient can lose all vision in the eye. In patients with the acute retinal necrosis syndrome, treatment without an antiviral agent can be fraught with serious difficulty. Patients who have presumed fungal endophthalmitis, particularly those who are intravenous drug abusers, can have one or more focal necrotizing lesion in the retina. This should lead to a strong suspicion of fungal endophthalmitis. Patients with toxoplasmosis in association with AIDS probably warrant being treated for the rest of their lives with antitoxoplasmosis therapy. Discontinuance of treatment after resolution of the lesion in an AIDS patient is fraught with serious danger and is almost universally associated with reactivation. Consequently, either a sulfa drug, clindamycin, pyrimethamine, or a combination thereof must be used.

ACKNOWLEDGMENTS

This work was supported by an unrestricted grant from Fight for Sight, Inc. (New York, NY), and by an unrestricted grant from Research to Prevent Blindness, Inc. (New York, NY).

Practical Atlas of Retinal Disease and Therapy, Second Edition
edited by William R. Freeman,
Lippincott–Raven Publishers, Philadelphia © 1997.

· 4 ·

Inflammatory Multifocal Chorioretinopathies

Lee M. Jampol

This chapter reviews a series of diseases characterized by multifocal lesions involving the retina and choroid. Some of these conditions are associated with white spots in the retina (for example, multiple evanescent white-dot syndrome [MEWDS] and birdshot chorioretinopathy). Others cause geographic white areas in the retina: serpiginous choroiditis and acute posterior multifocal placoid pigment epitheliopathy. Other conditions are associated with multifocal choroiditis, including multifocal choroiditis with panuveitis and punctate inner choroidopathy. Also reviewed are other miscellaneous multifocal chorioretinopathies, including acute macular neuroretinopathy, acute zonal occult outer retinopathy, diffuse unilateral subacute neuroretinitis, acute retinal pigment epitheliitis, acute retinal necrosis, large cell lymphoma of the retina, and unilateral acute idiopathic maculopathy.

MULTIPLE EVANESCENT WHITE-DOT SYNDROME

MEWDS (Figs. 1–4) is an idiopathic inflammatory disease producing unilateral or occasionally bilateral visual loss. The disease has been reported only in young patients (between the ages of 11 and 47; average, 26 years). There is a strong female predominance (38 of the first 48 cases reported in the literature). The disease is characterized by white dots at the level of the deep retina or pigment epithelium. These dots are usually scattered in the paramacular area and may be confluent. As one approaches the equator or as one approaches the fovea, the dots become less dense. There is often an associated granularity to the macula, consisting of multiple, tiny, yellow–orange dots in the macula. There is evidence of inflammation, which may vary from just a few cells in the vitreous to severe vitreous infiltration. Retinal vascular sheathing and disc edema may be seen. The

disease is often unilateral, although it is sometimes asymmetrically bilateral, with marked involvement in one eye and very mild involvement in the second eye. It is rarely symmetrically bilateral. MEWDS usually presents with visual loss, but another presenting complaint is photopsias in the involved eye, and often a temporal scotoma is detected that corresponds to a markedly enlarged blind spot. The exact mechanisms for visual loss in patients with MEWDS are not clear, but could include the macular changes, optic nerve dysfunction, diffuse retinal dysfunction, or other mechanisms. Visual field testing often reveals an enlarged blind spot or rarely other optic nerve visual field defects. The enlarged blind spot is usually absolute, with steep margins suggesting retinal rather than optic nerve dysfunction as the cause of the scotoma. The white spots usually do not obviously cluster around the disc, and the exact cause of this peripapillary retinal dysfunction is not clear [indocyanine green (ICG) angiography does sometimes show peripapillary clustering of hypofluorescent lesions].

In reviewing the first 48 cases in the literature, 6 were bilateral and 42 were unilateral. Vision ranged from 20/15 to 20/300 in the involved eye. Some patients demonstrate multiple recurrences in both eyes, but the visual outcome is still good in these cases. Further testing in MEWDS patients often reveals an abnormal electroretinogram and an abnormal early receptor potential. Fluorescein angiography shows leakage from disc capillaries, retinal capillaries, and at the level of pigment epithelium. Tiny hyperfluorescent points cluster at the level of the RPE in a leakage area corresponding to some of the white dots. The macula may or may not show hyperfluorescence or leakage despite the granularity. With time, the retinal vascular leakage and disc capillary leakage diminish and the white spots become much less apparent. There may be residual retinal pigment epithelial abnormalities, but usually surprisingly very little in the way of retinal pigment epithelial window defects.

L.M. Jampol, M.D.: Department of Ophthalmology, Northwestern University Medical School, Chicago, IL 60611.

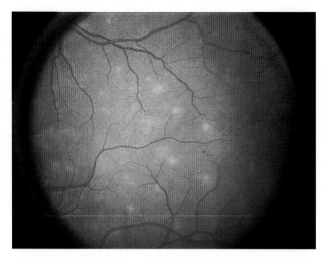

FIG. 1. The temporal periphery of the eye demonstrates the classic white dots in a patient with multiple evanescent white-dot syndrome.

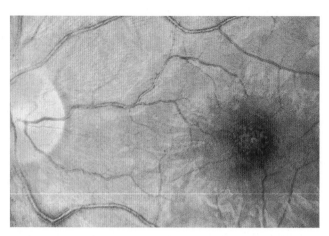

FIG. 3. The characteristic granularity to the fovea is well shown in this close-up view of the macula.

Some patients may develop focal chorioretinal scars that may be peripapillary areas posterior, or peripheral. ICG angiography shows focal areas of hypofluorescence with more lesions seen than are appreciated clinically. The ICG angiogram returns to normal as the white spots fade.

The etiology of MEWDS remains uncertain. A similarity in symptoms to multifocal choroiditis (which is described later) has been noted, with photopsias and enlarged blind spots. Whether MEWDS and multifocal choroiditis represent different diseases or different manifestations of a similar etiologic agent remains uncertain. Gass has suggested that MEWDS, multifocal choroiditis, acute macular neuroretinopathy, and acute zonal occult outer retinopathy (AZOOR) may be etiologically related. (This is discussed in the section on AZOOR). Very often, patients with MEWDS have had symptoms of a "viral syndrome" prior to the onset of symptoms, yet no infectious or immunologic cause has as yet been defined.

No therapy is necessary for MEWDS because the patients show a dramatic recovery in visual acuity as well as in the electroretinogram and early receptor potential. There is a visual recovery to virtually normal levels over a period of 1–10 weeks. In addition, the enlarged blind spot and other visual field defects often improve. The white spots and disc edema disappear, leaving behind mild or no pigmentary irregularity. The macula never returns to normal appearance, although the granularity may diminish. The vascular sheathing and vitreal cells decrease.

Rare instances of choroidal neovascularization following

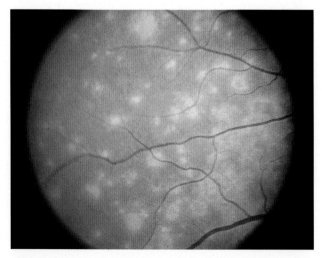

FIG. 2. A case of multiple evanescent white-dot syndrome. The multiple white dots are becoming confluent in areas. There is marked vitreous inflammation.

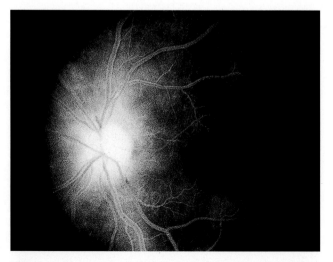

FIG. 4. A fluorescein angiogram in the late phase in a patient with multiple evanescent white-dot syndrome showing staining of the disc, and staining and leakage at the level of pigment epithelium.

MEWDS have been reported. This may account for some instances of apparent idiopathic choroidal neovascularization (the white spots are gone). In addition, in two cases, an association of MEWDS with acute macular neuroretinopathy has been described. It is uncertain why these apparently different disorders should occur in the same patient.

A syndrome of acute idiopathic blind spot enlargement has been described in young women with an enlarged blind spot associated with no disc edema. Several authors have suggested that this syndrome represents a subset of patients with MEWDS. These patients may not have white spots, or the white spots may already have resolved by the time the patients are seen with the enlarged blind spots.

MULTIFOCAL CHOROIDITIS

Multifocal choroiditis with panuveitis (Figs. 5–11) is a common inflammatory disease characterized by a variable amount of intraocular inflammation, with the development of multiple foci of choroiditis in the eye. These foci may be clustered in the posterior pole, in the peripheral retina, or both. One study described a subgroup of young myopic women who had small foci of choroiditis in the macula associated with small serous detachments. These patients showed recurrences and the subsequent development of choroidal neovascularization. This group of patients was called punctate inner choroidopathy. Other authors have described patients with multifocal choroiditis involving the posterior pole or periphery associated with a variable amount of vitreous inflammation and again a tendency to develop choroidal neovascularization. Central vision was lost due to the choroidal neovascularization or the choroiditis. Whether punctate inner choroidopathy and multifocal choroiditis are the same

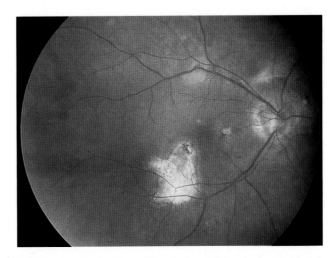

FIG. 6. A patient with multifocal choroiditis who has had multiple subretinal neovascular membranes. Note the peculiar disc. The lesion inferotemporal to the fovea is a laser scar. Some other areas represent choroidal neovascularization that has spontaneously involuted. Multiple small chorioretinal scars are seen.

disease or are two or more distinct diseases is uncertain. Patients with multifocal choroiditis often develop subretinal fibrosis. Some patients have subretinal scar tissue in a circular ring around the optic nerve. In a small group of patients, a tremendous amount of subretinal fibrosis occurs, with virtual destruction of all vision in the eye. These patients, in our experience, often have tiny foci of choroiditis acutely. It is uncertain whether this is the same disease or a distinct entity.

Many patients with multifocal choroiditis appear to respond to systemic or periocular corticosteroid therapy, with resolution of the serous detachments and an improvement in the amount of inflammation. Whether this is helpful in preventing choroidal neovascularization is unclear. Whether the

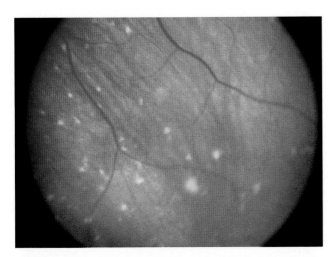

FIG. 5. Multifocal choroiditis with small discrete lesions in the midperiphery. These are inactive.

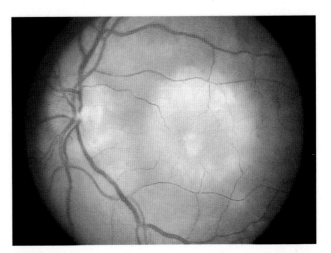

FIG. 7. A patient with a very active exudative maculopathy caused by multifocal choroiditis. There is neurosensory detachment in the macula.

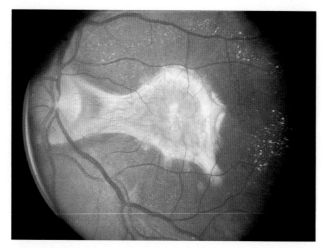

FIG. 8. Following corticosteroid therapy, there has been rapid resorption of the subretinal fluid with some residual subretinal exudate. Fibrovascular tissue is seen under the macula and surrounding the disc.

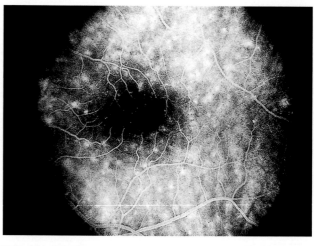

FIG. 10. A fluorescein angiogram from the patient in Fig. 9, demonstrating small hyperfluorescent acute lesions.

long-term outcome is affected by corticosteroid therapy is uncertain. It is also unclear whether steroid therapy would work on patients with punctate inner choroidopathy. Patients with subretinal fibrosis do seem to respond to corticosteroids, although relapses may occur with diminished doses of steroids. Laser photocoagulation has been used successfully to treat choroidal neovascularization, but these vessels not uncommonly spontaneously involute. It has been suggested that Epstein–Barr virus may be a cause of the multifocal choroiditis syndrome, but this has not been confirmed by other groups. Therapy (for example, antiviral drugs like acyclovir) beyond the use of corticosteroids has not been systematically evaluated. One patient of ours was treated with intravenous acyclovir without apparent benefit.

ACUTE MACULAR NEURORETINOPATHY

Acute macular neuroretinopathy (Figs. 12 and 13) is a multifocal chorioretinopathy that was initially described in 1975. This disease occurs in young adults, mostly women, and may be unilateral or bilateral. The patients sometimes have had a preceding viral illness. They complain of decreased vision and multiple paracentral scotomas. The results of eye examination are normal, except for the presence of multiple petal-shaped or round lesions in the parafoveal areas that are often a darker red than the surrounding areas. Sometimes, the lesions may appear brownish or orange. A fluorescein angiogram is usually normal. Careful visual field testing shows scotomas corresponding to the active lesions

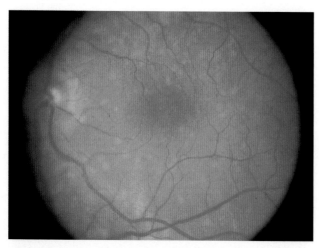

FIG. 9. A patient with multifocal choroiditis with subretinal fibrosis demonstrating multiple small white lesions at the level of the choroid.

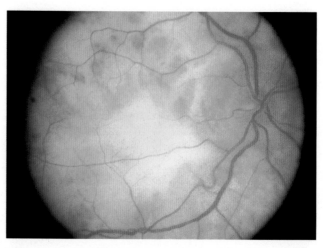

FIG. 11. The opposite eye of the patient in Fig. 9, demonstrating massive subretinal fibrosis with large lacunar areas of subretinal scarring.

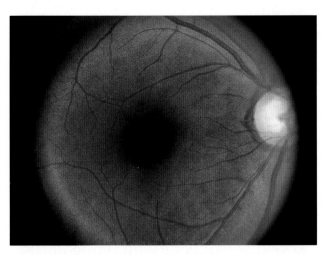

FIG. 12. A black patient with acute macular neuroretinopathy demonstrating dark-appearing petaloid lesions surrounding the fovea.

and sometimes an enlarged blind spot. Findings on electroretinography are normal. During the subsequent follow-up, patients may show a gradual improvement in vision and a decrease in the size of the paracentral scotomas. Retinal lesions become less apparent but usually do not disappear.

The exact level of the retinal lesions remains controversial, and the origin remains unknown. The possibility of an association with intravenous administration of sympathomimetic compounds (for example, ephedrine) has been raised, and it has been suggested that perhaps the lesions represent paracentral infarcts of the inner retina. During the acute phase, however, no cotton-wool spots have been noted. We have seen one patient who showed multiple recurrences in both eyes. A possible relationship with MEWDS and multifocal choroiditis has been suggested (see AZOOR).

ACUTE ZONAL OCCULT OUTER RETINOPATHY

In 1993, Gass reported 13 young, mostly female patients with the onset of peripheral loss of retinal function in large areas, which sometimes was contiguous with the blind spot. These patients are included in this discussion, although they do not have white spots in the retina, because Gass has suggested that AZOOR may be part of the same disease spectrum as MEWDS, multifocal choroiditis, and acute macular neuroretinopathy. AZOOR patients initially have a normal fundus appearance, despite the loss of outer retinal function, but later develop retinal arteriolar narrowing, chorioretinal atrophy, and pigment clumping (Figs. 14 and 15). Some patients have a relentless downhill course, whereas others seem to stabilize. The patients reported by Gass did not have inflammation and did not have white spots or punched-out chorioretinal lesions. They did, however, have photopsias and large peripheral retinal scotomas.

Because of the similarity of the symptoms and the age and gender (young and female) to patients with MEWDS, multifocal choroiditis and acute macular neuroretinopathy, Gass has hypothesized that MEWDS, multifocal choroiditis, acute macular neuroretinopathy, acute idiopathic blind spot enlargement, and AZOOR represent parts of the spectrum of one disease or at least somehow are related to each other. An alternative view has been put forward in a recent editorial suggesting that these syndromes are distinct clinically, although they have overlapping symptoms and, at times, clinical findings. The similarities and differences between these various syndromes have recently been reviewed by Jampol and Wiredu (see Bibliography).

BIRDSHOT RETINOCHOROIDOPATHY

Birdshot retinochoroidopathy (vitiliginous choroidopathy) is a unilateral (rare) or bilateral (common) disease seen

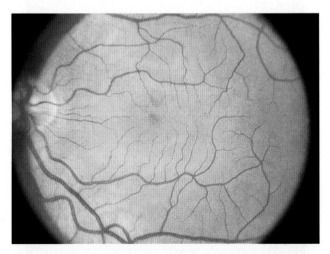

FIG. 13. A white patient with acute macular neuroretinopathy demonstrating small circular and petaloid lesions surrounding the fovea. This patient has had multiple recurrences in both eyes.

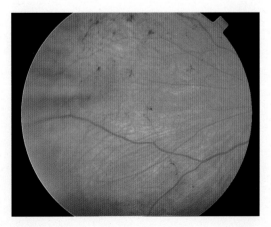

FIG. 14. The nasal periphery of a healthy patient with acute zonal occult outer retinopathy and progressive temporal field loss shows atrophy of retinal pigment epithelium, pigment clumping, and arteriolar narrowing.

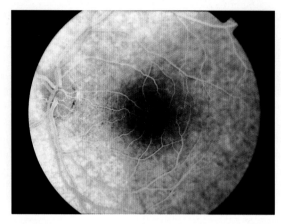

FIG. 15. The fluorescein angiogram shows hypofluorescence from pigmentary atrophy that extends posteriorly.

in middle-aged patients (Fig. 16). They may present with complaints of floaters, night blindness, or blurring of vision related to cystoid macular edema. The diagnosis requires the presence of marked vitreous cellular infiltration. In addition, the patients have multiple, birdshotlike areas scattered about the posterior pole of both eyes. These lesions may be yellow, gray, or white. They appear to be at the level of the deep retina or choroid. In association with this, the patients may show cystoid macular edema, retinal vascular sheathing, retinal arteriolar narrowing, and marked leakage of fluorescein from disc and posterior pole capillaries. In many cases, the electroretinogram is diminished and color vision is abnormal. The optic nerve may be pale. In about 90% of cases, birdshot retinochoroidopathy is associated with HLA A29. The patients may show evidence of sensitization of their

lymphocytes to S antigen, and it has thus been suggested that the disease represents an autoimmune reaction against one's own retinal antigens. The differential diagnosis includes pars planitis, other uveitis syndromes, reticulum cell sarcoma (large cell lymphoma—see below), and senile vitritis. Because of the visual loss from cystoid macular edema, corticosteroids and cyclosporine have been used. These are effective in reducing inflammation, but when they are tapered or discontinued, the macular leakage usually relapses. This can be a very difficult disease to treat. Some patients have a progressive course, whereas at other times birdshot retinochoroidopathy may have an indolent course not requiring much therapy.

SERPIGINOUS (GEOGRAPHIC) CHOROIDITIS

Serpiginous (geographic) choroiditis (Figs. 17–21) is a chronic recurring disease usually seen in patients between the ages of 30 and 70. There is no associated systemic disease. The choroiditis eventually becomes bilateral, although patients initially present with symptoms in only one eye. The lesions may be present in the macula or may begin in the peripapillary area. The acute lesions are characterized by geographic or irregular white "edematous" areas at the level of the retinal pigment epithelium and choroid. There is often associated vitreous cellular reaction. There may be a mild anterior chamber reaction. The lesions evolve over several weeks or months into atrophic scars with pigmentary mottling and a variable amount of atrophy of the pigment epithelium and choroid. Recurrences invariably are seen, with new lesions usually occurring adjacent to old healed lesions. Patients with the macular presentation may have abrupt loss of vision

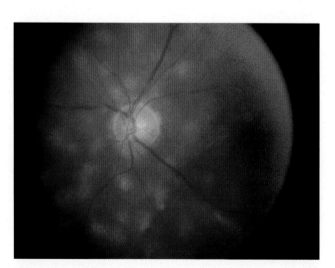

FIG. 16. A patient with birdshot chorioretinopathy demonstrating multiple lesions surrounding the disc.

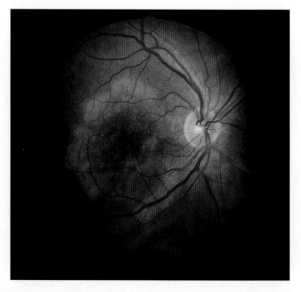

FIG. 17. An acute lesion of macular serpiginous choroiditis.

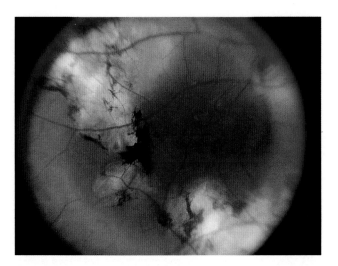

FIG. 18. Recurrence in a patient with serpiginous choroiditis adjacent to multiple old scars.

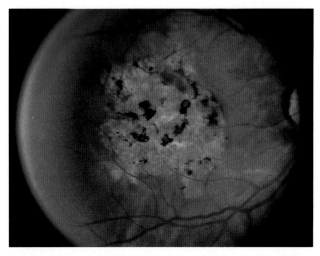

FIG. 20. Old chorioretinal scarring in the macula of a patient with active macular serpiginous choroiditis in the other eye.

as their first sign, whereas patients with peripapillary lesions may have far-advanced disease before they become symptomatic because of involvement of central vision. Eventually, the whole posterior pole may be involved by widespread chorioretinal atrophy from recurrent episodes. Choroidal neovascularization is seen as a complication in many patients and may itself contribute to loss of central vision.

A fluorescein angiogram in patients with acute serpiginous choroiditis is very characteristic in that it shows darkening in the area of acute lesions. This may be related to blockage by swollen opaque pigment epithelium or hypoperfusion of the underlying choriocapillaris. As the lesions heal, there is variable atrophy of pigment epithelium and

choroid. At this stage, the fluorescein angiograms show window defects or absence of choroidal perfusion. Recurrences are in a serpentine fashion.

The etiology of serpiginous choroiditis remains unknown. There is still some debate, but most retinal specialists do feel that this disease is sensitive to corticosteroids. Systemic corticosteroid therapy or periocular steroids result in more rapid resolution of the acute lesion, and maintenance of a certain level of systemic therapy may be useful in preventing recurrences when central vision is threatened. Recently, acyclovir has been tried, but the value of this treatment remains uncertain. Some investigators are using immunosuppressive therapy to prevent relapses. The differential diagnosis of serpig-

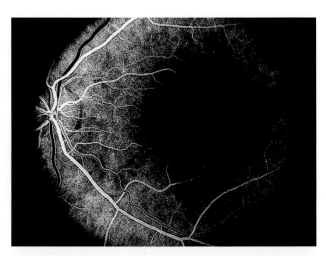

FIG. 19. An early-phase fluorescein angiogram from a patient with acute macular serpiginous choroiditis showing hypofluorescence.

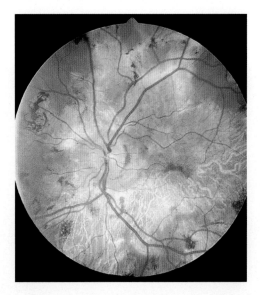

FIG. 21. The end stage of serpiginous choroiditis showing destruction of the whole posterior pole.

inous choroiditis includes acute posterior multifocal placoid pigment epitheliopathy (which is discussed later). In addition, the inactive lesions in the fundus may resemble ocular histoplasmosis, multifocal choroiditis, or myopic chorioretinal degeneration.

Serpiginous choroiditis is invariably a bilateral disease; however, the condition usually is active in only one eye at a time, and in patients who have bilaterally active lesions, the diagnosis of acute posterior multifocal placoid pigment epitheliopathy should be considered. In addition, patients who have previously been diagnosed as having acute posterior multifocal placoid pigment epitheliopathy who have recurrences probably have serpiginous choroiditis.

ACUTE POSTERIOR MULTIFOCAL PLACOID PIGMENT EPITHELIOPATHY

Acute posterior multifocal placoid pigment epitheliopathy (APMPPE) (Figs. 22–24) is an inflammatory disease seen in young patients who have geographic areas of whitening of the outer retina in the posterior pole of both eyes (occasionally unilateral). There is often associated visual loss. The patients are usually healthy, although they may show signs of a viral infection and have a mild meningoencephalitis, as manifested by headaches and by cells and protein in the spinal fluid. Urinary changes have been noted, and rarely systemic vasculitis or a cerebral vasculitis may accompany the condition. Rare cases of cerebral vasculitis from APMPPE have even been fatal.

The bilateral visual loss is often abrupt and can reduce vision to the level of 20/200. With time, however, the patient's visual acuity gradually returns, although the vision may be permanently diminished in a minority of cases. The acute lesions are white, but as they heal they show granularity with

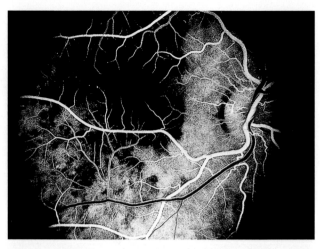

FIG. 23. This fluorescein angiogram demonstrates a large area of hypofluorescence due to either hypoperfusion of the choroid or blockage.

pigmentary loss and hypertrophy. Fluorescein angiography during the acute stages shows blockage of the underlying choroidal fluorescence by swollen retinal pigment epithelium or choroidal hypoperfusion. ICG angiography also shows hypofluorescence from hypoperfusion or blockage. Although APMPPE and serpiginous choroiditis show similarities, the differences between the two diseases are that (1) serpiginous choroiditis usually shows more severe atrophy of the retina and choroid and has multiple recurrences, (2) APMPPE is usually a single episode with healing and visual recovery, and (3) APMPPE is rarely if ever associated with choroidal neovascularization, whereas this is not unusual with serpiginous choroiditis. In a few cases, it maybe difficult or impossible to distinguish between these two diagnostic possibilities.

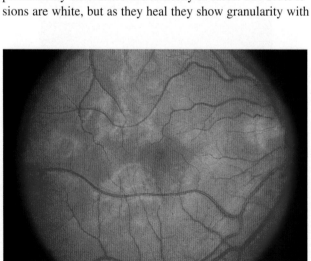

FIG. 22. A young patient with acute posterior multifocal placoid pigment epitheliopathy. Multiple lesions are seen scattered around the posterior pole.

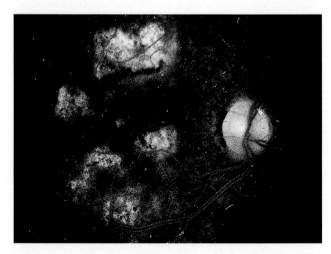

FIG. 24. The late phase of the fluorescein angiogram shows foci of staining of the acute lesions.

Most retinal specialists do not feel that therapy (corticosteroids) is indicated for APMPPE. They feel that the natural history is excellent and this is not necessary.

DIFFUSE UNILATERAL SUBACUTE NEURORETINITIS

Diffuse unilateral subacute neuroretinitis (Figs. 25 and 26), which was initially described as "the unilateral wipe-out syndrome," is an inflammatory disease seen in young patients. During the acute phase, patients present with a unilateral uveitis, including vitreous cells, mild anterior chamber reaction, and often papillitis. Disseminated small white spots may be present deep in the retina. Subsequently, patients have a chronic course of inflammation, but show progressive optic atrophy, arteriolar attenuation, and the development of pigmentary irregularity in the fundus. The inflammation and white spots eventually disappear. Patients may be left with an eye that looks like unilateral retinitis pigmentosa, with vitreous cells, a pale disc, attenuated arterioles, and diffuse bone spicule pigmentation. Some patients show circular pigmented chorioretinal scars in the peripheral retina.

Recent work has suggested that this syndrome is probably caused by an intraocular nematode, and at least two different species have been implicated: *Baylisascaris procyonis* (a roundworm in raccoons) and *Ancylostoma caninum*. During the active phase, the worm is present in the eye, often in the subretinal space. The worm migrates, leaving acute inflammatory areas of retinal whitening and later subtle pigmentary changes and reaction. Toxins or an immune response cause progressive visual loss, optic atrophy, arteriole changes, and pigmentary atrophy. By the time patients note visual loss, no worm may be seen. A careful search for the worm should be undertaken during the acute phase, because destruction of the worm with the laser or in some cases removal of the

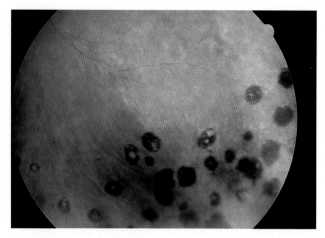

FIG. 26. The same patient as in Fig. 21 also demonstrates multiple black lesions in the midperiphery.

worm from the eye may prevent further visual loss. Corticosteroids may suppress the inflammation, but probably do not prevent long-term changes in the eye. Antihelminthic drugs like thiabendazole or ivermectin may be helpful if the worm cannot be located.

ACUTE RETINAL PIGMENT EPITHELIITIS

Acute retinal pigment epitheliitis (Fig. 27) was described in 1972. Young adults were reported with acute visual loss that could be minimal or down to the level of 20/200. Patients were seen with unilateral or bilateral involvement. Results of the eye examination were normal, except for discrete clusters of small brown or greyish spots (usually 2–4 spots in the involved macula). The spots were often surrounded by a

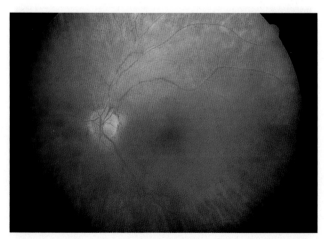

FIG. 25. A young woman with diffuse unilateral subacute neuroretinitis demonstrating arteriolar attenuation and pigmentary changes in the midperiphery.

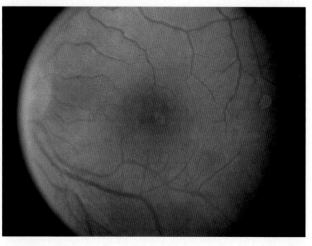

FIG. 27. Acute retinal pigment epitheliitis demonstrating several small yellowish lesions near the fovea.

yellow or white halo. Fluorescein angiography during the acute phase showed hypofluorescence, and the surrounding halo appeared normal or slightly hyperfluorescent. Results of electrophysiologic testing, including electroretinogram and visual evoked response, were normal. The electro-oculogram was subnormal in several cases. Over a 6- to 12-month period, central visual acuity returned to normal. The lesions became less prominent with time.

Whether this represents a true entity remains uncertain, although several subsequent publications have described patients with this disease. No therapy is indicated in view of the good outcome.

ACUTE RETINAL NECROSIS SYNDROME

The acute retinal necrosis syndrome (Fig. 28) was initially described in the Japanese literature by Urayama as Kirisawa's uveitis. The patients had unilateral or bilateral uveitis, including severe vitreous cellular reaction and subsequently the development of necrotizing retinitis. The patients showed anterior chamber reaction with marked flare and cells, keratic precipitates, synechiae, vitritis, and the retinitis. Associated with the necrotizing retinitis are large areas of vascular sheathing, vascular occlusion, retinal infarction, and hemorrhages. When first described, this entity was idiopathic and seen only in healthy people. A similar syndrome has now been described in immunosuppressed patients, including AIDS patients. Acute whitening of the retina and pigment epithelium is noted, usually in the peripheral retina, although some cases can begin in the midperiphery or even the macula. In some patients, there is choroidal involvement with serous elevation of the retina. When the macula or optic nerve is involved, vision is lost. Subsequently, the retinitis heals with mottled pigmentation,

but many of the patients develop vitreoretinal traction with tractional or rhegmatogenous retinal detachments. Standard buckling surgery or vitrectomy to repair these detachments is often unsuccessful. Silicone oil may improve the surgical success rate.

Although this disease was initially of unknown cause, subsequent work has shown that is usually associated with herpes zoster, although occasionally other herpes viruses like herpes simplex may be involved. Standard therapy should include antiviral therapy, usually high-dose intravenous acyclovir. Systemic corticosteroids can be used to treat inflammation in the eye. In an attempt to prevent the subsequent development of retinal detachment, some authors have tried a barrier of photocoagulation or even prophylactic buckling or vitrectomy. Aspirin and other anticoagulants have been tried to diminish the vascular occlusive component. At present, antiviral therapy and corticosteroids combined with very close observation and early retinal detachment surgery seem the best therapy.

PROGRESSIVE OUTER RETINAL NECROSIS

In patients with AIDS, a particularly virulent form of retinal necrosis is seen, which has been called progressive outer retinal necrosis (PORN) (Fig. 29). This syndrome, thought to be caused by the zoster virus, has a rapid, progressive course of retinal necrosis with either centripetal extensions of small, peripheral lesions or peripheral lesions in association with macular lesions progressing toward each other to involve the entire retina. When the fovea is involved, the reddish color of the fovea may give it an appearance of a cherry red spot. At the time of presentation, eyes demonstrate mimimal clinical signs of inflammation. These patients have a relentless downhill course of retinal necrosis and often develop rheg-

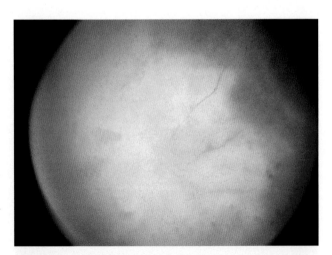

FIG. 28. The classic appearance of acute retinal necrosis with retinal whitening and scattered intraretinal hemorrhages, as well as vascular obstruction.

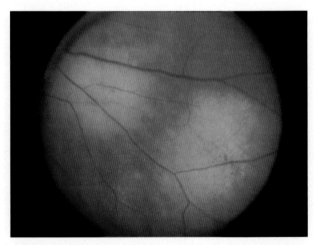

FIG. 29. This AIDS patient has outer retinal necrosis with no involvement of overlying retinal circulation.

matogenous retinal detachments with loss of vision, often to the level of no light perception. Acute retinal necrosis tends to have full-thickness involvement of the retina, with an occlusive retinal vasculitis. PORN appears to be deeper, without obvious involvement of the retinal circulation.

The results of treatment of patients with PORN have been very disappointing. Acyclovir appears to be of little value in most patients. Attempts have been made to treat the disease with other antiviral agents, including combination foscarnet and acyclovir or foscarnet and ganciclovir. Recent data suggest that therapy with ganciclovir or combination foscarnet and ganciclovir may reduce visual loss in patients with PORN. Other newer antiviral agents, such as cidofovir, are also being tested. Aggressive surgical intervention, including laser photocoagulation, pars plana vitrectomy with silicone oil, or gas tamponade, appears to improve the chances for retaining some vision in these eyes.

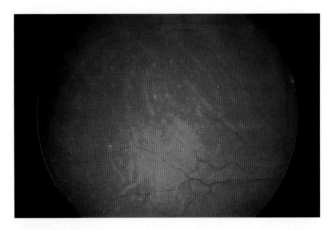

FIG. 30. White spots on the outer retina in a patient with infiltration of large cell lymphoma.

LARGE CELL (NON-HODGKIN'S) LYMPHOMA

Ocular non-Hodgkin's lymphoma is usually a disease of middle-aged and older people. Although it may begin unilaterally, almost all cases eventually become bilateral. It can evolve with or without evidence of associated systemic (visceral) disease or its more common association, central nervous system lymphoma. Immune dysfunction predisposes patients to the development of large cell lymphoma. Although large cell lymphoma can involve the iris, choroid, vitreous, and optic nerve, we have included this entity here because of its ability to present as small white spots in the retina (Fig. 30) that may resemble MEWDS and other entities in this discussion. Patients presenting in this way complain of painless blurred vision, floaters, or other vague visual symptoms. Vitreous cellular involvement is frequently seen and, in some cases, anterior segment cells may be seen as well. The characteristic findings in the fundus include solid pigment epithelial masses, which can be yellow, white, or orange. They can enlarge and become confluent, or they may show spontaneous resolution. At times, retinal whitening from infiltration may resemble necrotizing retinitis and vasculitis and can produce retinal vascular occlusion. In some cases, small whitish spots or dots may be seen in the outer layers of the retina. Other findings that may be seen include optic nerve swelling, areas of choroidal atrophy, and chorioretinal scarring. The white spots, in our experience, usually grow, so that they no longer resemble MEWDS, but more clearly represent tumor infiltration. By this time, substantial visual loss may have occurred. Most patients with this ocular form of disease develop progressive central nervous system disease as well.

Aggressive radiation therapy in combination with chemotherapy may improve survival, which previously has been poor. These patients often die within 2–3 years of diagnosis.

UNILATERAL ACUTE IDIOPATHIC MACULOPATHY

The last disease entity to be described is not a multifocal disease, but is a new inflammatory disease included in the differential diagnosis of other entities discussed in this chapter. This newly recognized entity, unilateral acute idiopathic maculopathy (Figs. 31–34), is seen in young adults who experience sudden, marked unilateral or rarely bilateral loss of vision following a flulike illness. The loss of vision is secondary to an exudative maculopathy, with a loss of vision to the level of 20/200 or less. There is a neurosensory detachment with irregular margins. There is also subretinal whitening or thickening at the level of pigment epithelium, below the neurosensory detachment. The lesions may be foveal (common) or extrafoveal. Many of the patients have small

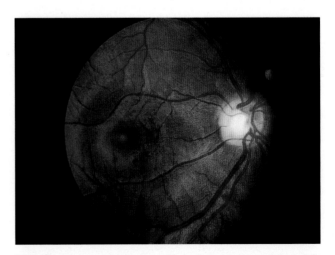

FIG. 31. A young woman with unilateral acute idiopathic maculopathy. There are several retinal hemorrhages, as well as neurosensory elevation.

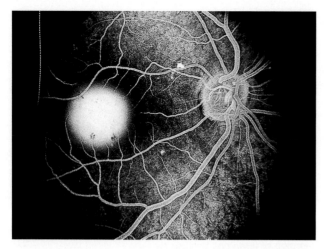

FIG. 32. The fluorescein angiogram of this patient demonstrates pooling of fluorescein in the subretinal space, as well as blockage by hemorrhage.

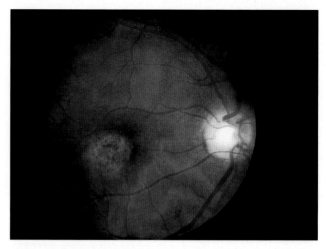

FIG. 34. The same patient as in Fig. 33. Several months later, the lesion has become more atrophic.

intraretinal hemorrhages that suggest subretinal neovascularization, but no neovascularization is present. Vitreous inflammatory cells may be seen. The fluorescein angiogram in these patients shows initial minimal subretinal hypofluorescence. In the late phases, however, there is consistently a pooling of fluorescein within the subneurosensory space and staining of the thickening at the level of the pigment epithelium.

Within a several-week period, patients show a rapid, spontaneous improvement in vision and a resolution of the neurosensory detachment. This often leaves behind a bull's eye-type lesion in the macula. No recurrences have been noted, but some patients have developed secondary choroidal neovascularization months after the resolution of their exudative changes. The visual outcome is excellent, except in those patients who develop choroidal neovascularization.

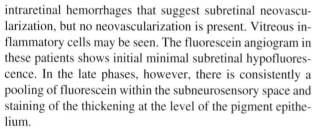

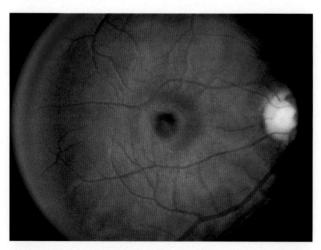

FIG. 33. The same patient as in Figs. 31 and 32, demonstrating rapid resorption of the subretinal fluid. This is 2 weeks later. There is a bull's eye lesion.

BIBLIOGRAPHY

Bos PJM, Deutman AF. Acute macular neuroretinopathy. *Am J Ophthalmol* 1975;80:573–584.

Dreyer RF, Gass JDM. Multifocal choroiditis and panuveitis. *Arch Ophthalmol* 1984;102:1176–1184.

Duker JS, Blumenkranz MS. Diagnosis and management of the acute retinal necrosis syndrome. *Surv Ophthalmol* 1991;35:327–343.

Gass JDM. Acute posterior multifocal placoid pigment epitheliopathy. *Arch Ophthalmol* 1968;80:177–185.

Gass JDM. Vitiliginous choriodoretinitis. *Arch Ophthalmol* 1981;99:1778–1787.

Gass JDM. Acute zonal occult outer retinopathy. *J Clin Neuroophthalmol* 1993;13:79–97.

Gass JDM, Braunstein RA. Further observations concerning the diffuse unilateral subacute neuroretinitis syndrome. *Arch Ophthalmol* 1983;101:1689–1697.

Jampol LM, Sieving PA, Pugh D, et al. Multiple evanescent white dot syndrome. I. Clinical findings. *Arch Ophthalmol* 1984;102:671–674.

Jampol LM, Wiredu A. MEWDS, MFC, PIC, AMN, AIBSE, and AZOOR: one disease or many? *Retina* 1995;15:373–378.

Krill AE, Deutman AF. Acute retinal pigment epitheliitis. *Am J Ophthalmol* 1972;74:193–205.

Mansour AM, Jampol LM, Packo KH, Hrisomalos NF. Macular serpiginous choroiditis. *Retina* 1988;8:125–131.

Tiedeman JS. Epstein–Barr viral antibodies in multifocal choroiditis and panuveitis. *Am J Ophthalmol* 1987;103:659–663.

Watzke RC, Packer AJ, Folk JC, Benson WE, Burgess D, Ober RR. Punctate inner choroidopathy. *Am J Ophthalmol* 1984;98:572–584.

Yannuzzi LA, Jampol LM, Rabb MF, et al. Unilateral acute idiopathic maculopathy. *Arch Ophthalmol* 1991;109:1411–1416.

Practical Atlas of Retinal Disease and Therapy, Second Edition
edited by William R. Freeman,
Lippincott–Raven Publishers, Philadelphia © 1997.

· 5 ·

Infectious Viral and Opportunistic Retinitis

Everett Ai

Infection with the human immunodeficiency virus (HIV) produces a derangement of cell-mediated immunity that results in disruption of multiple organ systems. Ocular findings are common in individuals with acquired immunodeficiency syndrome (AIDS) and involve both the anterior and posterior segments of the eye. Anterior involvement includes tumors of the periocular tissues, microvascular changes in the conjunctiva, and a variety of external infections. Posterior segment manifestations include a microvascular disorder of the retina known as noninfectious AIDS retinopathy. Numerous infections of the retina and choroid may also be seen. New therapeutic regimens have been found to be of benefit in many of these conditions and, as a result, prompt and accurate diagnosis may enable the institution of appropriate therapy with subsequent preservation of vision.

Systemic infection with HIV predisposes the retina, choroid, and optic nerve to a variety of disorders that may be broadly divided into two categories: those associated with noninfectious etiologies and an expanding group of secondary opportunistic infections.

NONINFECTIOUS MANIFESTATIONS

Retina

The clinical spectrum of noninfectious AIDS retinopathy includes cotton-wool spots, microaneurysms, retinal hemorrhages, telangiectatic vascular changes, and capillary nonperfusion. These microvascular changes are the most common retinal manifestation of AIDS and are clinically apparent in about 70% of affected individuals. They are also seen in approximately 40% of patients with AIDS-related complex and in approximately 1% of individuals with asymptomatic HIV infection.

Cotton-wool spots occur in approximately 50%–60% of AIDS patients and have been found to be the earliest and most consistent finding of noninfectious AIDS retinopathy (Fig. 1A). These spots represent infarcts of the nerve fiber layer and are no different than cotton-wool spots seen in other systemic medical disorders (Fig. 1B). However, they are occasionally responsible for the presence of small symptomatic visual defects in patients with AIDS. In addition, they can be confused with early cytomegalovirus (CMV) retinitis lesions, although cotton-wool spots can be differentiated by their smaller size, superficial location, lack of progression, and evanescent nature.

Hemorrhages are less commonly found than cotton-wool spots and are estimated to occur in about 20% of patients with AIDS and in about 3% of patients with AIDS-related complex. They may involve both the nerve fiber layer and deeper retina, and appear as flame-shaped and dot and blot hemorrhages (Fig. 2).

Telangiectatic vascular changes are also seen in patients with AIDS and are often associated with microaneurysms (Fig. 3). Associated with these changes may be areas of capillary nonperfusion. We have seen two nondiabetic patients with AIDS who developed small tufts of disc neovascularization (Fig. 4). These findings were confirmed by fluorescein angiography (Fig. 5). None of these patients have developed vitreous hemorrhages or required treatment for these findings.

Central retinal vein and artery occlusions have also been reported in patients with AIDS and usually are similar in appearance to those seen in individuals with other types of vascular disease (Fig. 6). Patients with CMV retinitis may also develop vascular occlusions in areas of active infection, and these usually appear as zones of white ghost vessel formation. In addition, an occasional individual may demonstrate a marked degree of retinal ischemia secondary to retinitis (Fig. 7). As a result, consideration should be given to testing for exposure to HIV in individuals with unexplained vascular occlusions.

Text continues on p 104.

E. Ai, M.D.: Retina Unit, California Pacific Medical Center; and Pacific Vision Foundation, California Pacific Medical Center, San Francisco, CA 94115

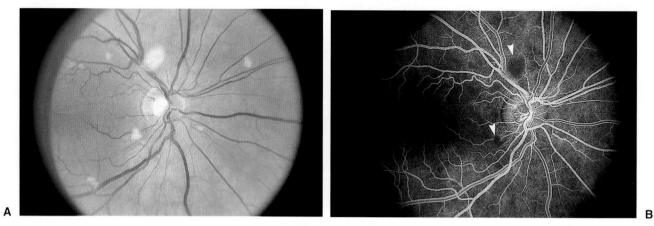

FIG. 1. Cotton-wool spots (**A**) are the most common retinal manifestation of AIDS. Fluorescein angiography (**B**) demonstrates early hypofluorescence (*arrows*) of these infarcts of the nerve fiber layer.

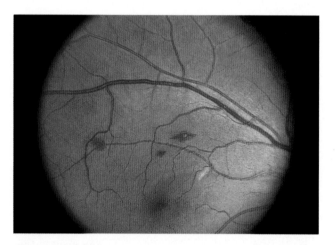

FIG. 2. Hemorrhages are also seen as part of noninfectious AIDS retinopathy.

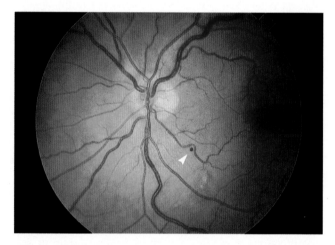

FIG. 3. Microaneurysms (*arrow*) may also constitute a manifestation of noninfectious AIDS retinopathy.

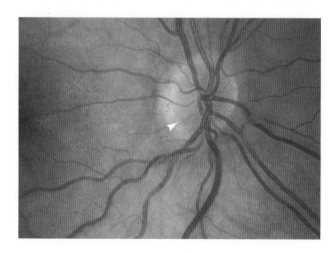

FIG. 4. This nondiabetic patient with AIDS developed neovascularization (*arrow*) overlying the inferotemporal portion of the optic disc.

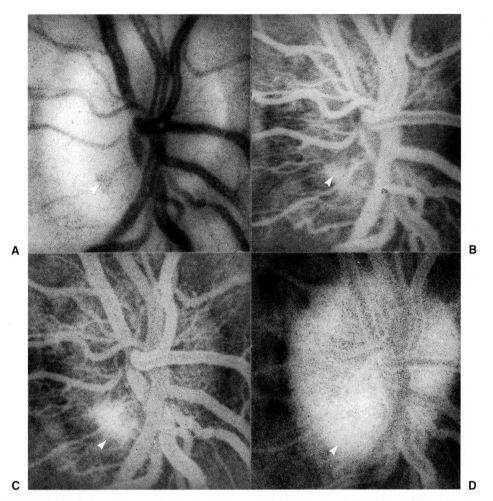

FIG. 5. Red-free (**A**) and sequential fluorescein angiographic images (**B–D**) reveal hyperfluorescence at the site of neovascularization (*arrows*).

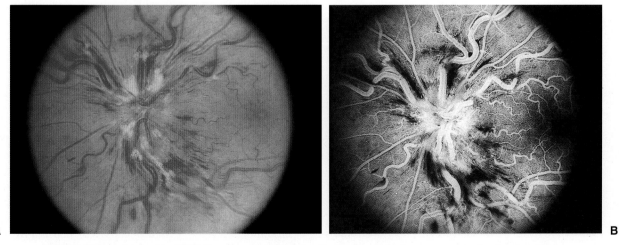

FIG. 6. This patient with AIDS developed a central retinal vein occlusion as seen in the fundus photograph (**A**) and fluorescein angiogram (**B**).

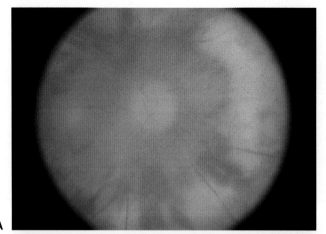

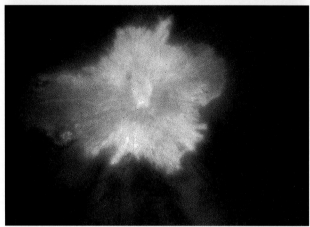

FIG. 7. This patient with retinitis (A) also demonstrated evidence of massive retinal ischemia as evidenced by the hypofluorescent zones surrounding the optic disc in his left eye (B). (Courtesy of Scarlette M. Wilson, M.D., Department of Ophthalmology, California Pacific Medical Center, San Francisco, CA.)

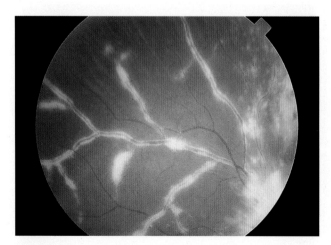

FIG. 8. Perivasculitis may be seen in association with CMV retinitis. This unusually severe example constitutes a variant of frosted branch angiitis.

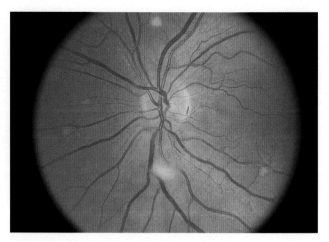

FIG. 9. The presence of somewhat full-appearing optic discs with small or absent cups is rather common in patients with HIV infection.

Retinal perivasculitis in the absence of CMV retinitis has also been reported in Africa, but is rare in the North American AIDS population. A clinical study of 200 patients with AIDS demonstrated no evidence of perivasculitis other than that associated with CMV retinitis (Fig. 8).

Optic Disc

Noninfectious optic nerve involvement in AIDS is far less common than involvement of the retina and includes papilledema, anterior ischemic optic neuropathy, and optic atrophy. Papilledema usually occurs in patients with AIDS and central nervous system (CNS) malignancies, and is secondary to increased intracranial pressure. Among the most prevalent intracranial tumors in individuals with AIDS are non-Hodgkin's and Burkitt's lymphomas. Kaposi's sarcoma may also occasionally result in metastatic CNS involvement. In addition, anterior ischemic optic neuropathy has been reported as an early manifestation of AIDS. A number of patients with AIDS present with slightly swollen, full-appearing discs with small or absent cups (Fig. 9). Evaluation for this finding has not revealed any neurologic abnormalities or evidence of other infectious processes, such as syphilis, and the etiology of these changes is not clear.

INFECTIOUS MANIFESTATIONS

An expanding list of infections of the retina and choroid have been reported to affect individuals with AIDS. Whereas a number of these infections can also be seen in immunocompetent individuals, it is important to remember that significant differences in the clinical presentation may be encountered in patients with AIDS. The degree of accompanying inflammation may be significantly lessened in AIDS patients, their response to therapy may take longer, and there is a greater chance of recurrent infection in immunodeficient individuals. Multifocal areas of infection, as well as bilateral

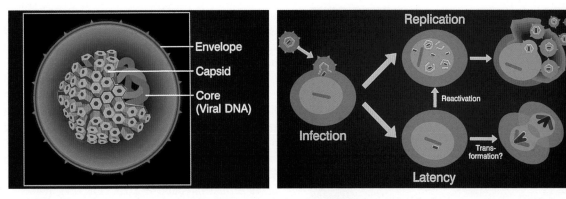

FIG. 10. CMV is a species-specific DNA virus belonging in the herpes family (structure shown in **A**). It demonstrates the biologic hallmark of the herpesvirus group in its capacity to reactivate (**B**). (Courtesy of Syntex Laboratories, Inc., Palo Alto, CA © 1989.)

infection, may be seen in individuals with AIDS. In addition, more than one infection may be present in the same eye. It is also important to consider that new, as yet undescribed, infections of the retina and choroid are likely to be seen in the future.

CYTOMEGALOVIRUS RETINITIS

CMV retinitis is the most common retinal infection in patients with AIDS. It has been observed in approximately 30% of affected individuals and may be the initial presenting sign of symptomatic HIV infection. It is a species-specific DNA virus classified in the herpes group of viruses (Fig. 10). Serologic studies indicate that previous exposure has occurred in approximately 80%–90% of middle-aged adults. However, disease affecting the eye tends to occur only in the developing fetus or in immunocompromised patients.

It is important to be familiar with the clinical features of CMV retinitis and to recognize the need to screen individuals with HIV at regular intervals mandated, in part, by the pa-

tient's CD4+ T-lymphocyte (CD4) counts. Most patients with HIV presenting with CMV retinitis have a CD4 count of less than 40 cells/mm^3. Although an occasional patient with a CD4 count in excess of 200 cells/mm^3 may develop CMV retinitis, this is not typical, and other causes of necrotizing retinitis, including *Toxoplasma gondii*, should be considered in the differential diagnosis. Patients with CD4 counts of less than 50 cells/mm^3 should have dilated indirect ophthalmoscopic fundus examinations every 2–3 months. A retrospective review demonstrated that, by 27 months, 42% of individuals meeting this criteria developed CMV retinitis. In addition, by 27 months, 26% and 15% of patients with a baseline CD4 count of 51–100 and 101–250 cells/mm^3, respectively, developed CMV retinitis. We screen patients with CD4 counts of 50–250 cells/mm^3 every 3–4 months and with CD4 counts of 250–500 cells/mm^3 every 5–6 months. It should be emphasized that there can be variability between CD4 measurements in the same individual, as well as a rapid downward trend in the count in some individuals.

CMV infection of the retina produces characteristic clinical findings due to viral invasion of retinal cells with resul-

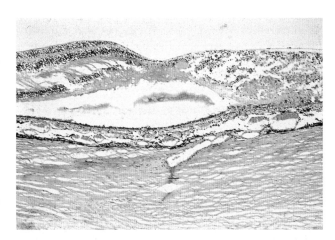

FIG. 11. CMV infection of the retina produces widespread retinal necrosis as seen on *right half* of this photograph. (Courtesy of William H. Spencer, M.D., Department of Ophthalmology, California Pacific Medical Center, San Francisco, CA.)

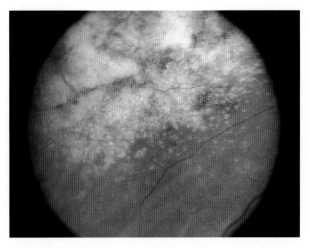

FIG. 12. CMV retinitis as manifested by the presence of multiple granular-appearing white dots with varying amounts of retinal hemorrhage.

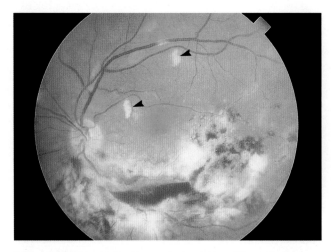

FIG. 13. CMV retinitis (*bottom*) should be differentiated from cotton-wool spots (*arrows*).

tant retinal necrosis (Fig. 11). Clinically, the lesions appear as multiple granular-appearing white dots with varying amounts of retinal hemorrhage (Fig. 12). Although they can be confused with cotton-wool spots, which may well be present in the same eye (Fig. 13), they can be distinguished by their tendency to enlarge and coalesce progressively over time (Fig. 14). They may be predominantly necrotic (white) in appearance (Fig. 15A) or accompanied by significant retinal hemorrhage (Fig. 15B). As areas of retinitis enlarge, they are often associated with broad regions of intraretinal hemorrhage and appear to follow the vascular arcades, resulting in an arcuate or triangular zone of infection (Fig. 16). Areas of active infection may also take on a characteristic linear appearance, seemingly following the retinal vessels or nerve fiber layer into the periphery (Fig. 17).

Actively infected regions of retinal tissue are gradually replaced after several weeks by atrophic tissue that has lost the capacity to support viral replication. The underlying retinal pigment epithelium demonstrates pigment loss and migration with increased visualization of the choroidal vasculature. Untreated cases of CMV retinitis typically demonstrate a leading edge of active white retinal infection with varying amounts of hemorrhage that spreads outward from a zone of chorioretinal atrophic change (Figs. 18–20). Other findings associated with CMV retinitis include perivasculitis, vascular attenuation, and vessel closure. In addition, vitritis and anterior uveitis, as well as papillitis, may be seen (Fig. 21).

Retinal detachments may be seen in conjunction with CMV retinitis. Whereas these may occasionally be exudative in nature, they are more typically rhegmatogenous (Fig. 22A,B) and usually involve cases of peripheral retinitis where retinal breaks occur either within the zone of necrotic retina or at the interface between necrotic and uninvolved retinal tissues. These detachments may occur during periods of active infection, as well as after the retinitis has been stabilized by antiviral therapy. However, retinal breaks in this setting may be extremely difficult to visualize because of

marked retinal thinning in areas of necrosis. It should also be kept in mind that proliferative vitreoretinopathy is often seen in association with these detachments. Fortunately, these detachments may respond to traditional scleral buckling and vitrectomy techniques (Fig. 22C). Whereas pneumatic retinopexy may be used in patients who are not surgical candidates, the long-term success rate of this procedure used in this setting has not been impressive (Fig. 23). In addition, control of active retinitis is critical for an anatomically successful surgical outcome. Vitrectomy and silicone oil injection are favored in those cases in which the risk of continued active retinal infection is great (Fig. 24). It increases the chance of reattachment with a single procedure and may maintain retinal apposition even in the face of active recurrent infection. For individuals in whom surgical intervention is not deemed to be appropriate, either cryopexy or photocoagulation therapy to the leading edge of the detachment may be helpful in slowing the progression of retinal detachment (Fig. 25).

Two antiviral agents have been successfully used in the treatment of CMV retinitis in AIDS patients. The first of these is ganciclovir [dihydroxy propoxymethyl guanine (DHPG)], which is a purine analogue similar in structure to acyclovir with the exception of an additional side-chain methoxyl group (Fig. 26). Its antiviral effect is due to competitive inhibition of viral DNA polymerase. Ganciclovir demonstrates activity against most of the human herpes viruses, including CMV, herpes simplex types 1 and 2, varicella–zoster, and Epstein–Barr virus. Typically administered intravenously, ganciclovir results in initial stabilization or improvement of CMV retinitis over a 2- to 3-week period in over 80% of treated patients (Fig. 27). If a patient has what appears to be CMV retinitis and the patient does not respond to intravenous therapy after 3–5 weeks of treatment, one should strongly consider the possibility that the retinitis is being caused by an etiologic agent other than CMV. However, the emergence of ganciclovir-resistant viral strains will undoubtedly change this treatment strategy in the future.

Intravenous therapy entails a 2- to 3-week induction period of twice-daily infusions at a rate of 5 mg/kg of body weight in individuals with normal renal function. Following this, a maintenance regimen is begun that consists of either a single daily dose at 5 mg/kg for 7 days/week or 6 mg/kg for 5 days/week. Patients on maintenance therapy should be monitored for neutropenia weekly, because intravenous medication has been shown to produce significant myelosuppression in at least one-third of treated patients. The neutropenia is often severe enough to necessitate temporary or permanent discontinuation of the drug. In addition, concurrent treatment of patients with ganciclovir and zidovudine [azidothymidine (also known as AZT), a thymidine analogue that inhibits HIV replication] may be difficult because of additive myelosuppressive effects. It has become common practice for ophthalmologists to diagnose and monitor the progress of CMV retinitis and to have other medical specialists provide

Text continues on p 111.

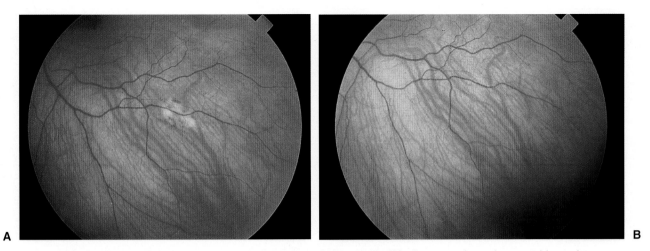

FIG. 14. This patient developed evidence of early CMV retinitis (**A**) after a previous photographic study taken 7 days earlier demonstrated no clinical evidence of infection (**B**).

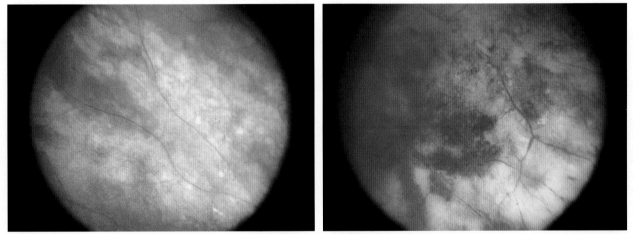

FIG. 15. CMV retinitis may be predominantly necrotic in appearance with few, if any, hemorrhages (**A**), or it can demonstrate a significant degree of accompanying retinal hemorrhage (**B**).

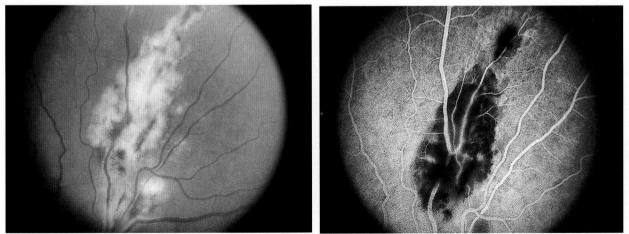

FIG. 16. Areas of CMV retinitis appear to follow the vascular arcades, often resulting in a wedge-shaped zone of retinal infection (**A**). Fluorescein angiography (**B**) demonstrates only mild fluorescein dye leakage at the site of infection.

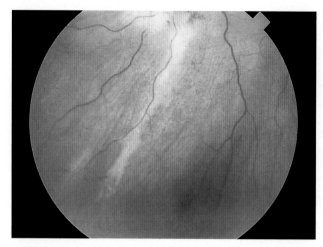

FIG. 17. CMV retinitis may demonstrate a characteristic linear pattern of progression as it extends into the midperiphery and far periphery.

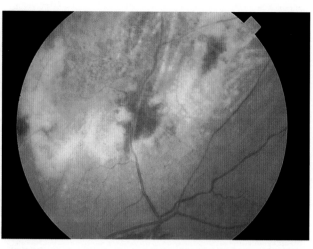

FIG. 18. CMV retinitis demonstrates a leading edge of active white infection with an advancing edge of small white granular dots that will later coalesce. Progression of the infection leaves behind a zone of chorioretinal pigmentary derangement as seen superiorly.

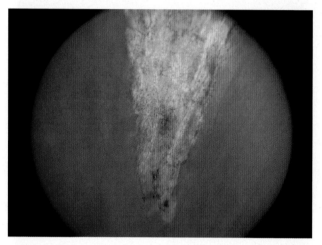

FIG. 19. The presence of a wedge-shaped zone of chorioretinal disruption in the eye of a patient with HIV disease should make one suspect the possible presence of prior CMV retinitis.

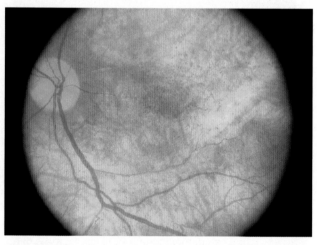

FIG. 20. End-stage CMV retinitis as manifested by widespread chorioretinal scarring, vascular attenuation, and optic atrophy. At this point, the retina is no longer able to support viral replication and no evidence of active infection may be visible.

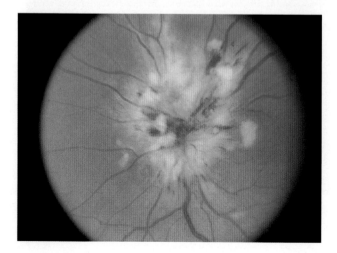

FIG. 21. CMV papillitis can usually be diagnosed by examining the peripapillary retina, as changes consistent with the presence of CMV retinitis in the surrounding tissues usually suggest the diagnosis.

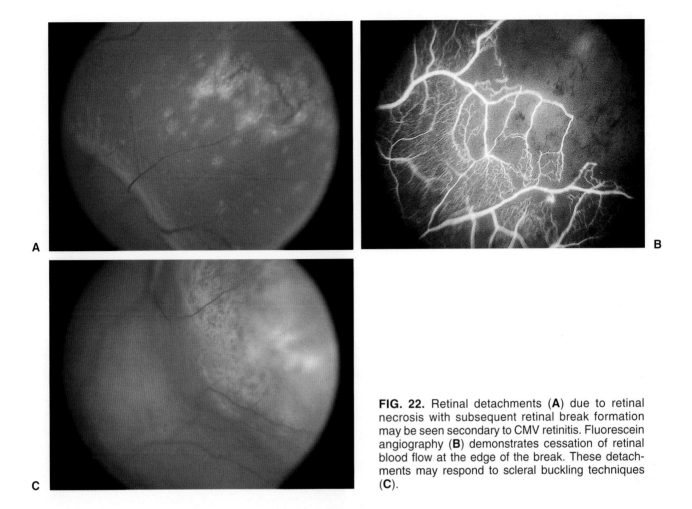

FIG. 22. Retinal detachments (**A**) due to retinal necrosis with subsequent retinal break formation may be seen secondary to CMV retinitis. Fluorescein angiography (**B**) demonstrates cessation of retinal blood flow at the edge of the break. These detachments may respond to scleral buckling techniques (**C**).

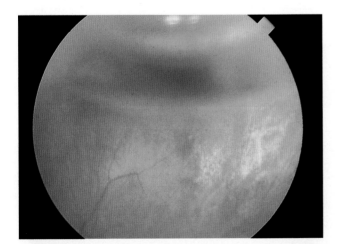

FIG. 23. Pneumatic retinopexy for CMV-related retinal detachments may be effective for a limited period of time, although the long-term success rate in patients with CMV retinitis does not appear to be very great.

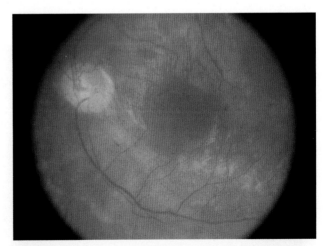

FIG. 24. Vitrectomy and silicone oil injection are the preferred treatments for those patients with complicated detachments secondary to CMV retinitis in whom the risk of continued active retinal infection is great. This retina remained attached despite the persistent presence of active CMV infection seen at the inferior margin of the anatomic fovea.

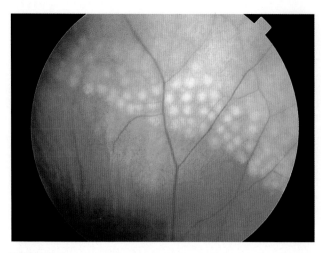

FIG. 25. Laser treatment may be helpful in slowing the spread of retinal detachment. It may also prove to be efficacious as prophylaxis for fellow eyes of patients with bilateral CMV retinitis and retinal detachment in one eye.

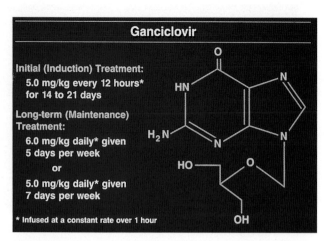

FIG. 26. Foscarnet (DHPG) is a purine analogue similar in structure to acyclovir. (Courtesy of Syntex Laboratories, Inc., Palo Alto, CA © 1989.)

Ganciclovir

Initial (Induction) Treatment:
5.0 mg/kg every 12 hours*
for 14 to 21 days

Long-term (Maintenance)
Treatment:
6.0 mg/kg daily* given
5 days per week
or
5.0 mg/kg daily* given
7 days per week

* Infused at a constant rate over 1 hour

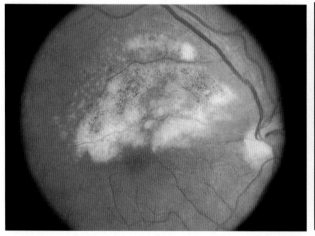
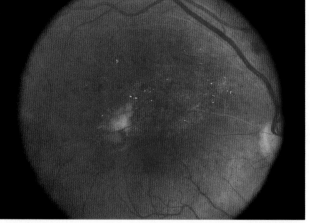

FIG. 27. A patient with CMV retinitis prior to treatment with ganciclovir (**A**) and 6 weeks later (**B**).

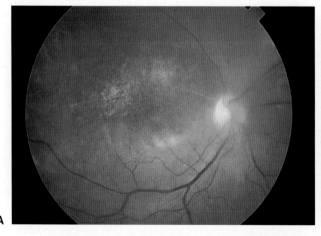
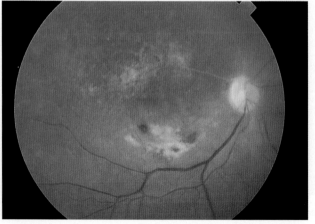

FIG. 28. The same patient as depicted in Fig. 27, but 7 months later. A zone of smoldering CMV retinitis can now be seen inferior to the anatomic fovea despite continued ganciclovir treatment (**A**). Two months later (**B**), the infection was noted to be quite active. The patient was very ill at this point and demonstrated progressive CMV retinitis despite continued ganciclovir therapy.

and monitor the patient's systemic response to anti-CMV medications. This team approach has been adopted because of the possibility of potentially severe drug side effects and the generally complex medical condition of affected individuals. It is critical that communication between the ophthalmologist and other medical personnel be kept open to allow close monitoring of the patient's ocular status.

Given that DHPG therapy has a lag period from onset of treatment to visible improvement in the retinal infection, it is not unusual to see no change in the infection after 1 week to 10 days of therapy. After 2–3 weeks, one may see less whitening of the infected tissue and beginning resolution of any accompanying hemorrhage. This is usually indicative of a positive response to therapy. However, treatment simply results in cessation of active retinitis, with resultant chorioretinal scarring and thinning of previously infected retina. CMV remains dormant within the retinal tissues at the margins of the involved areas, and infection will relapse after several weeks if therapy is discontinued. As a result, indefinite maintenance therapy is required for AIDS patients with CMV retinitis. However, temporary cessation of intravenous ganciclovir therapy may not result in significant progression of the retinitis as long as intravenous therapy is restarted within a 1- to 2-week period. Intravenous therapy with ganciclovir also provides protection against infection in the fellow eyes of individuals with unilateral infection and causes regression of foci of CMV infection elsewhere in the body. In addition, an oral preparation of ganciclovir may be used for maintenance therapy following 2 or 3 weeks of standard intravenous induction treatment. Oral therapy is best suited for individuals with limited zones of retinitis, and treatment consists of 1- to 1.5-g doses administered three times daily.

Up to 50% of individuals on intravenous maintenance therapy will eventually show progression of CMV retinitis and may require reinduction doses of the medication. Disease progression during maintenance therapy is often due to inadequate drug dosing, but may also occur in patients with satisfactory drug levels when advanced HIV infection or concurrent systemic infections cause increased impairment of the immune system. In addition, viral resistance to ganciclovir therapy may occur, resulting in "breakthrough" of CMV infection. This is an increasingly common and serious problem that is likely to become even more frequent due to longer survival times of patients.

An alternative to ganciclovir for treatment of CMV retinitis is foscarnet (trisodium phosphonoformate), a drug that selectively inhibits viral DNA polymerase and has been shown to be active in vitro against all human herpes viruses. It also has activity against HIV, which makes it particularly interesting. Like ganciclovir, it is administered intravenously and requires indefinite maintenance therapy. Induction doses are typically 90 mg/kg for patients with normal renal function given twice per day for 2–3 weeks. This is then followed by maintenance doses of 120 mg/kg once daily.

Foscarnet differs from ganciclovir in that it has no known myelosuppressive action. As such, it may be used concurrently with zidovudine (azidothymidine). However, foscarnet may produce increases in serum creatinine, has been shown to result in reversible renal failure, and may result in CNS side effects. Nevertheless, it does appear to be equally effective as ganciclovir in the management of CMV retinitis. Foscarnet has also been a useful alternative in the treatment of those patients with recurrent CMV infection who do not respond to increased doses of ganciclovir. Perhaps most importantly, foscarnet was recently shown to prolong life expectancy by 50% in patients with CMV retinitis. This is probably due to its anti-HIV effect. For this reason, its use will become more frequent.

Of particular importance is the prompt recognition of recurrent CMV retinitis. Its appearance differs sufficiently from that of untreated retinitis such that it may go undetected for long periods of time. Early recurrences appear as subtle white or grey zones of retinitis with little hemorrhage that usually, but not always, occur at the margins of previously active infection (Fig. 28A). Extremely subtle recurrences may be detected by looking for enlarging areas of ghost vessel formation, signifying continuing retinal necrosis with subsequent vascular occlusion. Patients may also report progressive field-of-vision loss or a darkening of vision. Of interest is the presence of foveal sparing, which is seen in virtually all cases of recurrent CMV retinitis in patients on anti-CMV therapy. The term foveal sparing refers to the fact that recurrent CMV retinitis spares or goes around the anatomic fovea as the retinitis progresses within the macula (Fig. 29). This allows preservation of central macular function for a longer period than might have been expected based on the proximity of the infection to the foveola alone.

Recurrent CMV retinitis in patients on treatment tends to "smolder" rather than actively progress. Nevertheless, they will continue to spread slowly, but inexorably, if the treatment regimen is not altered. A particularly ominous sign is seen when smoldering retinitis reaches the optic disc. Reinduction doses of anti-CMV medication will often lead to inhibition of these recurrent lesions. Therapy may consist of

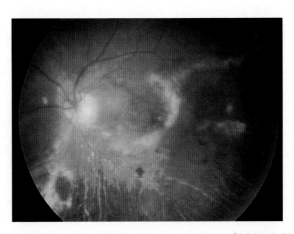

FIG. 29. Foveal "sparing" pattern of recurrent CMV retinitis, which typically spares the anatomic fovea for a prolonged period.

twice-daily induction doses of either ganciclovir or foscarnet given for 2–3 weeks, depending on the severity of the recurrence and its proximity to the fovea and/or optic disc. This should then be followed by maintenance doses of medication that are at least 10%–25% greater than the patient was on when the retinitis recurred. Retinitis progression may recur again, however, and eventually necessitate alternative modes of treatment. Patients with recurrent infection that is active in appearance (characterized by the presence of moderate retinal whitening with significant accompanying hemorrhage) have an especially poor ocular prognosis, even with increased doses of medication (Fig. 28B). Accordingly, combined therapy consisting of daily infusions of both ganciclovir and foscarnet, or an alternating formula of foscarnet and ganciclovir maintenance therapy, may be considered. Ganciclovir and foscarnet have different mechanisms of action for inhibition of viral DNA polymerase, and there may be an in vitro synergy between the two medications. Nevertheless, combined toxic effects of the medications and the increased time needed for medication administration may limit use of this therapeutic regimen.

ALTERNATIVE THERAPIES

Treatment of CMV retinitis with intravitreal drug injections has been shown to be efficacious. A dose of 200 μg results in intravitreal levels that are above the minimum inhibitory concentration of most CMV isolates. However, the half-life of intravitreal ganciclovir is only 13 hours, and induction injections 2–3 times per week for 2–3 weeks, followed by weekly injections indefinitely, is a major disadvantage of this therapy. In addition, intravitreal injections do not prevent infection in uninvolved fellow eyes and have no effect on systemic CMV infection. As a result, this mode of therapy may be best suited for patients with recurrent progressive CMV retinitis that is unresponsive to maximal systemic medication.

Our protocol for intravitreal anti-CMV therapy involves the use of ganciclovir 2,000 μg in 0.05 ml given intravitreally 2–3 times per week for 3 weeks, followed by once-a-week maintenance intravitreal injections. Alternatively, foscarnet may be used and is given intravitreally at a dose of 2,400 μg in 0.05 ml twice per week for 3 weeks, followed by once-a-week maintenance injections. It is performed as an outpatient procedure, and the protocol is as outlined. Topical anesthetic is given and the conjunctiva cleansed with a povidone swab. Xylocaine 2% with epinephrine is injected subconjunctivally in the temporal quadrant, and a circular conjunctival impression is made with a syringe hub at the margin of the cornea. Because the hub of all Luer-Lok (but not tuberculin) syringes measure 4 mm in diameter, the posterior border of the circular impression approximates the pars plana. A syringe with a 30-gauge, 0.5-inch needle is used for injecting the medication, usually in a volume of 0.1 ml. An indirect ophthalmoscopic examination is performed to monitor the central retinal artery and to check for vitreous

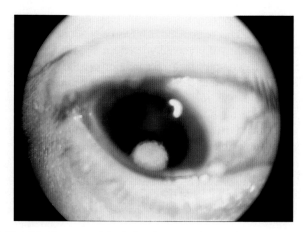

FIG. 30. The ganciclovir implant positioned in the vitreous cavity following surgical placement.

hemorrhage or retinal detachment. Complications of intravitreal injection include endophthalmitis (0.6%), vitreous hemorrhage (3%), retinal detachment (8%), and optic atrophy (8%). However, the latter two findings may, in part, be secondary to the retinitis itself and not the injections.

The ganciclovir intraocular device or implant also plays a role in therapy, possibly in conjunction with oral CMV prophylaxis for the fellow eye and for protection against systemic infection. It consists of a 6-mg pellet of ganciclovir that is 2.5 mm in diameter and coated with 10% polyvinyl alcohol, which is permeable to ganciclovir (Fig. 30). A suturing strut is attached to one edge of the pellet, and the pellet is then sealed on three sides by ethyl-vinyl acetate, which is impermeable to ganciclovir. The resultant sustained linear drug release provides 3 or 6 months (depending on pellet construction) of anti-CMV activity. The surgical technique involves a conjunctival peritomy in the inferotemporal quadrant followed by a 5.5-mm pars plana incision located 4.0 mm posterior to the limbus. A limited vitrectomy without infusion is performed through the incision as well as at the wound site to remove prolapsed vitreous. The suturing strut of the implant is trimmed to approximately 1 mm in length, and a double-armed 9-0 mersilene suture is passed and locked through both edges of the strut. The implant is carefully placed into the vitreous cavity, and the preplaced 9-0 mersilene is sutured to the sclera and tied. The sclerotomy is then closed with a continuous 8-0 nylon suture.

Finally, cidofovir represents a new class of acyclic nucleoside phosphonate analogue with a broad spectrum of anti-DNA viral activity. It can be administered intravenously (in conjunction with probenecid to prevent renal toxicity) or intravitreally and demonstrates an extended antiviral effect with either mode of administration. Accordingly, it will undoubtedly play a future role in CMV retinitis treatment.

TOXOPLASMOSIS RETINOCHOROIDITIS

Toxoplasma gondii is a protozoan parasite occurring in active and encysted forms. In contrast to the well-demarcated

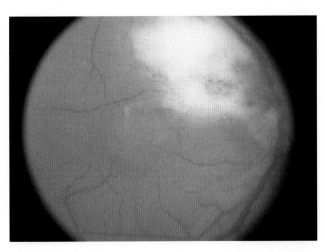

FIG. 31. Toxoplasmic retinochoroiditis in a patient with AIDS. The area of infection is more intensely white in appearance and accompanied by less retinal hemorrhage than usually seen with CMV retinitis.

nature of toxoplasmosis infection in immunocompetent individuals, AIDS patients may demonstrate evidence of multifocal disease with less vitritis than is usually encountered in immunocompetent individuals. Bilateral involvement is also not unusual, and proliferative vitreoretinopathy may accompany later stages of the disease (see also Chapter 3 by A.H. Friedman).

Toxoplasmosis retinochoroiditis may be confused with other forms of retinitis, but is differentiated by the presence of intense, almost "fluffy"-appearing areas of retinal whitening with varying amounts of vitritis (Fig. 31). In addition, there is usually less accompanying retinal hemorrhage than is seen with untreated CMV retinitis. Fluorescein angiography usually demonstrates more leakage in active toxoplasmosis infection than seen in patients with CMV infection. Of note is the fact that toxoplasmosis quite commonly involves the CNS in AIDS patients, resulting in neurologic manifestations in approximately 10% of patients with AIDS.

Laboratory studies for the evaluation of AIDS patients with suspected toxoplasmosis have been relatively unreliable. Antibody titers in patients with toxoplasmosis have demonstrated conflicting results, and increasing serum antibody titers in AIDS patients with CNS toxoplasmosis may not be detectable. A therapeutic trial with antitoxoplasmosis medications or an endoretinal biopsy may be appropriate in patients with a confusing clinical presentation.

As is the case with CMV retinitis, indefinite antitoxoplasmosis therapy may be necessary in some individuals to prevent recurrences. We generally start with *triple therapy* (pyrimethamine–sulfonamides–corticosteroids). Pyrimethamine (Daraprim) is given with an initial loading dose of 100 mg on the first day, followed by 25 mg twice a day for 4–6 weeks. *Triple sulfa* (sulfadiazine) is given as a 4-g loading dose on the first day, followed by 1 g four times per day for 4–6 weeks. Prednisone may also be given if warranted by the presence of accompanying inflammation.

When indicated, 80–100 mg/day may be administered orally for 7–10 days, with rapid tapering thereafter. These dosages are adjusted according to the response of the infection to treatment; leukocyte and platelet counts must be monitored on at least a weekly basis.

SYPHILITIC UVEITIS

Treponema pallidum organisms may accompany the HIV as a sexually transmitted disease, resulting in a strong epidemiologic link between these two entities. Given this association, it has been suggested that all patients with HIV infection be tested for syphilis and vice versa (see also Chapter 3 by A.H. Friedman).

Posterior segment syphilitic involvement in patients with concurrent HIV infection has been well documented. Findings may be highly variable and include chorioretinitis, perivasculitis, intraretinal hemorrhage, papillitis, and panuveitis (Fig. 32). Ocular involvement may be unilateral or bilateral, and is associated with evidence of CNS infection in up to 85% of patients. In addition, one-third of patients with both ocular and CNS infection manifest symptomatic neurosyphilis. This high correlation between neurosyphilis and ocular involvement supports the current recommendation of lumbar puncture and cerebrospinal fluid evaluation in patients with ocular syphilis who are seropositive for HIV.

Due to the variety of manifestations seen in ocular syphilis, laboratory studies may be helpful in reaching the appropriate diagnosis. The most reliable studies are the serum fluorescent treponema antibody absorption test and the microhemagglutination assay, both of which provide evidence of past luetic infection and may remain positive for years. The rapid plasma reagin (RPR) test is positive in 99% of cases of secondary syphilis, but its sensitivity is lower in tertiary disease. One case of RPR-negative secondary syphilis in an HIV-positive patient has been described, and an AIDS patient with syphilitic neuroretinitis and a negative

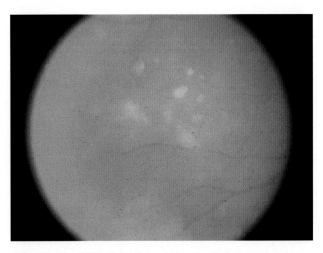

FIG. 32. Syphilitic infection of the posterior segment may present as a chorioretinitis with vitritis and panuveitis.

RPR has been reported. The RPR is ordinarily confirmed with either the serum fluorescent treponema antibody absorption test or the microhemagglutination assay to avoid false positives. Cerebrospinal fluid evaluations with determinations of protein and glucose levels, leukocyte counts, and a Venereal Disease Research Laboratory test have a high degree of accuracy in the diagnosis of neurosyphilis.

Multiple reports suggest that syphilis in HIV-positive individuals runs a more rapid and aggressive course than in seronegative patients. One comparison of HIV patients with immunocompetent patients with ocular syphilis demonstrated that the HIV-positive group had more extensive ocular disease. This, in addition to the strong association of neurosyphilis with ocular syphilis in HIV-positive individuals, provides support for the increased severity of syphilitic manifestations in the HIV-infected population.

Antibiotic regimens as recommended by the Centers for Disease Control for treatment of syphilis in immunocompetent patients may not be appropriate for patients who are HIV positive. Several HIV patients have been reported to develop recurrent syphilitic infection after treatment of primary or secondary lues with 2.4 million units of intramuscular benzathine penicillin. Administration of intravenous penicillin for longer durations has resulted in visual improvement in HIV-positive patients with syphilis. It has been recommended that all HIV-positive patients with ocular syphilis be treated with the antibiotic regimen (12–24 million units of aqueous penicillin G intravenously for a minimum of 10 days) suggested by the Centers for Disease Control for patients with concurrent neurosyphilis and HIV infection. However, one patient has been reported to have received intravenous penicillin (24 million units daily) for 10 days and yet presented 14 months later with recurrent syphilis. Current recommendations for the treatment of syphilis in AIDS patients will undoubtedly be modified as more experience is gained in the management of this disorder.

FUNGAL RETINITIS AND VITRITIS

Immunosuppressed patients, especially individuals with indwelling catheters, have long been known to be at risk for systemic fungal infection with endogenous ocular involvement. Typical candidal lesions appear as fluffy white "mounds" (Fig. 33) that are frequently bilateral, located at the surface of the inner retina, and often extend into the vitreous. There is usually an overlying vitritis, and there may be vitreous abscesses.

Amphotericin B has been used for candidal infections in non-AIDS patients. This drug may be administered intravenously with success, but has potentially severe side effects. Intravitreal administration of amphotericin B (5 μg) has been reported to result in resolution of candidal chorioretinitis after a single injection. Other antifungal agents, including 5-fluorocytosine and ketoconazole, have been used successfully in the treatment of, or as adjuvant therapy for,

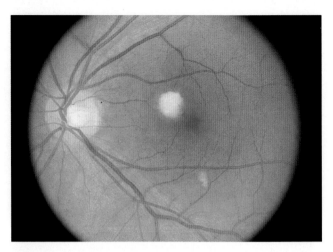

FIG. 33. Candida retinitis in a patient with candida septicemia.

candidal retinitis in non-AIDS patients. Vitrectomy may also be a useful adjunct in the management of intraocular candidal infection.

Despite the present relative infrequency of candida retinitis in AIDS patients, increasing numbers of cases can be expected as more patients undergo placement of indwelling catheters for intravenous antiviral treatment (see also Chapter 3 by A.H. Friedman).

ENDOGENOUS BACTERIAL RETINITIS

Several cases of AIDS patients with endogenous bacterial retinitis have been reported. Two patients were seen with a slowly progressive retinitis characterized by the presence of multifocal, yellow–white retinal lesions with surrounding subretinal fluid and exudate. Retinal biopsy of one patient revealed the presence of gram-positive bacteria on histologic examination. Both patients responded to doxycycline therapy. Two cases of endogenous *Staphylococcus epidermidis* ocular infection have also been described in AIDS patients. One case presented as an inflammatory choroidal mass and the other as a diffuse uveitis. Biopsy of the choroid and vitreous demonstrated the organism on stain and culture. Bacterial chorioretinitis and uveitis, although rare, should be considered in AIDS patients with posterior segment infection unresponsive to treatment for suspected viral, fungal, or protozoan etiologies.

ACUTE RETINAL NECROSIS AND PROGRESSIVE OUTER RETINAL NECROSIS

Acute retinal necrosis (ARN) is a rapidly progressive viral uveitis that was first reported as a new clinical syndrome in 1971. The first case report of this disorder in an AIDS patient appeared in 1985. Acute retinal necrosis is characterized initially by peripheral retinal whitening that progresses

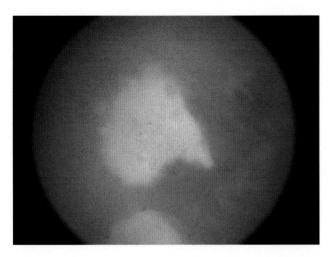

FIG. 34. Acute retinal necrosis in a patient with AIDS. Two foci of infection with fairly well-defined margins can be seen. Note paucity of accompanying retinal hemorrhages.

to necrosis over several days (Fig. 34). As the process continues, retinal whitening and necrosis expand and typically involve the entire peripheral retina in untreated cases. In later stages, scattered intraretinal hemorrhages may be seen, and retinal detachments with proliferative vitreoretinopathy commonly occur. Associated ocular findings include vascular occlusion, optic disc edema, anterior uveitis, vitritis, and scleritis. In addition, patients may demonstrate bilateral involvement.

Several viral pathogens have been associated with ARN. Varicella–zoster has been the most frequently implicated virus in this disorder. Viral antibodies have been described postmortem in eyes with ARN, and the virus itself has been detected in the vitreous of one eye. In addition, serum anti-varicella–zoster antibodies has been found to be elevated in patients with ARN, and transsynaptic spread of varicella virus through the CNS has been reported.

Herpes simplex and CMV have also been associated with ARN to varying degrees. Herpes simplex particles have been demonstrated in retinal biopsy specimens of non-AIDS patients with ARN. Immune complexes with herpes simplex antigen have been documented in the eye and serum of one patient. These data suggest that ARN may be caused by multiple viral pathogens. Nevertheless, all of these suspected agents are in the herpes family.

Acyclovir has been successfully used in the treatment of non-AIDS patients with ARN. This drug inhibits DNA replication and is active against most herpes viruses except CMV. To lessen retinal involvement and limit the potential for retinal detachment, patients with ARN should be placed on parenteral acyclovir immediately on diagnosis. Intravenous acyclovir has been used successfully at 1,500 mg/m²/day in three divided doses, and regression of the retinal lesions is usually seen approximately 4 days after initiation of therapy in immunocompetent individuals. Treatment for 10 days to 2 weeks is the usual recommendation, and antiplatelet therapy

and steroid treatment may be added as indicated. If patients have been previously receiving acyclovir or if retinitis is fulminant, many retina specialists use combination foscarnet and ganciclovir.

To provide a basis for appropriate therapeutic intervention, endoretinal biopsy has been proposed for differentiation of CMV retinitis from ARN in difficult cases. In suspected ARN cases unresponsive to acyclovir, CMV should be suspected, and treatment with ganciclovir, which has activity against most herpes viruses, should be considered.

A particularly virulent form of ARN in patients with AIDS has been termed progressive outer retinal necrosis. While this has been referred to as "PORN," some find this term objectionable and it may be simply considered ARN in AIDS. Features of this syndrome include

1. Multifocal deep retinal lesions
2. Lack of granular borders
3. Perivascular sparing or clearing (Fig. 35)
4. Minimal or no intraocular inflammation
5. Very rapid progression
6. High incidence of retinal detachment
7. Generally poor visual prognosis

A characteristic finding of this entity is primary involvement of the outer retina, shown by William Freeman to be secondary to varicella–zoster involvement of both the neurosensory retina and the retinal pigment epithelium. Given the very rapid progression and the poor visual outcome, one should consider prompt initiation of treatment with intravitreal injections of foscarnet or ganciclovir, followed by intravenous therapy, and use of other therapeutic agents as indicated.

Management of retinal detachment in ARN may be difficult because of the presence of proliferative vitreoretinopathy and widespread retinal necrosis. The incidence of retinal detachment in HIV-positive patients with ARN is quite high, with one study reporting 75% of patients progressing to reti-

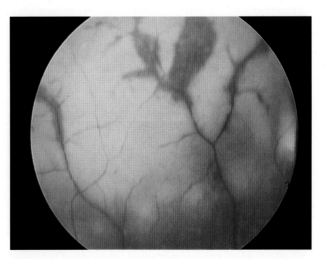

FIG. 35. Progressive outer retinal necrosis demonstrating perivascular "sparing" or "clearing."

nal detachment despite antiviral therapy. Nevertheless, vitrectomy with silicone oil instillation can be used and results in anatomically successful reattachment in a high percentage of cases. The very guarded visual prognosis in the setting of AIDS, however, should be remembered. Prophylactic laser treatment surrounding areas of retinal necrosis may also be helpful in decreasing the incidence of retinal detachment.

CRYPTOCOCCUS CHORIORETINITIS

Cryptococcus neoformans is a yeast that rarely causes human disease, but is a common cause of opportunistic infection in immunosuppressed patients. CNS involvement with cryptococcus in AIDS patients often results in meningitis with secondary ocular findings. Choroiditis and chorioretinitis from cryptococcus infection have also been reported in AIDS patients and appear to be associated with CNS involvement.

Typical cryptococcal lesions are located in the choroid and retina, and appear as multiple discrete yellowish spots varying in size from 500 to 3,000 μm in diameter. Associated findings include perivascular sheathing, vitritis, and anterior uveitis. Papilledema may be present due to increased intracranial pressure from meningitis (Fig. 36). Visual loss may occur and is thought to be due to cryptococcal involvement of afferent tissues, including the optic nerve, chiasm, and tract.

Specific treatment of cryptococcal chorioretinal disease in AIDS patients has yet to be described. Therapy for cryptococcal meningitis in immunosuppressed patients has included amphotericin B and 5-fluorocytosine. The combination of these two drugs has been successfully used to treat cryptococcal chorioretinitis in immunocompetent adults. Ketoconazole has also been used with 5-fluorocytosine and demonstrates synergistic activity against the cryptococcus organism.

PNEUMOCYSTIS CHOROIDITIS

Pneumocystis carinii is an unusual protozoan that exhibits some fungal characteristics. It is the cause of pneumocystis pneumonia, the most common opportunistic infection in patients with AIDS. This pneumonia is potentially life-threatening and occurs as the initial manifestation of AIDS in 63% of HIV-positive patients. As a result, many individuals with AIDS undergo aerosolized pentamidine treatment as a prophylaxis. While effective in the prevention of pneumonia, such therapy appears to allow the dissemination of pneumocystis elsewhere in the body. In 1987, histopathologic examination of autopsy eyes obtained from a patient with AIDS and disseminated pneumocystis revealed areas of choroidal thickening and exudate that harbored the characteristic cysts of *Pneumocystis carinii*.

Clinical reports of pneumocystis choroiditis first appeared in late 1988 and early 1989. One study reported the cases of three patients with AIDS, each of whom manifested an unusual choroidopathy and who later died from complications of pneumocystis pneumonia. Autopsy of the globes of these patients revealed multiple infiltrates involving the choroid and choroidal vessels. Light and electron microscopy demonstrated the presence of pneumocystis organisms in these infiltrates. Another study reported the case of a 43-year-old AIDS patient who developed a bilateral choroidopathy with no initial evidence of systemic infection who later developed pneumocystis pneumonia. A transscleral choroidal biopsy was performed, and typical pneumocystis organisms were seen within the choroidal lesions on electron microscopy.

Pneumocystis choroiditis is characterized clinically by the presence of multiple choroidal lesions, usually bilateral, that appear pale yellowish white and are typically one-half to two disc diameters in size (Fig. 37). The lesions are generally round or ovoid and may coalesce to form large regions of

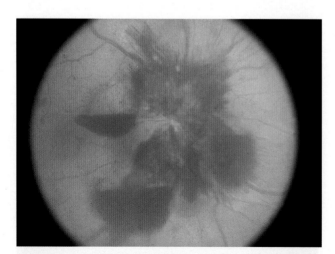

FIG. 36. A patient with cryptococcal meningitis and multiple subhyaloid hemorrhages demonstrating layering out of the red blood cells.

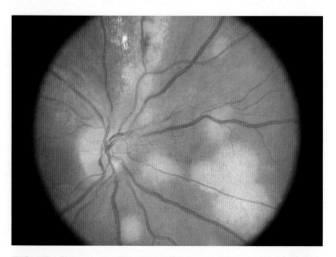

FIG. 37. Pneumocystis choroiditis appearing as multiple yellow choroidal lesions seen nasal to the optic nerve head. Note focus of CMV retinitis superior to the optic disc.

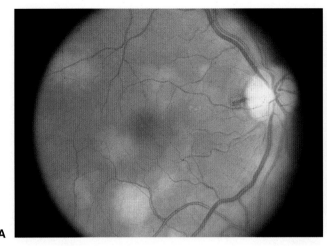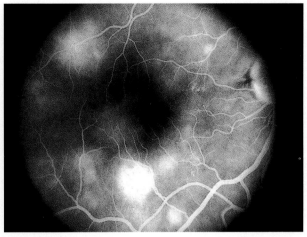

FIG. 38. Pneumocystis choroiditis in the macula (**A**). Fluorescein angiogram (**B**) demonstrates late fluorescein staining of lesions.

confluent involvement with resultant choroidal necrosis. If this process involves the foveal area, visual symptoms may result, but this has not been well studied. Fluorescein angiography of the choroidal lesions reveals early hypofluorescence and late staining with minimal evidence of dye leakage (Fig. 38). Of note is the almost total lack of an associated inflammatory response in the retina, vitreous, and anterior segments of these patients. A similar choroidal appearance may be seen in early cryptococcal chorioretinitis, but this entity is typically accompanied by an active vitritis.

COMMON PITFALLS

One of the pitfalls in the diagnosis and management of infections of the retina and choroid in individuals with AIDS is the mistaken assumption that cotton-wool spots represent foci of early infection (Fig. 39). Many individuals have been treated with anti-CMV medications for the presence of cotton-wool spots. Such treatment will have no effect on cotton-wool spot formation and subjects the patient to significant drug side effects. The natural history of cotton-wool spots should be kept in mind, because these lesions will fade over several weeks, and new lesions will appear over time with or without the concomitant administration of anti-CMV therapy.

Another common error in patient management relates to duration of anti-CMV therapeutic trials. Once the decision is made to treat individuals with CMV retinitis, it is critical to keep in mind the lag phase between the initiation of therapy and the first clinical signs of improvement. Early signs may occur in as short a period as 1 week in patients with mild infection. Some individuals, however, with massive areas of retinal necrosis and extensive hemorrhage may take at least 3–4 weeks to show definite evidence of clinical improvement. As a result, if one is convinced that CMV is the cause of retinal infection, treatment should not be altered until at least 4–6 weeks of adequate doses of medication have been given. Some individuals with CMV retinitis have mistakenly been switched to antitoxoplasmosis medications after only 2–3 weeks of anti-CMV treatment. Improvement of infection was then seen during week 4 (after one individual had been started on antitoxoplasmosis therapy). This gave the mistaken impression that the patient was responding to the antitoxoplasmosis medications. However, these patients deteriorated in the ensuing weeks and were eventually restarted on anti-CMV therapy. In general, careful photographic documentation will always enable one to detect signs of progression or improvement of infection at an earlier point (2–3 weeks) and with more certainty.

One of the most common pitfalls is the failure to diagnose correctly the presence of recurrent smoldering CMV retinitis and to institute aggressive anti-CMV treatment (Fig. 40). Again, evidence of vascular occlusions in the midperiphery,

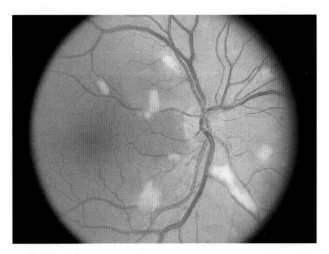

FIG. 39. Cotton-wool spots do not represent foci of early infection and should not be treated with anti-CMV therapy.

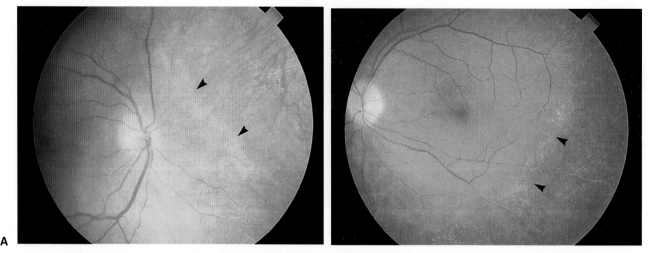

A

B

FIG. 40. One of the greatest pitfalls in the management of CMV retinitis is failure to recognize and aggressively treat smoldering CMV retinitis. Bands of subtle white retinal opacification that represent infection can be seen nasal to the optic disc (**A**) and temporal to the macula (**B**) (*arrows*).

especially if accompanied by contracting visual fields, should alert one to the possible presence of recurrent infection. Breakthrough of CMV retinitis needs to be considered, and testing for DHPG-resistant strains of CMV undertaken, if feasible. Because testing for DHPG resistance may take 1–2 months, it is important to consider such testing as soon as one first begins to suspect an inadequate response to therapy.

Pitfalls in the management of patients with viral retinitis and opportunistic infections of the retina and choroid include the mistaken treatment of noninfectious AIDS retinopathy with anti-CMV medications, failure to appreciate the time course necessary for appropriate medications to demonstrate clinical efficacy, and failure to diagnose and aggressively treat recurrent CMV infection. As we understand more about these complex infections, improved visual results will occur, with a concomitant improvement in the quality of lives of affected individuals.

SUMMARY

The posterior segment manifestations of HIV infection are many and varied. Numerous infections of the retina and choroid have been reported in patients with AIDS. The increasing longevity of individuals with HIV disease will undoubtedly result in greater numbers of patients presenting with opportunistic infections. Fortunately, many of these infections are now treatable. As a result, it is important that these infections be recognized early so that appropriate therapy can be instituted. It should be kept in mind that the underlying immunosuppression of affected individuals may modify the clinical presentation of a given infection and may also affect the patient's response to treatment. In addition, these infections may occur in combination, rendering diagnosis and therapeutic intervention more difficult. Recognition of these facts, and familiarity with the appropriate treatments available, will help to prevent vision loss in affected individuals and improve their quality of life.

BIBLIOGRAPHY

Ai E, Wong KL. Ophthalmic manifestations of AIDS. *Ophthalmol Clin North Am* 1988;1:53.

Freeman WR, Lerner CW, Mines JA, et al. A prospective study of the ophthalmologic findings in the acquired immune deficiency syndrome. *Am J Ophthalmol* 1984;97:133–142.

Holland GN, Buhles WC Jr, Mastre B, Kaplan HJ. A controlled retrospective study of ganciclovir treatment for cytomegalovirus retinopathy. *Arch Ophthalmol* 1989;107:1759–1766.

Jabs DA, Green WR, Fox R, et al. Ocular manifestations of acquired immune deficiency syndrome. *Ophthalmology* 1989;96:1092–1099.

Rao NA, Zimmerman PL, Boyer D, et al. A clinical, histopathologic, and electron microscopic study of *Pneumocystis carinii* choroiditis. *Am J Ophthalmol* 1989;107:218–228.

Practical Atlas of Retinal Disease and Therapy, Second Edition
edited by William R. Freeman,
Lippincott–Raven Publishers, Philadelphia © 1997.

· 6 ·

Diagnosis and Treatment of Posterior Uveal Tumors

James J. Augsburger

Posterior uveal tumors comprise a broad spectrum of benign and malignant intraocular neoplasms and related lesions arising within or secondarily involving the choroid, ciliary body, or both. The best known and most important of these tumors is unquestionably the posterior uveal malignant melanoma. In this chapter, we review the clinically determinable differential diagnostic features of posterior uveal malignant melanomas and several simulating tumors and consider currently available therapeutic options for each specific entity.

Before we begin our review of the specific tumors, let's take a moment to consider how posterior uveal tumors are detected and characterized to arrive at a diagnosis. Tumor-related symptoms such as blurred vision, flashes and floaters, ocular redness, and discomfort may or may not be present but are rarely sufficient to suggest the presence of a posterior uveal tumor. Consequently, a posterior uveal tumor is detected in most affected patients when they undergo a complete ophthalmic physical examination. That examination usually includes slit-lamp biomicroscopy of the anterior segment and indirect ophthalmoscopy of the ocular fundus.

Following detection of a possible posterior uveal tumor, the clinician must examine the affected eye and observed lesion comprehensively and systematically. The purpose of this examination is to enable the examiner to identify those characteristics of the observed lesion or lesions that are important for differential diagnosis. Evaluable clinical features that can be assessed by ophthalmic physical examination include the number and sizes of lesions, their anatomic sites, their colors, their cross-sectional shapes, and their effects on adjacent ocular tissues. The examiner is encouraged to make a detailed fundus drawing showing the lesion or lesions of interest and the pertinent localizing fundus landmarks. Such

an exercise is intended to ensure that the examiner has thoroughly evaluated all pertinent aspects of the lesion before arriving at a working diagnosis.

Once a fundus lesion has been detected and characterized by ophthalmic physical examination, the examiner can arrange for appropriate ancillary diagnostic evaluations, including studies such as B-scan ultrasonography and standardized A-scan ultrasonography, fluorescein angiography, and indocyanine green angiography. One should realize that such tests are supplements to clinical diagnosis but are not usually independently diagnostic.

Now let's begin our minireviews of posterior uveal malignant melanoma and several important simulating tumors in its differential diagnosis.

POSTERIOR UVEAL MALIGNANT MELANOMA

The posterior uveal malignant melanoma is a primary malignant intraocular neoplasm arising from melanocytes in the choroid or ciliary body. It is the most common malignant primary intraocular neoplasm in the white race, having a cumulative lifetime incidence of approximately 1 in 2,000 to 1 in 2,500 in that racial group. It is much less common in the black race and has an intermediate frequency in other racial groups. It is rare in persons younger than 30 years of age but increases in frequency with each passing decade.

Ophthalmoscopic Appearance of Tumor

The typical posterior uveal malignant melanoma (Fig. 1) appears as a solid, dark-brown to golden-brown subretinal mass that is circular to oval in basal configuration and either

J.J. Augsburger, M.D.: Oncology Unit, Retina Service, Wills Eye Hospital, Department of Ophthalmology, Jefferson Medical College, Thomas Jefferson University; and Department of Ophthalmology, Philadelphia, PA 19107

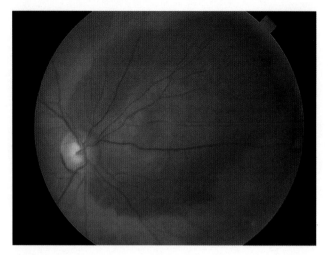

FIG. 1. Darkly melanotic juxtapapillary choroidal melanoma in a 65-year-old woman.

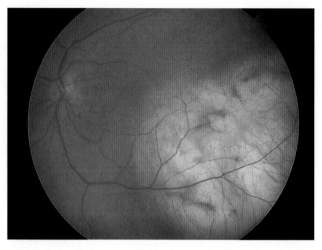

FIG. 3. Amelanotic choroidal melanoma (proven by fine-needle aspiration biopsy) in a 60-year-old man.

biconvex (75%–80%) or mushroom shaped (15%–20%) in cross section. Prominent clumps of orange pigment (lipofuscin) are frequently visible on the surface of darkly pigmented tumors (Fig. 2) but are not so obvious on the surface of clinically amelanotic ones (Fig. 3). The mushroom-shaped cross-sectional contour of some posterior uveal malignant melanomas (Fig. 4), which occurs when the tumor has broken through Bruch's membrane and formed a prominent apical subretinal nodule, is virtually pathognomic for this tumor. In some cases, the nodular eruption through Bruch's membrane becomes so pronounced that it totally obscures any view of the tumor base. In such instances, especially if the tumor nodule is hypomelanotic, the melanomatous nature of the tumor may be missed initially. Occasional posterior uveal melanomas are geographic in basal configuration and multinodular in cross-sectional shape.

Associated Clinical Features

Many eyes containing a posterior uveal malignant melanoma have an associated nonrhegmatogenous retinal detachment (Fig. 5). The subretinal fluid in such eyes is usually clear and shifting (that is, it moves to a dependent intraocular position with changes in the eye–head position). Some eyes, particularly ones containing a tumor that has erupted through Bruch's membrane and invaded the retina, have subretinal and intravitreal hemorrhage (Fig. 6). In occasional cases, the intraocular bleeding is so extensive that the fundus and tumor cannot be visualized. In such eyes, an imaging study such as B-scan ultrasonography or magnetic resonance imaging may be needed to detect the tumor.

Posterior uveal malignant melanomas involving the ciliary body frequently stimulate the development of dilated

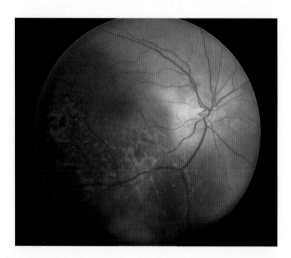

FIG. 2. Geographic, darkly melanotic, submacular choroidal melanoma with overlying prominent clumps of orange pigment.

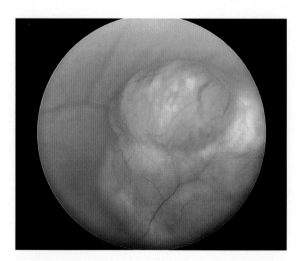

FIG. 4. Choroidal malignant melanoma with apical nodular eruption through Bruch's membrane in a 64-year-old man.

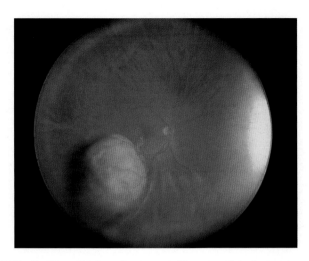

FIG. 5. Choroidal melanoma with associated nonrheg-matogenous retinal detachment inferiorly.

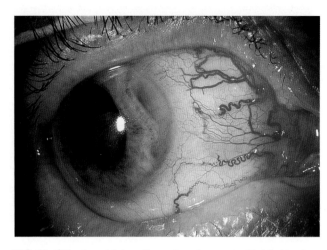

FIG. 7. Ciliochoroidal malignant melanoma with iris involve-ment and prominent episcleral "sentinel" blood vessels.

episcleral "sentinel" blood vessels (Fig. 7). Such tumors oc-casionally extend transclerally to form melanotic tumor nod-ules in the ciliary body region (Fig. 8). Transillumination of eyes containing a malignant melanoma of the ciliary body, peripheral choroid, or both using a right-angled transillumi-nator usually shows a well-defined tumor shadow on the overlying sclera. This tumor shadow can be helpful in deter-mining the full basal extent of such a tumor.

Ancillary Diagnostic Tests

Ultrasonography

Ultrasonography is frequently helpful in the differential diagnosis of posterior uveal malignant melanomas. *B-scan ultrasonography* shows the cross-sectional shape of the tu-mor (Figs. 9A and 10A), reveals the presence of nonrheg-matogenous retinal detachment that might have been over-looked ophthalmoscopically (Figs. 9A and 10A), and identi-fies nodular foci of posterior extrascleral tumor extension when present. *Standardized A-scan ultrasonography* shows the internal reflectivity pattern of the lesion (Figs. 9B and 10B), and A-scan biometry measures the maximal thickness of the mass. B-scan of a biconvex nodular posterior uveal malignant melanoma (Fig. 9A) usually shows the tumor to be homogeneous and relatively sonolucent (dark) in com-parison to the overlying sclera and adjacent orbital fat. Prominent intralesional large blood vessels with flowing blood can frequently be demonstrated during dynamic scan-ning. On standardized A-scan, such a tumor typically ex-hibits a pattern of high-amplitude surface reflectivity fol-lowed by internal echoes of rapidly decreasing amplitude down to a very low level (Fig. 9B). B-scan of a mushroom-

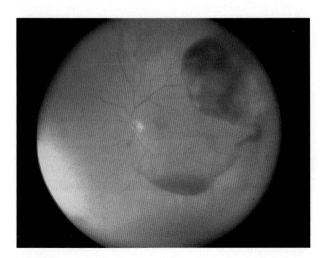

FIG. 6. Choroidal malignant melanoma with intralesional and preretinal vitreous hemorrhage.

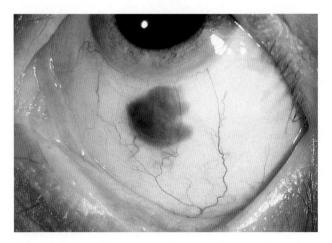

FIG. 8. Darkly melanotic episcleral extension of ciliary body melanoma in a 59-year-old woman.

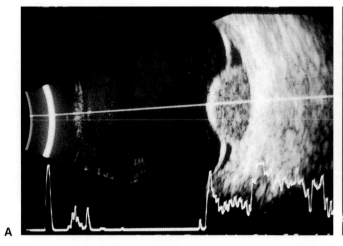

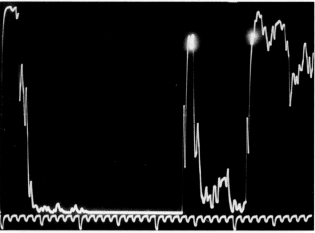

FIG. 9. Ultrasonography of nodular choroidal melanoma. **A:** B-scan showing the biconvex cross-sectional shape of the tumor, relative lesion sonolucency, and associated retinal detachment. **B:** Standardized A-scan of the same lesion showing low-amplitude internal reflectivity.

shaped posterior uveal malignant melanoma (Fig. 10A) usually shows the apical cap of tumor tissue to be relatively sonoreflective (bright) while the basal portion of the tumor retains the characteristic relative sonolucency. Standardized A-scan of such a tumor (Fig. 10B) typically shows high-amplitude internal reflectivity corresponding to the apical nodule but characteristic low-amplitude internal reflectivity corresponding to the tumor base.

Fluorescence Angiography

Both fluorescein angiography and indocyanine green angiography are currently in widespread use for characterization of suspected posterior uveal malignant melanomas.

Fluorescein angiography of the typical melanotic choroidal melanoma (Fig. 11) shows the lesion to be relatively hypo-fluorescent throughout early frames of the study. Any prominent clumps of orange pigment on the surface of the lesion tended to show pseudofluorescence throughout the study. Because choroidal melanomas are fed by large-caliber choroidal blood vessels, the intrinsic vasculature of the tumor gradually becomes fluorescent in most cases, resulting in leakage of fluorescein into the subretinal space overlying the tumor by the late frames. In amelanotic melanomas evaluated by fluorescein angiography (Fig. 12), a characteristic finding is a relatively well-defined large vessel intratumoral pattern in the early phase frames with the superimposed retinal vascular pattern overlying it. This has sometimes been referred to as the "double circulation pattern" of choroidal

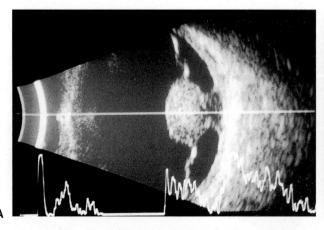

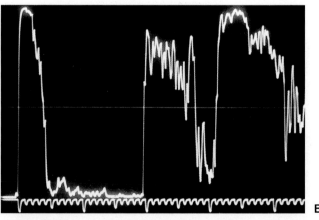

FIG. 10. Ultrasonography of mushroom-shaped choroidal melanoma. **A:** B-scan showing the characteristic mushroom cross-sectional shape of the tumor, relative apical brightness and basal sonolucency within the tumor, and associated retinal detachment. **B:** Standardized A-scan of the same tumor showing high-amplitude internal reflectivity corresponding to the apical portion of the tumor and low-amplitude internal reflectivity corresponding to the basal region.

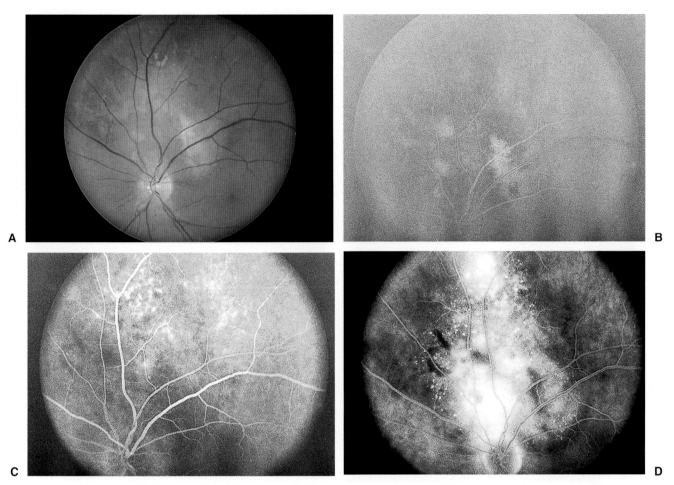

FIG. 11. Fluorescein angiogram of choroidal melanoma. **A:** Darkly melanotic superior juxtapapillary choroidal tumor with overlying clumps of orange pigment. **B:** Early laminar venous phase frame showing hypofluorescence of most of the tumor and faint pseudofluorescence corresponding to some of the pigment clumps. **C:** Full venous phase frame showing mottled hypofluorescence and hyperfluorescence corresponding to the lesion. **D:** Late phase frame showing sustained basal margin hypofluorescence, central superficial hyperfluorescence, and multifocal punctate hyperfluorescent dots on the surface of the lesion.

melanomas. In most melanomas, there is a characteristic pattern of multifocal punctate late hyperfluorescence on the surface of the lesion (Fig. 11) that has been regarded as being due to staining of cystic retinal pigment epithelium and sensory retina overlying the tumor.

Indocyanine green angiography of posterior uveal malignant melanomas (Fig. 13) usually reveals more prominent intralesional vasculature in the early frames than is apparent on a corresponding fluorescein angiogram. Most darkly melanotic choroidal melanomas tend to remain relatively hypofluorescent throughout the angiogram, but overlying serous subretinal fluid usually becomes intensely fluorescent by the late phase frames. In contrast, most lightly melanotic melanomas become diffusely and intensely hyperfluorescent by the last phase frames. Because indocyanine green angiography has been used much less frequently than fluorescein angiography in the evaluation of suspected posterior uveal

malignant melanomas and simulating lesions, its relative value in differential diagnosis is currently uncertain.

Other Ancillary Diagnostic Studies

Computed tomography (CT) is capable of demonstrating choroidal and ciliary body melanomas (Fig. 14). Most of the lesions appear just slightly hypodense relative to orbital fat. Furthermore, most choroidal and ciliary body melanomas show prominent contrast enhancement on CT. Unfortunately, CT is not particularly effective at distinguishing uveal melanomas from large simulating lesions that might also cause enhancement. Consequently, it has a lesser role in differential diagnosis than ultrasonography and fluorescein angiography.

Magnetic resonance imaging (MRI) has also been used as

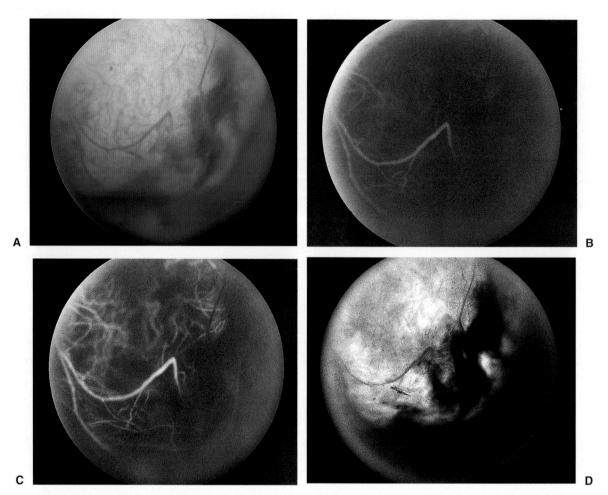

FIG. 12. Fluorescein angiogram of choroidal melanoma. **A:** An amelanotic, bizarrely vascularized nodule of choroidal melanoma that has erupted through Bruch's membrane, with associated superficial hemorrhage. **B:** Retinal arterial phase frame showing fluorescence of some intralesional vascular channels. **C:** Venous phase frame showing more prominent intralesional vasculature. **D:** Late phase frame showing superficial hyperfluorescence of the lesion, except where it is blocked by overlying blood.

a differential diagnostic test for some suspected posterior uveal malignant melanomas. The typical melanoma appears somewhat hyperintense (bright) relative to dark vitreous on the T1-weighted images and hypointense (dark) relative to bright vitreous on the T2-weighted images (Fig. 15). About 95% of choroidal and ciliary body melanomas appear to show this pattern. The few that do not tend to be clinically amelanotic, necrotic, or otherwise atypical. Most choroidal malignant melanomas also show gadolinium enhancement.

Color Doppler imaging has recently been used in several centers to characterize posterior uveal melanomas in terms of their intralesional macrovascular pattern. Almost all untreated posterior uveal malignant melanomas have prominent intralesional blood vessels with active blood flow demonstrable by this technology. Because intralesional vascular pulsations can usually be identified on conventional dynamic B-scan and A-scan ultrasonography, the actual differential diagnostic value of color Doppler imaging in such cases remains uncertain.

The *P-32 test* is a diagnostic test based on the expected unequal uptake of intravenously injected radioactive phosphorus (^{32}P) in a posterior uveal malignant melanoma versus in normal uvea. In this test, the radionuclide is administered 24–72 hours prior to testing, which uses a specially designed probe that has a small β-particle counting window. The window of the probe is positioned on the sclera overlying the presumed tumor, and the number of β-particles emitted over a specified time interval (usually 30 seconds to 1 minute) are counted. If the tumor is located at or behind the ocular equator, placement of the probe tip over the tumor requires a conjunctival incision and dissection of the subconjunctival connective tissues down to bare sclera. After a count has been obtained at the site of the tumor, the probe window is repositioned on the sclera overlying an uninvolved but otherwise comparable region of the eye (the "control site"). The difference between the count over the tumor minus the count over the control site divided by the count over the control site and then multiplied by 100 (to express the value as a percentage)

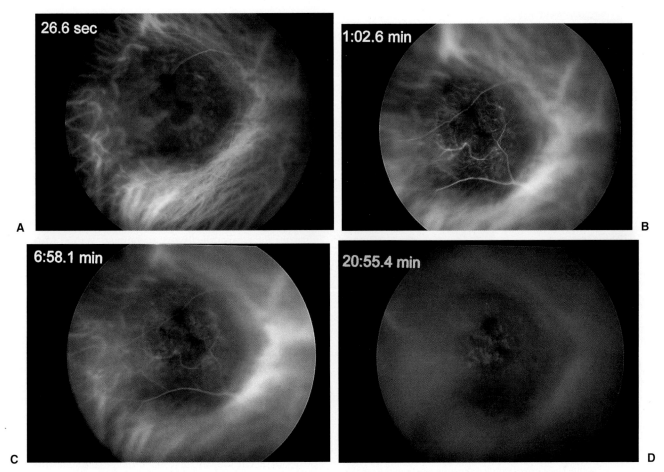

FIG. 13. Indocyanine green angiogram of melanotic choroidal malignant melanoma. **A:** Retinal arterial phase frame showing hypofluorescent choroidal tumor with intralesional blood vessels. **B:** Venous phase frame showing increased prominence of intralesional vasculature. **C:** Recirculation phase frame showing decreased prominence of retinal and intralesional blood vessels. **D:** Late phase frame showing persistently hyperfluorescent central intralesional blood vessels, mild hyperfluorescence of surrounding shallow subretinal fluid, and persistent hypofluorescence of the remainder of the tumor.

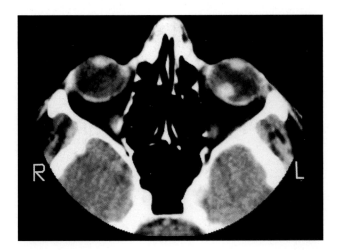

FIG. 14. Computed tomographic scan of mushroom-shaped choroidal melanoma of the left eye.

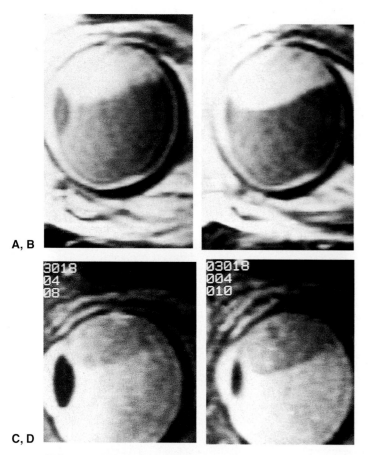

A, B

C, D

FIG. 15. Magnetic resonance image of ciliochoroidal melanoma. The tumor appears bright (hyperintense) relative to the dark vitreous on the T1-weighted images (**A,B**) and dark (hypointense) relative to the bright vitreous on the T2-weighted images (**C,D**).

is the result of the test. A result greater than 50% is generally considered "positive" (that is, consistent with a posterior uveal malignant melanoma), and a result greater than 100% is usually regarded as "strongly positive." Although the P-32 test used to be performed with great regularity in some ophthalmic centers, it is rarely employed today. Reasons for the decreased use of this technique include the nonspecific nature of the result (it is usually positive with any malignant uveal tumor), frequent "positive" results in eyes containing large benign tumors, and rupture of Bruch's membrane overlying the tumor and intraocular bleeding caused by indentation of the eye wall with the probe.

Radionuclide scanning of eyes containing a suspected posterior uveal malignant melanoma has been used in several centers in recent years. The current methodology entails intravenous injection of technetium-99m labeled monoclonal antibodies to uveal malignant melanoma cells followed in 6–16 hours by radionuclide scanning with a wide-field gamma camera. Unfortunately, scans of this type frequently fail to detect the tumor (that is, to distinguish it from background noise) and uniformly yield images of very poor resolution compared with B-scan, CT, and MRI.

Biopsy

In patients with a posterior uveal tumor that could be a posterior uveal malignant melanoma but has at least some atypical features, one must ultimately consider the option of biopsy to confirm or rule out the suspected diagnosis prior to recommending treatment. In the 1950s, several groups evaluated *incisional biopsy* and curettage of suspected posterior uveal malignant melanomas through scleral incisions made directly over the tumor. Unfortunately, the morbidity associated with such attempts was so high (a higher rate of mortality than expected and a very high rate of extraocular tumor growth following the biopsy) that these methods were appropriately abandoned. In the late 1970s and early 1980s, *fine-needle aspiration biopsy* techniques started to be applied to selected intraocular tumors, including some suspected posterior uveal malignant melanomas. This methodology required development of new techniques and the assistance and expertise of cytopathologists to interpret the specimens. Furthermore, experience to date has not been associated with any detectable increased risks of extraocular tumor seeding and metastasis compared with "background levels." Today, fine-needle aspiration biopsy is used in many ocular oncology centers to evaluate posterior uveal tumors in which the clinical diagnosis based on physical examination findings and ancillary test results is not certain beyond reasonable doubt.

Two general methods of fine-needle aspiration biopsy of posterior uveal tumors have been developed. The first approach is the *direct transcleral method*. In this technique, the surgeon usually prepares a lamellar scleral bed over the tumor, punctures the inner scleral layers with the tip of the biopsy needle, and then guides the needle tip directly into the underlying tumor (Fig. 16). When the needle is removed, the lamellar scleral flap is secured tightly with interrupted nylon sutures. The second technique is the *indirect transvitreal method*. In this technique, the surgeon creates a partial thickness sclerotomy in an appropriate meridian in the pars plana

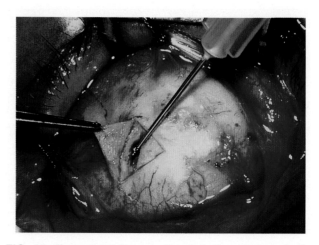

FIG. 16. Transcleral fine-needle aspiration biopsy of ciliochoroidal tumor.

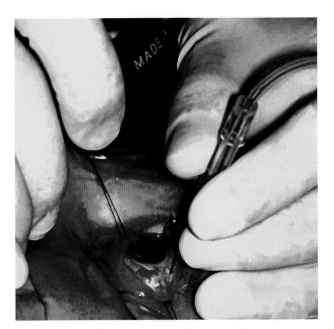

FIG. 17. Transvitreal fine-needle aspiration biopsy of choroidal tumor.

region, punctures the inner scleral layers, underlying uvea and pars plana epithelia with the tip of the needle, guides the needle tip through the vitreous to the surface of the tumor, punctures the overlying retina, and impales the tumor with the needle tip (Fig. 17). Passage of the needle tip in this technique is monitored visually using either an operating microscope or an indirect ophthalmoscope. When the needle is withdrawn, the surgeon closes the sclerotomy tightly with interrupted permanent sutures. In both methods, the device that I use to generate the suction force is usually a 10- or 20-ml sterile syringe. This syringe is never attached directly to the biopsy needle but rather is attached to a sterile flexible connector tubing that links it to the needle. Use of such a tubing ensures that the act of generating the suction force by pulling out abruptly on the plunger of the syringe will not cause inadvertent displacement of the needle tip in the eye during the biopsy. In both methods, biopsy needles of various calibers can be used; however, my colleagues and I have concluded that a 25-gauge needle probably provides the best combination of shaft rigidity and lumen size for most biopsies of posterior uveal tumors. For tumors thicker than 3 mm, I generally use a straight needle (Fig. 18A). For tumors thin-

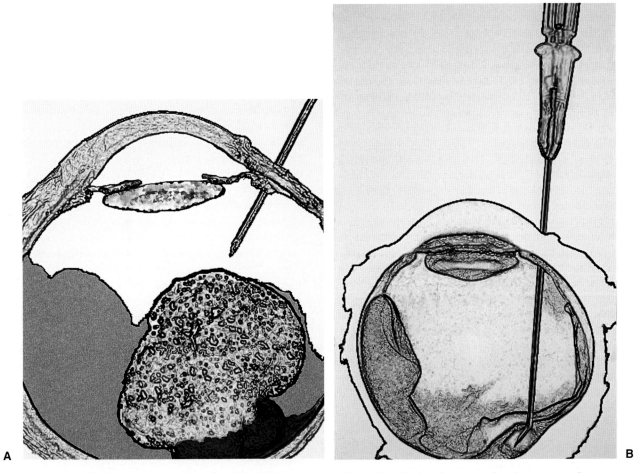

A   B

FIG. 18. Schematic cross-sectional images of eyes containing choroidal melanomas, showing route and needle type. **A:** Straight-needle technique. **B:** Bent-needle technique.

ner than 3 mm, however, I always use a needle that is bent to approximately 30°–60° relative to its shaft at a point about 2–3 mm from the its tip (Fig. 18B).

In my opinion, there are two valid indications for performing a fine-needle aspiration biopsy on a suspected posterior uveal malignant melanoma. The first indication is "major diagnostic uncertainty." By this, I mean that malignant melanoma is the leading diagnosis (that is, the prebiopsy probability that the tumor in question is a genuine malignant melanoma, as estimated by a clinician experienced in the differential diagnosis of intraocular tumors, is greater than 50%) but that a simulating lesion of some type cannot be excluded with an acceptable degree of clinical certainty (that is, the prebiopsy probability of such a simulating lesion is estimated to be substantially greater than 5%). The second indication is "request for pathologic confirmation of the presumed diagnosis by an informed patient prior to consenting to recommended therapy." This latter indication is most applicable when the recommended management is enucleation of the affected eye and the eye is minimally symptomatic and retains good visual acuity.

Most suspected posterior uveal melanomas that are 2 mm or more in thickness can be biopsied successfully. The thinner the tumor, however, the greater is the probability of an insufficient aspirate for cytologic diagnosis. In my experience to date with over 200 clinical fine-needle biopsies of solid intraocular tumors between 1982 and 1995, about 15% have produced an insufficient specimen for cytodiagnosis. However, of the biopsies that obtained a sufficient aspirate, the cytopathologic diagnosis has been shown in cytologic–histopathologic correlation studies to be accurate in over 95% of cases. False-positive results have been extremely rare, and the occasional false-negative results have typically occurred when low-grade melanomas with cohesive cells were biopsied.

Aspirates of suspected posterior uveal malignant melanomas obtained by fine-needle aspiration biopsy can be processed in several ways. Some cytopathologists like to spray the aspirated cells onto a clean glass slide, fix the cells with a cytofixative spray, and stain and examine the slides within minutes after the procedure. Other cytopathologists prefer to suspend the aspirated cells in isotonic saline solution, add a fixative to the suspension, vacuum the fluid containing the suspended fixed cells through a Millipore filter, and stain and examine the filters within 6–12 hours after the procedure. The former technique allows the surgeon to proceed with definitive therapy, if appropriate, immediately after receipt of the pathologic diagnosis, while the eye is still anesthetized. The latter technique requires that the patient be sent home following the biopsy and then informed by telephone of the pathologic diagnosis and its implications for treatment.

Therapy

Once one has identified a choroidal or ciliary body tumor and has concluded that it is likely to be a posterior uveal ma-

lignant melanoma, one must discuss the findings and diagnosis with the patient and advise him or her of the prognostic implications of the tumor for sight in the affected eye and survival. One must also discuss all pertinent available treatment options with the patient and explain their recognized potential benefits versus risks and potential complications.

Factors Influencing Therapeutic Recommendation

A number of factors must be taken into account when arriving at a therapeutic recommendation for a specific patient. These include size and location of the tumor, activity of the tumor (that is, has growth been documented?), associated effects of the tumor on adjacent tissues, vision in the affected eye, vision in the fellow eye, general health and age of the patient, and psychological status of the patient. The recommendation for a 95-year-old patient who has a small juxtapapillary choroidal malignant melanoma nasal to the optic disc in one eye and severe visual loss caused by macular degeneration in the fellow eye is likely to be quite different from the recommendation for a healthy 30-year-old individual who has an asymptomatic medium-sized ciliochoroidal malignant melanoma in one eye and no visual impairment or physical problems in the fellow eye.

Baseline Systemic Medical Evaluation ("Metastatic Search")

Before any intervention is instituted for the ocular tumor, a comprehensive systemic baseline evaluation must be undertaken to search for metastatic uveal malignant melanoma. This evaluation should include at least a general physical examination (looking for hepatomegaly and subcutaneous nodules), blood studies for liver enzyme levels (particularly lactate dehydrogenase and γ-glutamyltranspeptidase), a chest x-ray, and some abdominal imaging study (usually CT, MRI, or ultrasound of the liver). If clinical metastasis is found concurrently with the diagnosis of the posterior uveal tumor, the ophthalmologist should try to be as conservative as possible with regard to the intraocular lesion. Once metastasis has developed, the median survival time in most series has been substantially less than 1 year and is usually in the range of 3–6 months. Various regimens of chemotherapy are known to be "effective" in improving median survival times, but the actual incremental difference in length of survival between treated and untreated patients is at most several months.

After determining that the patient has no detectable metastatic disease, the clinician must discuss management options with the patient. As most ophthalmologists know, currently available management options for patients with a suspected posterior uveal malignant melanoma range from enucleation to no treatment at all. Such a wide spectrum of management options for a single type of tumor usually means that (1) all of the methods are effective, (2) none of the methods is effective, or (3) currently available evidence is confusing. For posterior uveal malignant melanomas, the latter of these three possibilities seems most correct.

Enucleation

I generally advise patients that enucleation or the tumor-containing eye is the standard treatment method for posterior uveal malignant melanomas throughout the world today. Enucleation has certainly been used for the longest period of time, and it has a well-characterized track record. Furthermore, a number of pathologic factors that can only be assessed by histopathologic study of the enucleated eye are important in terms of predicting a patient's survival prognosis. The most important of these histopathologic factors include the cell type of the tumor (as assessed by the modified Callender classification), the measured size of the tumor in the pathology laboratory, and evidence of extrascleral tumor extension. Additional pathologically evaluable prognostic factors include the number of epithelioid cells per high-power field, the number of mitotic figures per high-power field, the number and complexity of vascular networks and loops within the tumor, the cytomorphometric score of the tumor, and the degree of pigmentation within tumor cells.

Although there is a generally held strong belief that enucleation is effective in preventing melanoma-related mortality, there is still considerable controversy about the actual impact of this surgery on the survival of patients with posterior uveal malignant melanoma. In 1978, Zimmerman and colleagues initially pointed out that a plot of the yearly postenucleation death rate of patients with choroidal and ciliary body melanoma had the following shape: there was a very low rate of tumor-related death within the first 6 months, an abrupt rise thereafter to a peak between years 2 and 3, and a slow subsequent decline over the next 10–12 years to reach an asymptotic low level by about postenucleation years 10–12. Zimmerman and colleagues recognized that this particular yearly death rate curve could be converted to a normalized, "Gaussian," bell shape by replotting length of survival on a logarithmic time scale rather than on a linear one. This curve is known as a lognormal yearly mortality curve. Zimmerman and colleagues inferred from the lognormal distribution of deaths that a biologic phenomenon acting at or near the time of enucleation is responsible for the observed mortality pattern. They hypothesized that this factor may be the dissemination of tumor cells at the time of enucleation. This hypothesis has come to be known as the Zimmerman–McLean hypothesis. Currently, this hypothesis remains controversial, but it has not been disproved.

In spite of concerns about the potential adverse effects of enucleation, there are still circumstances in which enucleation is almost certainly warranted. These include a blind, painful eye due to tumor (Fig. 19), a tumor too large to be managed by any other method, and a circumpapillary melanoma causing marked visual loss.

Enhanced Enucleation

Because of the concern about the potential adverse effects of enucleation suggested by Zimmerman and colleagues, a number of clinicians have recommended modifications of the standard enucleation procedure. One of these modifications is the so-called "no touch" enucleation technique. In this technique, the surgeon uses a specially designed cryoring to freeze the surface of the globe at the site of the posterior uveal tumor. Some type of insulating material must be placed between the cryoprobe and adjacent orbital soft tissues to avoid incorporating those tissues in the ice ball. Once the tumor appears completely frozen, the surgeon elevates the globe by using the cryoapparatus and then cuts the optic nerve. Unfortunately, this technique can only be applied in practice to tumors that would probably not have to be managed by enucleation. If the tumor is circumpapillary, no cryoprobe can cover it completely. If the tumor is very large, getting both the insulating material and the cryoprobe into place almost certainly requires more manipulation than does conventional enucleation. Other modifications of the enucleation procedure intended to avoid tumor dissemination at the time of enucleation include a *manometric procedure* (use of a manometric system for normalizing the intraocular pressure throughout the enucleation) and an *injection procedure* (injection of an expansile gas or a noncompressible liquid that elevates the intraocular pressure abruptly and collapses all the choroidal veins). The postulated benefits of these modified enucleation methods have never been confirmed by comparative clinical survival data.

Pre-enucleation Radiation Therapy

An alternative method of enucleation in which the surgery is coupled with supplemental treatment is the use of preop-

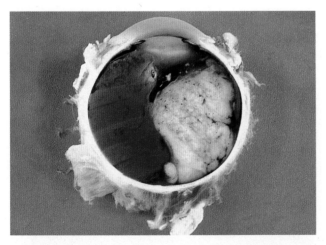

FIG. 19. Large, relatively amelanotic choroidal melanoma with massive hemorrhagic retinal detachment in an enucleated globe; this eye was removed because it was blind and painful.

erative oculo-orbital external beam radiation therapy. The most commonly employed method of pre-enucleation ocular irradiation employs conventional external beam radiation therapy delivered by means of a linear accelerator. The total dose of radiation delivered to the eye and orbit is 20 Gy in fractional doses of 4 Gy each over an elapsed duration of 5–8 days. Unfortunately for the proponents of this technique, preliminary comparative survival studies of patients managed by simple enucleation versus enucleation with presurgical ocular radiotherapy have shown no appreciable beneficial effect of this treatment on survival.

Periodic Monitoring Without Intervention ("Observation as Management")

The most conservative alternative to enucleation is periodic monitoring of the tumor without intervention unless a predetermined threshhold is reached (Fig. 20). Observation as management seems appropriate for patients with a very small tumor that might be either a benign nevus or a small malignant melanoma and also for elderly or systemically ill patients with a definite malignant melanoma that is growing slowly. Current evidence suggests that a judicious interval of periodic observation until convincing tumor growth is documented does not substantially worsen the survival of patients compared with that of promptly treated patients. Unfortunately, most of what we know about the impact of observation comes from patients with relatively small or dormant-appearing tumors that are probably not representative of the entire spectrum of patients with posterior uveal malignant melanomas.

A number of clinically determinable features of small melanocytic choroidal tumors have been found to be prognostic of tumor enlargement. These factors include tumor size (the larger the tumor, the more likely the lesion is to enlarge) and the presence of prominent clumps of orange (lipofuscin) pigment on the tumor, serous subretinal fluid associated with the tumor, and abruptly occurring visual symptoms related to the tumor. In contrast, the presence of prominent drusen on the surface of the lesion and prominent clumps of retinal pigment epithelial pigment on the surface of the tumor are predictive of lesion dormancy. If one decides to monitor a patient with a melanocytic choroidal tumor, one should make the determination about how soon to reevaluate the lesion and how frequently to repeat the examinations over time based on the number of worrisome features of the tumor at the time of initial examination.

Of course, documentation of lesion enlargement is not sufficient to ensure that a presumably melanocytic posterior uveal tumor is a malignant melanoma. Benign nevi have frequently been documented to enlarge. The clinician must take into account not only whether the lesion enlarges but also how much it enlarges and how long it takes to do so. Certainly, the more a tumor grows over a relatively short time, the greater the concern should be about that lesion's malignant potential.

Photocoagulation and Laser Therapy

Photocoagulation is a treatment option that is applicable to the occasional patient with a thin choroidal melanoma (thickness usually 3 mm or less) in an eye with clear optical media (Fig. 21). Conventional photocoagulation consists of a series of treatment sessions in which intense, overlapping, light-induced burns are produced in and around the tumor to disrupt the tumor cells and occlude its choroidal vascular supply. Either a xenon arc photocoagulator or a laser (argon green, krypton red, or dye laser) can be used as the source of the light flashes. The margins of the tumor are usually treated at the initial session, and the more central portions of the tumor are then treated during subsequent sessions. Treatment should be continued until there is no tumor residue detectable by ophthalmoscopy and ultrasonography.

In recent years, I have modified my method of photocoag-

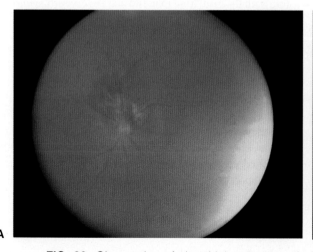
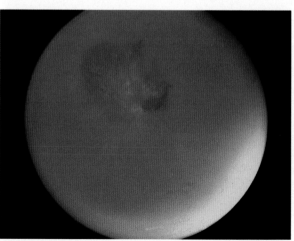

A **B**

FIG. 20. Observation of choroidal melanoma. **A:** The initial appearance of superior juxtapapillary choroidal melanoma. **B:** The same lesion 18 months later, with enlargement in all basal directions.

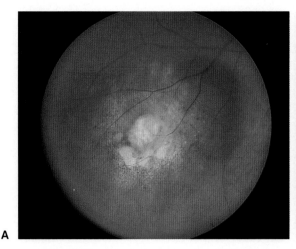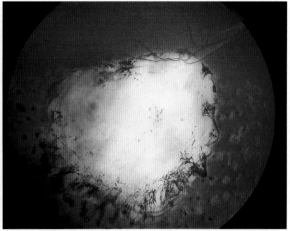

A   B

FIG. 21. Photocoagulation of choroidal melanoma. **A:** Small choroidal melanoma prior to treatment; the melanotic portion of the tumor had been documented to be growing. **B:** The same lesion 6 years following photocoagulation. The atrophic scar corresponds to the treated tumor. Scattered photocoagulation burns are evident peripheral to the treated lesion.

ulation considerably. Instead of using a xenon arc photocoagulator or a slit-lamp laser and generating intense burns with high power settings and brief exposures (that is, less than 0.5 second), I now use an indirect ophthalmoscope laser (usually argon green, occasionally diode) almost exclusively and employ relatively low power settings (typically 200–400 mW) of long duration (several seconds) in the continuous wave mode. I do not try to whiten the retina instantaneously but rather create a slowly developing, confluent, gray–white burn over the course of 3–10 seconds. At the initial session, I still direct my treatment to the margin of the tumor rather than to the central region of the mass. I try to create a confluent gray–white burn about 2–3 spot diameters wide completely around the base of the tumor. The intensity of the marginal burn is intended to be sufficient to block all choroidal blood vessels. I usually wait 2–4 weeks and then proceed with a second session, reinforcing the basal marginal treatment initially and then proceeding with encroachment onto the peripheral aspect of the tumor. At a third session, another 4–6 weeks later, I again treat the basal marginal zone and tumor periphery and then treat the central portion of the tumor directly. I then determine whether to use any additional laser therapy based on the response of the tumor to this treatment. If treatment is successful, one ends up with an intensely white, flat chorioretinal scar corresponding to the original tumor site (Fig. 21).

Problems with photocoagulation include creation of an absolute scotoma corresponding to the area of treatment, preretinal fibrosis with retinal wrinkling, chorioretinal or choroidovitreal neovascularization with preretinal or intravitreal hemorrhage, and complicated retinal detachment. Moreover, some tumors that initially appear to have been treated effectively eventually continue to grow and must then be managed by additional photocoagulation or an alternative method. The most bothersome aspect of photocoagulation is that there is no currently available evidence telling us how effective it is in terms of patient survival relative to enucleation or any other method of therapy.

Radiation Therapy

Two methods of focal irradiation are currently in use as treatment for posterior uveal malignant melanomas. The most commonly used method of radiotherapy is *episcleral radioactive plaque therapy.* In this method, one uses a radioactive device (plaque) that is secured with sutures to the sclera directly exterior to the choroidal or ciliary body tumor. Plaques of various radioisotopes, including cobalt 60, ruthenium 106, iridium 192, and iodine 125, have been used in this country and abroad during the past 25 years. At this time, iodine-125 shielded plaques are the most commonly used plaques in the United States. Plaque placement entails accurate localization of the tumor margin by a combination of ocular transillumination and indirect ophthalmoscopy, followed by securing of the radioactive device to the sclera immediately over the marked zone. The plaque is generally left in place until an apical dose of approximately 80–100 Gy has been delivered, usually over a duration of approximately 4–7 days. Because of the dose distributions inherent in plaque radiation therapy, the base of the tumor always receives a substantially greater dose than does the tumor apex. In the United States, most radiation oncologists dealing with plaque therapy attempt to limit the basal dose to approximately 450 Gy. In contrast, some of our European colleagues using ruthenium-106 applicators frequently treat the sclera to a dose of more than 900 to 1,000 Gy.

The second method of radiotherapy for posterior uveal melanomas is *charged particle beam irradiation.* This method employs a cyclotron capable of generating a beam of collimated protons or helium ions that can be directed into the eye and at the entire tumor. The treatment requires pre-

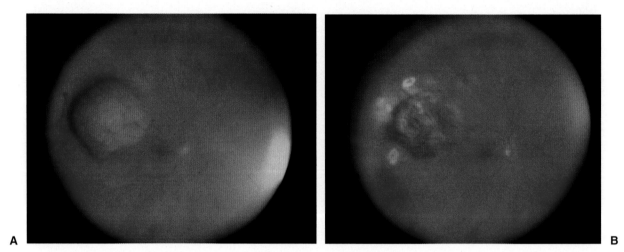

FIG. 22. Episcleral plaque radiation therapy of choroidal melanoma. **A:** Pretreatment appearance of choroidal melanoma. **B:** Regressed tumor 18 months following plaque therapy.

liminary localization of the margins of the tumor and marking of those margins with inert, radiopaque tantalum rings. The treatment is generally given in five outpatient sessions over a 5- to 7-day interval. In this method of treatment, the tumor receives a uniform dose of radiation that is delivered at a high dose rate.

Some, but certainly not all, choroidal and ciliary body melanomas exhibit pronounced clinical tumor regression following plaque radiotherapy or charged particle beam irradiation (Fig. 22). The "average" posterior uveal melanoma in my experience shrinks to about 30%–50% of its initial thickness but changes little if at all in basal dimensions following treatment. In occasional cases, a melanoma that extends to the fovea prior to treatment even regresses with basal retraction away from the foveola; such a regression pattern is sometimes associated with a remarkable although often temporary recovery of vision. Absorption of subretinal fluid that

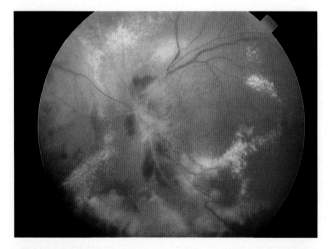

FIG. 23. Radiation retinopathy and papillopathy 3 years following episcleral plaque therapy of nasal juxtapapillary choroidal melanoma.

is present at the time of treatment commonly occurs within several months after plaque treatment, and the resultant retinal reattachment is frequently accompanied by visual improvement in the treated eye.

Unfortunately, a large proportion of patients treated by plaque radiotherapy or charged particle beam irradiation eventually develop radiation retinopathy, radiation optic papillopathy, or even radiation-induced ocular ischemia (Fig. 23). This latter problem can, in turn, lead to neovascularization of the iris and neovascular glaucoma, which may result in a blind painful eye that requires enucleation. Radiation cataract also occurs in a substantial proportion of patients, particularly those with a very large tumor, a ciliary body tumor, or both; however, cataract extraction can be performed and can result in a favorable visual outcome in such cases, provided that the optic disc and macula are healthy.

As nice as it is to see rapid, complete local tumor regression following tumor irradiation, it has been shown that a rapid, pronounced local tumor response is actually an unfavorable prognostic indicator of the patient's chance for long-term, melanoma-free survival. Several studies performed in the past decade have shown that patients who show rapid, complete local tumor regression following tumor irradiation are more likely to develop and die of metastatic disease than are patients with relatively slow and less complete local tumor shrinkage.

Unlike the experience with observation, photocoagulation, and laser therapy, there is a considerable amount of comparative survival data on enucleated versus irradiated patients with posterior uveal melanoma. All currently published, nonrandomized comparative survival studies of irradiated versus enucleated patients that excluded patients who would not have been candidates for radiation therapy and included multivariate statistical adjustment for recognized intergroup differences in baseline clinical prognostic covariables have shown similar 5- to 10-year rates of melanoma metastasis, melanoma-specific mortality, and all-cause mortality. Subgroup analyses based on patients with equivalent baseline prognostic indices have also shown no significant survival advantage of enucleation over plaque radiotherapy.

There are a number of theoretical advantages of charged particle beam irradiation over plaque radiotherapy in terms of uveal melanoma management. These advantages include homogeneity of dose, limitation of undesired radiation to normal tissues adjacent to the basal margins of the tumor, high dose rate, dose fractionation, and higher radiation biologic effectiveness of charged particles relative to photons. The only currently available clinical information that pertains to the actual relative effectiveness of charged particle beam therapy and plaque therapy, however, comes from the University of California–San Francisco, where a prospective study of helium ion beam therapy versus iodine-125 plaque therapy has been performed. That study identified some intergroup differences between the plaque and charged particle beam-irradiated patients in terms of the frequencies of specific complications, such as neovascular glaucoma and radiation retinopathy; however, the total vision loss rates of the two groups were quite similar. In addition, the two treatments were similarly effective in terms of local tumor control *except* for juxtapapillary tumors; for tumors of in this specific location, charged particle beam irradiation was substantially more effective than plaque therapy. In spite of this difference, melanoma-specific mortality rates in the two groups were essentially equivalent.

Microsurgical Resection

Microsurgical tumor resection with preservation of the eye is a therapeutic option that can be considered, in my opinion, for relatively healthy, reasonably young patients with a rather sizable choroidal or ciliary body melanoma that tends to be quite thick relative to its basal diameter. Three different approaches have been employed. The first technique to be used with even limited regularity in a few centers was *eye-wall resection*. In this technique, full-thickness sclera, the tumor along with a marginal zone of uninvolved choroid, ciliary body, or both around the lesion, and the underlying retina are excised as a single piece. The defect is then closed with a button of donor sclera. If possible, laser therapy, cryotherapy, or both are performed around the margins of the tumor prior to surgery to create a strong chorioretinal adhesion and reduce the blood supply to the area. Preexistent retinal detachment is generally considered to be a contraindication to such a procedure.

More recently, a number of individuals have used *lamellar scleral resection*. In this method, originally developed by Foulds and colleagues in Scotland, a deep lamellar scleral flap is created overlying the entire tumor and extending several millimeters beyond the detectable margins of the lesion. Once the flap has been raised, the inner lamellar scleral fibers and uvea around the tumor are incised, and the entire tumor with the adherent inner scleral lamellae and a marginal rim of normal uvea is removed, leaving the underlying retina intact (if possible). The procedure is performed with the patient under hypotensive general anesthesia. At the conclusion of the procedure, the lamellar scleral flap is repositioned and sutured securely. If necessary, a pars plana vitrectomy can be done to facilitate tumor removal and remove intravitreal blood that sometimes accumulates during the procedure. If the tumor is removed completely without tearing or substantially cutting the underlying retina, the retina will go back into place normally in spite of the defect in the retinal pigment epithelium (Fig. 24).

An uncommon technique for excision of posterior uveal melanomas is *endoresection*. In this procedure, the surgeon performs a complete vitrectomy and then makes a retinotomy that is flipped over to expose the tumor. The tumor is removed piecemeal by using specially designed vitrectomy instruments, and intense endolaser therapy is performed to the sclera corresponding to the base of the lesion to obliter-

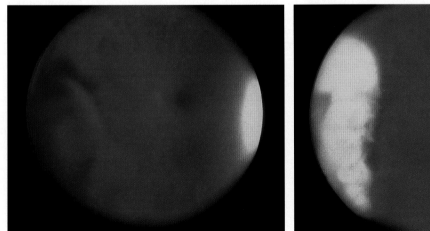
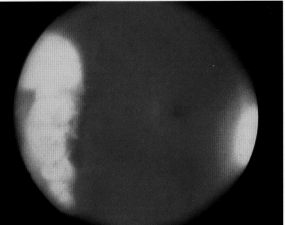

FIG. 24. Microsurgical resection of ciliochoroidal melanoma. **A:** The appearance of ciliochoroidal tumor before surgery. **B:** The same eye 5 years after resection; the retina is still fully attached.

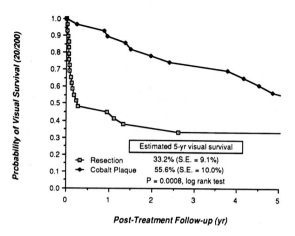

FIG. 25. Comparative visual preservation rates after microsurgical tumor resection versus cobalt-60 plaque radiation therapy (30 matched patients in each group).

ate any residual tumor cells and provide hemostasis. The retina is then repositioned, and the vitreous cavity is filled with silicone oil to prevent postoperative retinal detachment.

Some eyes that tolerate microsurgical tumor excision by eye-wall resection or lamellar resection retain or regain excellent visual acuity (several patients in my own personal experience have 20/40 visual acuity or better). On the other hand, over half of the eyes subjected to such surgery, especially for a relatively large tumor, develop posttreatment proliferative vitreoretinopathy leading to total retinal detachment or phthisis bulbi. Approximately one-fourth of eyes undergoing resection eventually come to enucleation because of surgical complications or concern about residual or recurrent tumor. If one compares posttreatment "visual survival curves" of eyes managed by tumor resection versus plaque radiotherapy (Fig. 25), one notes that there is a much more rapid drop-off in the eyes managed by resection but a flattening of the visual survival curve for such eyes after the first year. In contrast, there is a slow decrement in the visual survival curve of the plaqued patients, which appears to cross the visual survival curve of the resected patients by about posttreatment years 7–10. I infer from this relative visual survival graph that elderly patients, those with relatively poor general health, and others for whom it seems appropriate to maximize length of visual survival at the possible expense of a lower ultimate probability of visual survival are more appropriately managed by plaque radiation therapy. In contrast, patients who are relatively young and others for whom it seems appropriate to maximize the long-term probability of visual preservation at the possible expense of a substantially higher probability of early severe visual loss are probably more appropriately managed by tumor resection.

Chemotherapy

At present, no chemotherapy regimen has been shown to have consistently favorable effects on metastatic uveal ma-

lignant melanoma. The most commonly employed conventional chemotherapy regimen at present (the "Finnish regimen") improves duration of survival only marginally in most patients. In patients with localized hematic metastasis, local arterial infusion chemotherapy has been used with limited success. No chemotherapy has ever been shown to be effective against intraocular posterior uveal malignant melanomas.

Immunotherapy

Although there is great interest in immunotherapeutic methods to treat various human malignancies, no such regimen has yet proven effective against human uveal malignant melanoma. In a randomized clinical trial of patients managed by enucleation, nonspecific immunostimulation with methanol extracted residue of bacillus Calmette–Guérin did not improve survival.

Photodynamic Therapy

Photodynamic therapy refers to administration of a photosensitizing agent followed by low-power laser exposures of wavelengths that stimulate the agent and produce intralesional heating and free radicals. Several different photosensitizers have been developed, but few patients have been treated by these various agents to date.

Hyperthermia

Hyperthermia refers to treatment of a tumor to a sustained intralesional temperature of approximately 42°–46°C for 10 minutes or longer. This form of therapy has been proven to be effective in experimental animal models of uveal melanoma, but it has not been used widely enough to date in humans with primary posterior uveal malignant melanoma to evaluate its effectiveness. Four different methods of elevating the intralesional temperature have been developed. *Ultrasonic hyperthermia* employs focused ultrasound beams to heat the tumor. *Microwave hyperthermia* and *ferromagnetic hyperthermia* both use a plaquelike device that becomes a heat source when it is exposed to an appropriate electromagnetic field. Finally, *transpupillary infrared laser hyperthermia* employs a specially modified diode laser beam at low power settings but long exposure times (typically 10–20 minutes) to heat the tumor. All of these methods are limited by the inability to measure temperature levels directly within intraocular tumors.

Combination Therapies

To increase the potential for local tumor destruction and simultaneously minimize the risk of complications related to individual methods of treatment, a few clinicians have developed therapeutic strategies that employ two treatment methods simultaneously. The most frequently employed combination therapy for posterior uveal melanomas is *thermoradiotherapy*. In this therapy, the tumor receives both focal tumor irradiation and hyperthermia simultaneously by means of a radioactive plaque that also serves as a microwave or ferromagnetic hyperthermia source.

Planned Sequential Therapies

For selected tumors, some clinicians have also developed therapeutic strategies that call for two distinct treatment methods to be used sequentially. The most commonly employed method of this type is planned sequential plaque radiotherapy and tumor laser therapy. This method is most likely to be used for tumors that extend to the optic disc margin or involve the macula, for which either plaque therapy or laser therapy alone is not particularly effective.

Prognosis

A patient's prognosis for survival following detection and treatment of a primary posterior uveal malignant melanoma is a function of many factors, including absence versus presence and extent of metastatic disease at the time of intraocular tumor detection, age at the time of treatment, size of the intraocular tumor, absence versus presence and extent of extrascleral tumor extension, absence versus presence of ciliary body involvement, and many pathologic features of the tumor (which will not be determinable unless the tumor is treated by enucleation of the eye or en bloc tumor resection). At present, there is no compelling scientific evidence that any form of locally effective treatment is substantially better than another in terms of prevention of metastatic disease or prolongation of survival.

CHOROIDAL NEVUS

The choroidal nevus is a benign neoplasm arising from uveal melanocytes in the choroid. It is unquestionably the

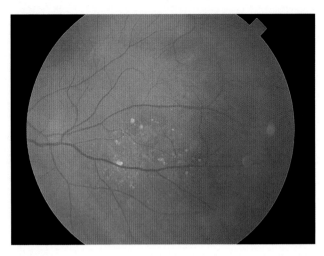

FIG. 27. Large but relatively ill-defined choroidal nevus with overlying drusen.

most common primary intraocular tumor. It has been estimated that upward of 10% of persons over the age of 50 have at least one choroidal nevus in one eye. Some posterior uveal nevi may be predisposed to undergo malignant change, but only about 1 in 4,000 posterior uveal nevi actually does so.

Ophthalmoscopic Appearance of Tumor

The typical posterior uveal nevus appears as a thin, gray to dark-brown lesion (Fig. 26) with indistinct margins that blend into the surrounding choroid. It is usually less than 5 mm in diameter and less than 1 mm thick, but occasional lesions of this type achieve a size greater than 7 mm in diameter and 2 mm thick. Drusen and retinal pigment epithelial pigment clumps are commonly present on the surface of nevi (Fig. 27). Occasional choroidal nevi have a "halo" appearance (Fig. 28) characterized by relatively typical brown to gray coloration centrally but yellow–orange coloration peripherally. By slit-lamp biomicroscopy, one can usually distinguish this intrinsic yellow–orange pigmentation of the lesion from the surface lipofuscin deposits that are common

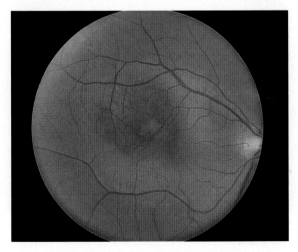

FIG. 26. Macular choroidal nevus.

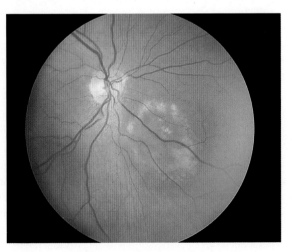

FIG. 28. "Halo" choroidal nevus.

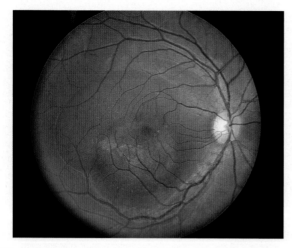

FIG. 29. Macular choroidal nevus with an overlying and surrounding blister of clear subretinal fluid. The lesion has not enlarged over 9 years of follow-up. Subretinal fluid reabsorbed spontaneously and has not recurred.

over melanomas. Although subretinal fluid associated with choroidal nevi is uncommon, it is important to be aware that some choroidal nevi are associated with accumulations of subretinal fluid over and around the lesion (Fig. 29). A fluid accumulation of this type is particularly common in association with macular choroidal nevi. The precise reason for the development of the fluid is not known.

Ancillary Diagnostic Tests

Fluorescein angiography of a choroidal nevus typically shows it to be hypofluorescent throughout the study, except for the overlying drusen that often will stain in the late frames. In eyes with subretinal fluid associated with the lesion, fluorescein angiography frequently reveals punctate sites of fluorescein leakage on the surface of the lesion as the probable source of the fluid. *Indocyanine green angiography* also shows most choroidal nevi to be hypofluorescent throughout the study.

B-scan ultrasonography of a typical choroidal nevus confirms the limited thickness of the lesion (in most cases, 1 mm or less) and shows relative internal sonolucency of the thin lesion but reveals no scleral invasion or transcleral extension. *Standardized A-scan* is rarely helpful because of the limited thickness of the lesion.

Natural History

Although most choroidal nevi appear to change minimally if at all over many years, some choroidal nevi enlarge unequivocally during follow-up. Minimal lesion enlargement that can be detected only after many years of follow-up is not nearly as worrisome, of course, as is pronounced lesion enlargement that occurs within just a few months. Subretinal fluid that develops in association with a choroidal nevus fre-

quently disappears spontaneously, so no laser therapy or other treatment to the leaking site or sites revealed by fluorescein angiography is generally advised unless the visual acuity is markedly impaired or the fluid does not resolve within 2–3 months.

Melanocytoma of Optic Disc

An important clinical variety of choroidal nevus that is occasionally seen in ophthalmic practice is the melanocytoma of the optic disc (Fig. 30). This lesion is really no more than a juxtapapillary choroidal nevus with intrapapillary extension. The typical lesion appears dark brown to almost black. The tumor can involve just a small portion of the disc or virtually the entire area of the optic nerve head. There is often an associated, relatively flat, juxtapapillary, typical choroidal nevus component. In some cases, the disc is highly elevated and the margins of the disc are blurred. Prominent visual field defects corresponding to the melanocytoma are occasionally encountered. If observed, such lesions tend to grow very slowly, if at all, during long periods of observation.

Management

Observation is the recommended management for all typical choroidal nevi. Atypical nevi (that is, lesions that one believes are benign nevi but are larger than typical nevi or have other worrisome features such as associated subretinal fluid or orange pigment clumps) must be documented and observed on a regular periodic basis to be certain that they are not actually small malignant melanomas. If a presumed nevus is extremely worrisome, fine-needle aspiration biopsy can be considered to establish the diagnosis pathologically and thereby guide subsequent patient management.

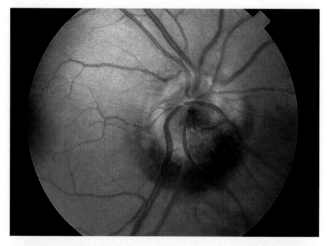

FIG. 30. Melanocytoma of the optic disc in a 42-year-old Hispanic woman.

METASTATIC CARCINOMA

Metastatic carcinoma to the posterior uvea is a malignant neoplasm of nonocular primary source that has involved the choroid or ciliary body via hematogenous dissemination and is now growing in that implantation site. It has been estimated to be the most common malignant intraocular tumor (at least in an autopsy population), although it is relatively uncommon as a clinical entity requiring treatment. It is undoubtedly the most important lesion in the differential diagnosis of a clinically hypomelanotic or amelanotic choroidal melanoma. The great majority of women and a smaller majority of men with such a lesion have a well-documented prior history of systemic cancer. However, a substantial proportion of patients, particularly men, have no prior history of cancer at the time of detection of a metastatic choroidal lesion; furthermore, approximately 15% of men presenting with a metastasis in this particular context never have an identified primary site, even though most of these patients eventually die of widespread disseminated metastasis.

Ophthalmoscopic Appearance of Tumor

The typical unifocal metastatic carcinoma to the choroid is a yellow to white choroidal mass (Fig. 31A). The usual lesion tends to be relatively flat compared with its basal dimensions. Occasional metastatic tumors are more nodular, however, having a shape similar to that of most choroidal melanomas. The retinal vasculature overlying a choroidal metastasis is usually normal. However, retinal detachment out of proportion to the size of the lesion is a characteristic feature of metastatic carcinomas. Although limited hemorrhage on the surface of the tumor or at its margins is observed occasionally in eyes containing a metastatic carcinoma, massive subretinal bleeding and intravitreal bleeding are distinctly uncommon. Bilateral, multifocal choroidal metastatic lesions are present in the eyes of about 20% of affected individuals (Fig. 32). This means, though, that about 80% of affected persons have only a single tumor in one eye. In a classic case with multifocal bilateral amelanotic choroidal lesions occurring in the context of a patient with

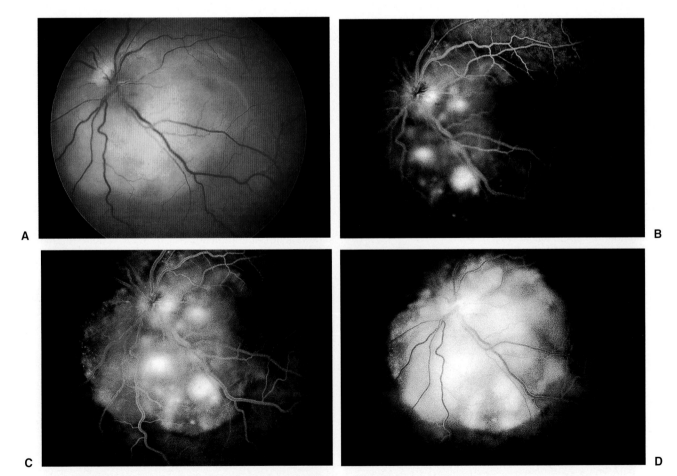

FIG. 31. Metastatic breast carcinoma to the choroid in a 53-year-old woman. **A:** Turbid subretinal fluid overlies the choroidal mass. **B:** Laminar venous phase frame showing multiple hyperfluorescent leak sites on the surface of the generally hypofluorescent tumor. **C:** Late venous phase frame showing expansion of leak sites and staining of the surface of the lesion. **D:** Late phase frame showing intense subretinal hyperfluorescence corresponding to the lesion.

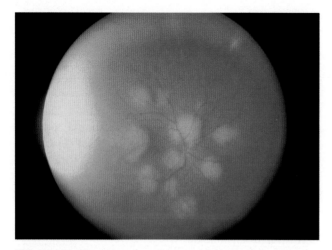

FIG. 32. Multifocal amelanotic choroidal lesions in a 59-year-old man with metastatic undifferentiated carcinoma of the lung.

known systemic cancer, the diagnosis usually poses no problem. However, in the more common unifocal unilateral presentation of metastatic carcinoma to the choroid, the differential diagnosis between amelanotic melanoma and unifocal metastatic carcinoma may be quite difficult.

Ancillary Diagnostic Tests

B-scan ultrasonography of a typical metastatic carcinoma shows the lesion to be relatively thin in relation to its basal diameters (Fig. 33A). Ultrasound almost never reveals anything resembling a mushroom shape with a metastatic carcinoma. Unlike a typical melanoma, a metastatic carcinoma characteristically appears almost as bright on B-scan as the orbital fat. On *standardized A-scan*, the typical metastatic carcinoma exhibits high-amplitude internal reflectivity throughout the entire lesion (Fig. 33B).

Fluorescence angiography is of limited value in the diagnosis of a metastatic carcinoma. On *fluorescein angiography* (Fig. 31), the typical lesion appears relatively hypofluorescent in the early frames, somewhat mottled with hypofluorescent and hyperfluorescent foci in the intermediate frames, and diffusely hyperfluorescent on the entire surface of the lesion with leakage of fluorescein into the overlying and surrounding subretinal space in the late frames. On *indocyanine green angiography*, a metastatic carcinoma to the choroid usually appears hypofluorescent and larger than its ophthalmoscopically estimated size in the early frames and diffusely hyperfluorescent in the late frames.

If a metastatic carcinoma is suspected, it is imperative that the patient undergoes a comprehensive metastatic evaluation prior to the initiation of ocular therapy. This evaluation should, at a minimum, include a comprehensive physical examination and diagnostic imaging studies (such as a chest x-ray, mammography, CT, MRI, and other studies as indicated), as well as a biopsy of accessible lesions. The patient's ultimate prognosis is more dependent on what is found on the systemic evaluation than on the extent of the tumor or tumors in the eye.

If the systemic evaluation fails to reveal any evidence of a primary cancer or other metastatic foci and yet metastatic carcinoma is still strongly suspected on the basis of physical examination findings and ancillary ophthalmic test results, one should probably consider the option of transvitreal or transscleral fine-needle aspiration biopsy. This technique was described in detail in the earlier section on choroidal malignant melanoma.

Treatment

Once one has established the diagnosis of metastatic carcinoma to the choroid, one must proceed with arrangements for management of the ocular lesion. Factors influencing the therapeutic recommendation in such patients include the

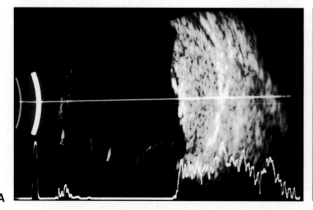
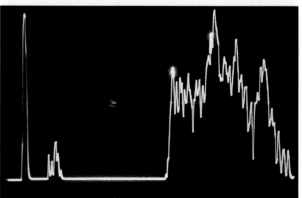

FIG. 33. Ultrasonography of breast carcinoma metastatic to the choroid. **A:** B-scan display shows a relatively bright (sonoreflective) matlike zone of choroidal thickening corresponding to the metastatic lesion. The retina is shallowly detached over the tumor and more bullously detached inferiorly. **B:** A-scan corresponding to the same lesion, showing high-amplitude internal reflectivity through the entire lesion.

clinicopathologic nature of the primary tumor; the usual responsiveness of such tumors to irradiation, chemotherapy, and hormonal therapy; the size of the tumor or tumors; the intraocular locations of the tumors; the laterality, number, and activity of the intraocular tumors; the presence and severity of associated ocular abnormalities; the visual status of the affected eye or eyes; and the general health and psychological status of the patient. If the tumor involves the macular region or the optic disc or is causing an extensive retinal detachment that is reducing visual acuity, *external beam radiation therapy* is generally recommended. In most patients, the target dose of radiation is in the range of 40–50 Gy in divided fractions over about 4 weeks. If the anterior segment is not involved, the radiation therapist can design treatment portals that will minimize exposure to the cornea and lens. In patients with tumors in an extramacular location not involving the optic disc and not associated with an extensive retinal detachment causing visual impairment, one may elect to initiate *chemotherapy* or *hormonal therapy*, assuming that such treatments are appropriate for the patient's systemic disease. In such a patient, one needs to monitor the tumor for regression or progression before concluding that the drug therapy is sufficient or advising supplemental external beam radiation therapy (Fig. 34). In a substantial portion of patients, both chemotherapy–hormonal therapy and ocular irradiation are required. In occasional patients with an isolated metastasis to the posterior uvea, one can use *episcleral plaque radiation therapy*. The actual procedure is the same as with choroidal melanoma treatment. The only difference is that the target dose is usually reduced to 40–50 Gy to the tumor's apex. Patients for whom this treatment is applicable should have limited or no other evidence of metastasis and no active residual primary neoplasm. Occasional patients with metastatic carcinoma to the posterior uvea present with a blind painful eye and associated retinal detach-

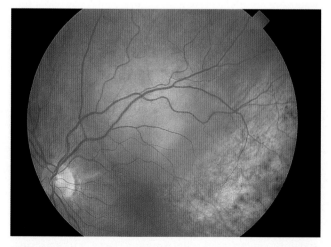

FIG. 34. Regressed macular lesion of breast carcinoma following external beam radiation therapy, but there is new tumor formation above the macula while on tamoxifen therapy 21 months after ocular irradiation.

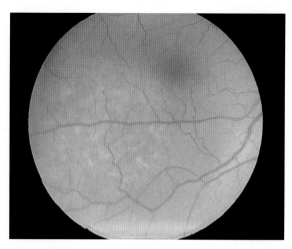

FIG. 35. Circumscribed choroidal hemangioma inferotemporal to the fovea in the right eye.

ment as a consequence of the tumor. In such patients, the only applicable method of management is usually *enucleation*.

Prognosis

The survival prognosis of patients with metastatic carcinoma to the choroid is generally poor. The median survival time for patients with metastatic cutaneous malignant melanoma to the choroid is only about 3 months, that for patients with metastatic lung cancer to the choroid is about 6 months, and that for patients with metastatic breast carcinoma to the choroid is approximately 1 year.

CIRCUMSCRIBED CHOROIDAL HEMANGIOMA

Circumscribed choroidal hemangioma is a benign neoplasm composed of large-caliber vascular channels lined by mature endothelial cells. It is probably congenital in most if not all cases, but many lesions of this type are not detected prior to middle age. There is no recognized racial or sex predilection for such tumors.

Ophthalmoscopic Appearance of Tumor

The typical circumscribed choroidal hemangioma is a poorly defined red–orange lesion located near the optic disc or macula (Fig. 35). Most lesions of this type are less than 7 mm in basal diameter and less than 3 mm thick, but larger ones are encountered occasionally (Fig. 36). If the fundus is examined by direct ophthalmoscopy, the lesion is frequently so indistinct that it is completely overlooked. It is much easier (although still often quite difficult) to detect lesions of this type by indirect ophthalmoscopy. Virtually all circumscribed choroidal hemangiomas are located posterior to the ocular equator, and most of them are located within 2 disc di-

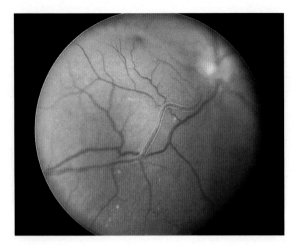

FIG. 36. Large circumscribed choroidal hemangioma involving the macula and the juxtapapillary choroid.

ameters from the optic disc margin, the foveola, or both. Many lesions of this type underlie the fovea and cause visual impairment on the basis of either chronic or recurrent serous subretinal fluid, cystic degeneration of the overlying retina, or both.

Ancillary Diagnostic Tests

Fluorescence angiography can be of great help in confirming the diagnosis of circumscribed choroidal hemangioma. On *fluorescein angiography*, the typical lesion shows very intense early hyperfluorescence of large-caliber intralesional vessels during the prearterial and arterial phase frames of the study (Fig. 37). Within just a second or two, the entire lesion becomes brightly hyperfluorescent, and it stays hyperfluorescent with gradual leakage of fluorescein into the overlying retina and subretinal space by the late frames. *In-*

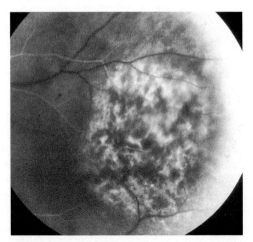

FIG. 37. Fluorescein angiogram of circumscribed choroidal hemangioma. Retinal arterial phase frame shows intense hyperfluorescence of multiple large-caliber vascular channels comprising the choroidal tumor.

docyanine green angiography also shows rapid filling of large-caliber intralesional blood vessels, followed by intense hyperfluorescence of the entire lesion within a few seconds; however, most circumscribed choroidal hemangiomas become generally hypofluorescent ("washed out") by the late phase frames.

Ultrasonography is also helpful in confirming the diagnosis of a circumscribed choroidal hemangioma. On *B-scan ultrasonography* (Fig. 38A), the typical lesion appears intensely sonoreflective (bright) and therefore difficult to distinguish from the adjacent sclera and orbital fat. On *A-scan ultrasonography* (Fig. 38B), the lesion exhibits very high-amplitude, broad-based intratumoral echo spikes.

Natural History

Although the size of most circumscribed choroidal hemangiomas remains clinically unchanged over many years of follow-up, some lesions of this type enlarge substantially over several years. Furthermore, the retinal pigment epithelium overlying a choroidal hemangioma sometimes undergoes pronounced fibrous metaplasia and occasionally becomes diffusely calcified. Some eyes containing a large circumscribed choroidal hemangioma develop a bullous exudative retinal detachment and progress to intractable secondary angle closure glaucoma.

Treatment

Because circumscribed choroidal hemangiomas are benign lesions, treatment is indicated only in an effort to restore or prevent progression of visual loss related to secondary retinal detachment and cystic retinal degeneration caused by the tumor. In most cases, I recommend *scatter laser photocoagulation* to the entire surface of the tumor (Fig. 39), generally using an argon green laser. This form of treatment usually leads to reabsorption of the subretinal fluid within a few weeks. Unfortunately, the fluid frequently reaccumulates within a few months. Additional treatment is usually required in such cases. If photocoagulation fails to produce retinal reattachment or if the retinal detachment becomes bullous, then I advise low-dose fractionated *external beam radiation therapy* to the affected eye. Treatment with as little as 1,200–1,500 cGy in 5–7 fractions over the course of 1–1.5 weeks is almost uniformly followed by slow reabsorption of the subretinal fluid over 3–6 months and partial flattening of the hemangioma. In most cases, the subretinal fluid does not reaccumulate following such treatment. With the exception of an occasional radiation-induced cataract, no significant long-term complications of such low-dose ocular radiation therapy have been encountered. Unfortunately, some eyes containing a large circumscribed choroidal hemangioma associated with a bullous secondary retinal detachment still come to *enucleation*, either because a choroidal malignant melanoma is suspected or because the

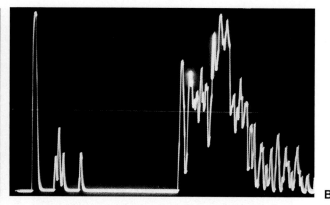

FIG. 38. Ultrasonography of circumscribed choroidal hemangioma. **A:** B-scan shows the lesion to be extremely bright (sonoreflective), with associated overlying and adjacent retinal detachment. **B:** A-scan ultrasound of the same lesion reveals high-amplitude, broad-based internal echo spikes.

eye becomes blind and painful on the basis of intractable secondary angle closure glaucoma.

PRIMARY INTRAOCULAR LYMPHOMA

An amelanotic fundus lesion that can occasionally enter the differential diagnosis of choroidal melanoma is the subretinal pigment epithelial infiltrate that occurs in some patients with primary intraocular lymphoma (diffuse large cell lymphoma, and "reticulum cell sarcoma"). This disorder is most common in individuals over the age of 50 and is substantially more frequent in women than in men. Central nervous system lymphomatous lesions are commonly associated with the ocular lesions.

Ophthalmoscopic Appearance of Tumor

The characteristic fundus lesion in this disorder is the geographic, yellowish white collection of cells occupying the

subretinal pigment epithelial space (Fig. 40A). The principal geographic lesions are often surrounded by multifocal satellite lesions. The lesions commonly have prominent clumps of black retinal pigment epithelial pigment on their surfaces, but they virtually never have any associated orange pigment clumps. Both eyes are occasionally affected. In addition, many patients with these characteristic subretinal pigment epithelial lesions also have diffuse intravitreal lymphoma cells (Fig. 41).

Ancillary Diagnostic Tests

If primary intraocular lymphoma is suspected, pathologic diagnosis is generally recommended. If there are prominent vitreous cells (Fig. 41), one can usually make the diagnosis by cytologic evaluation of a vitreous specimen obtained by *pars plana vitrectomy*. If there are characteristic subretinal pigment epithelial lesions but a paucity of vitreous cells, one can alternatively establish the diagnosis by transvitreal *fine-*

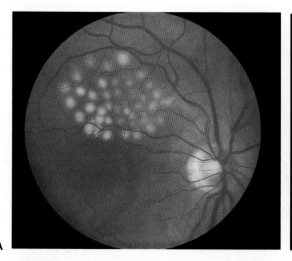

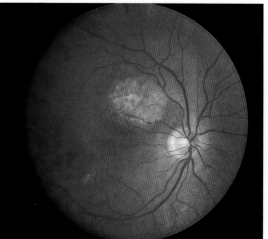

FIG. 39. Grid laser photocoagulation for circumscribed choroidal hemangioma. **A:** Immediate postlaser appearance of circumscribed choroidal hemangioma with shallow serous subretinal fluid in the macula. **B:** The same lesion 4 1/2 years later, showing resolution of subretinal fluid and whitish discoloration of the surface of the tumor.

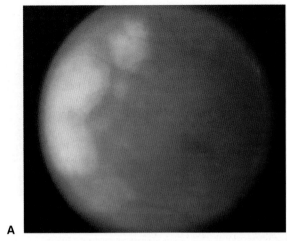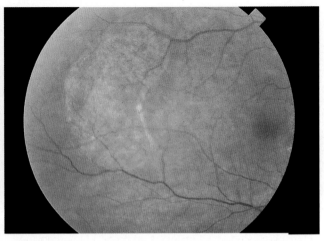

A B

FIG. 40. Diffuse large cell lymphoma ("reticulum cell sarcoma"). **A:** Whitish, geographic, subretinal pigment epithelial infiltrates of lymphoma cells prior to irradiation and chemotherapy. **B:** The same lesion 1 month following external beam radiation therapy and the start of systemic chemotherapy.

needle aspiration biopsy. Unfortunately, many reported cases of primary intraocular lymphoma are not diagnosed until the eyes are studied at autopsy.

Natural History

Infiltration of the retina and choroid by lymphoma cells generally causes progressive loss of visual function. However, the individual geographic subretinal pigment epithelial lesions frequently wax and wane spontaneously over time. The reason for this fluctuation is unknown.

Treatment

The proper treatment for patients with ocular reticulum cell sarcoma without central nervous system or visceral manifestations of lymphoma is controversial. Most patients are

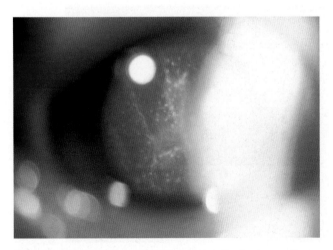

FIG. 41. Primary intraocular lymphoma ("reticulum cell sarcoma"). The slit-lamp photograph shows prominent intravitreal cells behind the lens.

treated by *external beam radiation therapy* to the affected eye or eyes (Fig. 40), and some are even given prophylactic external beam radiation therapy to the brain and spinal cord in the absence of documented central nervous system involvement. Obviously, those patients who have central nervous system involvement or systemic visceral lymphoma will require *chemotherapy* as well as irradiation to affected sites. The precise approach to therapy usually must be made on a case-by-case basis, depending on the extent and sites of disease.

CHOROIDAL OSTEOMA

The choroidal osteoma is an unusual benign posterior uveal tumor composed of mature bone. It is rarely if ever congenital and usually does not become apparent until the second or third decade of life. About 90% of these lesions occur in young adult women, and approximately 20% of cases are bilateral. The stimulus for formation of such tumors is unknown, but virtually all affected individuals have normal levels of serum calcium and phosphorus and no evidence of hyperparathyroidism or similar disorders.

Ophthalmoscopic Appearance of Tumor

The classic choroidal osteoma is a juxtapapillary or circumpapillary, golden to orange, platelike lesion with well-defined pseudopodlike margins (Fig. 42). The choroid peripheral to the affected zone appears unremarkable. A prominent pattern of interlacing choroidal blood vessels is commonly noted on the surface of the osteoma. A lesion that involves the macular region frequently causes marked disruption of the overlying retinal pigment epithelium and sensory retina, and often gives rise to subretinal neovascularization in the macular region (Fig. 43).

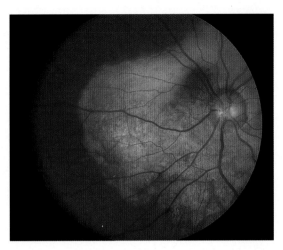

FIG. 42. Circumpapillary choroidal osteoma in a 35-year-old woman.

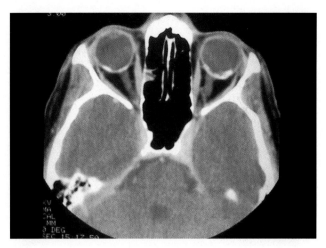

FIG. 44. Computed tomographic scan of choroidal osteoma. The axial view shows bilateral posterior eye-wall bony plate.

Ancillary Diagnostic Tests

B-scan ultrasonography of a choroidal osteoma reveals a densely reflective, platelike lesion in the posterior choroid. *Computed tomography* also reveals the bone density and platelike configuration of these tumors and is particularly dramatic in bilateral advanced cases (Fig. 44).

Natural History

Choroidal osteomas have been documented to enlarge slowly in most affected patients. Some patients who appear to be affected unilaterally at the time of initial diagnosis eventually develop a similar lesion in the fellow eye. In many patients, the choroidal osteoma eventually extends beneath the fovea and causes macular photoreceptor degeneration with resultant severe, uncorrectable visual loss.

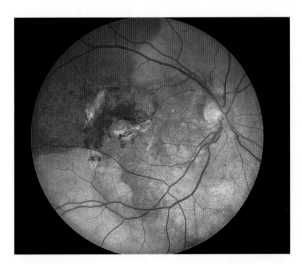

FIG. 43. Macular choroidal neovascular membrane lesion associated with circumpapillary choroidal osteoma in a 29-year-old woman.

Treatment

Because choroidal osteomas are benign, intervention is only required to treat potentially correctable causes of reduced visual acuity. The most common cause of potentially treatable visual impairment is choroidal neovascularization in the macular region. If the subretinal neovascularization is extrafoveal in location, one can treat it with focal laser therapy just as one does choroidal neovascularization in age-related macular degeneration. Unfortunately, the choroidal neovascularization in many cases is ill defined, subfoveal, or both.

UNIFOCAL RETINAL PIGMENT EPITHELIUM HYPERTROPHY

Unifocal hypertrophy of the retinal pigment epithelium is a melanotic fundus lesion that is occasionally mistaken for a posterior uveal malignant melanoma. The lesion consists of a well-circumscribed region of relatively uniform enlargement (hypertrophy) of retinal pigment epithelial cells that are densely packed with melanin granules. It appears to be congenital in most if not all affected individuals.

Ophthalmoscopic Appearance of Tumor

The typical unifocal hypertrophy of the retinal pigment epithelium is a well-circumscribed, dark gray to black, nummular fundus lesion (Fig. 45). Its margins tend to be well defined and smooth, and there is often "pseudoshadowing" around the margins that gives the impression of sloping elevation (Fig. 46). If one performs indirect ophthalmoscopy with scleral depression on an eye containing a lesion of this type, one will usually appreciate that the tumor is virtually flat. Discrete depigmented foci (lacunae) are often noted within a unifocal hypertrophy of the retinal pigment epithe-

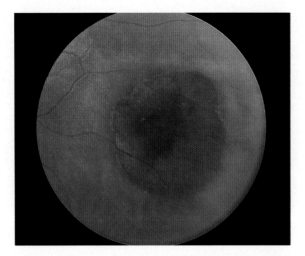

FIG. 45. Unifocal hypertrophy of retinal pigment epithelium.

lium. In some cases, almost the entire lesion becomes depigmented by expansion and coalescence of the lacunae.

Ancillary Diagnostic Tests

Fluorescein angiography of a unifocal hypertrophy of the retinal pigment epithelium usually reveals blockage of the choroidal fluorescence corresponding to the pigmented portion of the lesion, and transmission of the choroidal fluores-

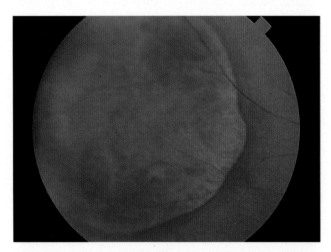

FIG. 46. Large unifocal hypertrophy of retinal pigment epithelium with marginal "pseudoshadowing."

cence and late scleral fluorescence corresponding to the lacunae. In most cases evaluated by fluorescein angiography, the overlying retinal vasculature appears normal.

Treatment

Although slight enlargement of a unifocal hypertrophy of the retinal pigment epithelium over several years is not uncommon, malignant transformation of a lesion of this type has not been documented. Consequently, no intervention is warranted for such tumors.

CONCLUSION

In addition to the neoplasms described, there are a number of nonneoplastic fundus lesions (mostly hematomas, fibrovascular proliferations, and inflammatory lesions) that can also simulate posterior uveal melanoma. The clinician who encounters a patient with an intraocular mass lesion that even remotely resembles a posterior uveal melanoma should always take that possibility very seriously. He or she should examine the fundus systematically, consider in detail the differential diagnostic features previously described in this chapter, and perform appropriate ancillary diagnostic studies, when indicated, to maximize the chance of arriving at the correct clinical diagnosis. Finally, if one is still not certain, one should obtain additional opinions from more experienced colleagues who are intimately familiar with the differential diagnosis of posterior uveal tumors.

BIBLIOGRAPHY

Augsburger JJ. Differential diagnosis of choroidal neoplasms. *Oncology* 1991;5:87–96.

Augsburger JJ. Fluorescein angiography of retinal and choroidal tumors. In: Tasman W, Jaeger EA, eds. *Foundations of clinical ophthalmology.* Philadelphia: Lippincott, 1991:chap 113A.

Augsburger JJ. Impact of enucleation on survival in posterior uveal melanoma: a reappraisal of the Zimmerman hypothesis. In: Laibson PR (Ed.). *The Year Book of Ophthalmology.* St. Louis, CV Mosby Co.; 1991:123–126.

Augsburger JJ. Intrauveal neoplasms. In: Podos SM, Yanoff M, eds. *Textbook of ophthalmology.* Philadelphia: Gower, 1991:chap 10–13.

Augsburger JJ, Schroeder RP, Territo C, Gamel JW, Shields JA. Clinical parameters predictive of enlargement of melanocytic choroidal lesions. *Br J Ophthalmol* 1989;73:911–917.

Shields JA, Augsburger JJ, Brown GC, Stephens RF. The differential diagnosis of posterior uveal melanoma. *Ophthalmology* 1980;87:518–522.

Practical Atlas of Retinal Disease and Therapy, Second Edition
edited by William R. Freeman,
Lippincott–Raven Publishers, Philadelphia © 1997.

· 7 ·

Retinal Complications of Cataract Surgery

Alexander Irvine

This chapter deals with the common retinal complications of cataract surgery—complications that every cataract surgeon hopes to prevent.

CYSTOID MACULAR EDEMA

Retinal specialists have found that the incidence of cystoid macular edema after cataract extraction seems to be decreasing for several reasons related to improved surgical technique. Cystoid macular edema was first described in association with vitreous adherent to the wound, either secondary to vitreous loss at cataract surgery or following later rupture of the hyaloid face with vitreous strands adhering to the wound. This vitreous to the wound seemed to exacerbate cystoid macular edema and accounted for many of the most serious and persistent cases. With modern microscopic techniques, including the use of extracapsular surgery and modern vitrectomy instruments for dealing with those cases where there is vitreous loss, the incidence of persistent vitreous strands to the wound has decreased markedly. This probably accounts for the decrease in the number of severe cases of cystoid edema that are seen.

Nonetheless, cystoid macular edema remains a major problem, and the cataract surgeon must understand it. When we study patients with cystoid macular edema and examine the disease through angiography, we are struck by the fact that the leakage comes primarily from the perifoveal capillaries and the capillaries of the optic nerve head (Fig. 1). Cystoid macular edema is essentially a disease of increased capillary permeability. There appears to be something about these perifoveal capillaries that makes them, like the capillaries on the disc, susceptible to this permeability change. It is unclear why these capillaries are so susceptible, but it is intriguing to note that the area where the greatest susceptibility to permeability changes seems to lie corresponds to that area where the internal limiting lamina is the thinnest. Over the disc and over the region of the fovea, the internal limit-

ing lamina is extremely thin, whereas it becomes much thicker further from the fovea. Thus, if one looks at the internal limiting lamina as a diffusion barrier, one can surmise that it may make those areas where it is thinnest more susceptible to inflammatory products that were diffusing through the vitreous from the anterior segment. The hypothesis that inflammatory products that affect vascular permeability travel through the vitreous to the retinal surface as a consequence of cataract surgery is one of the oldest explanations of cystoid macular edema, and the more we learn about prostaglandins and other substances released by inflammation, the more it seems to fit.

If one thinks of cystoid macular edema as being simply an increased permeability in the perifoveal capillaries, then one can better understand a number of the factors that work to provoke it. The first such factor is inflammation, and anything that causes anterior segment and vitreous inflammation increases the tendency to cystoid macular edema. Hypertension also increases the tendency to cystoid macular edema (Fig. 2). As soon as the permeability in the perifoveal capillaries rises, if we increase the pressure head in those capillaries, leakage is increased. Finally, diabetes also increases capillary permeability. Hypertension, diabetes, and inflammation all work together to cause increasing amounts of leakage. Thus, diabetics (reviewed below) have a greater tendency to develop aphakic or pseudophakic cystoid edema, as do hypertensive patients. When we consider cataract surgery per se in the pathogenesis of cystoid macular edema, we must concentrate on the inflammation factor. In trying to decrease the tendency to cystoid macular edema, cataract surgeons must minimize the tendency for inflammation in the anterior segment and minimize the ease of diffusion of any inflammatory products that might pass from the anterior segment posteriorly to the surface of the retina. Surgeons can do this in several ways. If an intact posterior capsule can be preserved, that is of value. If surgeons can avoid any irritation of the iris by the intraocular lens or by vitreous and chronic irritation, this will also be helpful.

A. Irvine, M.D.: Department of Ophthalmology, University of California, San Francisco, CA 94143

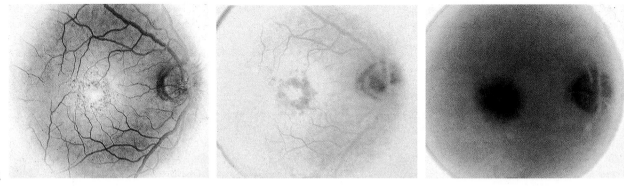

A   **B,C**

FIG. 1. Early (**A**), middle (**B**), and late (**C**) fluorescein angiograms showing cystoid macular edema. The fluorescein angiogram shows clearly that the leakage seems to come from the perifoveal capillary net as well as the vessels on the disc.

Obviously, surgeons must prevent vitreous adherence to the wound. If one reviews the "vitreous syndrome," where cystoid macular edema was first described, and sees how vitreous to the wound behaves, some of the factors that tend to cause inflammation in an aphakic eye can be better understood. Figure 3 shows an area where vitreous has adhered to the wound, and one may note that endothelial cells grow down along that vitreous strand and lay down collagen much like a Descemet's membrane. With time, a very firm membrane develops and contracts, pulling the iris up toward the wound. Thus, the thin strand of vitreous to the wound that may occur at surgery or later with delayed rupture of the hyaloid face develops into a very tough contractile strand that puts tension on the iris and distorts it. This can lead to inflammation, given that the rest of the vitreous body is placing traction on the iris each time the eye moves. In Fig. 4, the vitreous adhering to the posterior surface on the iris has developed a cellular membrane along the anterior hyaloid face. Contraction along that membrane has pulled the pigmented

posterior surface of the iris forward, showing the contractile force that the vitreous face can have on the iris even when it is not adherent to the wound. In the extracapsular situation, we must realize that often the capsule becomes adherent to the posterior surface of the iris and the vitreous can become adherent to that capsule. Again, we have vitreous placing traction on the iris with movement of the eye. Figure 5 shows the posterior capsular adherence to the posterior surface of the iris. We can see how firmly that adherence develops and see why a small capsulotomy with "in-the-bag" placement might seem preferable in terms of avoiding vitreocapsular adherence and traction on the iris.

Do we have any evidence to support this concept that not only vitreous to the wound but also vitreous adherent to the capsule and iris may be important in causing cystoid macular edema? If we review the multicenter collaborative controlled study of vitrectomy in eyes with chronic aphakic cystoid macular edema and vitreous to the wound, we see that vitrectomy was indeed effective in decreasing cystoid macu-

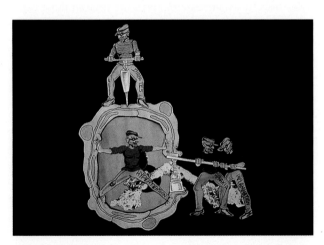

FIG. 2. Multiple factors have an additive effect on retinal capillary permeability.

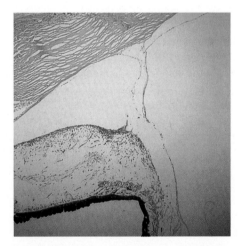

FIG. 3. Endothelial cells grow along the vitreous strand to the wound and lay down new collagen that contracts and pulls the iris up toward the wound. One can see the posterior vitreous in addition is adherent so that movement of the vitreous would pull on the iris as well as on the wound.

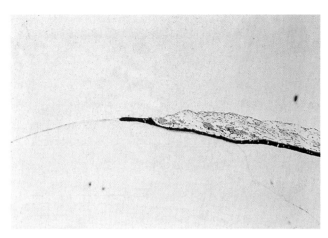

FIG. 4. An intact hyaloid face has become adherent to the iris, and cells have proliferated on its surface with contraction pulling the posterior pigmented layer of the iris toward the center of the pupil.

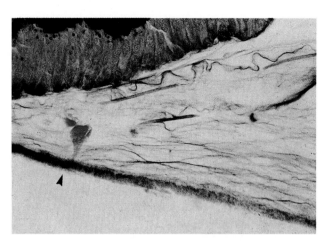

FIG. 6. The dense compact layer forming the anterior hyaloid (*arrow*). This is more of a diffusion barrier than the thin zonules anterior to it.

lar edema in these patients but, most interestingly, it showed that vitrectomy done through the pars plana, severing both the vitreous adherence to the back of the iris and vitreous adherence between the iris and the wound, was more effective than vitrectomy done through the limbus, only cutting the vitreous out of the anterior segment. Thus, the first principle we learn regarding how to decrease the incidence of cystoid edema after cataract surgery is that we must decrease the tendency for vitreous to adhere either to the wound or to the iris, and thereby decrease the tendency for vitreous traction on the iris, which can produce inflammatory stimuli.

When we consider inflammatory stimuli traveling from the anterior segment posteriorly, this may seem at first like a far-flung hypothesis. The important question is whether there really is any significant barrier to diffusion of inflammatory substances from the anterior segment to the posterior segment and how cataract surgery affects that barrier. When intracapsular cataract surgery was the norm, occasionally pa-

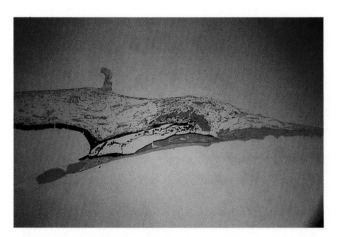

FIG. 5. The marked adherence of lens remnants and posterior capsule to the iris. Vitreous in turn is adherent to this capsule and thus secondarily to the iris.

tients did very well following cataract surgery, but several weeks later would suddenly develop a red and painful eye. The only change detectable clinically was that the anterior hyaloid face had been intact and was then seen to be ruptured. Somehow the rupture of the anterior hyaloid face seemed to lead to a brief period of definite inflammation. When we look at the hyaloid face histologically, it is, in fact, a significant barrier to diffusion. This has been proven, and Fig. 6 shows the thickness of the anterior hyaloid face that presents the real diffusion barrier. It is not the so-called zonular ligament that is the diffusion barrier but, rather, the intact anterior hyaloid face. Keeping the structure intact is the prime goal if one is to decrease the transport of any inflammatory substances from the anterior segment posteriorly to the retina. In fact, if there were some way that the cataract surgeon could perform a yttrium–aluminum–Garnet (YAG) posterior capsulotomy without disturbing the anterior hyaloid face, most of the secondary complications of that capsulotomy could probably be avoided. Unfortunately, such selective ablation does not seem feasible at the current time.

We have discussed the importance of what happens to the vitreous face in cataract surgery and in decreasing the tendency to cystoid macular edema. Another factor is the intraocular lens. If we look at some of the initial intraocular lenses, we see how certain lenses can cause inflammation. Anterior chamber lenses, particularly if they are slightly out of position so as to imbricate the iris root, will produce some irritation and reaction (Fig. 7). Obviously, older iris-fixed lenses could cause a good deal of inflammation, which was seen well on angiograms of the iris. The lens would strike against the iris with ocular saccades, resulting in focal fluorescein leakage. Even with posterior chamber lenses in the sulcus, one can sometimes see that the lenses strike against the back of the iris and cause loss of iris pigment (Fig. 8). On the other hand, a posterior chamber lens placed truly in the

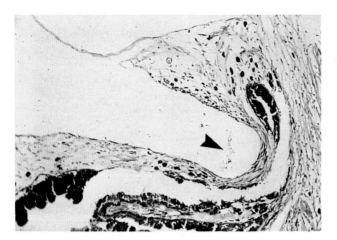

FIG. 7. The area of indentation of the iris root (*arrow*) by an anterior chamber lens haptic. There are macrophages with engulfed pigment surrounding this area.

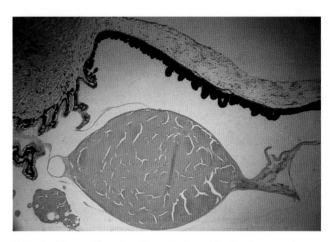

FIG. 9. Here with a haptic well placed in the bag, one sees no affect on the overlying iris or ciliary body.

bag causes amazingly little change in the overlying iris (Fig. 9). Miyake and colleagues conducted extremely important studies in which they performed anterior chamber fluorophotometry several months following cataract extraction. They compared intracapsular and extracapsular cataract extraction and extracapsular cataract extraction with either anterior chamber lenses or posterior chamber lenses. What they found was that, even in the extracapsular extractions, the anterior chamber lenses caused more vascular permeability than did the posterior chamber lenses. Among the anterior chamber lenses, the open loops caused less leakage than did the closed loops. With the posterior chamber lenses, Miyake and colleagues showed that the placement of the lens in the capsular bag caused the least fluorescein leakage and was better than placement of the lens in the ciliary sulcus. This correlates well with what we have been showing in histologic studies. Placement of the lens in the bag with the anterior capsular opening relatively small and without capsule

and vitreous adherence to the iris is certainly the most physiologic and seems to cause the least permeability change.

The modern cataract surgeon does seem to be producing less severe and persistent cystoid macular edema. This is due to the improved microscopic techniques, both in preventing vitreous loss and in dealing with it when it occurs. Even without vitreous adherent to the wound, we must realize that vitreous adherence to the capsule and iris can produce chronic inflammation. To minimize that, one wants to preserve an intact posterior capsule, avoid adherence to the iris, and avoid vitreous adherence to the capsule and iris. If one can do this, a relatively physiologic situation is created where there is no chronic irritation that will prolong cystoid macular edema. It may be fallacious to consider the trauma of the surgery itself as the cause of cystoid macular edema. Cystoid macular edema tends to come on weeks following the surgery. It is not the trauma of the surgery itself but rather the conditions that the surgery produces, leading to persis-

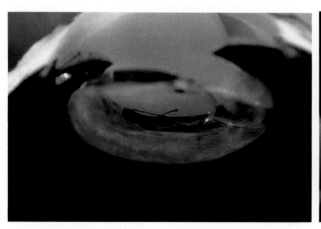

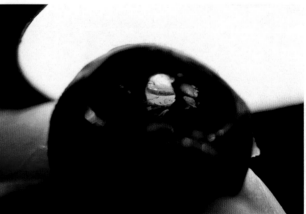

FIG. 8. A: Posterior chamber lens placed with one haptic in the bag (*left*) but the other in the sulcus (*right*). **B:** A view of the eye transilluminated shows the haptic that is placed in the sulcus (*right*) has rubbed the pigment off the back surface of the iris.

tent low-grade irritation and inflammation, that cause chronic cystoid macular edema. These conditions usually relate to vitreous adherence to iris, capsule, or wound.

When surgeons understand that it is this chronic irritation and inflammation in the anterior segment that causes inflammatory factors to pass posteriorly to affect the permeability of the perifoveal capillaries and cause cystoid macular edema, the treatment for cystoid macular edema will be directed at cutting down on those factors. We have discussed how one can do that best with surgery if one can maintain an intact posterior capsule and place the intraocular lens in the bag. Even with the best intentions, however, we do have some cases of cystoid edema that develop and persist. How can one treat these patients? One must try to minimize any exacerbating conditions, such as hypertension or diabetes, that may be playing a role, but anti-inflammatory drugs of one type or another must be used. Subtenons periocular steroids are often effective, sometimes only temporarily but at times it seems one can break the cycle of inflammation. After two or more monthly steroid injections, the inflammation sometimes will not return, and the cystoid macular edema will remain regressed. Nonsteroidal anti-inflammatory agents, such as ketorlac, are effective, as has been shown by Flach and his colleagues in a study done on the nonsteroidal anti-inflammatory agents, and these are often used topically in conjunction with either topical or subtenons steroids. Only in those cases that do not respond to such medical treatment do we search for areas of abnormal vitreous adherence that might be attacked surgically.

DIABETIC RETINOPATHY AND CATARACT SURGERY

Having discussed the way in which cataract surgery increases retinal vascular permeability, we should turn to the problem of cataract surgery in diabetic individuals. It is crit-

ical that every cataract surgeon realize the increase in risk to diabetic patients. Diabetes most often causes loss of vision by producing macular edema. Because diabetes causes increased capillary permeability and leakage in the macula and, as we have discussed, cataract extraction causes macular edema by increased vascular permeability, diabetes and cataract extraction, when combined, are synergistic. All too often, retinal surgeons are faced with patients like the 61-year-old diabetic discussed here (Fig. 10). This patient had been diabetic only 10 years and was felt to have only background diabetic retinopathy in each eye preoperatively. Vision was 20/60 in the left eye preoperatively. The patient then underwent cataract extraction. Vision was 20/25 immediately following cataract surgery, but by 6 months postoperatively it was reduced to 20/200. Review of the fluorescein angiograms from the two eyes shows that there is not very much difference between the two eyes in the early stage of the angiogram. Here, we see the number of microaneurysms, but in the late stages of the angiogram there is severe leakage in the aphakic left eye, leading to marked cystoid edema (Fig. 11). Thus, cataract extraction did this patient a great disservice by increasing capillary leakage and thus reducing vision from 20/60 to 20/200 in the left eye. This common problem must be recognized by cataract surgeons. In diabetic patients, we see this problem of increased risk of cystoid macular edema with either intracapsular or extracapsular cataract extraction and even with posterior chamber intraocular lenses and an intact posterior capsule. It is likely that everything that was just mentioned in the discussion of cystoid macular edema holds true in an exaggerated form in diabetic patients. Everything must be done to decrease the tendency for inflammation of the anterior segment. If a cataract is to be extracted and an intraocular lens is to be placed, a posterior chamber lens placed in the capsular bag is certainly the operation of choice. Even in this ideal situation, however, there is some increase in vascular permeability that

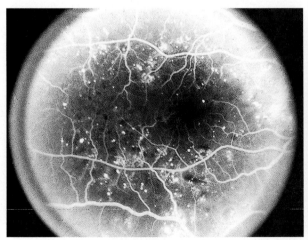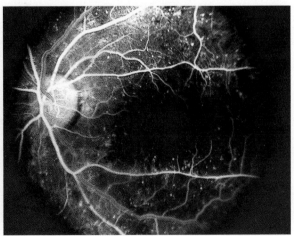

FIG. 10. In the early stages in the angiogram of this diabetic patient who recently underwent cataract surgery in the left eye, the degree of retinopathy in the right (**A**) and left (**B**) eyes seems approximately equal.

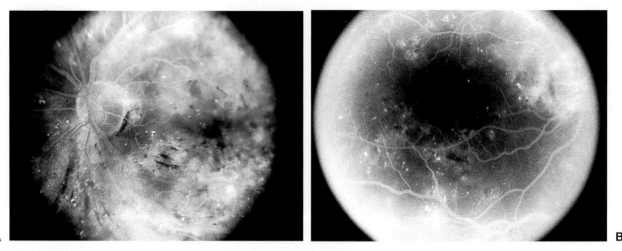

FIG. 11. In the late stages of the angiogram, we see that the left eye (**A**) after cataract extraction has much more leakage and has developed severe macular edema, whereas the capillaries in the right eye (**B**) leak much less.

synergizes with the preexistent diabetic increase in vascular permeability. This can lead to a disastrous visual result. Patients who have been led to expect improvement in vision after cataract surgery may have a real decrease due to chronic, persistent macular edema. In these cases, it does make sense to attempt to treat the diabetic contribution to that macular edema with focal laser photocoagulation, but all too often that is unsuccessful.

Sometimes the increased permeability caused by cataract extraction when coupled with diabetes is highlighted by marked lipid deposition, as seen in the patient represented in Figs. 12 and 13. This patient underwent an extracapsular cataract extraction with posterior chamber lens placement in the left eye. Both eyes prior to surgery seemed to have minimal background retinopathy, as seen in the right eye (Fig.

12). Postoperatively, the left eye developed a marked lipid deposition throughout the retina and severe cystoid macular edema, as seen on the fluorescein angiogram (Figs. 12 and 13). Some diabetics, particularly if hypertensive or having hyperlipidemia, will develop this type of lipid deposition when cataract extraction adds one more stimulus to increase vascular permeability. When it occurs, it strikingly illustrates the increased leakage and permeability to larger molecules in the aphakic or pseudophakic eye.

In addition to the problem of the marked increase in cystoid macular edema in diabetics, we see another severe complication. All too often elderly diabetics who are felt to have "mild background retinopathy" develop rubeosis irides unexpectedly and rapidly after cataract extraction or after a secondary YAG capsulotomy. The explanation is that these are

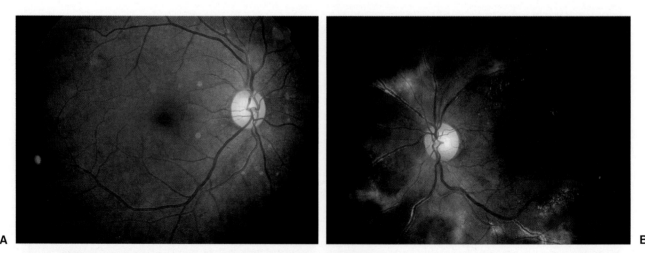

FIG. 12. The right (**A**) and left (**B**) eyes of a 58-year-old woman who had been diabetic only 6 years. She had an extracapsular cataract extraction with an anterior chamber intraocular lens placed in the left eye 6 months ago and now has vision that has fallen in that left eye to 20/50, whereas it was 20/20 shortly after cataract extraction.

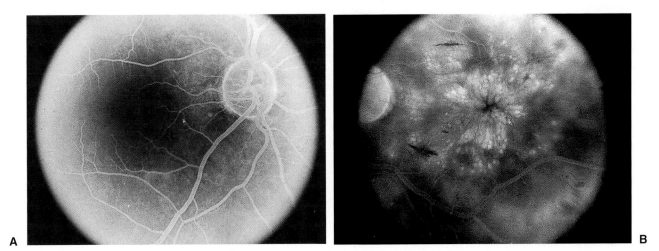

FIG. 13. Fluorescein angiograms of patient in Fig. 12, comparing the right (**A**) and left (**B**) eyes with marked leakage in the left eye compared with the right eye. This is also illustrated by the marked lipid exudation in the left eye (Fig. 12B) as compared with the right eye (Fig. 12A).

elderly patients who have had a posterior vitreous detachment and have rather extensive capillary nonperfusion. They do not show it by the development of retinal neovascular proliferans, however, because the vitreous has detached; therefore, they appear to have only mild background retinopathy. After the posterior capsule is ruptured, allowing free diffusion of neovascular factors from the posterior chamber anteriorly, this posterior area of capillary nonperfusion causes rapid development of rubeosis irides and neovascular glaucoma. Figure 14 shows a patient who was felt to have "mild background retinopathy" prior to cataract extraction and then rapidly developed rubeosis irides just a few

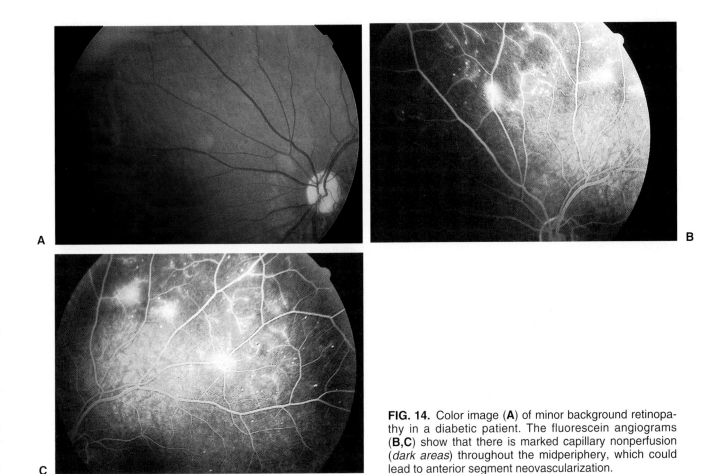

FIG. 14. Color image (**A**) of minor background retinopathy in a diabetic patient. The fluorescein angiograms (**B,C**) show that there is marked capillary nonperfusion (*dark areas*) throughout the midperiphery, which could lead to anterior segment neovascularization.

weeks after a YAG posterior capsulotomy. The color photograph shows relatively little retinopathy. The fluorescein angiograms shows that in the midperiphery there is marked capillary nonperfusion, which is not suspected when looking at the color photograph of the posterior pole, especially if one is looking preoperatively through a moderate cataract. Therefore, it is often best to do a wide-field fluorescein angiography or, if necessary, fluorescein angioscopy, to look at the midperiphery and determine the amount of capillary nonperfusion before considering cataract extraction in diabetic patients. It is critical that cataract surgeons appreciate the increased risk in the diabetic patients, not just in the obvious patients with proliferative disease who may develop a traction retinal detachment following a cataract extraction, but also in the subtle patients who appear to have just mild background diabetic retinopathy and who may develop severe loss of vision following cataract extraction due to either cystoid macular edema or rubeosis irides. (See also Chapter 10 by E. Ai and Chapter 11 by H. Lewis and G. Sanchez.)

RETINAL DETACHMENT

The next complication of cataract extraction to be discussed is retinal detachment. Similar to the situation with cystoid macular edema, the incidence of retinal detachment has also decreased with the advent of modern microsurgical techniques. Nonetheless, the basic factors causing retinal detachment following cataract surgery seem not to have been changed. There is still marked increase—almost a 100-fold increase—in the incidence of retinal detachment following cataract extraction. It is important to consider why this is so.

When retinal surgeons study aphakic or pseudophakic retinal detachments, three types of breaks are found to cause those detachments. First are typical tears at an area of vitreoretinal adherence posterior to the normal vitreous base, such as are seen in patients with lattice degeneration. This is the same type of break that is found in phakic retinal detachments. In the composite diagram (Fig. 15), we see that type of break at the 10:30 position behind the equator. The second kind of break, one that is more peculiar to aphakic or pseudophakic detachment, is the very tiny horseshoe tear that occurs right along the white with the pressure line that indicates the posterior edge of the vitreous base. There are often a number of such tiny tears along this line in the aphakic or pseudophakic eye. It is easy to understand the larger tear that occurs at an area of abnormal vitreoretinal adherence behind the vitreous base, for when the vitreous detaches all of the weight of the vitreous is pulling on the one area as the vitreous is pulled one way or the other with ocular rotation. These multiple small tears at the vitreous base in areas where there is no abnormal vitreoretinal adherence seem to imply a stronger force. Below we will consider why the aphakic eye or pseudophakic eye causes greater traction on the vitreous base than does the phakic eye. The third type of break is illustrated in our composite diagram at the 4:00 position, with

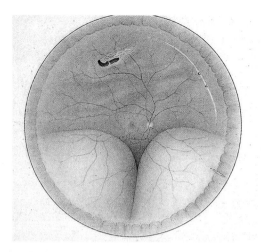

FIG. 15. In this composite drawing are the three types of retinal breaks seen in retinal detachment following cataract extraction. The typical tear behind the vitreous base at an area of abnormal vitreal retinal adherence, such as lattice, is at the 10:30 position. The two typical "aphakic breaks," which are small horseshoe tears along the posterior edge of the vitreous base, are at the 2:00 position. The tiny round atrophic break within the vitreous base is just behind the meridional complex at the 4:30 position.

a tiny atrophic round hole lying at the back of a meridional fold within the vitreous base. In a phakic eye, an atrophic round hole within the vitreous base would not cause a retinal detachment, for the vitreous base has a high enough hyaluronic acid content that the vitreous is solid there and fluid will not go through a small hole. This situation changes in the aphakic eye: the vitreous becomes more liquid and therefore may pass through a tiny hole at or near the ora. This can lead to retinal detachment.

We have discussed three types of retinal breaks. That leads to a discussion of three factors that account for the marked increase in the incidence of retinal detachment in aphakia or pseudophakia. First, there is a decreased hyaluronic acid concentration. Second, there is the loss of the mechanical "hold" that the lens has on the vitreous and by which the lens imparts motion to the vitreous and relieves vitreoretinal traction. Finally, there is the increased incidence of posterior vitreous detachment after cataract extraction. These are the three factors; they are somewhat interrelated but we will discuss each in order to understand why, even with the most modern techniques of cataract surgery, a markedly increased incidence of retinal detachment still occurs following cataract surgery.

Osterlin was a biochemist as well as an ophthalmologist who studied the vitreous after cataract extraction and showed that the vitreous concentration of hyaluronic acid dropped markedly after cataract extraction if the posterior capsule was ruptured. After either an intracapsular cataract extraction or an extracapsular cataract extraction with a posterior capsulotomy, the hyaluronic acid leeched out of the vitreous cavity into the anterior chamber and then passed out through the trabecular meshwork. Osterlin first studied human autopsy eyes in unilateral aphakes and found a marked decrease in hyaluronic acid content in the aphakic as opposed to the phakic eye. He then studied monkeys and showed that extracapsular lens extraction with posterior capsulotomy led to a marked decrease in hyaluronic acid content. If the posterior capsule was left intact, however, that did not occur. Osterlin was the first to suggest that the tiny atrophic holes within the vitreous base became dangerous in a patient after cataract extraction, because the hyaluronic acid content in the vitreous cortex at the vitreous base was so decreased that the liquefied vitreous passed through those holes and caused retinal detachment. We see that principle illustrated in Fig. 16. Osterlin showed that there was a three- to fourfold decrease in the hyaluronic acid content at the vitreous base following cataract extraction. Figure 16 shows such a threefold decrease, so liquefying the vitreous that it can now go through a break and cause elevation and detachment.

Not only does liquefication of the vitreous tend to open peripheral breaks, but also it increases the incidence of or speeds the development of posterior vitreous detachment. Aphakia dramatically increases the incidence of posterior vitreous detachment. Several autopsy studies have shown that either intracapsular cataract extraction or extracapsular cataract extraction with posterior capsulotomy leads to essentially a doubling of the incidence of posterior vitreous detachment. The incidence was increased from approximately 40% to 80% in these autopsy series.

To illustrate the importance of posterior vitreous detachment in the production of pseudophakic or aphakic retinal detachments, Hovland studied 100 bilateral aphakes who presented with a fresh unilateral retinal detachment. He carefully studied the vitreous in the fellow eye and then followed that eye. He found that, if the fellow eye already had a vitreous detachment without a tear, the incidence of later retinal detachment was extremely low (one of 42 patients), whereas if the second eye had not yet developed a vitreous detachment, the incidence of a later retinal detachment was much

higher (eight of 32); this was a significant difference ($p = 0.01$). A similar study was done in Israel by Friedman and Neumann, who looked at the vitreous in nonmyopic aphakic eyes and found that patients in whom a posterior vitreous detachment was present on initial examination did not tend to develop new tears. If there was no posterior vitreous detachment on the initial examination, as they followed those patients and the patients developed vitreous detachments, they had a high incidence of fresh tears. Thus, both these longitudinal studies of aphakic patients have shown that it is, indeed, at the time of posterior vitreous detachment that the retinal tears and retinal detachments tend to occur in aphakes, just as they do in phakic patients.

In aphakic or pseudophakic eyes, posterior vitreous detachment is not only twice as common, but it also has more of a tendency to cause tears and detachment. Why? This brings us to the second type of break that we initially discussed: tiny horseshoe breaks that occur along the ridge at the posterior border of the vitreous base. Why these tears tend to occur at this point where there is no abnormal vitreoretinal adherence but just the normal long ridge of adherence is an important question. One would think that it would require greater than the usual force to produce tears at this normal vitreous base.

A.C. Hilding was a physicist who studied the vitreous forces on the retina with rotation of the globe. He was the first to point out that the lens plays an important role in reducing vitreoretinal traction. He likened the vitreous to a gel filling the center of a hollow sphere. He noted that when rotating the sphere rapidly, the gel tended to lag behind and did not rotate with the sphere, just as the vitreous gel in the eye tends to lag when the extraocular muscles rotate the globe with saccades. However, he determined that if one put a slight indentation in the wall of that sphere, then as one rotated the sphere that indentation would push on the gel, carry much of the weight of the gel, and cause it to rotate along with the sphere. In the same way, he concluded the lens carries much of the weight of the vitreous and thus tends to re-

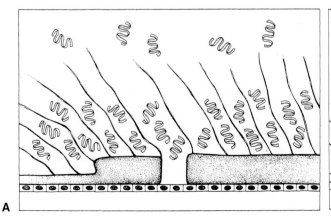

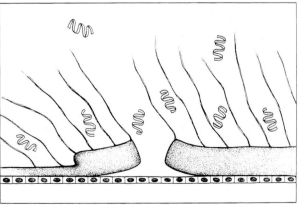

A B

FIG. 16. The hyaluronic acid concentration as shown by the spirals is decreased from normal (**A**) to one-third (**B**) following cataract extraction, thus making the vitreous base liquid enough that fluid can go through the break and begin to detach the surrounding retina.

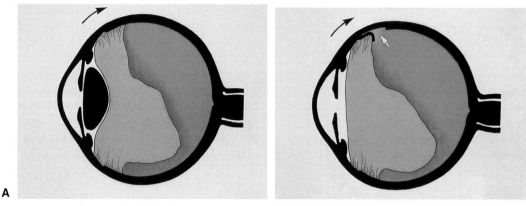

A   B

FIG. 17. With rapid saccades and rotation at the globe, the vitreous tends to lag behind. **A:** The lens protruding in the vitreous helps to move it along and takes some of the pull off the vitreoretinal interface at the vitreous base. **B:** In the aphakic eye, all of the weight of the vitreous is placed at the vitreoretinal interface, and thus a small tear (*white arrow*) is produced at the posterior edge of the vitreous base.

duce vitreoretinal traction at the vitreous base. Without the lens, as the sphere rotates, all of the inertial force of the vitreous is put on that vitreoretinal interface (Fig. 17). Thus, in aphakic eyes with a posterior vitreous detachment, all of the weight of the vitreous pulls on the vitreous base, explaining the multiple tiny, aphakic breaks that tend to occur there in

aphakes and pseudophakes (Figs. 17 and 18). We can thus review Fig. 15, showing the three types of breaks that tend to occur in pseudophakic or aphakic detachments and consider these in conjunction with the three major factors that increase the incidence of retinal detachment following cataract extraction. These are the decreased hyaluronic acid concen-

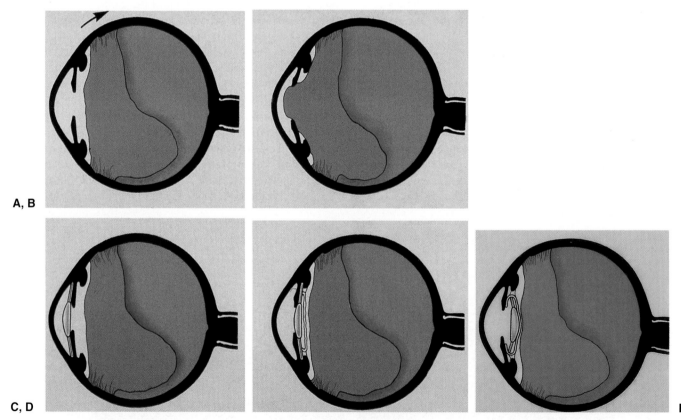

A, B

C, D   E

FIG. 18. Whether an intracapsular or an extracapsular procedure is done and whether an intraocular lens is present or not do not seem to have much effect on the pull of the vitreous at the vitreoretinal interface (**A–D**). Only in a situation (**E**) where a lens actually protrudes posteriorly into the vitreous will it help to move that vitreous and take some of the weight of the vitreous off the vitreous base with saccades.

tration that permits passage of fluid through preexisting small atrophic holes in the vitreous base and also leads to posterior vitreous detachment, the marked increase in vitreous detachment, and finally the fact that when the lens is removed its "hold" on the vitreous is removed, so that the full weight of the vitreous pulls on the remaining vitreoretinal attachments.

For cataract surgeons, this means that the goal should be to decrease the incidence of detachment by leaving the posterior capsule intact. Unfortunately, in approximately 50% of cases, the posterior capsule opacifies to the point where a capsulotomy is required and thus all the hazards just mentioned come into play. We need a method to keep the capsule clear and intact or need to find some way to make a capsulotomy without disturbing the anterior hyaloid face. Even with the capsule and hyaloid face intact, however, if we remove the lens we remove that protuberance into the vitreous and the lens' hold on the vitreous. Therefore, we have increased traction on the vitreous base or on any abnormal vitreoretinal adherences behind the base. To eliminate this, one would want an intraocular lens that not only would maintain a clear posterior capsule but also would bulge back into the vitreous to the same degree that the normal lens did. Thus, a lens with posterior convexity and with anteriorly angulated loops would seem most desirable (Fig. 18E).

In addition to understanding these basic principles, whereby cataract extraction increases the tendency to retinal detachment by its effects on the vitreous, cataract surgeons must realize that certain eyes are much more prone to detachment whether phakic or aphakic. Highly myopic eyes have a far greater tendency to retinal detachment whether phakic or aphakic, and making such myopic eyes aphakic or pseudophakic does markedly increase their tendency to develop retinal detachment. This is a critical fact, especially when we consider the high incidence of cataracts in high myopes and the proposal by some surgeons to remove even clear lenses in high myopes as a means of alleviating myopia. (See also Chapter 13 by H. Lincoff and I. Kreissig.)

PHOTOTOXICITY

The final retinal complication of cataract extraction that we will discuss is phototoxicity or phototoxic maculopathy. This is a condition that is commonly unrecognized because it can be very subtle on fundus examination and may be asymptomatic. This is illustrated in the photograph of Fig. 19, where one easily recognizes the small hypertensive hemorrhage inferotemporal to the fovea, but one must look very carefully to recognize the mild pigment changes just above the fovea. The accompanying fluorescein angiogram (Fig. 19B) brings these pigment changes out much more obviously, and a visual field (Fig. 20) shows that there is a striking defect corresponding with those pigmentary changes. It is only with a high degree of suspicion, however, that one will recognize this change. The fundus change can be variable, depending on the severity of the phototoxic insult and the patient's tendency to produce pigment. Most cases are quite subtle; on the other hand, some cases are more striking, such as is seen in Fig. 21, with marked pigment change just below the fovea. The elliptical or rectangular shape of the lesion is typical for those lesions produced by an operating microscope with a horizontally aligned light filament. On the other hand, a microscope with a round fiberoptic source may produce a lesion such as that seen in Fig. 22, with a round burn adjacent to the fovea.

As was the case with retinal detachment, one must understand the etiology of phototoxic maculopathy before one can decide the best means to avoid it. One must realize that phototoxicity is not the same as a photocoagulation burn; rather it is a true toxic lesion. Visible light interacts with certain molecules, such as cytochrome molecules in mitochondria, and its absorption there leads to the production of oxygen radicals that, in turn, cause cellular damage and, if sufficient, cellular death (Fig. 23). When one considers phototoxic maculopathy as a chemical/toxic reaction, one can understand some of the factors involved. One can divide the factors producing phototoxic maculopathy into minor and ma-

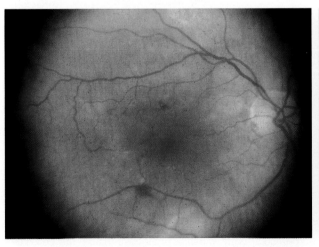 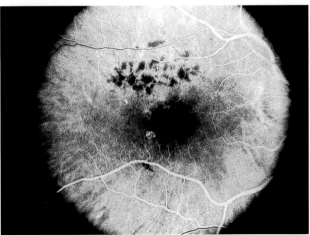

A B

FIG. 19. The pigment changes above the fovea from phototoxic maculopathy are subtle on the color image (**A**) but are brought out much more on the fluorescein angiogram (**B**).

OD

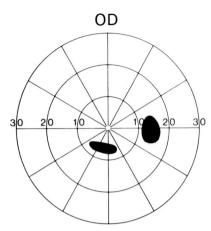

FIG. 20. The field loss corresponding to Fig. 19. Isopters: 3/2,000.

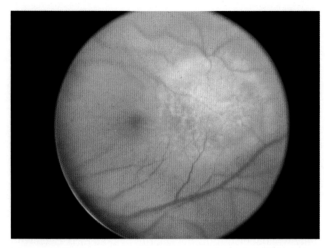

FIG. 22. A large round lesion is produced by the round fiberoptic illuminator of an operating microscope. Microscopes that illuminate the retina via a filament bulb will produce a linear or elliptical lesion.

jor factors. These are minor or major only insofar as surgeons can use them to influence the incidence of phototoxic maculopathy. The minor factors are the wavelength of the light, oxygen tension, and temperature. As for wavelength, it has been shown that the retina is most sensitive to the shortest wavelengths. The shortest wavelengths carry the most energy and produce more oxygen radicals. It has been shown that the retina is six times more sensitive to wavelengths in the 315-nm ultraviolet range than to wavelengths of 440 nm (blue) or longer. This has led to the use of yellow filters to block light that is less than 400 or 410 nm in some microscopes. This does not, however, seem to play a major role clinically. In our studies on monkeys, we found that the presence or absence of one of these commercial filters did not make a major difference in the threshold duration needed to produce a retinal lesion. This seemed to be primarily because

the Zeiss operating microscope has a spectrum of transmission that emits very little light that is less than 410 nm.

Theoretically, oxygen tension has been seen to be important, and clinically it has been shown that, with general anesthesia, anesthesiologists often use over 90% oxygen and can increase the oxygen tension in the tissues severalfold. This

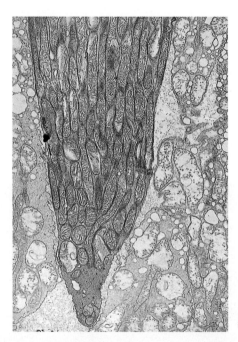

FIG. 23. The mitochondria of the photoreceptors may be one area of photon absorption where oxygen radicals are released and cause damage due to microscope phototoxicity. If too many mitochondria are damaged, the cell dies, as we see in the cells on either side of this cone. However, in this particular cone within a phototoxic lesion, the cell has survived and the mitochondria now appear healthy 2 months following phototoxic exposure.

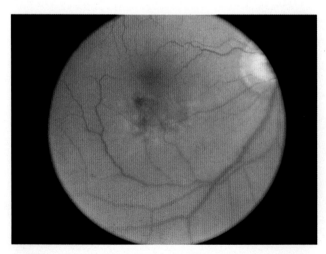

FIG. 21. A patient with dense pigmentation of the retina by a microscope-induced phototoxic lesion below the fovea.

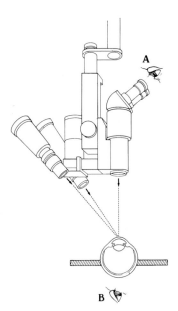

FIG. 24. The albino rabbit eye is placed in the hole on a table so one can view it either through the operating microscope as in **A** or from below as in **B**. Note that this microscope has both a coaxial illuminator and two side illuminators.

would have a theoretical effect of increasing phototoxicity. When we studied this in monkeys, we found that, in fact, lesions were more severe in those monkeys exposed under high oxygen conditions. Similarly, a very slight increase in temperature increases the photochemical toxic reaction.

These "minor" factors should be understood by surgeons. Just as the wavelength can be affected by filters, tissue oxygen tension can be affected by the oxygen concentration given by nasal cannula or via general anesthesia, and the retinal temperature might be altered by an irrigating solution. Nonetheless, the effects of these are relatively minor, as compared with the major factors that surgeons can influence. These major factors are the time of retinal exposure, tilt of

the microscope, and intensity of the microscope illumination. These three are the major factors through which surgeons can reduce the risk of phototoxic maculopathy. When considering the duration of exposure, it is critical that one understands the focal nature of the exposure from the operating microscope light. The optical system of the eye focuses the illuminating source of the microscope onto the retina. Although the surgeon sees a diffuse illumination of the anterior segment, the retina is exposed to a very small focal area of intense illumination. We demonstrated this through a simple experiment, wherein an albino rabbit eye was placed on a table with a small hole, the eye just fitting in that hole. This allowed us to view the eye from the front surface with the operating microscope to get the surgeon's view of illumination, and to view the backside of the eye from under the table to see the actual illumination of the retina (Figs. 24 and 25). When this is done, the surgeon's view through the microscope shows broad, even illumination of the anterior segment with a diffuse red reflex; whereas, when one looks at the retina from the backside of the eye, one sees a focal area of illumination from each of the illuminating sources on the microscope. When one talks about the time of exposure with the operating microscope, it is the time that the microscope is focused at one particular point on the retina that is critical, not the duration of the operation. The next point that one must realize is the very sharp threshold for structural photochemical damage. The eye is designed to process light, and below a certain threshold, light will cause no structural damage. That is a very sharp threshold. When we performed experiments with one particular microscope on a group of monkeys, we found that with either a 30-minute, 15-minute, or a 7½-minute exposure we obtained reproducible lesions. When we reduced exposure from 7½ to 4 minutes, however, no lesions occurred. Two 4-minute exposures 5 or 10 minutes apart to the same area produced a lesion essentially the same as if we had given 8 minutes of continuous exposure. We found that, with phototoxicity, repeated exposures

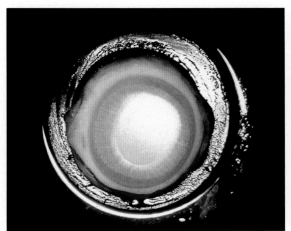
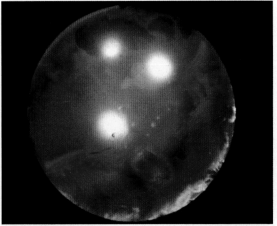

FIG. 25. A: Operating microscope view (see Fig. 24A) from the surgeon's viewpoint. Diffuse illumination of the anterior segment with a clear red reflex. **B:** View from under the table and the focal retinal illumination by each of the three microscope illuminators.

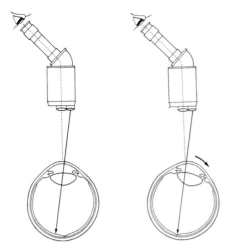

FIG. 26. A: With the microscope straight up and down and centered over the cornea, the illuminating filament is imaged just superior to the fovea. **B:** If the eye is rotated down with a superior rectus suture or the microscope is rotated (eyepieces tilted toward the surgeon), then the illuminating element will be focused on the center of the fovea, producing a visually significant burn.

within a period of hours are additive. This is a property of the photochemical nature of the lesion, as opposed to a simple thermal or photocoagulation burn. In terms of the time of exposure, if the illuminating filament is left at maximal intensity on one area of the retina, it probably requires only somewhere between 4 and 10 minutes to produce permanent structural damage in the human eye.

The tilt of the microscope is the second major factor in producing photochemical microscope burns. The illuminating system is slightly off axis from the viewing system, so that if the viewing system is centered on the cornea, the illuminating system will strike the retina 5°–6° above the foveola (Fig. 26). Now, however, if one has a superior rectus su-

ture in the eye and tilts the eye slightly downward, then the illuminating system will strike directly on the fovea (Fig. 26B). Conversely, if one tilts the microscope slightly toward oneself, one also moves the image of the illuminating element downward striking the fovea. It is true that the lutea pigment near the center of the fovea seems to offer some degree of protection, so that the lesions sometimes tend to just spare the foveola or allow recovery of the foveola (Fig. 27); however, this is not always the case. In addition to paracentral scotomas, permanent loss in visual acuity may result from a phototoxic lesion. Some surgeons have tilted the microscope and the eye downward in an attempt to deflect the image of the illumination system to strike the retina well below the macula. Unfortunately, in order to tilt either the microscope or the eye sufficiently to focus light more than 15° off axis (more than approximately 9° below the fovea), one loses the red reflex (Fig. 28). Therefore, the zone of safety is small, and surgeons must realize that, if a good red reflex is seen, the illuminating element is focused within 9° of the foveola. Another common error is to assume that, if one moves that microscope toward the superior limbus, one will be moving further away from the fovea and be safe. This assumption is made because surgeons know that the illumination strikes above the fovea when the microscope is not tilted and is centered on the cornea. In fact, the eye as an optical system has a prismatic effect so that, when one moves off center and moves the microscope superiorly, the illuminating element is deflected inferiorly, striking the fovea (Fig. 29). One must understand how tilting and moving the microscope affects the focal area of illumination on the retina and try to keep that area of illumination away from the fovea. Most importantly, however, one must not depend on tilt alone for, if there is a good red reflex, the light is close to the center of the fovea.

We now come to the final major factor in avoiding microscope burns on the retina: illumination intensity. This is the single most important factor for surgeons and the single fac-

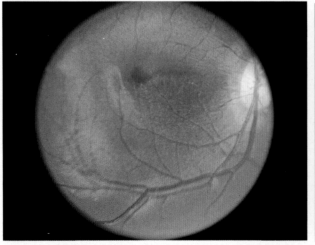

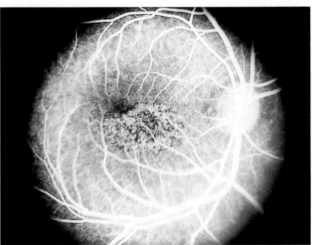

FIG. 27. A,B: The tendency of the phototoxic lesions to spare the very center of the fovea.

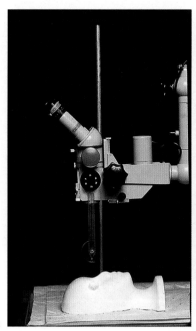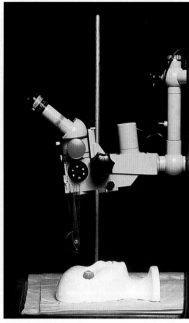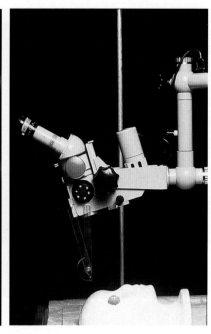

A   B, C

FIG. 28. Images show the microscope at 0° (**A**), 6° (**B**), and 15° (**C**) measured tilt. Notice the large amount of tilt required to reach 15° (so that the light is focused in a safe area 9° below the fovea). More tilt causes loss of the red reflex. If a red reflex is seen, the illuminating element is focused on the retina within 9° of the foveola.

tor over which they have the greatest control. There is a common tendency to use the operating microscope at maximum intensity, and since surgeons have a wide range of light adaptation, we can use it that way but should not. We must educate the operating-room personnel and take care ourselves to see that the microscope illumination is set only as high as is needed for good visualization. On our microscope, we have both a high setting and a low setting and then a rheostat to adjust the illumination within each of those settings. We rarely use the high setting and usually do not have the rheostat at maximum even in the low setting. By halving the illumination intensity, one doubles the threshold time of exposure required to produce a phototoxic lesion. It should be stressed that this is the single most important and simplest maneuver that surgeons can perform to decrease the risk of phototoxicity. All of the other factors—ranging from the minor factors of wavelength of light, oxygen tension, and temperature to the major factors of time of illumination and tilt of the microscope—are outweighed by this factor of illumination intensity. When one understands these factors, one will take other steps. One will ensure that the time of exposure is reduced by covering the cornea when it is not necessary to see a red reflex. One should be aware of where the tilt is placing the illumination on the retina, and most of all, one should use only the light intensity that is needed. Some surgeons have gained false confidence from noting that the majority of reported cases of phototoxicity have been cases operated on by residents and cases in which the cataract surgery took more than 1 hour. These surgeons feel that, because

they are more experienced, they need not consider phototoxicity. It is true that any surgeon taking a long time and leaving the microscope in one position for a long time is more apt to produce a phototoxic lesion, but the cases we have been recognizing recently have not come from the residents, but rather from some of the most experienced surgeons. The residents have been made aware of the dangers of phototoxicity and are taking the appropriate steps to prevent it. It is now the unusual case—such as the combined penetrating kerato-

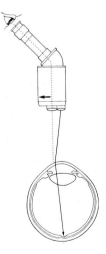

FIG. 29. If the microscope is moved away from the center of the cornea toward the superior limbus, the optical system of the eye has a prismatic effect that deflects the light back inferiorly toward the fovea.

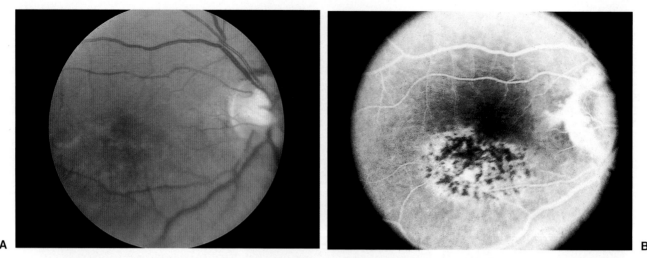

FIG. 30. A: This patient has 20/25 vision, but multiple visual complaints following placement of a secondary posterior chamber intraocular lens sutured to the iris. The surgeon suspected cystoid macular edema, but fluorescein angiography (**B**) showed macular phototoxicity.

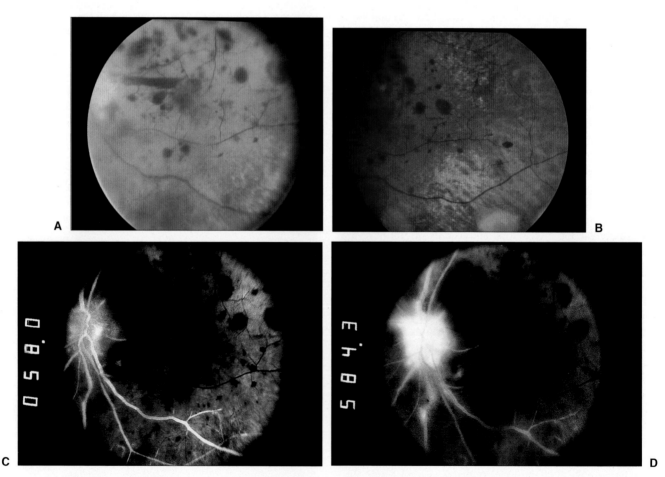

FIG. 31. A tunnel incision and single stitch wound closure were used in cataract surgery and posterior chamber lens implantation. Subconjunctival gentamycin was used. **A:** The fundus appearance on the first day; retinal hemorrhages are most prominent in the posterior pole. **B,C:** Early and late fluorescein angiogram frames with sharply demarcated vessel occlusion and late staining and leakage of retinal vessels and the optic nerve head.

plasty and intraocular lens placement, or the replacement of one intraocular lens with another—that is sometimes associated with unexpected phototoxicity at our institution. One of our most skilled and experienced anterior segment surgeons performed a secondary lens implantation, placing an iris-sutured posterior chamber intraocular lens in a 65-year-old patient (Fig. 30). Postoperatively, the patient had a visual acuity of 20/25 and yet complained. The surgeon suspected cystoid macular edema, but the fluorescein angiogram showed a typical phototoxic lesion. The paracentral scotoma interfered with visual function, despite the good single-letter Snellen acuity.

Thus, even the most experienced surgeons need to be aware of the danger of phototoxicity from the operating microscope and should be especially wary of it in the difficult and unusual case that requires a longer duration with the microscope focused over the center of the cornea or pupil. Thus, with phototoxicity, as was the case with cystoid macular edema and retinal detachment, to prevent the problem surgeons must first understand it. Surgeons must ensure that the illumination setting on the microscope is only as high as is needed for good visualization and be aware of where the tilt is placing the illumination. One must minimize the time that the area around the macula is illuminated by covering the cornea at any time when a red reflex or visualization through that cornea is not necessary. It is worth considering the role of oxygen and limiting nasal oxygen or high concentrations in general anesthesia to when they are needed and perhaps using a filter to eliminate the short wavelengths; however, these latter factors are not nearly as important as the time and intensity of the exposure. Surgeons should not be lulled into a false sense of security because a yellow filter is in the operating microscope.

AMINOGLYCOSIDE RETINAL TOXICITY

Aminoglycoside retinal toxicity, albeit rare, is one of the most severe retinal complications of cataract surgery. It is seen not only with inadvertent penetrations of the sclera by the needle but also has been seen in some cases where a true subconjunctival injection seemed to force a small amount of gentamycin (or amikacin) through a well-closed cataract wound (either with or without sutures). The tunneled wounds of today have a valvelike action that enables them to resist high intraocular pressures without leaking, but that may not resist the external pressure and distortion of a subconjunctival injection. If one is injecting 40 mg/ml gentamycin subconjunctivally, only 0.01 ml needs to squeeze

through the wound to result in a toxic dose. Gentamycin is heavier than water and tends to settle right on the macula of a supine patient. Because of the danger, gentamycin is no longer used as a routine postoperative antibiotic at our institution.

The following case illustrates the danger. The 64-year-old woman had lost central vision in her right eye from a macular hole around 1989. Vision in the left eye gradually fell to best corrected 20/80 due to cataract. She underwent phacoemulsification cataract surgery with posterior chamber lens implantation through a small tunnel incision. The wound was closed with a single stitch. Gentamycin was injected subconjunctivally after lifting the conjunctiva with a toothed forceps. All went smoothly until the bandage was removed on the first postoperative day, and she had only peripheral finger-counting vision.

The fundus photographs (Fig. 31) show complete occlusion of all retinal vessels in the macular region, with scattered hemorrhages. Fluorescein angiography reveals the characteristic sharply demarcated area of vessel occlusion restricted to the posterior pole. Unfortunately, nothing can be done for cases such as this, other than to try to limit their occurrence by being aware of the danger.

BIBLIOGRAPHY

Brod RD, Olson KR, Ball SF, Packer AJ. The site of operating microscope light induced injury on the human retina. *Am J Ophthalmol* 1989;107:390.

Flach AJ, Jampel LM, Weinberg D, et al. Improvement in visual acuity in chronic aphakic and pseudophakic cystoid macular edema after treatment with topical 0.5% ketorlac tromethamine. *Am J Ophthal* 1991;112:514.

Freedman Z, Neumann E. Posterior vitreous detachment after cataract extraction in non-myopic eyes and the resulting retinal lesions. *Brit J Ophthal* 1975;59:451.

Hilding AC. Normal vitreous: its attachments and dynamics during ocular movement. *Arch Ophthalmol* 1954;52:497.

Hilding AC. Alterations in the form, movement, and structure of the vitreous body in aphakic eyes. *Arch Ophthalmol* 1954;52:699.

Hovland KR. Vitreous findings in fellow eyes of aphakic retinal detachment. *Am J Ophthal* 1978;86:350.

Jaffe GJ, Burton TC. Progression of nonproliferative diabetic retinopathy following cataract extraction. *Arch Ophthalmol* 1988;106:745.

MacDonald HR, Irvine AR. Light-induced maculopathy from the operating microscope in extracapsular cataract extraction and intraocular lens implantation. *Ophthalmology* 1983;90:945.

Miyake K, Asakura M, Kobayashi H. The effect of intraocular lens fixation on the blood aqueous barrier. *Am J Ophthalmol* 1984;98:451.

Osterlin S. On the molecular biology of the vitreous in the aphakic eye. *Acta Ophthalmol* 1977;55:353.

Osterlin S. Macromolecular composition of the vitreous in the aphakic owl monkey eye. *Exp Eye Res* 1978;26:77.

Practical Atlas of Retinal Disease and Therapy, Second Edition
edited by William R. Freeman,
Lippincott–Raven Publishers, Philadelphia © 1997.

• 8 •

Branch and Central Retinal Vein Occlusions

Daniel Finkelstein

BRANCH RETINAL VEIN OCCLUSION

Diagnosis

Retinal branch vein occlusion (Fig. 1) presents a pathognomonic fundus appearance in its acute phase because of the segmental distribution of intraretinal hemorrhage that generally respects the horizontal raphe. Along with central retinal vein occlusion (Fig. 2), branch and central venous occlusions represent the second most common cause of retinal vascular disturbance in patients (second only to diabetic retinopathy).

Branch retinal vein occlusion (Fig. 3) usually occurs in the age range from 50 to 70 years, with about half of the patients having systemic hypertension, but this is not much different from the rate of hypertension in a control group of this age. In idiopathic branch retinal vein occlusion, the occlusion always occurs at an arteriovenous crossing site, suggesting that some mechanical aspect of the crossing predisposes the eye to the occlusion. In the acute phase of the disease, for the first 6–9 months, there is usually significant intraretinal hemorrhage that on occasion may become subretinal, preretinal, or vitreal. When the intraretinal hemorrhage occurs in the fovea (as seen in Fig. 3), it may be responsible for a spontaneous totally reversible visual loss if there is no other cause of visual loss, such as macular edema or capillary nonperfusion.

In the chronic phase of the branch vein occlusion, after resorption of intraretinal hemorrhage, vascular collaterals (Fig. 4) are often apparent, along with the segmental capillary abnormalities of dilatation and/or nonperfusion in a segmental pattern that will persist for the remainder of the patient's life as a pathognomonic sign that a branch retinal vein occlusion has occurred.

Numerous previous investigators (Table 1) have studied the natural history of the complications of branch vein occlusion, primarily vision loss from macular edema and vitreous hemorrhage from neovascularization, along with laser photocoagulation management of these complications. These studies laid the groundwork for a randomized clinical trial from 1978 to 1985 (Table 2) that established the efficacy of laser photocoagulation for the improvement in visual acuity that had been lost to macular edema and for the lessening of neovascularization and vitreous hemorrhage.

Therapy

For the management of vision loss from macular edema, as demonstrated by fluorescein angiogram (Fig. 5A,B), the Collaborative Branch Vein Occlusion Study demonstrated that grid laser photocoagulation placed over the region of dilated and leaking capillaries (as demonstrated in Fig. 5C,D) could lessen edema and improve visual acuity. When the argon laser was used, this grid laser photocoagulation produced a medium white burn in such a pattern as demonstrated in Fig. 6. When foveal and macular landmarks are not clear, patients are treated in several sittings, maintaining a safe distance from the foveal avascular zone until laser pigmentation and repeat fluorescein angiography can establish more discrete landmarks for safer further photocoagulation. The Collaborative Branch Vein Occlusion Study demonstrated that patients treated in this fashion were twice as likely as controls to improve in visual acuity, with 65% of the treated patients improving as compared with 37% of the controls.

In summarizing the guidelines for laser management of macular edema with vision loss secondary to branch vein occlusion, the study emphasized that one should wait for foveal and macular hemorrhage to clear prior to consideration of laser therapy, with this period usually lasting at least 3–6 months. During this interval, clearing of the hemorrhage will permit residual foveal hemorrhage to absorb, providing a more accurate evaluation of acuity. When the hem-

Text continues on p 166.

D. Finkelstein, M.D.: Wilmer Eye Institute, Johns Hopkins Hospital, Baltimore, MD 21205

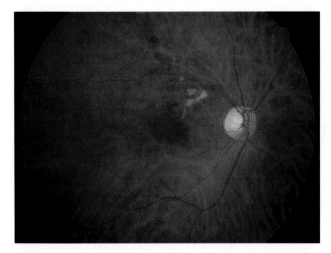

FIG. 1. Fundus photograph of acute, superotemporal retinal branch vein occlusion demonstrating the pathognomonic pattern of segmental intraretinal hemorrhage.

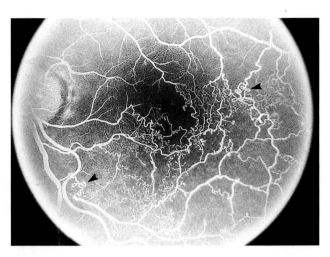

FIG. 4. Fluorescein angiogram of branch retinal vein occlusion demonstrating collateral formation (*arrows*).

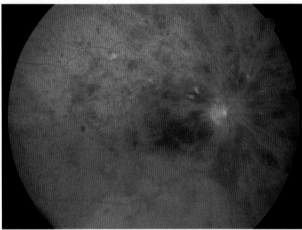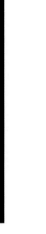

FIG. 2. Fundus photograph of acute central retinal vein occlusion demonstrating diffuse intraretinal hemorrhage with dilated and tortuous retinal veins.

TABLE 1. *Investigators who contributed important information regarding the natural history and treatment of branch vein occlusion*

Archer	l'Esperance
Blankenship	Michels
Clement	Margargal
Coscas	Newell
Gass	Okun
Gitter	Patz
Gutman	Schatz
Hayreh	Shilling
Henkind	Wetzig
Joffe	Wise
Kelley	Yannuzzi
Kohner	Zegarra and others
Krill	

TABLE 2. *Institutions participating in the Collaborative Branch Vein Occlusion Study, a randomized clinical trial, 1978–1985*

Bascom Palmer, Miami, Florida
  John Clarkson, M.D.
Estelle Doheny, Los Angeles, California
  Stephen Ryan, M.D.
Illinois Eye and Ear Infirmary, Ingalls Memorial Hospital, Chicago, Illinois
  David Orth, M.D.
Retina Associates, Boston, Massachusetts
  Clement Trempe, M.D.
Wilmer Institute, Baltimore, Maryland
  Daniel Finkelstein, M.D.

FIG. 3. Fundus photograph of acute, superotemporal retinal branch vein occlusion demonstrating the pathognomonic pattern of segmental intraretinal hemorrhage.

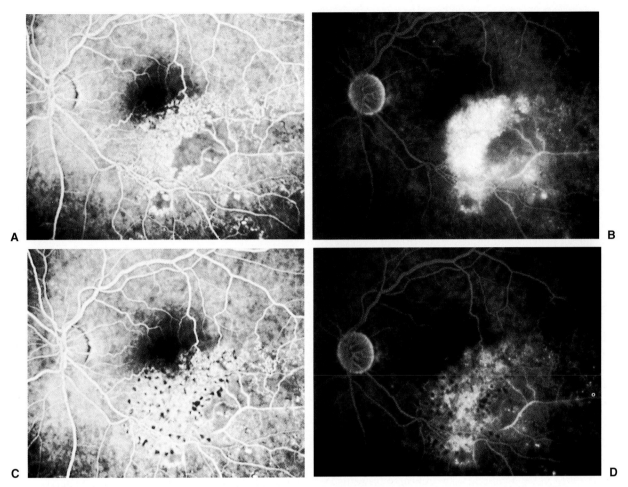

FIG. 5. A: Transit fluorescein angiogram of inferotemporal branch vein occlusion demonstrating macular dilated capillaries. **B:** Fluorescein angiogram, late phase, demonstrating fluorescein leakage and cystoid accumulation involving the fovea. **C:** Fluorescein angiogram, transit phase, demonstrating the pattern of grid laser photocoagulation. **D:** Fluorescein angiogram, late phase, demonstrating lessened macular edema.

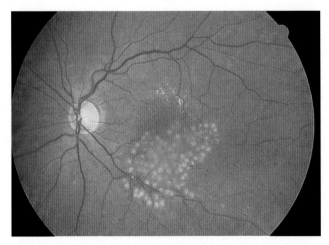

FIG. 6. Fundus photograph demonstrating the pattern of grid laser photocoagulation, immediately after treatment.

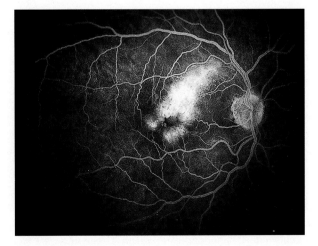

FIG. 7. Fluorescein angiogram, late phase, demonstrating prominent macular edema with cystoid edema accumulation involving the fovea.

orrhage has absorbed, high-quality angiography can then be attained that would otherwise be obscured by overlying intraretinal hemorrhage. In addition, photocoagulation is contraindicated directly over intraretinal hemorrhage because the intraretinal hemorrhage will absorb the photocoagulation rather than the desired absorption by pigment epithelium.

The Branch Vein Occlusion Study guidelines also state that the fluorescein angiogram must show macular edema with foveal edema and vision of 20/40 or worse. Both the doctor and the patient must be satisfied that the vision is stable or worsening and not improving. The doctor and the patient must remember that complications of treatment can occur, that improvement of visual acuity is small, on average, and that not all patients will improve. The Branch Vein Occlusion Study presented no evidence that there is a need to treat patients early in the course of the disease, and the Branch Vein Occlusion Study results suggest that patients with systemic hypertension and edema lasting more than 1 year are most likely to benefit from laser photocoagulation. A review of the original study provides further details of laser management of macular edema. It is important to emphasize the need for high-quality angiography demonstrating dilated macular capillaries resulting in definite foveal edema (Fig. 7) prior to consideration of laser photocoagulation.

The fluorescein angiogram in Fig. 8 demonstrates capillary nonperfusion, rather than capillary leakage producing foveal edema, as a cause of vision loss. Nonperfusion is seen as a darker area in the angiogram due to loss of the retinal capillary network that, when present, gives the angiogram a grey appearance. In the late phase of the angiogram in patients with significant nonperfusion, as demonstrated in Fig. 9, there is a small amount of fluorescein leakage at the border of nonperfused and perfused retina, as there always is

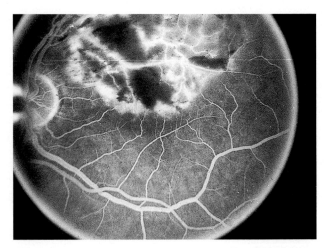

FIG. 9. Fluorescein angiogram, late phase, demonstrating macular nonperfusion with mild fluorescein leakage at the border of the perfused and nonperfused zone.

acutely in such situations; but this edema will spontaneously resolve, the vision will continue to remain reduced from the nonperfusion, and laser photocoagulation will be of no benefit. It is important to reemphasize that when there is intraretinal hemorrhage in the acute phase of the occlusion (Fig. 10), during the first several months, fluorescein angiography will not demonstrate sufficient details of the macular region to be helpful.

It is not understood how grid laser photocoagulation and its absorption at the level of the pigment epithelium lessen macular edema from branch vein occlusion and improve visual acuity. When Wilson and colleagues studied the effect of grid photocoagulation on the retinal vasculature of the normal rhesus monkey (as shown in Fig. 11), they demonstrated that the retinal capillaries narrowed weeks following the laser photocoagulation, suggesting an indirect effect of

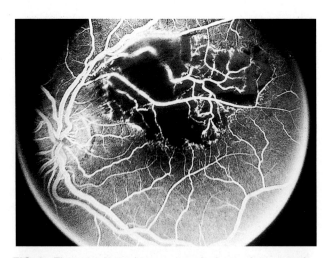

FIG. 8. Fluorescein angiogram, transit phase, demonstrating macular capillary nonperfusion, which is seen as a *dark black* area in the angiogram.

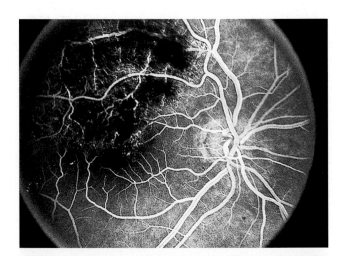

FIG. 10. Fluorescein angiogram, late transit phase, demonstrating blockage of fluorescein detail by intraretinal hemorrhage. Blockage from blood appears dark and should not be confused with nonperfusion; examination of color photograph or the patient will help to distinguish these two entities.

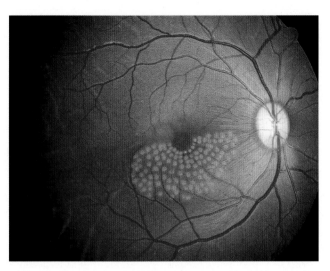

FIG. 11. Color photograph demonstrating grid laser photocoagulation in rhesus monkey, immediately after treatment.

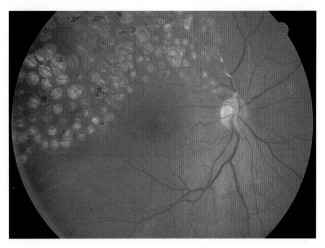

FIG. 13. Fundus photograph demonstrating involution of disc neovascularization following scatter photocoagulation of superotemporal branch vein occlusion.

the photocoagulation, perhaps as an autoregulation of the retinal vessels because the outer retina was destroyed by the laser photocoagulation. With the retina therefore thinned and the retinal vessels closer to the choroid, one could suggest the hypothesis that autoregulatory narrowing of the retinal vasculature might decrease retinal blood flow and thereby decrease retinal edema. Other mechanisms, such as an increase in the pumping capacity of the pigment epithelium, have also been suggested.

Neovascularization secondary to ischemic branch vein occlusion is an important complication that may cause vitreous hemorrhage, retinal traction, and other vision-threatening problems. Neovascularization was recognized prior to the branch vein occlusion study and scatter photocoagulation, as demonstrated in Fig. 12 over the ischemic retina for the management of retinal neovascularization, was felt to be beneficial. The consequent involution of the neovascularization, as

demonstrated in Fig. 13, was often apparent. The Collaborative Branch Vein Occlusion Study demonstrated that 50% of large branch vein occlusions are nonperfused, that 50% of nonperfused patients with branch vein occlusion will develop neovascularization, and that 50% of those with neovascularization will develop vitreous hemorrhage. However, if scatter laser photocoagulation is placed throughout the ischemic segment prior to the development of neovascularization, the onset of neovascularization can be reduced by 50%. If scatter photocoagulation is applied after the onset of neovascularization, the likelihood of vitreous hemorrhage is reduced by 50%. Consequently, the Branch Vein Occlusion Study recommended scatter laser photocoagulation in the affected ischemic segment at the first sign of disc or peripheral neovascularization. It is important to realize that the collaterals that form so commonly in branch vein occlusion can mimic the appearance of neovascularization. Figure 14

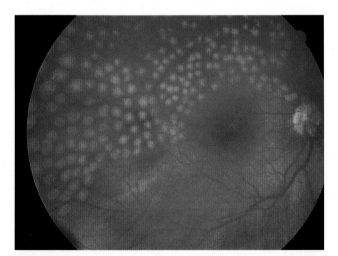

FIG. 12. Fundus photograph demonstrating scatter laser photocoagulation of branch vein occlusion with secondary disc neovascularization, immediately after treatment.

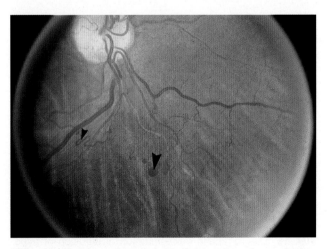

FIG. 14. Fundus photograph of branch vein occlusion demonstrating both collaterals (*small arrow*) and neovascularization (*large arrow*).

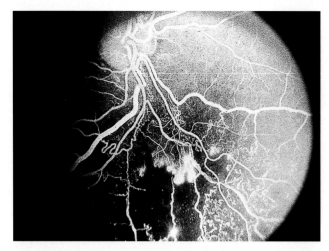

FIG. 15. Fluorescein angiogram, late transit phase, demonstrating leakage of fluorescein from neovascularization, without leakage from collaterals.

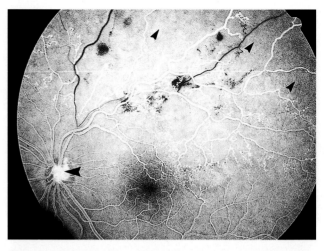

FIG. 17. Fluorescein angiogram demonstrating peripheral capillary nonperfusion (*small arrows*) associated with disc neovascularization (*large arrow*) in branch vein occlusion.

shows that it may be difficult to determine which vascular abnormality represents collaterals and which represents true neovascularization in some eyes.

Fluorescein angiography can be helpful not only in determining the extent of macular edema and nonperfusion, but also in distinguishing between collaterals and neovascularization. Neovascularization leaks fluorescein profusely, whereas collaterals either do not leak or only stain minimally, as demonstrated in Fig. 15. The present concept regarding the development of neovascularization in branch vein occlusion is that the ischemic retina liberates an angiogenic material that diffuses away from the area of ischemia and produces neovascularization as diagramed in Fig. 16. It is presumed that scatter photocoagulation changes the ischemic area in such a way that the stimulatory factors are reduced. No clinical situation provides a more vivid demon-

stration of the distant effect of ischemia on neovascular growth than cases such as the branch vein occlusion demonstrated in Fig. 17, in which peripheral ischemia is associated with the growth of neovascularization from a normal area of retina at the optic nerve head.

It is important for ophthalmologists contemplating laser photocoagulation to realize that although complications are rare in experienced hands, numerous complications can occur. For example, as demonstrated in Fig. 18, when photocoagulation is improperly applied over intraretinal hemorrhage, the surface of the retina is disturbed because of absorption of laser energy by blood causing excess inner retinal coagulation. A resultant preretinal fibrosis can be produced that can significantly reduce vision, as demonstrated in Fig. 19, where retinal vessels are seen as being distorted by epiretinal fibrous proliferation.

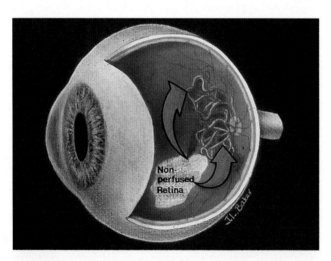

FIG. 16. Diagrammatic representation of diffusion of hypothetical angiogenesis factor from an ischemic retina.

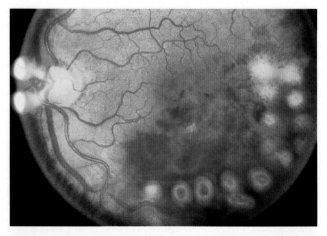

FIG. 18. Fundus photograph demonstrating improper laser photocoagulation technique in which light energy absorption has occurred in areas of intraretinal hemorrhage rather than by the pigment epithelium.

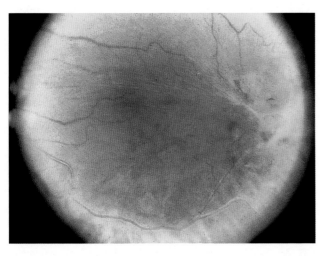

FIG. 19. Fundus photograph demonstrating preretinal fibrosis (*yellow* tissue) resulting from photocoagulation absorbed by surface retinal hemorrhage as a complication of improper laser photocoagulation. Retinal striae are seen (*arrows*) through the fovea.

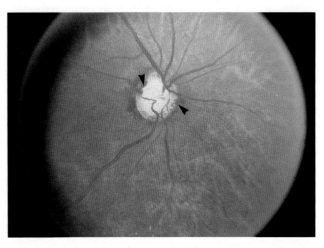

FIG. 21. Fundus photograph of central retinal vein occlusion in chronic phase demonstrating collateral vessels (*arrows*) on the disc.

CENTRAL RETINAL VEIN OCCLUSION

Diagnosis

Central retinal vein occlusion is easy to diagnose in its acute phase because of the scattered intraretinal hemorrhage along with dilated and tortuous retinal veins, as shown in Fig. 20. In the acute phase, this is a unilateral condition. When intraretinal hemorrhage is seen scattered in both fundi, one should consider systemic hyperviscosity syndromes and conduct whole blood viscosity and related studies to rule out such diseases. When the intraretinal hemorrhage occurs primarily in the far peripheral fundus, often in a blot fashion, one should consider carotid insufficiency. Glaucoma and diabetes appear to increase the risk of developing central vein occlusion.

In the chronic phase of central vein occlusion, after resorption of intraretinal hemorrhage, collaterals are often seen at the optic nerve head, as demonstrated in Fig. 21. On occasion, depending on the extent of macular involvement, one may identify a pigmented spot in the fovea (as demonstrated in Fig. 22).

It is important to distinguish between two types of central vein occlusion because these two types have quite different natural histories. The perfused form of central vein occlusion (Fig. 23), as demonstrated by the fluorescein angiogram in Fig. 24, is also termed nonischemic, partial, incomplete, impending, or venous stasis and is likely to have less intraretinal hemorrhage and visual acuity of 20/400 or better. When vision loss occurs or persists, the cause of the vision loss is often macular edema. The other type of central vein occlusion, as demonstrated by the fluorescein angiogram in Fig. 24, is ischemic in nature and has also been termed complete,

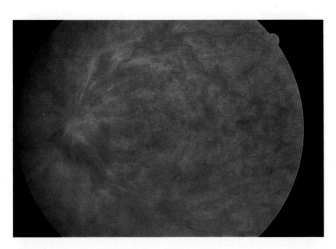

FIG. 20. Fundus photograph of central retinal vein occlusion in acute phase demonstrating diffuse intraretinal hemorrhage with dilated and tortuous retinal veins.

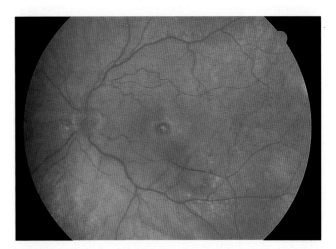

FIG. 22. Fundus photograph of central vein occlusion in chronic phase demonstrating macular pigmentation.

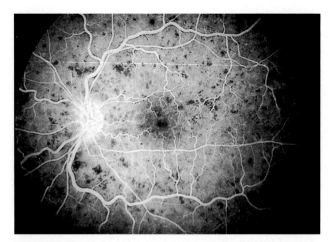

FIG. 23. Fluorescein angiogram of central vein occlusion, demonstrating perfused fluorescein pattern.

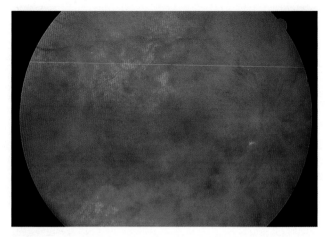

FIG. 25. Fluorescein angiogram of central retinal vein occlusion demonstrating the ischemic fluorescein pattern with large areas of nonperfusion.

nonperfused, severe, or hemorrhagic. The vision is likely to be 20/400 or worse.

The term "papillophlebitis" probably best refers to a collection of disease entities in which there is optic nerve edema with variable surrounding hemorrhagic involvement, dilation of the veins, and relatively good vision in a young, healthy adult with a good prognosis. It is suspected that the entity of "papillophlebitis" may include certain cases of optic neuritis or optic vasculitis, as well as cases of typical central vein occlusion in a young person. At this stage of our knowledge, it does not appear that "papillophlebitis" is used to represent a single distinct entity; as such, it is a term that probably should be dropped.

Recently, the nationwide collaborative Central Vein Occlusion Study Group reported baseline and early natural history information on 728 eyes with a central vein occlusion. Of particular importance was the observation that 16% of perfused eyes developed evidence of ischemia (10 or more

disc areas of nonperfusion) by the time of the first 4-month follow-up visit. In addition, of eyes that had too much intraretinal hemorrhage to judge perfusion status on the fluorescein angiogram, 83% developed evidence of an ischemic central vein occlusion.

Therapy

In the acute phase of a central vein occlusion, when there is significant intraretinal hemorrhage, as demonstrated in Fig. 26, it is frequently difficult to determine the status of capillary perfusion on the fluorescein angiogram (Fig. 24). Since the natural history report of the Central Vein Occlusion Study Group showed that 86% of such eyes are ischemic, these eyes should be evaluated frequently, every few weeks, watching for the development of iris neovascularization. To study the natural history of the complications of cen-

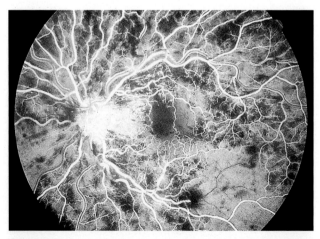

FIG. 24. Central retinal vein occlusion fluorescein angiogram demonstrating difficulty in determining capillary perfusion status because of intraretinal hemorrhage.

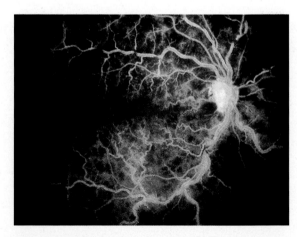

FIG. 26. Fundus photograph of acute central retinal vein occlusion with marked intraretinal hemorrhage that may prevent adequate visualization of capillary perfusion status on fluorescein angiography.

TABLE 3. *Participants in the collaborative Central Vein Occlusion Study who are ow recruiting patients*

John Clarkson, M.D., Study Director
  Miami, Florida
Daniel Finkelstein, M.D.
  Baltimore, Maryland
Clement Trempe, M.D.
  Boston, Massachusetts
David Orth, M.D.
  Chicago, Illinois
Froncie Gutman, M.D.
  Cleveland, Ohio
Lawrence Singerman, M.D.
  Cleveland, Ohio
George Bresnick, M.D.
  Madison, Wisconsin
Gabriel Coscas, M.D.
  Paris, France
Michael Klein, M.D.
  Portland, Oregan
John Clarkson, M.D.
  Reading Center, Miami, Florida
Argye Hillis, M.D.
  Coordinating Center, Scott and White Memorial Hospital,
    Temple, Texas
Donald Everett, M.D.
  National Eye Institute

tral vein occlusion, macular edema, and iris neovascularization, and to study the efficacy of laser photocoagulation for the management of these complications, a collaborative clinical trial was developed (Table 3). This clinical research study, like the previous branch vein occlusion study, was sponsored by the National Eye Institute. One branch of the Central Retinal Vein Occlusion Study examined the efficacy of panretinal photocoagulation (PRP) (Fig. 27) for the management of iris neovascularization. In comparing prophylactic PRP for ischemic vein occlusion with PRP at the first sign of iris neovascularization, the study group found that it seemed advantageous to perform PRP only after iris neovascularization first appears, because the response of early iris neovascularization to PRP in regressing is excellent; in addition, PRP at this stage will eliminate the need for prophylactic treatment of the many eyes that would never develop iris neovascularization.

To evaluate the efficacy of macular grid photocoagulation (Fig. 28) in preserving or improving central visual acuity in eyes with macular edema, the Central Vein Occlusion Study Group randomized eyes to grid treatment or observation if macular edema was documented on fluorescein angiography and visual acuity was 20/50 or worse. There was no difference between treated and untreated eyes in visual acuity at any point during the follow-up period. However, treatment clearly reduced angiographic evidence of macular edema. The results of this macular edema aspect of the randomized trial did not support a recommendation for macular grid photocoagulation. There was a suggestion of possible benefit in younger patients, but there were not enough patients younger than the age of 65 to differentiate this group sufficiently from the entire study group.

Ancillary studies within the Central Vein Occlusion Study include data regarding the electroretinogram, the relative afferent pupillary defect, and presumed retinal venous pressure; data from these ancillary studies and data regarding macular fundus features and the occurrence of occlusions in the fellow eye continues in preparation.

There is no firm research data to indicate that any systemic therapy or anticoagulation can provide prophylaxis or benefit.

Recently, McAllister and Constable provided evidence that the laser production of chorioretinal anastomosis between a blocked vein and the choroid may improve visual outcome. Further investigations of this promising technique need to be undertaken.

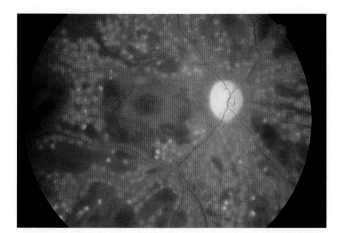

FIG. 27. Fundus photograph of panretinal photocoagulation for management of iris neovascularization secondary to ischemic central vein occlusion, immediately after treatment.

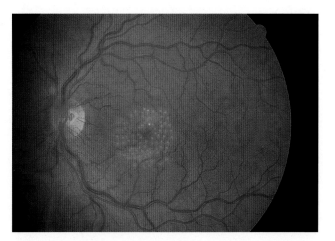

FIG. 28. Fundus photograph demonstrating the grid pattern of laser photocoagulation for the management of macular edema secondary to central vein occlusion, immediately after treatment.

BIBLIOGRAPHY

Branch Vein Occlusion Study Group. Argon laser photocoagulation for macular edema in branch vein occlusion. *Am J Ophthalmol* 1984;98:271–282.

Branch Vein Occlusion Study Group. Argon laser scatter photocoagulation for prevention of neovascularization and vitreous hemorrhage in branch vein occlusion: a randomized clinical trial. *Arch Ophthalmol* 1986;104:34–41.

Central Vein Occlusion Study Group. Baseline and early natural history report: the Central Vein Occlusion Study. *Arch Ophthalmol* 1993;111:1087–1095.

Central Vein Occlusion Study Group M Report. Evaluation of grid pattern photocoagulation for macular edema in central vein occlusion. *Ophthalmology* 1995;102:1425–1433.

Central Vein Occlusion Study Group N Report. A randomized clinical trial of early panretinal photocoagulation for ischemic central vein occlusion. *Ophthalmology* 1995;102:1434–1444.

Finkelstein D, Clarkson JG. Retinal vessel bypass: a promising new clinical investigative procedure [Editorial]. *Arch Ophthalmol* 1995;113:421–422.

Finkelstein D, Clarkson J, and the Branch Vein Occlusion Study Group. Branch and central retinal vein occlusions. In: *Focal points 1987: clinical modules for ophthalmologists;* vol 5, module 12.

Gutman FA. Evaluation of a patient with central retinal vein occlusion. *Ophthalmology* 1983;90:481–483.

Hayreh SS. Classification of central retinal vein occlusion. *Ophthalmology* 1983;90:458–474.

Kearns TP. Differential diagnosis of central retinal vein obstruction. *Ophthalmology* 1983;90:475–480.

Klein ML, Finkelstein D. Macular grid photocoagulation for macular edema in central retinal vein occlusion. *Arch Ophthalmol* 1989;107:1297–1302.

Kohner EM, Laatikainen L, Oughton J. The management of central retinal vein occlusion. *Ophthalmology* 1983;90:484–487.

McAllister IL, Constable IJ. Laser-induced chorioretinal venous anastomosis for treatment of nonischemic central retinal vein occlusion. *Arch Ophthalmol* 1995;113:456–462.

Orth DH, Patz A. Retinal branch vein occlusion. *Surv Ophthalmol* 1978;22:357–376.

Wilson DJ, Finkelstein D, Quigley HA, Green WR. Macular grid photocoagulation: an experimental study on the primate retina. *Arch Ophthalmol* 1988;106:100–105.

Practical Atlas of Retinal Disease and Therapy, Second Edition
edited by William R. Freeman,
Lippincott–Raven Publishers, Philadelphia © 1997.

• 9 •

Macular Degeneration and Related Disorders

Neil M. Bressler

DRUSEN AND RETINAL PIGMENT EPITHELIUM ABNORMALITIES

The non-neovascular features of age-related macular degeneration (AMD) include the presence of drusen and abnormalities of the retinal pigment epithelium (RPE). *Drusen* are yellow, round spots that are found predominantly in the center of the macula (Fig. 1A–C). Drusen represent an abnormal, diffuse thickening of the inner aspect of Bruch's membrane (Fig. 1D). Material mostly composed of wide-spaced collagen, with 100- to 110-nm periodicity, may collect between the plasma membrane and basement membrane of the RPE. This material, which may be 2–5 μm thick and is termed *basal laminar deposits* (Fig. 1E,F), may represent the earliest pathology of AMD or, more likely, is an aging phenomenon. Additional thicker material (7–15 μm thick) containing numerous 0.2- to 1.0-μm round-to-oval vacuoles, fine electron-dense material, and 30- to 55-nm randomly oriented collagen fibers may collect just external to the innermost aspect of the basement membrane of the RPE (just external to basal laminar deposits) and may lead to diffuse thickening of the inner aspect of Bruch's membrane. This material, which is termed *basal linear deposits* (Fig. 1E,F), may be unique to AMD rather than just an aging phenomenon. Presumably, as this material accumulates focally, or as RPE cells become depigmented in focal areas overlying this diffuse thickening, or as areas of the diffuse thickening of the inner aspect fracture from the remaining outer aspect of Bruch's membrane, the drusen become apparent clinically. The presence of large drusen typical for AMD usually have ill-defined, indistinct amorphous borders and may be referred to as soft drusen clinically. These drusen may predispose the eye to RPE atrophy or ingrowth of neovascularization from the choriocapillaris. Pinpoint yellow spots at the level of the RPE (less than 64 μm in size) probably represent lipoidal degeneration of individual RPE cells.

The significance of lipoidized RPE as a marker for AMD is not known.

RPE abnormalities include the development of atrophy and pigment clumps at the level of the RPE. Focal clumps of pigment or areas of focal hyperpigmentation (Fig. 1A) correlate histologically with clumps of pigmented cells in the subretinal space or in the outer layers of the retina. Atrophy, which may become geographic, is a circumscribed area of RPE loss, generally in the macular region. Visual acuity usually is impaired as the fovea becomes involved, because photoreceptor loss and atrophy of the choriocapillaris often accompany the RPE atrophy.

Areas of geographic atrophy secondary to AMD appear to develop and spread in one of two ways. In one scenario, areas of reticular RPE depigmentation and hyperpigmentation around the perimeter of the fovea (Fig. 2A) gradually become replaced by areas of geographic atrophy, often in a horseshoe fashion around the central fovea (Fig. 2B). Eventually, the horseshoe closes, yielding the bull's-eye pattern that may spare central fixation for many years until ultimately the fovea itself becomes involved. In the second scenario, areas of large, confluent soft drusen (Fig. 3A) evolve to multifocal areas of geographic atrophy (Fig. 3B).

At present, only low-vision aids can be offered as treatment for patients with non-neovascular AMD in whom visual loss has developed because atrophy involves the central macular region. One small prospective randomized trial with very limited follow-up (less than 24 months) suggested that zinc was associated with a retardation of visual loss when zinc-treated patients were compared with patients who took placebos. However, the authors of that study cautioned that because of the pilot nature of the study and possible side effects of long-term oral zinc administration, widespread use of zinc for AMD was not warranted. The difference in visual loss between the zinc-treated patients and the patients who

Text continues on p 176.

N.M. Bressler, M.D.: Retinal Vascular Center, Wilmer Ophthalmological Institute, Johns Hopkins University School of Medicine and Hospital, Baltimore, MD 21205-2010.

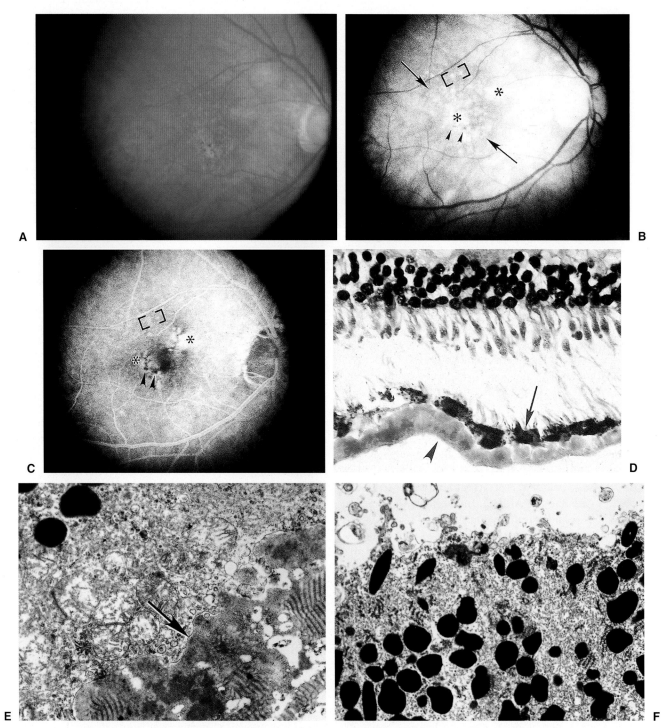

FIG. 1. Drusen and abnormalities of the retinal pigment epithelium (RPE). The color fundus photograph (**A**) and the red-free photograph (**B**) show numerous soft drusen (*between the arrows*), predominantly larger than 63 μm (for example, the drusen *between the brackets*). There are focal areas of hyperpigmentation (*arrowheads*) and focal areas of mottled hypopigmentation (*asterisks*). **C:** Frame from the early phase of the angiogram of the eye depicted in A and B. Some large drusen show slight staining (*between the brackets*). Mottled areas of hypopigmentation demonstrate more staining (*asterisks*), and focal areas of hyperpigmentation show blocked fluorescence (*arrowheads*). **D:** Area of diffuse thickening of the inner aspect of Bruch's membrane (*arrowhead*) with normal RPE and photoreceptors (periodic acid–Schiff, ×520), as well as areas of hypopigmentation (*left of the arrow*). Drusen are visualized in areas corresponding to regions where hypopigmented RPE is overlying the diffusely thickened Bruch's membrane or where localized detachment of RPE and basal linear deposit have occurred in an eye with diffuse basal linear deposit. (*continued*)

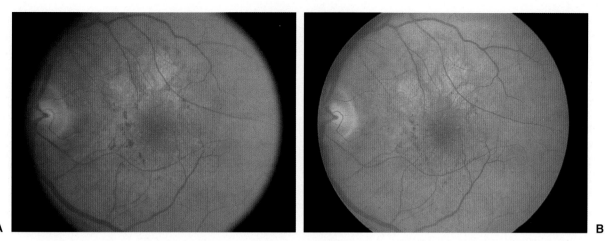

A B

FIG. 2. Geographic atrophy of the retinal pigment epithelium. **A:** The well-demarcated area of hypopigmentation with greater visibility of underlying choroidal vessels represents geographic atrophy. In addition, areas of reticular hypo- and hyperpigmentation around the perimeter of the fovea become replaced by additional areas of geographic atrophy (**B**).

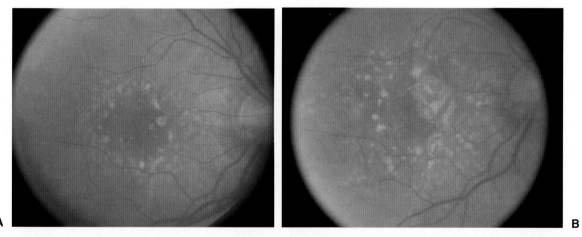

A B

FIG. 3. Geographic atrophy. Multifocal areas of large, confluent soft drusen (**A**) evolve to multifocal areas of geographic atrophy (**B**).

FIG. 1. *(Continued)* **E:** Macular area of the left eye with basal laminar deposit mostly composed of wide-spaced collagen located between the plasma membrane (*arrow*) and basement membrane (*arrowhead*) of the RPE (main figure and **inset**). A thick layer of electron-dense vesicles and amorphous material (basal linear deposit, *asterisk*) is located external to the RPE basement membrane in the inner aspect of Bruch's membrane (original magnification, ×11,000; inset, ×58,000). **F:** Macular area of the left eye with RPE, and a thin layer of basal laminar deposit composed mostly of wide-spaced collagen (*between the arrows*) located between the plasma membrane and basement membrane (*arrowhead*) of the RPE. The thick layer of electron-dense vesicular and membranous material (basal linear deposit, *asterisk* and **inset**) is located in the inner aspect of Bruch's membrane (original magnification, ×5,700; inset, ×1,500). (Courtesy of W.R. Green, M.D., Wilmer Ophthalmological Institute and *Retina* 1994;14: 130–142.)

were given placebo was greatest in cases that were followed for 12–18 months after study entry. The difference in treatment effect continued, but was less marked, with just 6 more months of follow-up (19–24 months). Without long-term follow-up, we do not know whether the effect of the zinc treatment will be temporary or actually become harmful by 36–48 months. Furthermore, the side effects of long-term zinc administration (10 years or more) in an older population are unknown. Finally, lens opacity was evaluated only subjectively in this clinical trial, so we do not know for certain whether the treatment benefit was because of an effect on progressive lens opacity, macular degenerative changes, neither, or both. Further information may be forthcoming in the Age-Related Eye Disease Study, sponsored by the National Eye Institute, in which the role of micronutrients in the progression of AMD and lens opacities will be evaluated. Until then, the treatment of patients with non-neovascular AMD should consist of education as to how they must monitor the visual acuity in each eye each day and contact the ophthalmologist promptly should they notice any sudden scotoma, metamorphopsia, or other change in vision that might herald the onset of choroidal neovascularization. In addition, low-vision aids should be made available as necessary.

CHOROIDAL NEOVASCULARIZATION

Clinical Features

Choroidal neovascularization (CNV) should be suspected in any patient (especially those over 65 with obvious drusen) who complains of metamorphopsia, central or paracentral scotoma, or any sudden, nonspecific change in central vision. These symptoms should alert the ophthalmologist to look for signs of CNV, including subretinal fluid, sub-RPE blood, subretinal lipid, elevation of the RPE, cystic changes to the sensory retina, or visualization of the choroidal neovascular vessels themselves. Fluorescein angiography should be performed and interpreted promptly to confirm whether CNV is the diagnosis and to determine whether photocoagulation is indicated. A fluorescein angiogram obtained with a 30° fundus camera that includes early-, mid-, and late-phase stereoscopic views of the macula is optimal in interpreting the location and extent of the CNV. On angiography, classic CNV will have a well-demarcated area of bright hyperfluorescence discerned during the early transit phase (Fig. 4A), with leakage in the late phase that often obscures the boundaries of the classic CNV (Fig. 4B) identified in the early phase of the angiogram. Occult CNV includes two patterns: fibrovascular pigment epithelial detachments (PEDs) and late leakage of an undetermined source. Fibrovascular PEDs demonstrate mottled, often speckled hyperfluorescence beneath irregular elevation of the pigment epithelium usually by 1 minute after dye injection (Fig. 5), with boundaries that may be well demarcated or poorly demarcated, followed by persistent staining or leakage of fluorescein at 10 minutes after dye injection. Late leakage of an undetermined source always has poorly demarcated boundaries, and the source of the late leakage does not correspond to an area of classic CNV or fibrovascular PED on review of earlier phases of the angiogram (Fig. 6). Other features that are important to recognize in determining whether laser treatment should be applied and where it should be applied include recognition of features that could obscure the boundaries of the CNV. The three most common features that may obscure CNV fluorescence are thick blood contiguous with CNV (Fig. 7); blocked fluorescence due to hyperpigmentation, fibrin, or fibrous tissue (Figs. 8 and 9); and serous (not fibrovascular) PED (Fig. 10).

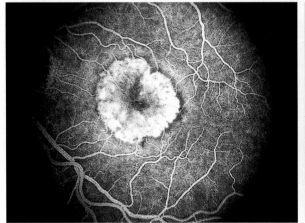
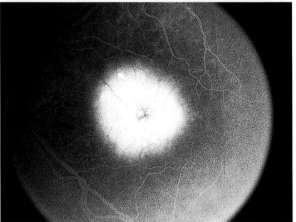

A

B

FIG. 4. Classic choroidal neovascularization (CNV). **A:** The early phase of the angiogram shows fluorescein leakage from well-demarcated CNV. **B:** The late phase of the angiogram shows pooling of dye in the subsensory retinal space, obscuring boundaries of CNV demarcated in the early phase of the angiogram. (Reprinted with permission of the American Medical Association from *Arch Ophthalmol* 1991;109:1242–1257.)

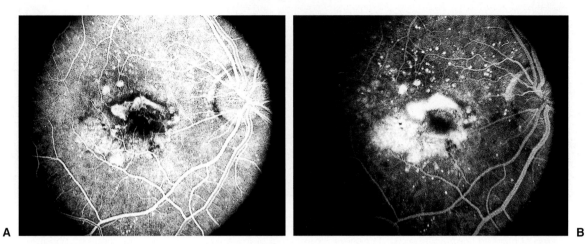

FIG. 5. Fibrovascular pigment epithelial detachment as a type of occult choroidal neovascularization (CNV). **A:** The early phase of the angiogram shows hyperfluorescence from classic CNV superior to the hypofluorescent laser scar and sharply demarcated hyperfluorescence of retinal pigment epithelium due to fibrovascular pigment epithelial detachment (indicative of occult CNV) temporal and inferior to the laser scar. **B:** The midphase of the angiogram demonstrates fluorescein leakage from both classic and occult CNV. (Reprinted with permission of the American Medical Association from *Arch Ophthalmol* 1991;109:1242–1257.)

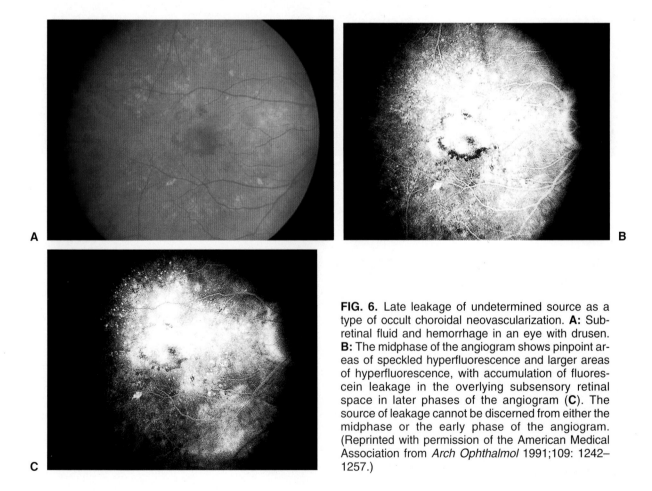

FIG. 6. Late leakage of undetermined source as a type of occult choroidal neovascularization. **A:** Subretinal fluid and hemorrhage in an eye with drusen. **B:** The midphase of the angiogram shows pinpoint areas of speckled hyperfluorescence and larger areas of hyperfluorescence, with accumulation of fluorescein leakage in the overlying subsensory retinal space in later phases of the angiogram (**C**). The source of leakage cannot be discerned from either the midphase or the early phase of the angiogram. (Reprinted with permission of the American Medical Association from *Arch Ophthalmol* 1991;109: 1242–1257.)

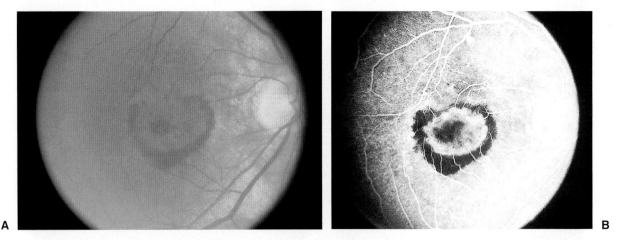

FIG. 7. Blood obscuring the boundaries of choroidal neovascularization (CNV). Fluorescence blocked by this blood (**A**) makes it impossible to determine whether, and to what extent, CNV extends under the area of blocked fluorescence (**B**). Therefore, boundaries of the entire lesion are determined by peripheral boundaries of fluorescence blocked by blood. (Reprinted with permission of the American Medical Association from *Arch Ophthalmol* 1991;109:1242–1257.

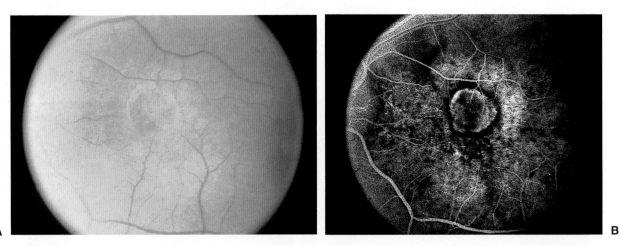

FIG. 8. Fluorescence blocked by scarring or pigment within fibrous tissue obscuring the boundaries of choroidal neovascularization. **A:** Color fundus photograph. **B:** The early phase of the angiogram shows blocked fluorescence obscuring the boundaries of choroidal neovascularization and corresponding to fibrous tissue noted in A. (Reprinted with permission of the American Medical Association from *Arch Ophthalmol* 1991;109:1242–1257.)

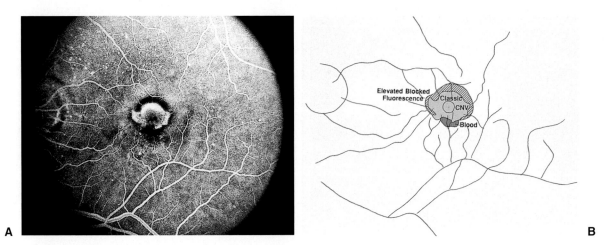

FIG. 9. Blocked fluorescence and blood obscuring boundaries of choroidal neovascularization (CNV). **A,B:** Hyperfluorescence of CNV is surrounded by fluorescence blocked by blood along the inferior edge, and fluorescence presumably blocked by hyperplastic pigment and/or fibrous tissue along the superior edge of CNV. (Reprinted with permission of the American Medical Association from *Arch Ophthalmol* 1991;109:1242–1257.)

178

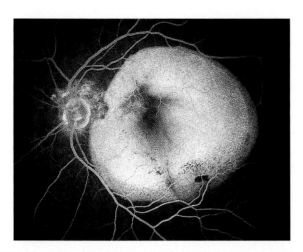

FIG. 10. Serous detachment of the retinal pigment epithelium (RPE) with uniform, smooth contours to the elevation of the RPE with uniform filling of dye beneath the detached RPE. Blocked fluorescence centrally may correspond to xanthophyll. Other blocked fluorescence along the inferior border of the pigment epithelial detachment corresponds to pigment clumping. Mottled hyperfluorescence contiguous to the temporal edge of the optic nerve may correspond to occult choroidal neovascularization.

Differential Diagnosis

CNV may be associated with a variety of pathologic entities. The presence of large, confluent drusen and/or abnormalities of the RPE (hyperpigmentation or atrophy) in either eye of a patient with CNV who is over 50 years of age will help to confirm the diagnosis of AMD. Similarly, the presence of peripapillary and peripheral focal atrophic areas of the RPE will help to confirm the diagnosis of the ocular histoplasmosis syndrome (OHS). Other common entities associated with CNV that ophthalmologists may detect include pathologic myopia, angioid streaks, optic nerve drusen, choroidal rupture, and, when no other pathology is seen, idiopathic causes. Identifying the underlying pathology associated with CNV assists ophthalmologists in determining whether laser treatment is indicated and in determining what the risks and benefits of that treatment will be. For example, if the CNV extends through the foveal center, treatment should be considered in selected cases associated with AMD in which the natural course may be extremely poor compared with laser treatment, which involves the fovea. On the other hand, subfoveal CNV secondary to OHS may not warrant consideration of photocoagulation treatment because the natural course probably is not as uniformly poor compared with cases of AMD and the natural course in OHS may not be significantly worse than lasering the fovea in those cases. Besides understanding what entities might be associated with CNV, ophthalmologists should be aware of the differential diagnosis of subretinal blood or fluid in which fluorescein angiography may identify a cause for the blood or fluid other than CNV. Subretinal blood may develop in as-

sociation with macroaneurysms, a lacquer crack in pathologic myopia, traumatic choroidal rupture, posterior vitreous detachment, choroidal tumors, or any retinal vascular disease (such as branch vein occlusion) in which intraretinal hemorrhage dissects into the subretinal space.

Subretinal fluid may be found in eyes with central serous chorioretinopathy, inflammatory conditions such as Harada's disease or posterior scleritis, uveal effusion with evidence of shifting fluid, or in association with choroidal tumors such as nevi, melanomas, cavernous hemangiomas, metastases, or osteomas.

Indications for Laser Treatment

For choroidal neovascular lesions that do not extend under the foveal center, laser treatment has been shown to decrease the risk of severe visual loss and should be considered when classic CNV is noted on angiography and the boundaries of the entire neovascular lesion and features that might be obscuring the boundaries are well demarcated. For subfoveal lesions studied by the Macular Photocoagulation Study (MPS) Group, where the CNV extends under the foveal center and where treatment will result in an immediate decrease in visual acuity, treatment usually is indicated only when the neovascular lesion is secondary to AMD, is well demarcated, and has evidence of classic CNV (although occult CNV also may be present). For new subfoveal lesions (with no prior laser treatment), the treatment benefit was greatest for small lesions (1 MPS disc area or less) with "good" or "moderate" visual acuity (20/160 or better) or medium-sized lesions (1–2 MPS disc areas) with "poor" visual acuity (20/200 or worse), and least for large lesions (2–3.5 MPS disc areas) with "good" or "moderate" visual acuity (20/160 or better). To assist in treatment recommendations, the MPS Group reported the various trends in treatment benefit for new subfoveal lesions in AMD based on the initial size in MPS disc areas (Fig. 11) and the initial visual acuity (Figs. 12 and 13). With this information, lesions in Group A (small lesions with visual acuity 20/125 or worse and medium-sized lesions with visual acuity 20/200 or worse) had a strong treatment benefit in which the risk of severe visual acuity loss always was greater in the untreated eyes. Lesions in Group B (small le-

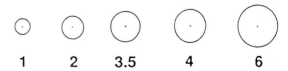

| 1 | 2 | 3.5 | 4 | 6 |

FIG. 11. The Macular Photocoagulation Study Reading Center disc area template consisting of five individual circles comparable to 1 MPS disc area (D = 4.5 mm), 2 MPS disc areas (D = 6.4 mm), 3.5 MPS disc areas (D = 8.4 mm), 4 MPS disc areas (D = 9.0 mm), and 6 MPS disc areas (D = 11.0 mm) as measured on a 30° fundus photograph assuming 3× magnification. The average disc diameter of 1.5 mm was used to calculate the diameters of the various disc area circles.

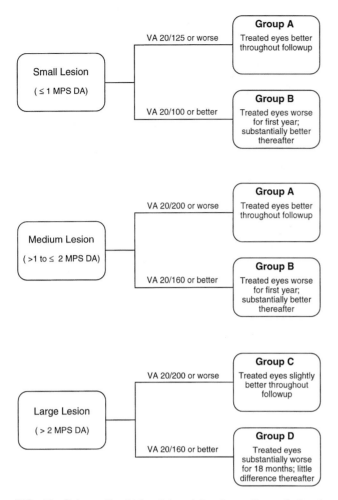

FIG. 12. Schematic aid for determining the pattern of visual loss in eyes with new subfoveal choroidal neovascularization. MPS, Macular Photocoagulation Study; DA, disc area; and VA, visual acuity. (Reprinted with permission of the American Medical Association from *Arch Ophthalmol* 1994;112: 480–488.)

sions with visual acuity 20/100 or better and medium-sized lesions with visual acuity 20/160 or better) had a moderate treatment benefit in which the risk of severe visual acuity loss was greater in untreated eyes beginning 1 year after study entry. Lesions in Group C (large lesions with visual acuity 20/200 or worse) had a small treatment benefit, so treatment usually is recommended for these lesions as well. Lesions in Group D (large lesions with visual acuity 20/160 or better) had no treatment benefit; treated eyes were worse than untreated eyes for 18 months, with little difference thereafter.

Treatment generally is not recommended for these Group D lesions. When these lesions were observed, a few eyes had loss of vision to 20/200 or worse, without a significant increase in size, so that the lesions met the criteria for Group C. Most lesions however, grew larger than 3.5 MPS disc areas, for which no treatment is recommended. Although eyes

with new lesions larger than 3.5 MPS disc areas were not eligible for this study, it is not likely that a treatment benefit would have been apparent if these lesions were included.

For recurrent subfoveal lesions (where prior laser treatment not involving the fovea had been applied and CNV recurred through the foveal center), the treatment benefit was not significantly different for larger (up to 6 MPS disc areas) versus smaller recurrent lesions or for lesions with "good" visual acuity (20/40–20/100), compared to "moderate" (20/125–20/160) or "poor" (20/200 or worse) visual acuity.

Because ophthalmologists treat many patients who have CNV secondary to AMD with the lesion already extending under the foveal center, and over half of the cases that have had prior laser treatment that did not extend under the foveal center develop recurrent CNV involving the foveal center, the results of the MPS trials on subfoveal lesions apply to a large number of patients that are likely to be treated by almost any ophthalmologist. Nevertheless, a variety of choroidal neovascular lesions do not meet these criteria and should not be considered for treatment at this time. For example, the benefits of laser treatment have not been proven for eyes with evidence of occult neovascularization without classic CNV (Fig. 14), lesions with poorly demarcated boundaries (Figs. 6 and 15), lesions with leakage from an undetermined source evident only on the late phase of the angiogram with no evidence of classic CNV (Fig. 6), lesions that are predominantly disciform scars that block fluorescence (Fig. 16), lesions with classic and occult CNV in which only the classic CNV was treated (Fig. 17), or subfoveal lesions that are larger than those studied by the MPS investigators. In fact, as just mentioned, findings from trials of laser treatment of subfoveal lesions in AMD suggest that eyes with poorly demarcated boundaries or lesions larger than 3.5 MPS disc areas at study entry probably will not gain any benefit from laser photocoagulation.

Indocyanine green (ICG) angiography has been used in cases of AMD that do not meet criteria on fluorescein angiography that likely would benefit from laser photocoagulation (because the lesions are too large, have poorly demarcated boundaries, or have occult CNV without evidence of classic CNV). In some cases, the late-phase frames on ICG angiography have demonstrated a well-demarcated plaque of fluorescence corresponding approximately to the area of occult CNV (and, if present, any component of classic CNV) identified on fluorescein angiography. Treatment of the areas corresponding to these plaques likely would not be beneficial because these lesions usually are larger than 3.5 MPS disc areas. As just described, photocoagulation of new subfoveal lesions larger than 3.5 MPS disc areas probably results in visual damage as great or greater than will occur without treatment.

In other cases, ICG angiography has demonstrated a "focal spot" of hyperfluorescence less than 1 MPS disc area in

Text continues on p 185.

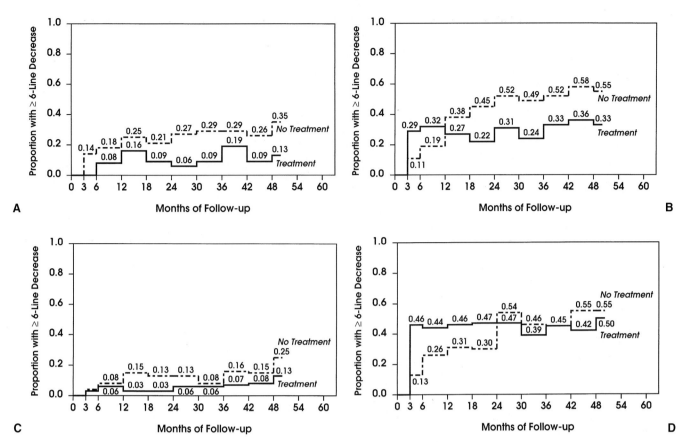

FIG. 13. The proportion of eyes in each group (from Fig. 12) with decreases in visual acuity of 6 or more lines from baseline at each specified time. (Reprinted with permission of the American Medical Association from *Arch Ophthalmol* 1994;112: 480–488.)

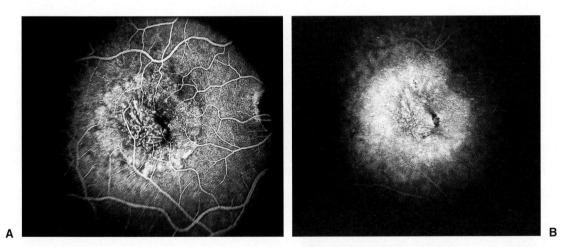

FIG. 14. A,B: Lesion with occult choroidal neovascularization (CNV) with well-demarcated boundaries, but no classic CNV. Benefits of laser treatment have not been proven for lesions such as this because no part of the lesion has classic CNV, even though boundaries of the entire lesion are well demarcated. (Reprinted with permission of the American Medical Association from *Arch Ophthalmol* 1991;109: 1242–1257.)

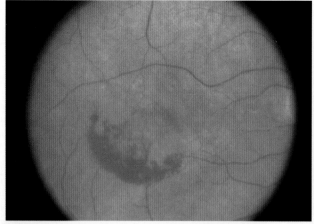

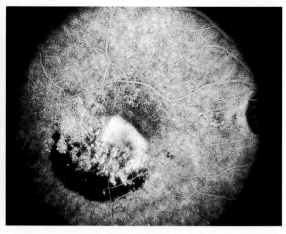

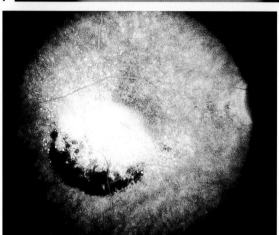

FIG. 15. Occult choroidal neovascularization (CNV) with poorly demarcated boundaries accompanied by classic CNV. **A:** Subretinal fluid and hemorrhage in an eye with drusen. **B:** The midphase of the angiogram shows classic CNV in the foveal center and speckled hyperfluorescence in an area of elevated retinal pigment epithelium (RPE) on stereoscopic pairs of photographs from the angiogram, which slopes gradually downward to surrounding flat RPE, so that sharp demarcation between elevated RPE (from fibrovascular pigment epithelial detachment) and flat RPE cannot be determined with certainty. Benefits of treatment have not been proven for lesions such as this; benefits have been shown only for lesions in which the borders of the entire lesion are well demarcated. **C:** The late phase of the angiogram shows other areas of leakage of undetermined source superior and nasal to the leakage from the classic CNV. (Reprinted with permission of the American Medical Association from *Arch Ophthalmol* 1991;109:1242–1257.)

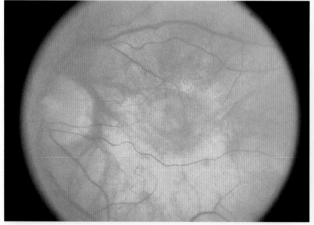

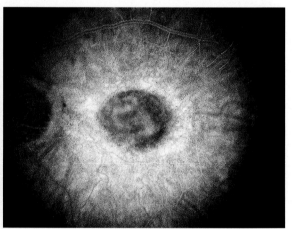

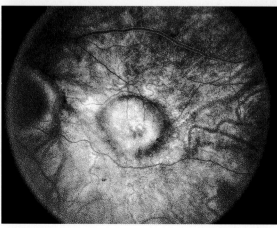

FIG. 16. Choroidal neovascularization (CNV) and scar in which fibrous tissue constitutes more than 25% of the entire lesion on color fundus photography (**A**). **B:** The midphase of the angiogram shows relatively blocked fluorescence (elevated on stereoscopic angiography) corresponding to fibrous tissue noted on the color photograph. Lesions such as this have not been shown to benefit by treatment as of this time; the lesion would not have been eligible for the Macular Photocoagulation Study trials of subfoveal lesions because the blocked fluorescence is larger (in area) than any CNV component in the eye. **C:** The late phase of the angiogram shows leakage from CNV centrally surrounded by fluorescence blocked by fibrous scar tissue. (Reprinted with permission of the American Medical Association from *Arch Ophthalmol* 1991;109:1242–1257.)

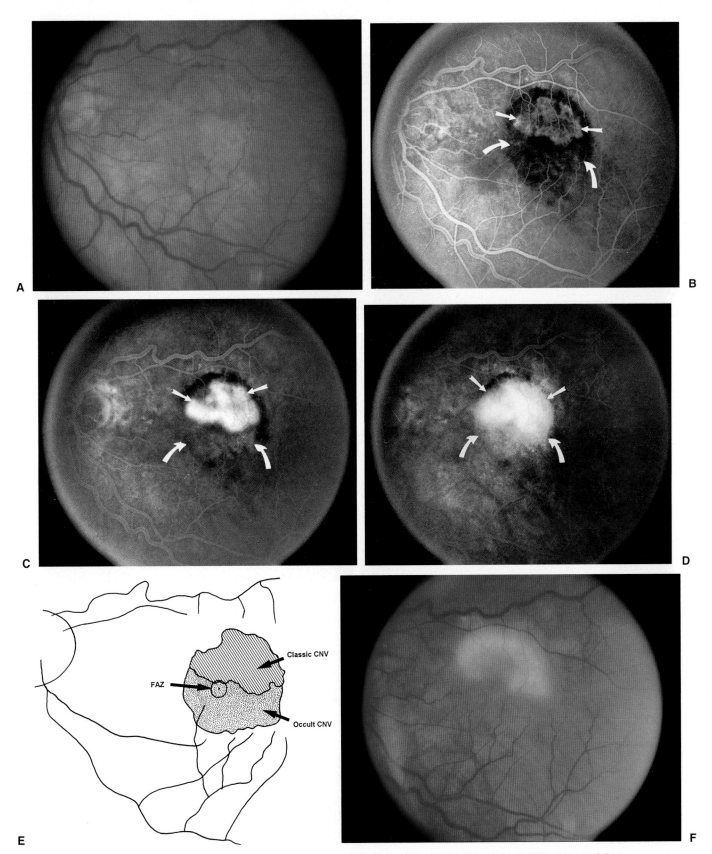

FIG. 17. The color photograph (**A**) and corresponding early (**B**), middle (**C**), and late (**D**) phases of the fluorescein angiogram show a lesion consisting of juxtafoveal classic choroidal neovascularization (CNV) (*straight arrows*) and subfoveal occult CNV (*curved arrows*). Identification of occult CNV is facilitated by observing stereoscopic frames of the angiogram in which irregular elevation of the retinal pigment epithelium, corresponding to the occult CNV, can be identified. The sketch (**E**) illustrates the extent of classic and occult CNV. Color photograph **F** shows laser photocoagulation of classic CNV component of lesion. The foveal side of treatment was less intense than required by the protocol. (*continued*)

183

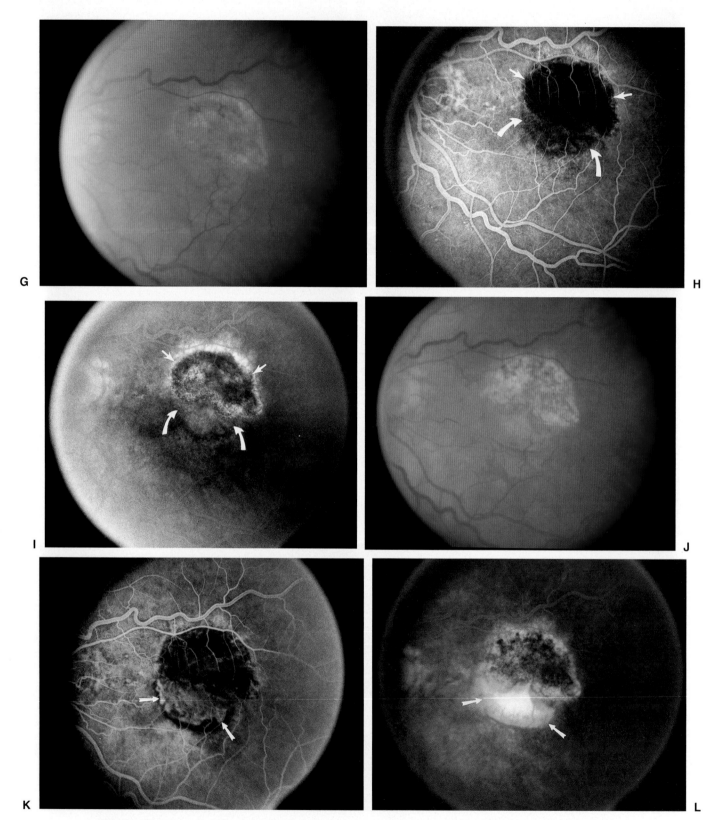

FIG. 17. *(Continued)* At 6 weeks after treatment, the color photograph (**G**) and early phase (**H**) and late phase (**I**) of the fluorescein angiogram show hypofluorescence of the treatment area (H and I, *straight arrows*) and persistent staining of occult CNV (*curved arrows*). At 3 months after treatment, the color photograph (**J**) and early phase (**K**) and late phase (**L**) of the fluorescein angiogram show classic CNV (*arrows*) occupying the area where untreated occult CNV was apparent previously, with continued growth of classic CNV surrounding the area of laser treatment 1 year after treatment [color photograph (**M**) and midphase fluorescein angiogram (**N**)]. (Reprinted with permission of the American Medical Association from *Arch Ophthalmol* 1996;114.

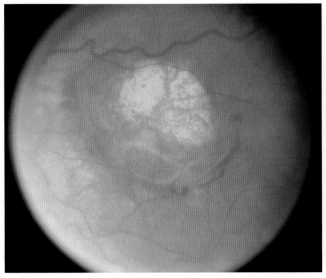
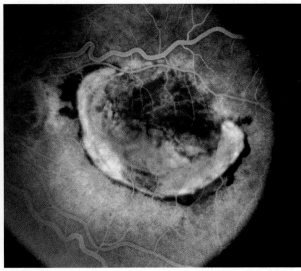

M

N

FIG. 17. *(Continued)*

size, usually not extending into the foveal center, and occasionally at an area where a retinal vessel dives externally toward the RPE. Case series evaluating laser photocoagulation of these focal spots have suggested that treatment of these lesions within a plaque of hyperfluorescence often does not result in resolution of subretinal fluid or in stabilization of vision. On the other hand, treatment of focal spots at the edge of an area of elevated retinal pigment epithelium was suggested to be beneficial in some cases by causing resolution of subretinal fluid, flattening of the area of RPE that was elevated prior to treatment, and stabilization of visual acuity. It is unknown, however, whether no treatment would have just as many (or more) instances of stabilized vision (since no controls, without treatment, were evaluated in these case series). Furthermore, these series had no standardized refraction or visual acuity measurements either before or after treatment; follow-up was limited in most cases and the outcome of cases lost to follow-up may have influenced the results.

Similar limitations apply to interpreting the results of the few case series in which ICG angiography was obtained in lesions in which a large area of hemorrhage potentially obscured CNV and in which ICG was used in an attempt to identify fluorescence from CNV that otherwise was not detected on fluorescein angiography. Although treatment of these areas of ICG fluorescence in selected cases resulted in resolution of subretinal fluid and hemorrhage with stabilization or improvement of vision, it is unknown how these cases would have fared if left untreated (certainly subretinal hemorrhage will clear without treatment) or whether successfully treated cases would have had stabilization or improvement of vision if a treatment plan was based on fluorescein angiography.

Therefore, there are no *strong* data to support treatment recommendations based on findings detected by ICG angiography. The data available suggest that selected cases should be considered for evaluation and treatment within the context of controlled clinical trials with an adequate sample size and follow-up.

Some of the most worthwhile information for determining the risks and benefits of laser treatment comes from randomized, clinical trials that evaluate how this treatment affects the natural course of the disease. However, the information from these studies can only be used as a strong guideline to assist ophthalmologists in deciding whether laser treatment should be recommended for particular patients. Patients should understand that the goal of treatment is to coagulate the neovascular lesion and prevent severe visual loss rather than to restore normal visual acuity. Furthermore, patients should be aware that the laser creates a permanent scotoma and, in cases in which treatment will involve the foveal center, patients also should be aware that treatment will cause an immediate decrease in visual acuity, although the decrease more often will be less than what might otherwise occur by 1 or 2 years should the lesions be left untreated. Finally, patients should be advised that the laser treatment does not necessarily prevent future neovascular complications either in the treated eye or in the other eye that could lead to additional visual loss.

Laser Treatment and Follow-up

Preparation

To reduce the possibility that the CNV has grown larger than that shown on the angiogram used to guide the boundaries of the treatment, an angiogram should be obtained preferably no more than 96 hours before treatment. Ideally, an angiogram obtained on the same day of treatment will minimize this possibility. Careful evaluation of vascular landmarks in the patient's fundus in comparison with landmarks concurrently viewed on a projection of a fluorescein angiogram during treatment should enable the ophthalmologist to identify the boundaries of the lesion with respect to these landmarks with confidence and accuracy. This evaluation should help to avoid inadvertent photocoagulation to areas of the retina that are not involved with the neovascular lesion, thereby avoiding inadvertent loss of visual acuity due to treatment of the retina not involved with part of the neovascular lesion.

Retrobulbar or peribulbar anesthesia should be used whenever the treating ophthalmologist judges that movement of the globe might compromise ability to obtain the end point of a uniform white laser burn and the ability to obtain adequate coverage of the lesion without unnecessarily damaging the uninvolved retina.

Retinal Area to Receive Laser Treatment

The immediate goal of treatment is to photocoagulate the entire area of the neovascular lesion. Additional areas of treatment in MPS protocols varied, depending on the location of the neovascular lesion. For extrafoveal lesions, addi-

tional treatment extended 100 μm beyond any adjacent blood, pigment ring circumferentially surrounding the lesion, or other blocked fluorescence surrounding the lesion. For juxtafoveal lesions, treatment was required to extend 100 μm beyond the neovascular lesion on the border away from the fovea, and 100 μm into any blood present on the foveal side if the hyperfluorescence from the neovascular lesion itself was 100 μm or further from the center of the foveal avascular zone. Otherwise, no additional treatment was administered beyond the hyperfluorescence from the CNV on the foveal side. For subfoveal lesions, treatment was to extend 100 μm beyond the peripheral boundaries of all lesion components except blood. Treatment was required to cover, but not necessarily extend 100 μm and beyond, areas of blocked fluorescence due to thick blood (Fig. 7 and Fig. 18). For recurrent neovascular lesions, treatment was to extend 300 μm into the previous treatment scar at the previous treatment scar–recurrent neovascular lesion interface (Fig. 19). Feeder vessels, when present in recurrent lesions, also received treatment that extended 100 μm beyond the

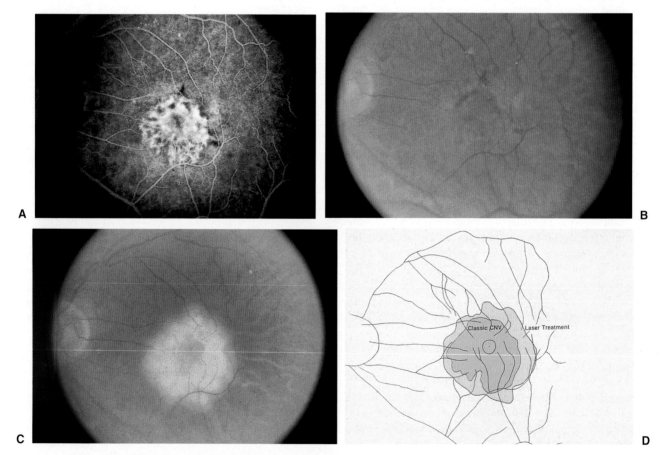

FIG. 18. A: The early phase of the fluorescein angiogram shows classic choroidal neovascularization with well-demarcated borders. Note the small area of blocked fluorescence along the superior and temporal borders of the lesion that correspond to small areas of blood seen on the color fundus photograph (**B**). **C:** The same lesion 12–48 hours after laser photocoagulation. Note the uniform whitening of the retina. **D:** The composite drawing made from the fluorescein angiogram (**A**) and the treatment photograph (**C**) demonstrates that heavy laser treatment (*yellow*) covered subfoveal choroidal neovascularization (*green*). (Reprinted with permission of the American Medical Association from *Arch Ophthalmol* 1991;109:1242–1257.)

lateral borders of the vessels and 300 μm radially beyond the base (origin) of the feeder vessel.

Treatment Parameters

The MPS protocol for treatment to the lesion boundaries specifies a 0.2- to 0.5-second treatment to a 200- to 500-μm spot. Photocoagulation is applied first to the border of the retinal area to be treated. The foveal side of the planned treatment is usually lasered first; subsequently, if any bleeding occurs during treatment, one need not be concerned about blood obscuring the foveal side of the border to be treated. The remaining boundaries of the area to be treated are then lasered. Finally, the remainder of the area to be treated is

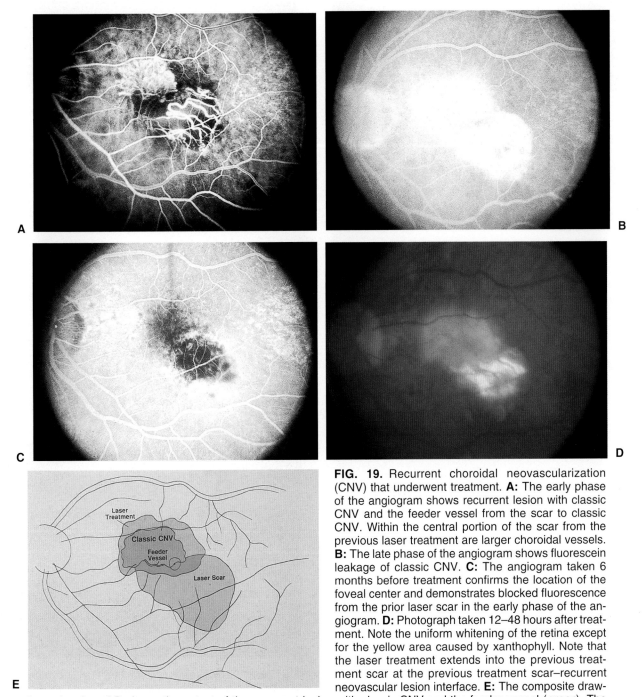

FIG. 19. Recurrent choroidal neovascularization (CNV) that underwent treatment. **A:** The early phase of the angiogram shows recurrent lesion with classic CNV and the feeder vessel from the scar to classic CNV. Within the central portion of the scar from the previous laser treatment are larger choroidal vessels. **B:** The late phase of the angiogram shows fluorescein leakage of classic CNV. **C:** The angiogram taken 6 months before treatment confirms the location of the foveal center and demonstrates blocked fluorescence from the prior laser scar in the early phase of the angiogram. **D:** Photograph taken 12–48 hours after treatment. Note the uniform whitening of the retina except for the yellow area caused by xanthophyll. Note that the laser treatment extends into the previous treatment scar at the previous treatment scar–recurrent neovascular lesion interface. **E:** The composite drawing using A and D shows the extent of the recurrent lesion with classic CNV and the feeder vessel (*green*). The drawing also shows the scar from the previous laser treatment (*light brown*) and the extent of the laser treatment (*yellow*). The treatment extends at least 100 μm beyond the CNV and at least 300 μm into the scar from the previous treatment (*orange*). (Reprinted with permission of the American Medical Association from *Arch Ophthalmol* 1991;109:1219–1231.)

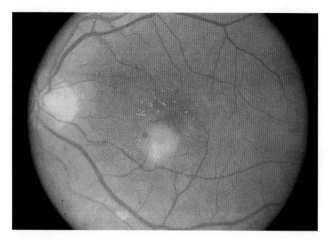

FIG. 20. Treatment intensity standard. The treatment protocol from the Macular Photocoagulation Study specified a uniform white burn at least as intense as the treatment standard. (Reprinted with permission of the American Medical Association from *Arch Ophthalmol* 1989;107:344–352.)

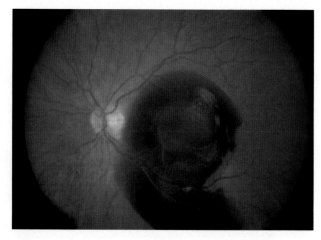

FIG. 21. Hemorrhagic detachment of the retinal pigment epithelium in which blood from a choroidal neovascular lesion is noted beneath or exterior to the retinal pigment epithelium.

lasered with overlapping burns of sufficient intensity to produce a uniformly white burn (Figs. 18 and 19).

Intensity of Laser Lesion

The desired end point for the intensity of the laser lesion is the creation of a uniformly white lesion. Ophthalmologists can achieve this end point either by applying initially white laser burns that meet or exceed the intensity illustrated by a standard photograph from the MPS or by applying lighter, gray–white laser spots that repeatedly overlap until the entire laser lesion is a uniform white treatment burn at least as white as the treatment intensity standard. Note that the published treatment intensity standard was the minimum treatment intensity that was recommended (Fig. 20).

PIGMENT EPITHELIAL DETACHMENTS AND RIPS

Retinal Pigment Epithelial Detachments in Age-Related Macular Degeneration

Various changes in AMD may result in RPE elevation or RPE detachment (RPED) as seen on stereoscopic biomicroscopic or angiographic evaluation. RPEDs secondary to AMD that may be readily recognized and that probably should be differentiated include (1) fibrovascular PEDs (an angiographic feature of occult CNV) as in Figs. 5 and 14, (2) elevated areas of RPE that block fluorescence caused by hyperplastic pigment and/or fibrous tissue as in Figs. 8 and 9, (3) serous RPEDs as in Fig. 10, (4) hemorrhagic RPEDs in which blood from a choroidal neovascular lesion is noted beneath or exterior to the RPE (Fig. 21), and (5) drusenoid

RPEDs in which large areas of confluent, soft drusen are noted (Fig. 22).

Elevated blocked fluorescence may be differentiated from fibrovascular PEDs and serous RPEDs, in that blocked fluorescence is noted within the area of elevated RPE throughout the angiogram. One of the more difficult differentiations is between fibrovascular PED (a type of occult CNV) and serous RPED (an angiographic feature in which the fluorescent pattern obscures one's ability to determine whether CNV is present within the area of the serous PED). Using descriptions from the MPS, fibrovascular PED (as a subset of occult CNV) has been distinguished from classic serous RPED, in that the former is slow filling with a stippled ap-

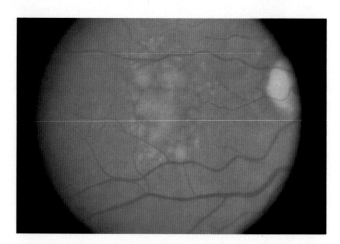

FIG. 22. Drusenoid retinal pigment epithelial detachment in which large areas of confluent, soft drusen are noted. On stereoscopic fundus photographs, the areas of drusen appear as elevated retinal pigment epithelium, presumably because this area represents fracturing of the diffusely thickened inner aspect of Bruch's membrane from the remainder of Bruch's membrane.

pearance to the surface of the RPE by the midphase of the angiogram and may have pooling of dye in the overlying subsensory retinal space in the late phase. However, the latter shows uniform bright hyperfluorescence in the early phase with a smoother contour to the RPE by the midphase and little, if any, leakage into the overlying sensory retinal space by the late phase.

A hemorrhagic RPED (Fig. 21) will block choroidal fluorescence as previously described for fluorescence blocked by hyperplastic pigment and/or fibrous tissue. In hemorrhagic RPEDs, however, the dark appearance on biomicroscopy caused by the moundlike collection of blood beneath the RPE will help to differentiate it from areas of elevated blocked fluorescence due to hyperplastic pigment and/or fibrous tissue. Occasionally, a hemorrhagic RPED may be mistaken for a choroidal melanoma; usually, though, hemorrhagic RPEDs will not echographically demonstrate the low internal reflectivity seen characteristically in choroidal melanomas.

The final feature of AMD that will appear as elevated or detached RPE is a drusenoid RPED (Fig. 22) or extensive areas of large confluent drusen. Drusenoid RPEDs can be distinguished from serous RPEDs in that drusenoid RPEDs will fluoresce faintly during the transit and do not progress to bright hyperfluorescence in the later phase of the angiogram. In contrast, serous RPEDs will fluoresce brightly in the early transit phase and remain brightly hyperfluorescent in the late phase. In addition, serous RPEDs usually will have a smoother, sharper boundary compared with drusenoid RPEDs. Drusenoid RPEDs can be distinguished from fibrovascular PEDs in occult CNV by noting that fibrovascular PEDs will show areas of stippled hyperfluorescence with persistence of staining or leakage within 5–10 minutes of dye injection. Detachments associated with large, soft, confluent drusen are usually smaller, more shallow, and more irregular in outline than serous RPEDs or fibrovascular PEDs. In addition, the drusenoid RPEDs often will have reticulated pigment clumping overlying the large, soft, confluent drusen.

Treatment of a serous RPED may be indicated when one is treating a subfoveal lesion and the RPED is a minor component of that lesion (that is, the area of the serous PED is smaller than the area of the CNV). In the MPS trials, fewer than 5% of the patients entered into the study had serous RPEDs. Most RPEDs in cases with AMD, and in our practice, have fibrovascular PEDs (Figs. 5 and 14), not serous PEDs (Fig. 10). Furthermore, the RPED should have well-demarcated boundaries so that the ophthalmologist knows where to treat and where not to treat the retina in order to cover the CNV in its entirety as well as areas that may be obscuring the boundaries of the CNV (including a serous PED). In this circumstance, laser treatment is applied to the entire area of CNV and the entire area of the serous PED since it is unknown whether the serous PED is obscuring additional CNV. Drusenoid RPEDs should not be included as a component to be treated in conjunction with subfoveal CNV, because this pattern is not suspected to be obscuring the boundaries of any CNV.

Most cases with serous RPEDs do not meet criteria for which treatment has been shown to be beneficial, because the boundaries of any CNV accompanying the serous PED usually are not well demarcated or because the CNV is not the major component of the lesion to be treated (that is, the area of CNV is less than the area of the serous RPED). No definitive treatment benefit has been shown for lesions that consist predominantly or entirely of an RPED; such lesions usually are observed unless classic CNV develops.

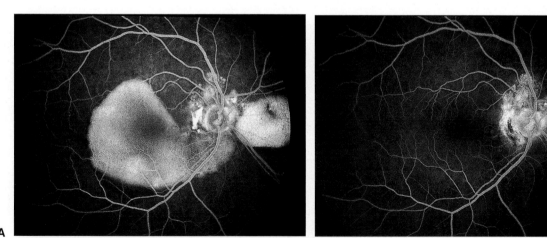

FIG. 23. Treatment of extrafoveal choroidal neovascularization (CNV) contiguous with serous detachment of the retinal pigment epithelium (RPE) in which the serous detachment extends through the foveal center, and only the CNV itself is treated. **A:** Pretreatment angiogram showing peripapillary CNV in an extrafoveal location contiguous to uniform smooth-contoured elevated RPE with uniform filling of dye corresponding to the serous detachment of the RPE temporal to the optic nerve, as well as a smaller detachment of the RPE nasal to the optic nerve. **B:** The angiogram 6 months after treatment shows staining of the laser scar on the temporal aspect of optic nerve, flattening of the RPE detachment temporally, and persistent peripapillary, poorly demarcated CNV and RPE detachment nasal to the optic nerve.

On rare occasions, patients will present with extrafoveal classic CNV contiguous to a serous RPED in which the serous detachment extends through the foveal center. In case reports about these lesions in which only the extrafoveal CNV is treated, the result is prompt flattening of the serous RPED with improvement of vision in selected cases (Fig. 23). Nevertheless, many of these patients have developed recurrent CNV, often within the area previously occupied by the RPED, with subsequent extensive scarring and visual loss. More often, classic extrafoveal CNV is associated with fibrovascular PED through the foveal center in which treatment of the extrafoveal CNV, alone, has not been shown to be of any benefit.

Tears or Rips in the Retinal Pigment Epithelium

An acute tear or rip in the RPE may occur spontaneously (Fig. 24) or during laser photocoagulation of a choroidal neovascular lesion. Visual acuity may fall precipitously, especially if CNV is present and has an opportunity to destroy foveal photoreceptors. In the absence of CNV, RPE tears through the fovea may be associated with preservation of good central visual acuity provided that the torn area, and not the scrolled-up RPE, underlies the foveal center. Angiography demonstrates early, bright, sharply demarcated hyperfluorescence within the torn region (Fig. 24B). Blocked fluorescence corresponding to heaped-up RPE will be noted at one side of the lesion. The bright hyperfluorescence presumably corresponds to fluorescein dye within the choriocapillaris that quickly leaks into the choroidal and scleral tissues, and is not blocked by pigment that is normally otherwise present within the overlying RPE. No leakage of dye is seen if no overlying sensory retinal detachment is present. The absence of a sensory retinal detachment over a tear in the RPE may be due to the higher osmotic pressure of the choroid compared with the subretinal space, which allows fluid to be removed rapidly from the subretinal space when the tight junctions of the RPE are absent and unable to prevent free movement of fluid.

MASQUERADES OF AGE-RELATED MACULAR DEGENERATION

A variety of maculopathies should be differentiated from CNV associated with AMD, especially since these other conditions have different prognoses from CNV associated with AMD. Most importantly, laser treatment is not indicated in these other conditions in the absence of CNV.

Basal Laminar Drusen

Patients with "basal laminar" drusen, also labeled cuticular drusen, may develop a pseudovitelliform detachment consisting of yellowish material at the level of the outer retina that may mimic the appearance of drusen associated with subretinal fluid from CNV. These unusual drusen, which correspond on clinicopathologic reports to an extremely thickened inner aspect of Bruch's membrane with overlying nodular excrescences, usually present as innumerable, small, uniformly sized, discretely round, slightly raised yellow subretinal lesions seen best with angiography in mid-

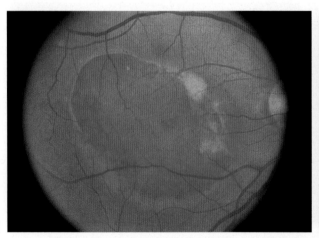
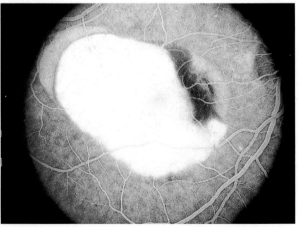

A   B

FIG. 24. Tear or rip of the retinal pigment epithelium (RPE). **A:** Color fundus photograph showing a large tear of the RPE, with the *orange* area representing tear. Nasal to the orange area is increased pigmentation from heaped-up RPE. **B:** The corresponding fluorescein angiogram shows bright, sharply demarcated hyperfluorescence within the torn region and blocked fluorescence corresponding to the heaped-up RPE at the nasal side of the lesion. (Reprinted with permission of the American Medical Association from *Arch Ophthalmol* 1990;108:1694–1697.)

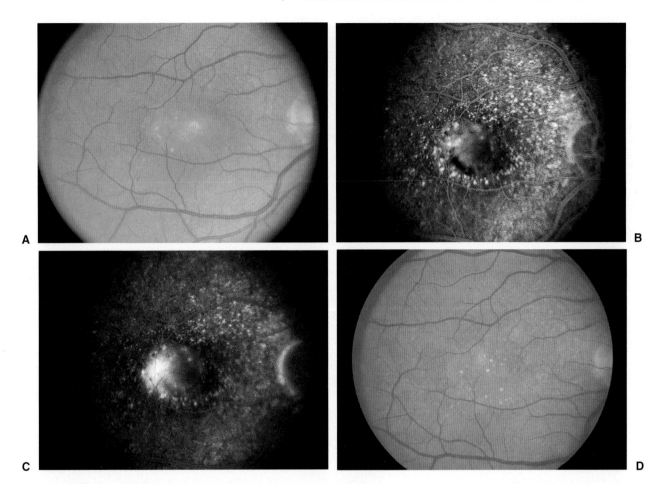

FIG. 25. Basal laminar or cuticular drusen. **A:** Innumerable, small, uniformly sized, discrete, round, slightly raised, yellow subretinal lesions throughout the posterior pole, as well as large, dull-yellow pseudovitelliform detachment in the center of macula. **B:** Angiography helps to highlight basal laminar drusen. In addition, hypofluorescence, presumably from the associated pseudovitelliform detachment, blocks the underlying fluorescence of the choriocapillaris. **C:** Progressive staining of pseudovitelliform detachment material becomes apparent in the middle and late phases of the angiogram. **D:** With time, the pseudovitelliform detachment can clear spontaneously often leaving discrete, large, yellow–white deposits.

dle-aged patients (Fig. 25). The yellowish material that may be mistaken for subretinal fluid from CNV appears to obscure details of the RPE, suggesting that it is present between the sensory retina and the RPE. On angiography, these detachments show early hypofluorescence (Fig. 25B), presumably due to the ability of the yellowish material to block the underlying fluorescence of the choriocapillaris. Progressive staining of the yellowish material becomes apparent in the middle and late phases of the angiogram (Fig. 25C), presumably due to the incompetence of the RPE's zonula occludnes, which fails to keep fluorescein from diffusing from the choriocapillaris to the subsensory retinal space, with subsequent staining of the yellowish material.

Because this hyperfluorescence may mimic CNV, one must recognize this appearance in order to avoid unnecessary photocoagulation of a pseudovitelliform detachment.

The natural course of these detachments can be spontaneous clearing (Fig. 25D), with extremely slow development of atrophy, or clearing associated with marked geographic atrophy. These pseudovitelliform detachments should be differentiated from true vitelliform detachments seen in Best's disease (in which the electro-oculogram will be abnormal) and from pattern dystrophies of the RPE that also may show pseudovitelliformlike detachments.

Patients with basal laminar or cuticular drusen have a diseased Bruch's membrane and are at risk of developing CNV. Therefore, careful scrutiny of any bright hyperfluorescence that appears to leak in these patients must be performed in order to determine whether the fluorescence is due to the presence of CNV or progressive staining of the pseudovitelliform detachment. Sometimes this differentiation is extremely difficult to make.

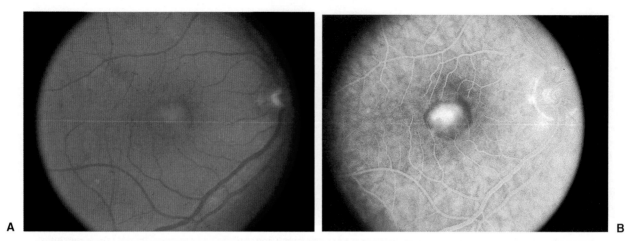

A

B

FIG. 26. Pattern dystrophy of the retinal pigment epithelium. **A:** Typical pattern dystrophy with greenish discoloration at the level of the retinal pigment epithelium surrounded by a dull-yellowish material termed a pseudovitelliform detachment. Angiography shows areas of blocked fluorescence, as well as very prominent staining and persistent hyperfluorescence in the later phases of the angiogram (**B**). If the boundaries of the hyperfluorescence on the early phase and midphase of the angiogram are compared carefully with the late phase, no leakage or spread of dye beyond the boundaries defined in the early and midphases can be detected in the late phase, confirming that these changes do indeed represent staining rather than leakage associated with choroidal neovascularization. Nevertheless, because of the moderately intense hyperfluorescence seen in the late phases of the angiogram, often in association with the pseudovitelliform detachment, these lesions may be mistaken for choroidal neovascularization secondary to age-related macular degeneration.

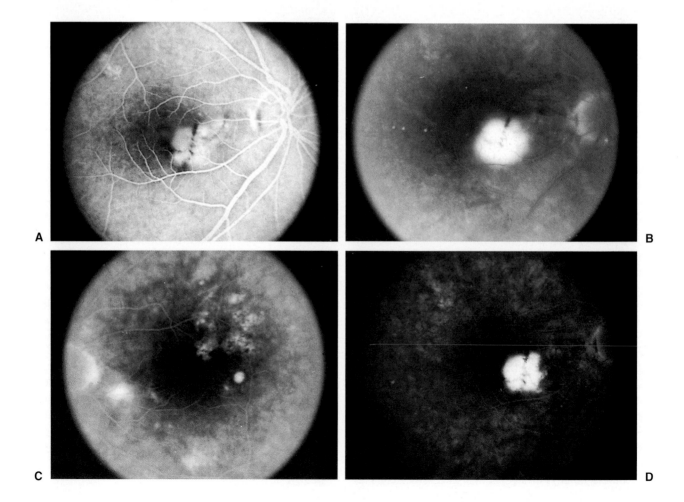

A

B

C

D

Pattern Dystrophy of the Retinal Pigment Epithelium

Patients with pattern dystrophy of the RPE (adult vitelliform dystrophy, adult-onset foveal pigment epithelial dystrophy, butterfly-shaped pigment dystrophy, or reticulated dystrophy of the pigment epithelium) will show a reticulated pattern of pigmentation, usually fairly symmetrical between the two eyes and often in the absence of more typical soft drusen (Fig. 26). These dystrophies may have a yellowish deposition at the level of the outer retina, often with a central area of greenish hyperpigmentation (sometimes seen best with transillumination of the yellowish material), and are occasionally surrounded by a petaloid pattern of hyperpigmentation more obvious on angiography (Fig. 26B).

Central Serous Chorioretinopathy

Occasionally, central serous chorioretinopathy will occur in patients over 65 years of age, suggesting that the source of the subretinal fluid could be CNV secondary to AMD. For example, the case shown in Fig. 27 presented with a somewhat flattened PED associated with subretinal fluid identified on fluorescein angiography. CNV secondary to AMD was suspected because the patient was 65 years old, had evidence of the RPED, and had subretinal fluid through the fovea (Fig. 27B). However, other features to suggest central serous chorioretinopathy included the presence of multifocal areas of mottled RPE atrophy in the fellow eye with otherwise normal appearing RPE (Fig. 27C), as well as the absence of soft drusen in both eyes. Furthermore, no evidence of classic CNV was noted, no evidence of fibrovascular PED was noted, and the uniform collection of fluid in the sensory retinal space was more typical for central serous than for late leakage of an undetermined source of occult neovascularization in AMD. Eyes with late leakage of an undetermined source from occult CNV in AMD usually have speckled hyperfluorescence associated with poorly demarcated areas of leakage in the middle and late phases of the angiogram. No treatment was recommended and, at the follow-up within 4 weeks, the subretinal fluid completely resolved (Fig. 27D) without atrophy or disciform scarring.

COMMON PITFALLS IN TREATING CHOROIDAL NEOVASCULARIZATION

The most common pitfalls in treating CNV probably include failure to recognize the presence of CNV, failure to recognize the entire extent of CNV, failure to cover the foveal side of CNV with laser treatment, failure to cover CNV with a laser of adequate intensity, and failure to recognize recurrent CNV following laser treatment.

Failure to Recognize the Presence of Choroidal Neovascularization

Failure to recognize the presence of CNV may occur when there are minimal signs of CNV. Unfortunately, cases with minimal signs of CNV may be cases that are most likely to have a significant benefit of treatment compared with no treatment. For example, the case in Fig. 28 represents an eye in which cataract surgery was contemplated because of decreased central visual acuity. An ophthalmologist who is looking for obvious areas of subretinal fluid or hemorrhage to determine whether CNV is contributing to decreased central visual acuity may not detect CNV in this eye. Only with careful contact-lens biomicroscopy using a thin-slit beam can one detect slight elevation of the sensory retinal vessels from the level of the RPE superonasal to the foveal center, with a loss of the normal concavity to the surface of the sensory retina in this area. Fluorescein angiography helped to confirm the presence of CNV in this eye (Fig. 28B).

Failure to Detect the Entire Extent of Choroidal Neovascularization

Failure to detect the entire extent of CNV may lead to erroneous management. Because the goal of treatment is to obliterate the neovascular lesion in its entirety, failure to identify a portion of the neovascular lesion may lead to incomplete coverage of the neovascular lesion, with subsequent persistent or recurrent neovascularization. For example, the early phase of the angiogram of the case in Fig. 29A suggests that only extrafoveal classic CNV is present, so one

Text continues on p 196.

FIG. 27. Central serous chorioretinopathy masquerading as choroidal neovascularization secondary to age-related macular degeneration. **A:** The early phase of the angiogram shows bright hyperfluorescence nasal to fovea. **B:** In late phases, subretinal fluid has collected beneath the sensory retina extending into the foveal center. Because the patient was 65 years old and had evidence of subretinal fluid through the fovea as well as detachment of the retinal pigment epithelium (RPE), corresponding to the bright area of hyperfluorescence nasal to the fovea in the early phase of the angiogram, choroidal neovascularization secondary to age-related macular degeneration was suspected. Multifocal areas of mottled RPE atrophy in the fellow eye (**C**) with otherwise normal-appearing RPE, as well as the absence of soft drusen in both eyes, suggest that these changes may be from central serous chorioretinopathy. No treatment was recommended and, within 4 weeks, the subretinal fluid completely resolved (**D**).

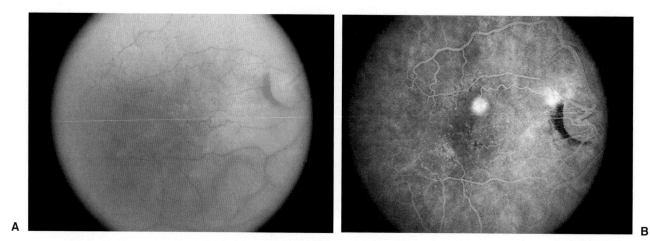

FIG. 28. Minimal signs of choroidal neovascularization in small lesions (**A**). Cataract surgery was contemplated because of some lenticular opacity in the presence of decreased vision. However, fluorescein angiography (**B**) revealed a small area of bright hyperfluorescence at the level of the retinal pigment epithelium that leaked in the late phase of the angiogram.

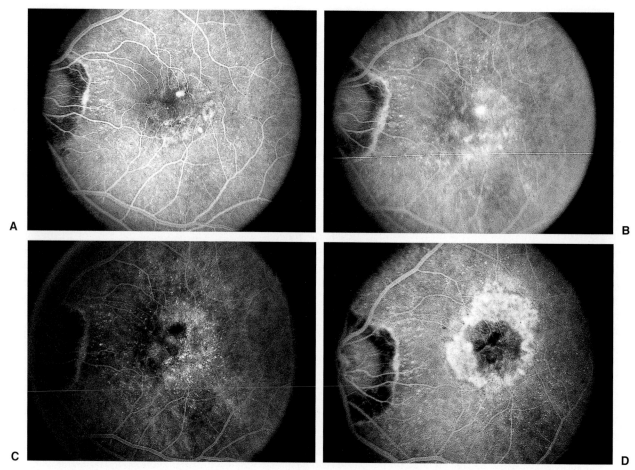

FIG. 29. Failure to detect the entire extent of choroidal neovascularization (CNV) from the early phase of the angiogram alone. **A:** The early phase of the angiogram suggests that only a small area of extrafoveal classic CNV is present, so one might erroneously consider treating this eye as an extrafoveal lesion only. Failure to look at stereoscopic frames from the middle and late phases of the angiogram (**B**) will lead to an inability to identify areas of occult CNV surrounding the CNV. Only the classic CNV was treated (**C**) and, at follow-up, disciform scarring developed in the area that was left untreated (**D**).

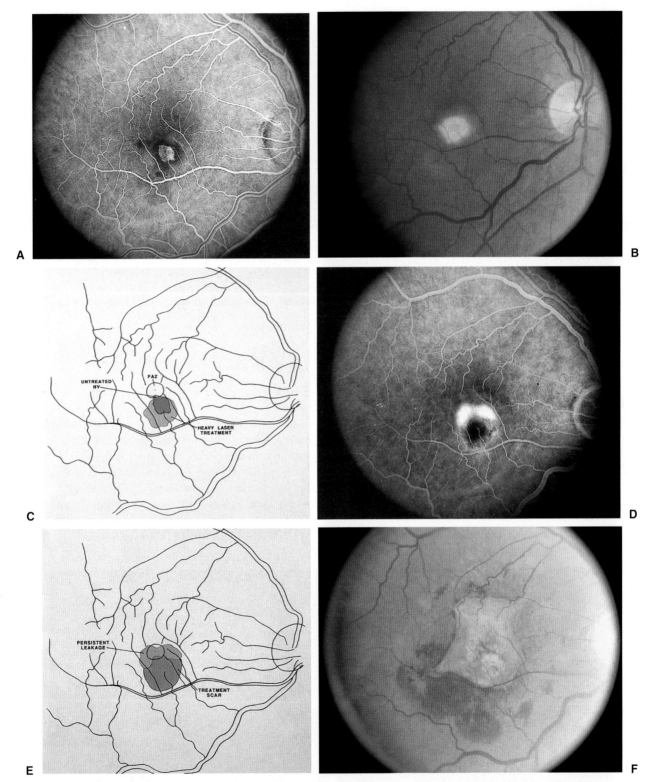

FIG. 30. Failure to cover choroidal neovascularization (CNV) completely with laser on the foveal side of lesion. **A:** Pretreatment angiogram of classic CNV. **B:** Posttreatment color photograph. **C:** Sketch made by superimposing the posttreatment photograph (B) on the pretreatment angiogram (A). The treatment is of adequate intensity, but the sketch shows that some of the CNV (*green*) is not covered by the heavy treatment (*orange*). **D:** The angiogram 6 weeks after treatment shows persistent leakage extending through the foveal center on the superior aspect of the scar corresponding to the area of incomplete treatment from 6 weeks previously. **E:** The sketch shows fluorescein leakage (*green*) in the area of incomplete treatment. **F:** One year after treatment, persistent leakage has resulted in extensive subretinal fluid, lipid, scarring, and severe visual loss. (Reprinted with permission of the American Medical Association from *Arch Ophthalmol* 1989;107:344–352.)

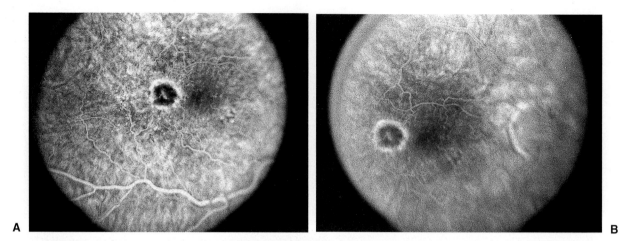

A   B

FIG. 31. Example of an eye with central leakage following treatment. **A:** The early phase of the angiogram shows some bright hyperfluorescence in the center of an area of blocked fluorescence corresponding to laser treatment scar. **B:** The late phase of the angiogram shows leakage from the area of bright hyperfluorescence noted in A, but this leakage does not extend beyond the boundaries of the laser scar (does not extend beyond the boundaries of the blocked fluorescence) and is considered central leakage. There is no evidence to suggest that treatment of central leakage is necessary to prevent a subsequent recurrence. Eyes with this change are no more likely to develop a recurrence than are eyes without central leakage.

might consider treating this eye as if it had an extrafoveal lesion. Failure to look at stereoscopic frames from the middle and late phases of the angiogram will lead to inability to identify areas of occult neovascularization surrounding the classic neovascularization. In the middle and late phases (Fig. 29B,C), areas of irregular elevation of the RPE identified by mottled hyper- and hypofluorescence probably represent fibrovascular tissue surrounding the classic CNV. Failure to laser the entire neovascular lesion may result in persistent occult neovascularization that could progress to

disciform scarring or atrophy in the areas that were untreated (Fig. 29D). Thus, to determine whether laser treatment is indicated and, if indicated, where the laser should be applied, one must identify the entire extent of the lesion. Areas of occult neovascularization often are not obvious from the early phases of the angiogram alone; careful scrutiny of stereoscopic frames from the middle and late phases of the angiogram is probably necessary to identify the entire extent of the lesion. As discussed earlier, treatment of just the classic CNV in an eye with classic and occult CNV has not been

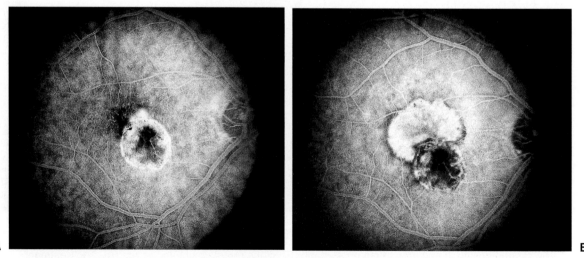

A   B

FIG. 32. The midphase fluorescein angiogram (**A**) shows well-demarcated fluorescence along the borders of a laser scar with additional bright hyperfluorescence and leakage at the superior edge of scar, indicative of recurrence. Failure to recognize and laser this recurrence resulted in progressive decreased visual acuity and a subsequent recurrent large growth within 6 weeks (**B**). Subsequent treatment required extensive ablation of the central macular area, which might not have been necessary had the recurrence been treated 6 weeks earlier (A) when it was relatively small.

shown to be beneficial when compared with observation of these lesions.

Incomplete Treatment of the Foveal Side

Data from the MPS have shown that eyes in which laser treatment did not cover the CNV completely on the foveal side (Fig. 30) or did not meet the required level of intensity (at least as white as shown in Fig. 20) had approximately three times the risk of developing persistent CNV within 6 weeks after treatment compared with eyes in which the CNV was covered completely by intense, confluent burns. Thus, it is essential not only to obtain a uniform white laser burn during treatment, but also to ensure that the extent of the intense confluent burns completely covers the extent of the CNV. This statement may be true especially for juxtafoveal lesions. Slight overtreatment may cover the lesion in its entirety and may be beneficial when compared with observation, but may lead to more visual loss when compared with covering the entire lesion without extensive overtreatment.

When CNV is not very close to the foveal center, it usually is not difficult for ophthalmologists who are experienced in treating CNV to extend laser treatment over the entire extent of the CNV. This is probably because there is little hesitancy in extending treatment slightly beyond the borders of the CNV in an effort to ensure adequate coverage when the CNV is far away from the foveal center. Slight extension of treatment should have little effect on the visual acuity because the treatment in these situations will not be affecting central foveal photoreceptors.

On the other hand, when treating a juxtafoveal lesion, even the most experienced ophthalmologists may be reluctant to treat too extensively on the foveal perimeter of the CNV. Excessive treatment in this situation could easily contribute to visual loss. On the other hand, failure to cover the CNV in its entirety could lead to increased persistence within 6 weeks following treatment (Fig. 30), as was shown in the MPS trials.

The development of persistent leakage within the confines of the scar (that is, where the leakage in the late phases of the angiogram does not extend beyond the boundaries of the laser-treated area as shown in Fig. 31) has been called "central leakage." Central leakage is not judged to require retreatment because it was shown not to be associated with subsequent recurrence (defined as leakage that extends beyond the periphery of the laser treated area and is associated with subsequent visual loss).

Failure to Identify Recurrent Choroidal Neovascularization

Failure to identify recurrences can result in significant loss of visual acuity. For example, for the case shown in Fig. 32A, the ophthalmologist failed to notice the development of bright hyperfluorescence, with leakage at the periphery of

the laser scar. Six weeks later, the patient returned with continued decreased visual acuity and a very large recurrence (Fig. 32B) for which treatment required extensive ablation of the central macular area. Such extensive treatment might not have been necessary had the recurrence been treated when it was relatively small.

SUMMARY

The ophthalmoscopic and angiographic features of AMD may have a variety of complex appearances. Recognition of these various presentations is critical in the management of these patients, especially now that treatment has been shown to be effective in selected cases of CNV secondary to AMD. Prompt recognition of these features is especially important, especially for lesions that extend through the foveal center, because treatment is most beneficial when the lesions are relatively small. Future investigations will help to determine the role of micronutrients, cellular biologic interventions, surgical interventions, preventive strategies, medical interventions, and transplantation in the management of AMD. Such a multidisciplinary approach will be necessary if we are to decrease the magnitude of blindness from this major cause of visual loss in the United States.

ACKNOWLEDGMENT

This work has been supported in part by a Research to Prevent Blindness Olga Keith Wiess Scholars Award to N.M.B.

BIBLIOGRAPHY

Bressler NM, Bressler SB. Preventative ophthalmology: age-related macular degeneration. *Ophthalmology* 1995;102:1206–1211.

Bressler NM, Bressler SB, Fine SL. Age-related macular degeneration. *Surv Ophthalmol* 1988;32:375–413.

Bressler NM, Silva JC, Bressler SB, Fine SL, Green WR. Clinicopathologic correlation of drusen and retinal pigment epithelial abnormalities in age-related macular degeneration. *Retina* 1994;14:130–142.

Bressler SB, Silva JC, Bressler NM, Alexander JA, Green WR. Clinico-pathologic correlation of occult choroidal neovascularization in age-related macular degeneration. *Arch Ophthalmol* 1992;110:827–832.

Chamberlin JA, Bressler NM, Bressler SB, et al., and the Macular Photocoagulation Study Group. The use of fundus photographs and fluorescein angiograms in the identification and treatment of choroidal neovascularization in the Macular Photocoagulation Study. *Ophthalmology* 1989;96:1526–1534.

Dyer DS, Brant AM, Schachat AP, Bressler SB, Bressler NM. Questionable recurrent choroidal neovascularization angiographic features and outcome. *Am J Ophthalmol* 1995;120:497–505.

Macular Photocoagulation Study Group. Krypton laser photocoagulation for neovascular lesions of ocular histoplasmosis: results of a randomized clinical trial. *Arch Ophthalmol* 1987;105:1499–1507.

Macular Photocoagulation Study Group. Persistent and recurrent neovascularization after krypton laser photocoagulation for neovascular lesions of ocular histoplasmosis. *Arch Ophthalmol* 1989;107:344–352.

Macular Photocoagulation Study Group. Krypton laser photocoagulation for neovascular lesions of age-related macular degeneration: results of a randomized clinical trial. *Arch Ophthalmol* 1990;108:816–824.

Macular Photocoagulation Study Group. Persistent and recurrent neovascularization after krypton laser photocoagulation for neovascular lesions of age-related macular degeneration. *Arch Ophthalmol* 1990;108:825–831.

Macular Photocoagulation Study Group. Argon laser photocoagulation for neovascular maculopathy after five years: results from randomized clinical trials. *Arch Ophthalmol* 1991;109:1109–1114.

Macular Photocoagulation Study Group. Laser photocoagulation of subfoveal neovascular lesions in age-related macular degeneration: results of a randomized clinical trial. *Arch Ophthalmol* 1991;109:1219–1231.

Macular Photocoagulation Study Group. Laser photocoagulation of subfoveal recurrent neovascular lesions in age-related macular degeneration: results of a randomized clinical trial. *Arch Ophthalmol* 1991;109:1232–1241.

Macular Photocoagulation Study Group. Subfoveal neovascular lesions in age-related macular degeneration: guidelines for evaluation and treatment in the Macular Photocoagulation Study. *Arch Ophthalmol* 1991;109:1242–1257.

Macular Photocoagulation Study Group. Laser photocoagulation of subfoveal neovascular lesions of age-related macular degeneration: updated findings from two clinical trials. *Arch Ophthalmol* 1993;111:1200–1209.

Macular Photocoagulation Study Group. Visual outcome after laser photocoagulation for subfoveal choroidal neovascularization secondary to age-related macular degeneration: the influence of initial lesion size and initial visual acuity. *Arch Ophthalmol* 1994;112:480–488.

Macular Photocoagulation Study Group. The influence of treatment coverage on the visual acuity of eyes treated with krypton laser for juxtafoveal choroidal neovascularization. *Arch Ophthalmol* 1995;113:190–194.

Macular Photocoagulation Study Group. Occult choroidal neovascularization: influence on visual outcome in patients with age-related macular degeneration. *Arch Ophthalmol* 1996;114 [*in press*].

Practical Atlas of Retinal Disease and Therapy, Second Edition
edited by William R. Freeman,
Lippincott–Raven Publishers, Philadelphia © 1997.

· 10 ·

Laser Treatment for Diabetic Retinopathy

Everett Ai

Diabetic retinopathy remains the leading cause of new blindness in the United States today, accounting for 5,800 new cases of legal blindness annually. In the last decade, major advances have been made in our understanding of the pathogenesis of this disorder. In addition, rapid evolution of therapeutic technology has resulted in earlier treatment and increasing control of this complex and challenging condition. The successful management of diabetic retinopathy is based on a clear understanding of the underlying pathogenic processes and timely therapeutic intervention. This chapter reviews the current management of diabetic retinopathy based on the results of these studies, an understanding of the underlying pathophysiologic processes, and clinical experience.

The ocular manifestations of diabetes mellitus comprise the same microvascular abnormalities that are found in other organs. Obstruction and leakage of retinal capillaries are the primary basis for the natural history of this disorder. Capillary closure and leakage result in early fundus changes referred to as *nonproliferative (or background) retinopathy.* Acceleration of these capillary abnormalities and progression of ischemia eventually affect adjacent arterioles, resulting in arteriolar closure and a clinical picture termed *preproliferative retinopathy.* These changes indicate the potential for rapid progression of the retinopathy. As the nonperfusion increases, a "vasoproliferative factor" is believed to be released from the ischemic retina. This diffusible substance induces the growth of new, abnormal blood vessels, a process termed *neovascularization.*

These new vessels herald the third, and final, stage of *proliferative retinopathy.* This cycle of capillary closure, ischemia, and neovascularization spreads throughout the retina. Management of diabetic retinopathy is based on recognizing and interrupting this cycle at each clinical stage.

PHOTOCOAGULATION IN DIABETIC RETINOPATHY

In 1960, photocoagulation for the treatment of diabetic retinopathy was first reported by Meyer–Schwickerath, who found that the treatment was ineffective in four cases of advanced proliferative retinopathy, but was followed by partial absorption of hard exudate in one eye with a circinate ring. In 1967, diabetic retinopathy was described by Duke–Elder as "not preventable" and "relatively untreatable." Since that time, advances in the understanding of diabetic retinopathy have enabled the development of new treatments directed at the preservation of sight. The Diabetic Retinopathy Study (DRS) of 1976 reported that visual loss in patients with high-risk proliferative diabetic retinopathy could be reduced by as much as 60% by the timely application of laser therapy. In 1985, the Early Treatment Diabetic Retinopathy Study (ETDRS) showed that focal photocoagulation therapy could reduce the risk of further vision loss in diabetic individuals with clinically significant macular edema (CSME).

LASER WAVELENGTH SELECTION

An ideal laser wavelength would be absorbed solely by the target tissue and would not be absorbed or scattered by the ocular media. Although no such single wavelength exists, essentially all individuals with diabetic retinopathy may be treated with an argon laser with laser wavelengths ranging from 488 nm to 514 nm. While green-only argon laser (514 nm) is preferred for full-scatter panretinal photocoagulation, it becomes a must when focally treating CSME, because green-only argon is well absorbed by melanin and hemoglobin and there is little inner retinal absorption of this wavelength. In addition, blue–green argon treatment results

E. Ai, M.D.: Retina Unit, California Pacific Medical Center; and California Pacific Vision Foundation, Pacific Medical Center, San Francisco, CA 94115

in a high degree of intraocular scatter as cataractous lens changes in the average 50-year-old patient requires three times the power at the cornea for an equivalent green-only argon retinal burn. In addition, due to xanthophyll absorption, the blue wavelengths (488 nm) contained in the blue–green laser result in a greater degree of inner retinal damage in the macula. Finally, there is also the concern that the blue wavelengths contained in the blue–green argon laser may pose a risk of retinal injury, from an accumulative standpoint, to the treating physician as well.

Alternative wavelengths may be helpful in treating cases of diabetic retinopathy complicated by opacities in the ocular media or advanced disease. Patients with vitreous hemorrhage may be more effectively treated with red krypton (647 nm) or dye red laser (610–640 nm), because of the better penetration through media opacities afforded by the red wavelengths as they represent the wavelengths with the least amount of scatter and are minimally absorbed by hemoglobin. They are a suboptimal choice, however, for pale fundi due to the lack of melanin pigment for absorption. They are also less visible because of their greater degree of absorption in the retinal pigment epithelium and choroid. Finally, use of the red wavelengths results in more complaints of pain, an increased incidence of accompanying hemorrhage, and possible choroidal edema due to deeper choroidal penetration. Dye yellow (560–580 nm) is safe for macular photocoagulation, because of the low level of accompanying light scatter and to the very low rate of absorption by xanthophyll pigments. Accordingly, it may also be used when treating focally for CSME. While the ETDRS primarily employed green-only argon laser for macular treatment (with one center using a blue–green argon), dye-yellow laser may enable more efficient closure of leaking microvascular abnormalities, because the yellow wavelengths are well absorbed by oxyhemoglobin, deoxyhemoglobin, and melanin. It is especially well suited for cases of CSME with marked retinal thickening, because it enables more effective treatment with lower laser powers. Nevertheless, one always has to titrate laser power carefully up to the desired end point of photocoagulation treatment based on the pathophysiology involved.

The experience in the United States with the diode laser for panretinal photocoagulation is limited. This laser emits continuous energy in the infrared wavelengths (810 nm) and likely has properties similar to krypton and dye red in its interaction with the retina, vitreous, blood, pigment epithelial, and choroidal layers of the eye. It is also likely to elicit more complaints of discomfort with treatment and may require retrobulbar anesthesia for panretinal photocoagulation.

PATHOPHYSIOLOGY OF NONPROLIFERATIVE DIABETIC RETINOPATHY

Nonproliferative (background) retinopathy is seen in 25% of all diabetic patients, and its prevalence has been shown to

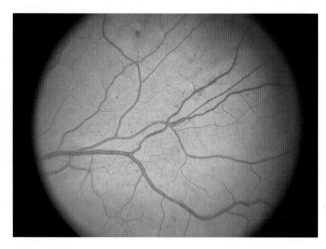

FIG. 1. Nonproliferative (background) retinopathy with microaneurysms and dot and blot hemorrhages.

be directly related to the duration of diabetes. Those patients who have had diabetes for 15 years or more have a 60% incidence of retinopathy. Nonproliferative retinopathy is the result of capillary closure and leakage. The underlying mechanism for this change is not known, but endothelial changes (basement membrane thickening and pericyte degeneration) have been demonstrated, and hemodynamic abnormalities (red blood cell and platelet aggregation) have been observed. Clinically, patients are asymptomatic and vision is normal (Fig. 1). Examination of the fundus reveals the presence of microaneurysms that represent a nonspecific response to ischemia (Fig. 2). These microaneurysms may leak plasma constituents that can later impinge on foveal photoreceptors and result in visual loss. Also seen are retinal hemorrhages that may be deep (dot and blot) or superficial (flame shaped).

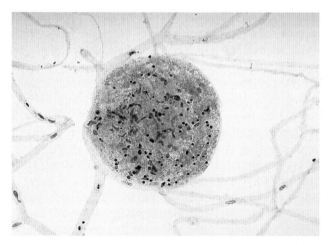

FIG. 2. Microaneurysm formation represents the first clinically visible manifestation of diabetic retinopathy and occurs adjacent to areas of capillary closure. (Courtesy of George H. Bresnick, M.D., University of Wisconsin, Madison, WI.)

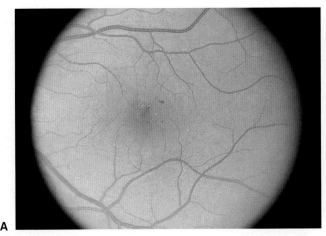
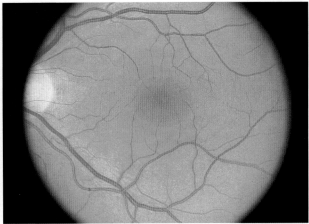

FIG. 3. Nonproliferative diabetic retinopathy and macular edema with hard exudate formation before (**A**) and after (**B**) improved control of blood glucose levels.

TREATMENT OF NONPROLIFERATIVE DIABETIC RETINOPATHY

The management of nonproliferative retinopathy is based on optimal medical control of diabetes. The effect of blood sugar control on the progression of retinopathy remains controversial, but there is accumulating evidence that both the rate and severity of retinal changes are favorably influenced by control of blood glucose levels (Fig. 3).

Another important part of the management of nonproliferative retinopathy is periodic examination of the fundus on a 4- to 6-month basis. It has been shown that the rate of microaneurysmal formation correlates with the rate of progression of the retinopathy. In addition, the presence of CSME, reviewed in the following sections, may indicate the need for therapeutic intervention.

PATHOPHYSIOLOGY OF PREPROLIFERATIVE DIABETIC RETINOPATHY AND MACULAR EDEMA

As the microvascular changes of capillary closure and leakage progress, ischemia impinges on the walls of the retinal arterioles. Damage to these vessels results in larger areas of nonperfusion and leakage of blood or plasma constituents through the defective endothelium. Clinically, the most obvious manifestation of arteriolar ischemia is the cotton-wool spot, an infarct of the nerve fiber layer (Fig. 4). The hallmark of preproliferative retinopathy is the presence of multiple cotton-wool spots, blot hemorrhages, intraretinal microvascular abnormalities, and venous beading (Figs. 5 and 6). The ETDRS accumulated considerable data on the natural history and rate of progression of diabetic retinopathy. One of the most clinically significant findings concerns the risk of progression from nonproliferative to proliferative retinopathy. Four severity levels of nonproliferative retinopathy were

defined. A 10-fold increase (5%–50%) was noted in the 1-year risk of developing proliferative retinopathy between the mildest and most severe levels (ETDRS, unpublished data presented at the American Academy of Ophthalmology, New Orleans, LA, 1989). The risk of progression was strongly related to four clinical findings: intraretinal microvascular abnormalities, increasing severity of intraretinal dot and blot hemorrhages, venous beading, and capillary nonperfusion on fluorescein angiography. The risk of progression to proliferative disease was not related to hard exudate deposits and only weakly related to the presence of cotton-wool spots.

With progression of the retinopathy, there is continued leakage from microaneurysms and defective small vessels. Fluid then accumulates within the retina and is seen clinically as retinal thickening. When this occurs within the central fovea, it is referred to as macular edema (Fig. 7). This complication occurs in approximately 10% of all diabetics

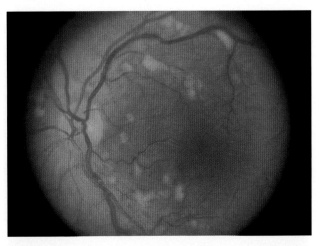

FIG. 4. Cotton-wool spots as a manifestation of retinal ischemia.

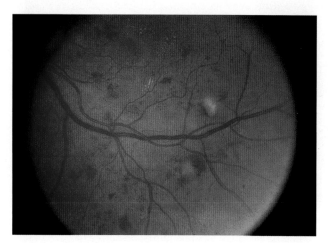

FIG. 5. Preproliferative retinopathy with multiple cotton-wool spots, blot hemorrhages, and intraretinal microvascular abnormalities.

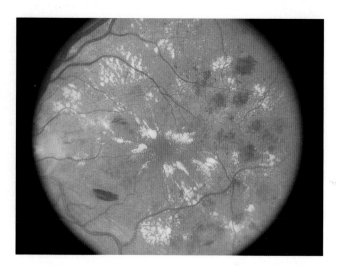

FIG. 7. Macular edema with hard exudate formation.

and, in those patients with diabetes for 20 or more years, the incidence increases to 25%. Cellular distortion due to macular edema may lead to visual loss. The impairment that results from fluid accumulation may be reversible, damage from chronic leakage and resultant hard exudate deposition is permanent. As a result, early treatment of this condition should be considered.

TREATMENT OF DIABETIC MACULAR EDEMA

The ETDRS has shown that photocoagulation for CSME reduces the risk of visual loss by 50% (Fig. 8). Laser treatment also increases the chance of visual improvement (Fig. 9), decreases the frequency of persistent macular edema, and is not accompanied by any major adverse side effects. Macular edema is defined as any retinal thickening or hard exudate deposits within one disc diameter of the center of the macula. Macular edema is termed *clinically significant* if

any one of three characteristics is present: (1) thickening of the retina within 500 μm of the center of the macula (Fig. 10), (2) hard exudates within 500 μm of the center of the macula if associated with adjacent retinal thickening (which may be outside the 500 μm limit) (Fig. 11), or (3) a zone of retinal thickening one disc diameter or larger within one disc diameter of the center of the macula (Fig. 12). Detection of macular edema is best accomplished by using a slit beam and a fundus contact lens. It can also be determined by analysis of stereo fundus photographs of the macula (Fig. 13).

Precise localization of hard exudate deposits and areas of retinal thickening can be achieved by using a grid developed by the ETDRS (Fig. 14). The three circles on the grid represent radii of 500, 1,500, and 3,000 μm. This grid may be placed over a standard 30° fundus photograph or red-free photograph in order to localize hard exudate deposits. It may also be used with the early images of the fluorescein angiogram to localize sites of leakage responsible for retinal thickening (Fig. 15).

The decision to treat diabetic macular edema is based on clinical and angiographic findings and is independent of the

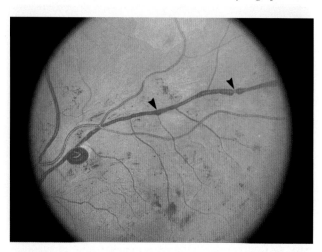

FIG. 6. Venous beading (*arrows*) in an eye with severe retinal ischemia.

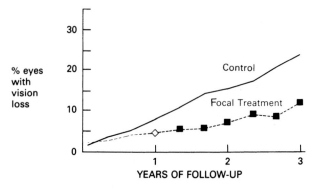

FIG. 8. Visual acuity results (all eyes with macular edema). Photocoagulation for clinically significant macular edema reduces the risk of visual loss by 50%.

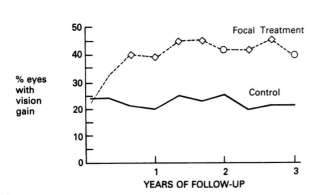

FIG. 9. Improvement in visual acuity (more than one line), initial acuity worse than 20/40. Laser treatment for clinically significant macular edema increases the chance of visual improvement.

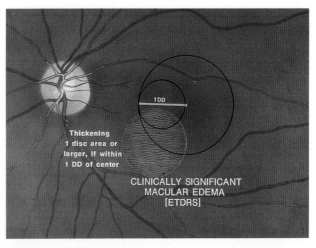

FIG. 12. Clinically significant macular edema defined as retinal thickening one disc area or larger in size if within one disc diameter of the center of the macula. ETDRS, Early Treatment Diabetic Retinopathy Study.

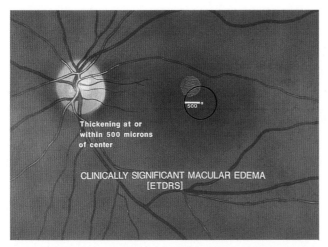

FIG. 10. Clinically significant macular edema defined as retinal thickening at or within 500 μm of the center of the macula. ETDRS, Early Treatment Diabetic Retinopathy Study.

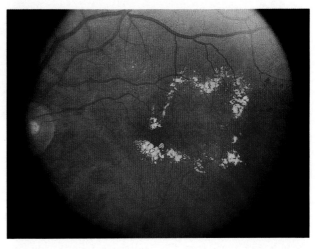

FIG. 13. Clinically significant macular edema with a circinate ring of hard exudate formation. Pretreatment photograph.

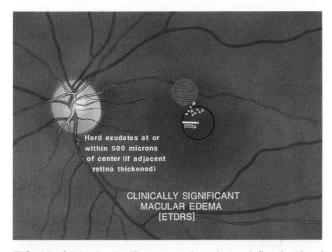

FIG. 11. Clinically significant macular edema defined as hard exudates at or within 500 μm of the center of the macula if there is adjacent retinal thickening. ETDRS, Early Treatment Diabetic Retinopathy Study.

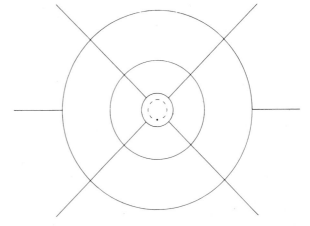

FIG. 14. Grid developed by the Early Treatment Diabetic Retinopathy Study that can be placed over a standard 30° fundus photograph. The three *solid circles* on the grid represent radii of 500, 1500, and 3000 μm.

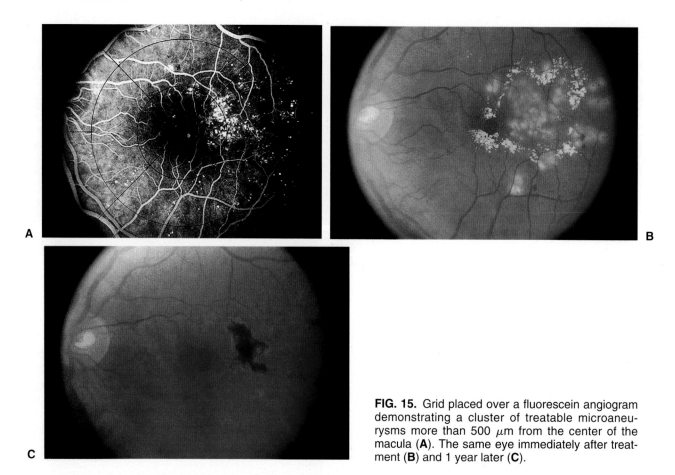

FIG. 15. Grid placed over a fluorescein angiogram demonstrating a cluster of treatable microaneurysms more than 500 μm from the center of the macula (**A**). The same eye immediately after treatment (**B**) and 1 year later (**C**).

patient's visual acuity. Careful analysis of the late-phase photographs of the angiogram serves to identify generalized areas of edema. Review of early frames allows one to determine whether the leakage is primarily focal in nature and secondary to leaking microaneurysms, or diffuse and due to generalized leakage from the capillary bed. Early- and late-phase photographs may also be projected at the time of treatment to aid in localization of the sites of leakage.

Focal laser therapy for CSME consists of (1) direct treatment to leaking microaneurysms, (2) grid therapy over all areas of diffuse leakage, and (3) grid treatment for capillary nonperfusion.

Direct treatment to leaking microaneurysms consists of the application of green-only argon (in preference to blue–green argon) photocoagulation to all leaking micro-

aneurysms in the areas between 500 and 3000 μm (two disc diameters) from the center of the macula (Table 1). Lesions between 300 and 500 μm from the center may be treated if previous treatment has been applied and CSME persists, vision is less than 20/40, and treatment is not likely to destroy the remaining perifoveal capillary network. Individual microaneurysms are treated with a spot size of 50–100 μm, with an exposure time of 0.1 seconds or less. Power is ini-

TABLE 1. *Parameters of focal treatment: direct photocoagulation*

1. 50–100 μm spot size
2. 0.1 second or less duration
3. Attempt to whiten or darken microaneurysms

Direct photocoagulation of leaking microaneurysms consists of the application of 50- and 100-μm spot size green-only argon applications to all leaking microaneurysms between 500 and 3,000 μg from the center of the macula.

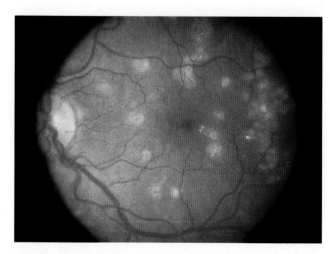

FIG. 16. Immediate posttreatment photograph of direct photocoagulation to leaking microaneurysms.

TABLE 2. *Parameters of focal treatment: grid pattern*

1. Less than 200-μm-diameter burn
2. Light (just above threshold) intensity burn
3. Spaced at least one burn width apart

Grid pattern photocoagulation consists of 100–200-μm spot size green-only argon applications of light intensity applied to all areas of diffuse leakage more than 500 μm from the center of the macula and 500 μm from the temporal margin of the optic disc.

tially set at 50 mW and slowly increased to obtain whitening or darkening of the microaneurysm at the minimum power setting (Fig. 16). When treating lesions within 500 μm of the center, a shorter exposure time of 0.05 second is recommended. Several laser applications to the same microaneurysm may be necessary to reach the desired therapeutic end point of whitening or darkening of the microaneurysm. This end point is rarely achieved with microaneurysms smaller than 40 μm. For these lesions, the end point is simply mild-to-moderate whitening of the adjacent retina, with care being taken to avoid rupturing Bruch's membrane.

Grid treatment to areas of diffuse leakage (or nonperfusion) is based on the identification of leakage in the middle and late frames of the angiogram unrelated to focal sites of leakage identified in the early frames. This leakage is secondary to permeability abnormalities within dilated capillaries. Grid treatment consists of placing 100- to 200-μm light burns at the level of the retinal pigment epithelium in areas of leakage that are more than 500 μm from the center of the macula and 500 μm from the temporal margin of the optic nerve (Table 2). Exposure time is 0.1 second or less, and one burn width is allowed between lesions.

Power settings are started at 10 mW and slowly increased to obtain a light gray–white lesion in the outer retina. The spot intensity should be above threshold, but significantly less intense than a panretinal photocoagulation burn (Fig. 17). In general, the spot should be just light enough so that it

can be barely visualized, a minimum criterion to achieve proper spacing between burns. In cases requiring a combination of direct and grid treatment, direct treatment should be administered first, followed by grid laser therapy. In this way, at least a partial "grid" of laser spots will be in place following the direct treatment, and this grid can then be completed with laser spots to all areas demonstrating diffuse leakage.

It should be emphasized that photocoagulation in the macular area involves interaction of light energy with luteal pigment that absorbs most strongly in the blue region. Argon green has been the most extensively studied wavelength for photocoagulation therapy of diabetic macular edema for this reason. In addition, argon laser has been available for ophthalmic use longer than krypton, dye, and diode lasers. The therapeutic effect of focal laser therapy for diabetic macular edema is far less dramatic than is panretinal photocoagulation for proliferative disease. For this reason, one must rely more heavily on the results of prospective randomized clinical trials in choosing treatment modalities. We therefore continue to use argon green for therapy of macular edema in diabetics, although dye yellow has the theoretical advantage of higher absorption by hemoglobin and may close microaneurysms more efficiently and with less energy absorption by the pigment epithelium and photoreceptor layers.

Before initiating focal photocoagulation, patients should be counseled about realistic expectations regarding visual outcomes. Most patients interpret the treatment as a means to regain vision damaged by macular edema. It is important to explain to patients that the visual acuity of only 15% of patients in the ETDRS actually improved (due, in part, to the fact that a number of patients had 20/20 or better vision at the time of therapy). The goal of treatment is to preserve the patient's current level of vision. This objective needs to be understood before treatment. Patients should also be advised that a period of 1–4 months is required for maximum resorption of fluid. If there is residual macular edema at 4 months, the fluorescein angiogram may be repeated and retreatment

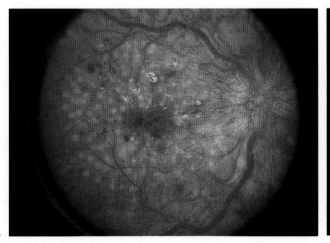
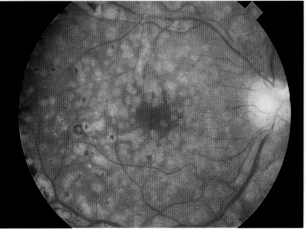

A   B

FIG. 17. Example of grid photocoagulation immediately following laser treatment (**A**) and 2 years later (**B**).

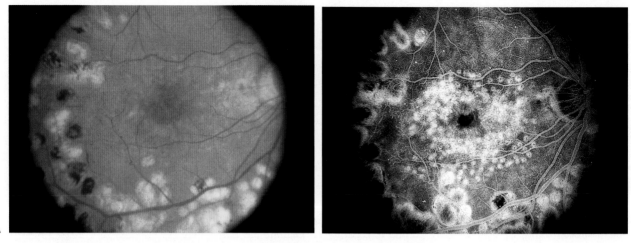

FIG. 18. Fundus photograph (**A**) and corresponding fluorescein angiogram (**B**) demonstrating a grid pattern of prior laser therapy applied to all areas of diffuse leakage. While persistent macular edema can be seen in this eye, no treatable lesions remain.

performed if "treatable" lesions are present. These consist of persistent leaking microaneurysms 500 μm from the center of the macula (or 300 μm from the center if vision is less than 20/40 and there is no perifoveal capillary dropout). Grid laser therapy can also be administered to areas of diffuse leakage 500 μm from the center of the macula if these areas have not previously been treated. Retreatment over areas previously lasered in a grid pattern is not recommended because excessive spread of laser scars may result (Fig. 18).

There is no level of visual activity decrease after which focal treatment is not warranted. Even eyes with the so-called lipemic retinitis form of diabetic retinopathy (Fig. 19) may benefit from restoration of a more stable physiologic state that may follow therapy. In addition, it has been our experience that most such eyes also require panretinal photocoag-

ulation therapy for concomitant proliferative disease or marked ischemia.

PATHOPHYSIOLOGY OF PROLIFERATIVE DIABETIC RETINOPATHY

The proliferative stage of diabetic retinopathy is characterized by the growth of abnormal new vessels and fibrous tissue in response to retinal ischemia. These proliferative new vessels are abnormal in their propensity to bleed into the vitreous cavity and obscure vision. These abnormal vessels also retain the potential for differentiation into fibroblasts, and proliferation of fibrous and vascular tissue may form firm adhesions at the interface between the retina and vitreous body (Fig. 20). As the vitreous undergoes syneresis and detachment over time, traction on the underlying retina may occur and result in a tractional retinal detachment.

FIG. 19. Lipemic retinitis with marked clinically significant macular edema and massive hard exudate formation. Focal laser treatment should still be considered for this eye in order to preserve as much of the remaining functional retina as possible.

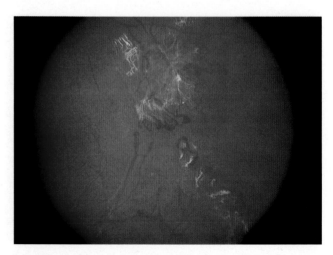

FIG. 20. Retinal neovascularization elsewhere in a patient with marked fibrovascular proliferation.

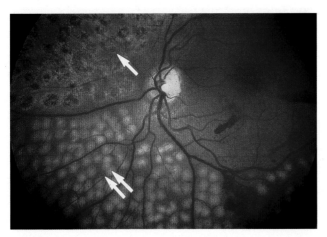

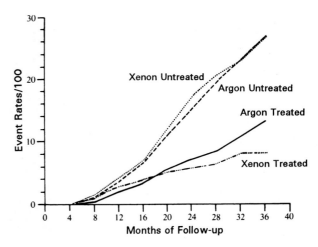

FIG. 21. Full-scatter panretinal photocoagulation therapy in a patient with high-risk characteristics. Note prior laser scars (*single arrow*) and fresh laser scars (*double arrows*). (Courtesy of the American Academy of Ophthalmology, San Francisco, CA.)

FIG. 23. Full-scatter panretinal photocoagulation therapy reduces the incidence of severe visual loss in patients with high-risk proliferative changes. Argon laser therapy is preferred over xenon photocoagulation therapy because of a lower incidence of side effects.

The proliferative stage of diabetic retinopathy is initially managed by laser photocoagulation (Fig. 21). The large areas of nonperfusion that result from arteriolar closure are thought to release a "vasoproliferative factor" that stimulates neovascularization (Fig. 22). The DRS demonstrated that the timely application of laser photocoagulation to eyes with high-risk proliferative changes reduces the incidence of severe visual loss and inhibits the progression of retinopathy (Fig. 23). Indications for the initiation of laser therapy according to the DRS include the following high-risk proliferative changes: (1) neovascularization of the disc (NVD; new vessels on or within one disc diameter of the optic disc)

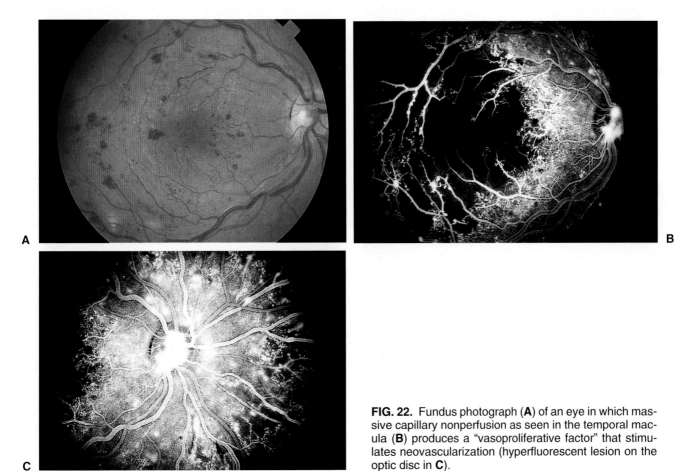

FIG. 22. Fundus photograph (**A**) of an eye in which massive capillary nonperfusion as seen in the temporal macula (**B**) produces a "vasoproliferative factor" that stimulates neovascularization (hyperfluorescent lesion on the optic disc in **C**).

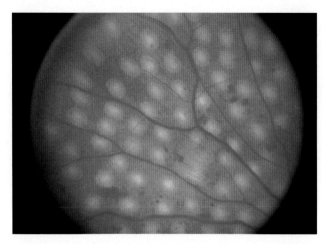

FIG. 24. Full-scatter panretinal photocoagulation therapy immediately following laser treatment.

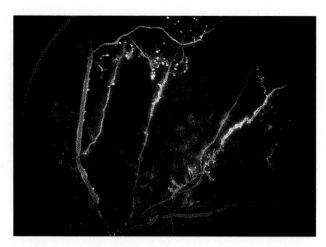

FIG. 26. Eyes with marked capillary nonperfusion as a manifestation of severe preproliferative retinopathy should be considered for full-scatter laser therapy. Almost no capillaries remain in the midperiphery of this eye.

greater than one-quarter of the disc area, (2) NVD with vitreous or preretinal hemorrhage, and (3) neovascularization elsewhere (NVE) greater than one-half of the disc area, with vitreous or preretinal hemorrhage. The ETDRS confirmed the finding of the DRS that panretinal photocoagulation for high-risk proliferative diabetic retinopathy was effective in reducing the risk of visual loss. The ETDRS also showed that eyes with less than high-risk proliferative retinopathy had relatively low rates of severe visual loss, regardless of whether photocoagulation treatment was applied early or deferred until the development of high-risk proliferative changes. In addition, full-scatter panretinal laser therapy (Fig. 24) was preferable to "mild scatter" treatment (Fig. 25) when therapy was indicated. The study concluded that it is safe to defer full-scatter laser treatment until the retinopathy approaches the high-risk stage, provided that careful follow-up can be maintained. However, this may not always occur

in practice and, as a result, it is conventional to consider photocoagulation therapy for eyes prior to the onset of high-risk proliferative changes once any definite neovascularization of the optic disc or retina is noted, especially if seen in conjunction with significant capillary nonperfusion. Eyes with rubeosis iridis or marked capillary nonperfusion (severe preproliferative retinopathy) should also be considered for laser treatment (Fig. 26). Patients under consideration for treatment with these findings are informed that waiting for the development of high-risk proliferative changes could result in ocular changes (vitreous hemorrhages or neovascular glaucoma) that could hinder future therapy.

TREATMENT OF PROLIFERATIVE DIABETIC RETINOPATHY

Full-scatter panretinal laser therapy consists of 500 μm blue–green argon laser applications with exposure times of 0.1 second, with power adjusted to obtain moderately intense white burns placed approximately one-half burn diameter apart. Treatment is placed two disc diameters above, temporal, and below the center of the macula and 500 μm from the nasal margin of the disc (Fig. 27). Treatment then extends peripherally to or beyond the equator, avoiding direct treatment of major retinal vessels and areas of fibrosis and chorioretinal scarring, if present. It is estimated that a total of 1,200–1,600 burns are required to complete panretinal scatter treatment in a given eye. However, some eyes may require more laser spots, and treatment should be tailored to each individual case.

Local photocoagulation of retinal NVE is also recommended. Treatment should be continued past the edges of the patch for 500 μm, but should not impinge on the papillomacular bundle nor come closer than 500 μm from the disc margin or one disc diameter from the center of the macula

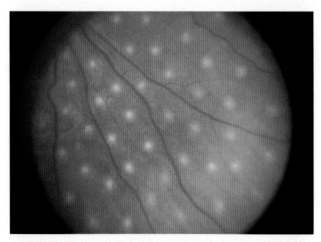

FIG. 25. "Mild scatter" photocoagulation treatment immediately following laser therapy. This form of treatment was evaluated in the Early Treatment Diabetic Retinopathy Study and found to be less effective than full-scatter therapy.

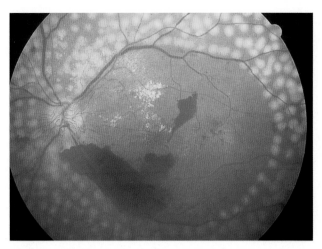

FIG. 27. Wide-field photograph of full-scatter panretinal photocoagulation therapy immediately following treatment for high-risk proliferative diabetic retinopathy.

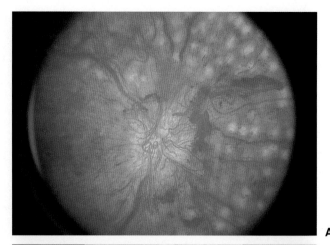

A

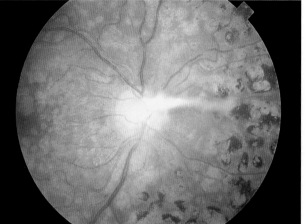

B

FIG. 29. This eye received follow-up treatment of persistent neovascularization of the disc (**A**) and demonstrated regression of the neovascularization with a residual fibrous scar (**B**) overlying the optic nerve head.

(Fig. 28). Treatment is placed confluently when patches of NVE are flat and no more than two disc diameters in size. A "local" full-scatter pattern is used when zones of NVE are located within 3,000 μm (two disc diameters) of the center of the macula. Such treatment should spare the area within 500 μm of the center of the macula and should utilize burns no larger than 200 μm in the zone between 500 and 1,500 μm from the center.

Follow-up treatment for persistent or recurrent NVE or NVD is recommended (Fig. 29). Small patches of NVE (less than two disc areas) should undergo direct confluent treatment. Because of the risk of producing choroidal connections to preretinal new vessels, treatment over scars is conducted only with caution, and strong burns with small spot sizes are avoided, especially over darkly pigmented scars. If it is apparent that there is additional room for scatter laser

spots between previous photocoagulation burns, additional "fill-in" treatment can also be delivered.

The ETDRS evaluated the effect of aspirin on diabetic retinopathy. All patients were randomly assigned to either two tablets of aspirin per day (a total daily dosage of 650 mg) or placebo. The study results indicate that aspirin does not affect vision in any way. It neither prevents the development of high-risk proliferative retinopathy nor increases the risk of vitreous hemorrhage. As a result, there is no reason for diabetic individuals to avoid taking aspirin in these quantities when it is needed for the treatment of other problems.

Follow-up treatment for NVD that develops for the first time following laser treatment, fails to regress, or recurs after initial regression consists of the application of additional scatter burns between prior treatment scars, anterior to them, or in the posterior pole (with care being taken to spare the area within 500 μm of the center of the macula and using burns no larger than 200 μm in the zone between 500 and 1,500 μm from the center) (Fig. 30). At least 500 additional scatter burns should be applied whenever the decision is made to add more scatter treatment to a previously treated

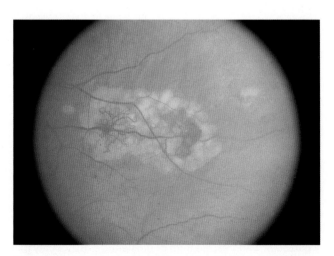

FIG. 28. Local photocoagulation of retinal neovascularization elsewhere should be continued past the edges of flat neovascularization for 500 μm.

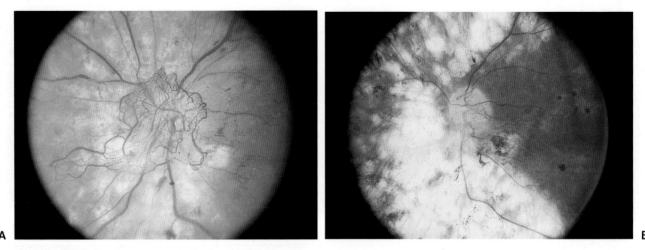

FIG. 30. This eye received additional laser therapy to treat persistent neovascularization of the disc (**A**). Even after such treatment, persistent fibrovascular proliferation can be seen (**B**).

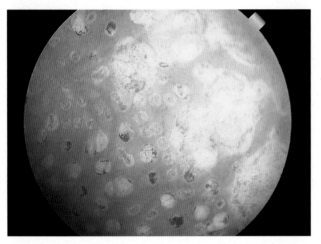

FIG. 31. Cryocoagulation therapy (seen on the *right* of figure) can be used to supplement previous full-scatter panretinal photocoagulation therapy.

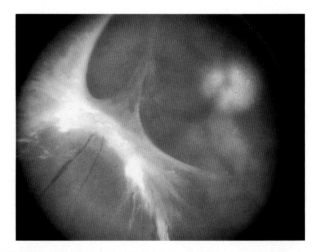

FIG. 32. Surgical intervention should be considered for patients with traction retinal detachments involving the macula.

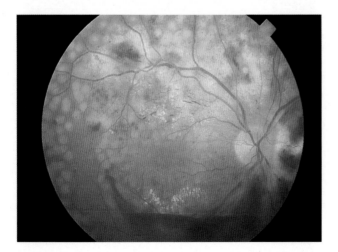

FIG. 33. Patients with AIDS and diabetes may demonstrate a particularly aggressive form of proliferative retinopathy that requires close monitoring and prompt laser therapy as indicated.

eye. Particular attention should also be given to those areas in which new vessels are growing and where laser scars are less tightly spaced. Individuals with marked neovascularization or significant areas of capillary nonperfusion as demonstrated by the presence of multiple occluded "ghost" retinal vessels may require the application of near-confluent laser burns throughout the midperiphery and far periphery. Treatment of the periphery may be facilitated by the use of cryocoagulation (Fig. 31) or laser indirect ophthalmoscopic techniques. One should pay particular attention to the area temporal to the macula where extensive capillary nonperfusion is commonly seen and where the posterior extent of the original scatter treatment is sometimes more than the prescribed two disc diameters from the center of the macula. If repeated vitreous hemorrhages or traction macular detachments occur despite laser treatment, surgical intervention should be considered (Fig. 32) (see also Chapter 11 by H. Lewis and G. Sanchez). Special attention is indicated for individuals with the acquired immunodeficiency syndrome (AIDS) and diabetes who may manifest a more "aggressive" form of diabetic retinopathy requiring particularly close monitoring and prompt laser therapy of treatable lesions (Fig. 33).

COMMON PITFALLS

A common pitfall in the management of background diabetic retinopathy is failure to identify CSME and institute timely photocoagulation therapy. As pointed out by the ETDRS, patients with CSME may qualify for treatment even when their level of visual acuity is 20/20 or better. Needless to say, some individuals who are visually asymptomatic and have good levels of vision may not be suitable candidates for such photocoagulation therapy. Nevertheless, the study results show that vision may be stabilized by laser therapy and that waiting until visual acuity decreases before instituting treatment may only allow vision to be stabilized at a lower level of acuity. As a result, patients should be adequately counseled as to the potential benefits and risks of treatment and therapy considered in all individuals who meet the treatment criteria.

In conjunction with the timely application of focal laser therapy, it is critical that the application of treatment be appropriate in pattern and intensity. It is important to keep grid laser spots as light in intensity as possible (just above threshold) to avoid initial overtreatment (Fig. 34) or future enlargement of laser spots with possible coalescence of the chorioretinal scars in the macula (Fig. 35). Great care must also be taken to avoid rupturing Bruch's membrane, which could result in the subsequent development of subretinal neovascularization. Finally, postlaser visits should include assessment for areas of persistent CSME with treatable lesions for which additional therapy may be warranted.

Another pitfall in the management of preproliferative dia-

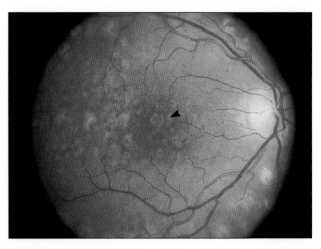

FIG. 34. Central focal laser spot (*arrow*) that was too high in intensity and placed too close to the center of the macula. Nevertheless, this patient maintained vision in the 20/16 range.

betic individuals is failure to consider institution of panretinal photocoagulation therapy because neovascularization of the optic disc or retina is not yet present. Patients with marked retinal ischemia without neovascularization may be at risk for the onset of rubeosis iridis and subsequent neovascular glaucoma, and should be considered for panretinal photocoagulation therapy. It is our experience that extreme capillary nonperfusion constitutes its own "high risk" sign in diabetic retinopathy and should be managed accordingly. In addition, individuals with signs of moderate-to-marked retinal ischemia without neovascularization who are unable or unwilling to return for routine follow-up visits may benefit from the early application of panretinal photocoagulation therapy. It should be noted that early treatment was not shown to be essential by the ETDRS, and any decisions re-

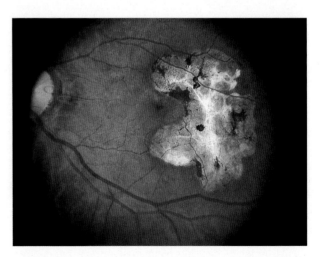

FIG. 35. Focal photocoagulation spots that are too high in intensity may run the risk of future coalescence of the laser scars as seen here.

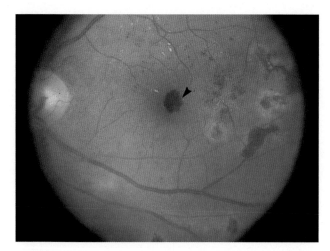

FIG. 36. This patient suffered an accidental laser application to the center of the macula, as evidenced by the spot of increased pigmentation in the center of the macula (*arrow*).

sults in failure to treat a portion of the retina that is prone to capillary nonperfusion and subsequent neovascularization (Fig. 37). Another potential pitfall is the failure to treat eyes aggressively with neovascularization and marked ischemia (Fig. 38).

It may be difficult to identify areas of recurrent or persistent retinal neovascularization following the application of panretinal photocoagulation therapy. As a result, careful examination utilizing direct and indirect ophthalmoscopy and the biomicroscope slit lamp with either a contact or hand-held fundus lens may be helpful in identifying zones of neovascularization requiring treatment. In addition, indirect ophthalmoscopy to visualize the far inferior periphery at each visit may be helpful in identifying small vitreous hemorrhages that may be either visually asymptomatic or have largely cleared by the time of the evaluation. Such a finding should prompt the examiner to look more closely for neovascularization and to consider performing fluorescein angiography or angioscopy.

garding panretinal photocoagulation therapy prior to the onset of high-risk characteristics should be made on an individual basis.

Pitfalls in the management of proliferative diabetic retinopathy include failure to apply panretinal photocoagulation therapy properly (Fig. 36) and failure to place panretinal photocoagulation scars to within two disc diameters (3,000 μm) temporal to the center of the macula in each eye. There is a tendency to try to avoid placing temporal laser spots "too close" to the macula. However, placement of laser spots outside the zone two disc diameters temporal to the macula re-

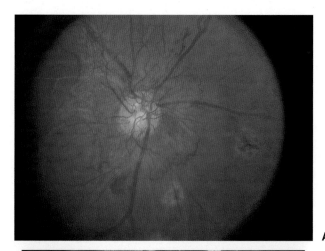

A

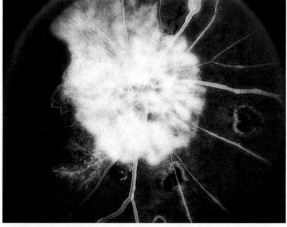

B

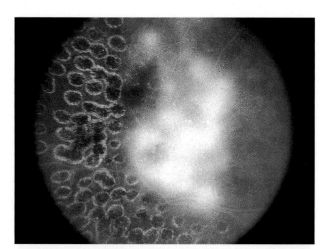

FIG. 37. Fluorescein angiogram demonstrates panretinal photocoagulation therapy that was placed much greater than two disc diameters (3,000 μm) temporal to the center of the macula. Areas of capillary nonperfusion (*dark areas* on the *right* of figure) did not receive laser photocoagulation and retinal neovascularization persisted, as evidenced by the area of hyperfluorescence.

FIG. 38. This patient with marked neovascularization of the disc (**A**) and massive capillary nonperfusion (**B**) was not treated aggressively enough, as evidenced by the sparsity of laser spots nasal to the optic disc. Persistent neovascularization of the disc with leakage remained after treatment (**B**).

SUMMARY

Advances in our understanding of the natural history and management of diabetic retinopathy represent a significant achievement in ophthalmology during the past decade. Effective methods of treatment are available for the two most frequent causes of visual loss: diabetic macular edema and proliferative diabetic retinopathy. A major challenge remains the timely application of therapy in the prevention and early treatment of these common complications of diabetes.

BIBLIOGRAPHY

Coonan P, Ai E. The early treatment of diabetic retinopathy. In: Ai E, Freeman WR, eds. *Ophthalmology clinics of North America: New developments in retinal disease.* Philadelphia: WB Saunders, 1990:359–372.

Diabetic Retinopathy Study Research Group. Photocoagulation treatment of proliferative diabetic retinopathy: the second report of Diabetic Retinopathy Study findings. *Ophthalmology* 1978;85:82–106.

Early Treatment Diabetic Retinopathy Study Research Group. Early treatment diabetic retinopathy: ETDRS report no. 4. *Int Ophthalmol Clin* 1987;27:265–262.

Early Treatment Diabetic Retinopathy Study Research Group. Techniques for scatter and local photocoagulation treatment of diabetic retinopathy: ETDRS report no. 3. *Int Ophthalmol Clin* 1987;27:254–264.

Early Treatment Diabetic Retinopathy Study Research Group. Treatment techniques and clinical guidelines for photocoagulation of diabetic macular edema: ETDRS report no. 2. *Ophthalmology* 1987;94:761–774.

Practical Atlas of Retinal Disease and Therapy, Second Edition
edited by William R. Freeman,
Lippincott–Raven Publishers, Philadelphia © 1997.

· 11 ·

Vitreoretinal Surgery for Complications of Diabetic Retinopathy

Hilel Lewis and German Sanchez

Pars plana vitrectomy for the management of complications of diabetic retinopathy was first performed by Machemer in 1970. Since then, significant advances in diagnosis and surgical techniques have occurred, and the indications for surgery have evolved (Tables 1 and 2).

Despite the success of vitreoretinal surgery in improving vision and preventing significant visual loss in a great number of patients, intraoperative and postoperative complications occur that can lead to severe visual loss. Therefore, the decision to offer surgery must be highly individualized, and the possibility to control the proliferative process and improve vision must be balanced against the risks of complications, reoperation, decreased vision, and complete loss of sight. The following factors should be considered prior to offering vitreoretinal surgery: visual acuity and severity of disease in the eye in which surgery is being considered, amount of prior photocoagulation, visual acuity and stability of the fellow eye, visual needs of the patient, anesthetic risk, and likelihood of developing severe postoperative complications.

The general objectives of vitreous surgery are (1) to reverse complications causing visual loss, and (2) to alter the course of the often progressive diabetic retinopathy by removing the posterior vitreous surface on which fibrovascular tissue grows.

VITREOUS HEMORRHAGE

Diagnosis

In eyes with clear cornea and lens, a vitreous hemorrhage is diagnosed with biomicroscopy and indirect ophthal-

moscopy. If the hemorrhage is recent, the bright red color of blood is characteristic (Fig. 1). However, vitreous opacification lacks a red color when the hemorrhage is old. Ultrasonography is required in all cases of severe diabetic vitreous opacification to determine the density and location of the hemorrhage, to identify areas of vitreoretinal adhesions and retinal detachment, and to determine whether the posterior hyaloid is detached.

Treatment

The information we have concerning the timing of vitrectomy for vitreous hemorrhage is derived from the randomized clinical trial known as the Diabetic Retinopathy Vitrectomy Study (DRVS). This study found that, in type I diabetic patients, vitrectomy performed within the first 6 months of a dense vitreous hemorrhage increased the chances of better visual acuity and improved the anatomic results (Fig. 1). The main advantages of early vitrectomy include (1) a better prognosis for recovery of vision, and (2) earlier recovery of vision in successful cases, which is particularly important if the vision in the fellow eye is poor.

The surgical technique consists of performing a three-port pars plana vitrectomy and endophotocoagulation. To prevent opacification of the lens, it is important to add 3 ml of dextrose without preservatives or antioxidants to the 500-ml infusion bottle of Balanced Salt Solution Plus. Initially in the vitrectomy, a small opening in the posterior hyaloid is made with the vitrectomy probe. Preoperative ultrasonography is useful in identifying the area where the hyaloid is separated and in determining whether subhyaloid blood is present. Once a small opening in the posterior hyaloid is made, the

H. Lewis, M.D.: Division of Ophthalmology, The Cleveland Clinic Foundation, Cleveland, OH 44195 and G. Sanchez, M.D.: Asociacion Para Evitar la Ceguera en Mexico, Mexico City, Mexico.

TABLE 1. *Indications for initial surgery*

	1974 (Aaberg)	1991 (Lewis)
Vitreous hemorrhage	70%	10%
Macular traction retinal detachment	20%	35%
Combined tractional-rhegmatogenous retinal detachment	10%	36%
Progressive fibrovascular proliferation	0%	8%
Diabetic macular edema and traction associated with posterior hyaloidal traction	0%	3%
Premacular hemorrhage	0%	3%
Anterior hyaloidal fibrovascular proliferation	0%	1%
Iris neovascularization in the presence of media opacification	0%	1%

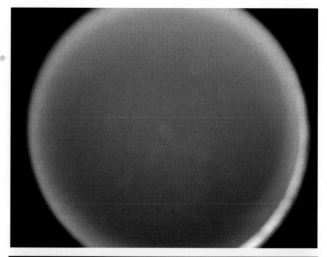

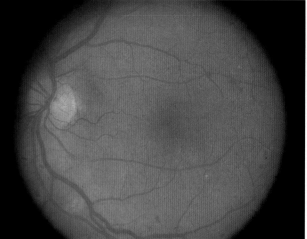

FIG. 1. A: Dense vitreous hemorrhage precluding visualization of the retina. Visual acuity: hand motions. **B:** Following vitrectomy and endophotocoagulation, the visual acuity improved to 20/30.

subhyaloid blood is evacuated by using a tapered extrusion needle, thus preventing stirring of subhyaloid blood that can interfere with intraoperative visualization. The entire posterior two-thirds of the vitreous gel and the posterior vitreous surface are then excised. If a posterior vitreous detachment is not present, the posterior hyaloid is separated from the retina by (1) engaging the hyaloid at the posterior pole adjacent to an area of fibrovascular proliferation, (2) grasping the posterior vitreous surface from the disc and pulling, or (3) incising the posterior hyaloid in an area of subhyaloid hemorrhage. If the vitreous hemorrhage is dense, the hemorrhagic basal vitreous gel is debulked to decrease the likelihood of the blood dispersing into the vitreous cavity in the postoperative period and resulting in decreased vision or hemolytic glaucoma. Finally, endophotocoagulation is applied in a

TABLE 2. *Indications for reoperation (Lewis) n = 30*

Vitreous cavity hemorrhage[a]	30%
Anterior hyaloidal fibrovascular proliferation[b]	16%
Severe fibrin response[c]	16%
Rhegmatogenous retinal detachment[d]	13%
Proliferative vitreoretinopathy[b]	6%
Neovascular glaucoma[e]	6%
Hemolytic glaucoma[a]	3%
Iris neovascularization and media oppacification[f]	3%
Fibrovascular ingrowth[b]	3%
Cataract[g]	3%

[a] Fluid/gas exchange or vitreous surgery.
[b] Vitreoretinal surgery.
[c] Injection of tissue plasminogen activator and fluid/gas exchange.
[d] Fluid/gas exchange and transpupillary photocoagulation or vitreoretinal surgery.
[e] Vitreous surgery, lensectomy (if phakic), and endocyclophotocoagulation.
[f] Lensectomy and endophotocoagulation.
[g] Extracapsular cataract extraction and placement of intraocular lens.

panretinal pattern unless adequate preoperative photocoagulation was performed.

Results

Vitreous surgery for diabetic vitreous hemorrhage results in improvement in visual acuity in up to 83% of cases, with 36% of eyes achieving a final vision of 20/40 or better.

PREMACULAR HEMORRHAGE

Definition

Some eyes with proliferative diabetic retinopathy develop a subhyaloid hemorrhage overlying the macula (Fig. 2). Although most of these hemorrhages clear spontaneously,

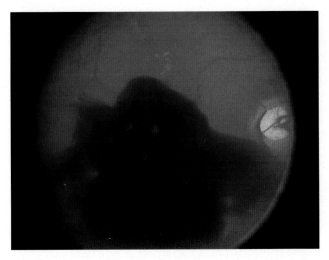

FIG. 2. Premacular hemorrhage. Blood is located in between the posterior vitreous surface and the inner retina.

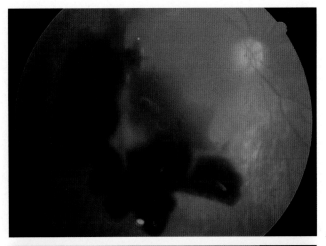

A

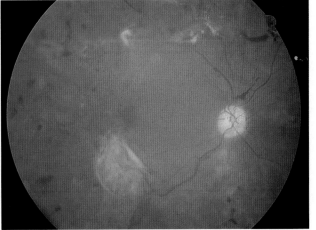

B

FIG. 4. Premacular hemorrhage. **A:** Dense premacular hemorrhage. Visual acuity: finger counting. **B:** Subhyaloid hemorrhage was evacuated during vitrectomy. Visual acuity is 20/25.

some of these eyes progress to develop premacular fibrosis (Fig. 3) or a traction macular detachment.

Treatment

To improve vision and in an attempt to prevent premacular fibrosis or traction macular detachment, early vitrectomy for large premacular hemorrhages has been suggested (Fig. 4). Eventually, prospective data from the DRVS will become available that will clarify the surgical indications and timing of premacular hemorrhages.

SEVERE AND ACTIVE FIBROVASCULAR PROLIFERATION

Definition

This condition is characterized by severe proliferative diabetic retinopathy with progression of extraretinal neovascularization and fibrous proliferation despite panretinal photocoagulation in eyes with good or useful vision (Figs. 5 and 6).

Treatment

In the early 1980s, the DRVS found that the natural history for eyes with severe fibrovascular proliferation was very poor. Recognizing the importance of vitreoretinal contact in the development of fibrovascular or neovascular proliferation, and knowing that once the vitreous gel is removed the disease process tends to stabilize, the DRVS evaluated the

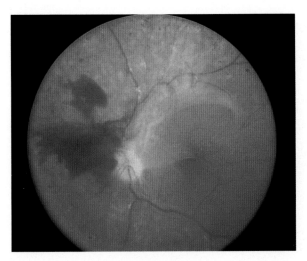

FIG. 3. Premacular fibrosis developed in an eye after spontaneous clearing of subhyaloid hemorrhage.

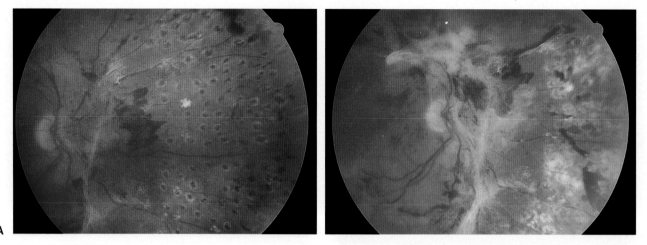

FIG. 5. Severe and active fibrovascular proliferation despite panretinal photocoagulation. **A,B:** Extensive fibrous and neovascular proliferation with subhyaloid hemorrhages in an eye treated with panretinal photocoagulation. Visual acuity is 20/50.

role of vitrectomy in eyes with extensive, active, neovascular, or fibrovascular proliferations and useful vision (better than 10/200). This study demonstrated that early vitrectomy can improve the prognosis for good vision without increasing the risk for poor vision.

Results

At the end of 48 months, 44% of eyes undergoing early vitrectomy achieved a visual acuity of 10/20 or better, compared with 28% of eyes undergoing conventional management. The greatest benefit was seen in patients with more severe retinopathy, particularly eyes with severe fibrous proliferation and moderately severe neovascularization. It is important to stress that, in these eyes with useful vision and advanced, active proliferative diabetic retinopathy, vitrectomy should not be used as an alternative to photocoagulation but

rather as an adjunct when there is progression of fibrovascular proliferation, despite panretinal photocoagulation.

TRACTION MACULAR DETACHMENT

Definition

The pathoanatomy of diabetic traction retinal detachment is complex and depends on the relationship between the posterior vitreous surface to the fibrovascular tissue and the retina. In severe diabetic retinopathy, the extraretinal neovascular and fibrovascular tissues grow along the posterior vitreous surface and occasionally into the vitreous gel. As the fibrovascular tissue contracts, the posterior hyaloid becomes taut and partially separates from the retina, creating anteroposterior traction on the remaining areas of vitreoretinal attachment. A trampolinelike configuration occurs when

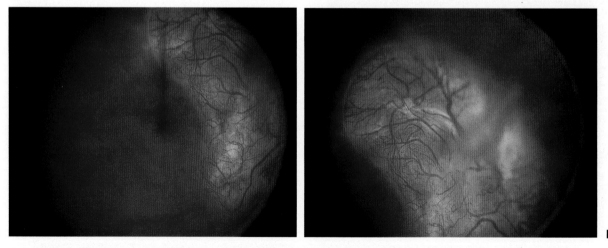

FIG. 6. Severe and active fibrovascular proliferation despite panretinal photocoagulation. **A,B:** Severe fibrous and neovascular proliferation despite treatment with panretinal photocoagulation. The macula is still attached, and visual acuity is 20/30.

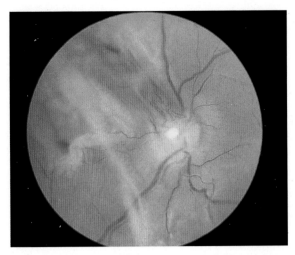

FIG. 7. Traction macular detachment with ectopia of the fovea due to tangential traction.

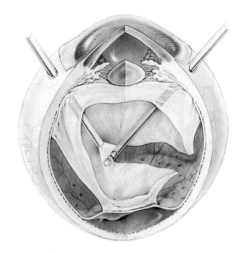

FIG. 8. Anteroposterior traction is released by removing the posterior hyaloid between the vitreous base and the posterior vitreoretinal attachments.

the posterior vitreous surface is separated in between the epicenters of fibrovascular proliferation. A table-top configuration occurs when the taut posterior vitreous surface is diffusely adherent to and detaches from the posterior retina. Tangential traction on the retina can also occur when the fibrovascular tissue growing along the inner retina contracts; in these cases, distortion or ectopia of the fovea occurs (Fig. 7). Frequently, the posterior vitreous surface is separated between the posterior vitreoretinal adhesions and the posterior border of the vitreous base.

Treatment

A traction macular detachment or ectopia of the fovea is a clear indication for vitreoretinal surgery, as long as the eye has visual potential. The general goals of surgery include (1) removing opacities causing visual loss, (2) removing the posterior vitreous surface on which fibrovascular tissue grows, (3) removing fibrovascular tissue, (4) releasing anteroposterior and tangential vitreoretinal traction, (5) obtaining hemostasis, and (6) minimizing complications. A variety of surgical techniques have been described to accomplish these goals. Because of the complex pathoanatomy of diabetic traction retinal detachments, no single technique can always be used.

Segmentation

Anteroposterior traction is released by excising the vitreous gel and circumferentially cutting the posterior vitreous surface where it is separated from the retina (Fig. 8). If there is no posterior vitreous detachment, the posterior vitreous surface can be separated by using the techniques discussed under the section on the treatment of vitreous hemorrhage.

The posterior vitreous surface in between areas of fibrovascular adhesions is then excised with the vitrectomy probe. Then, the fibrovascular tissue is divided into separate islands by using vertical cutting scissors. In areas where the fibrovascular tissue covers the entire posterior retina, the dissection begins temporal to the macula, placing the blades of the vertical cutting scissors in between the retina and the fibrovascular tissue and cutting across the horizontal raphe and around the optic nerve head (Fig. 9). Segmentation continues by making radial incisions in a posterior-to-anterior dissection, thus leaving only small islands of fibrovascular tissue (Figs. 9–11). Bleeding is frequently a problem during membrane segmentation, because the neovascular tissue is cut far away from its site of origin. Intraoperative hemorrhage is stopped by increasing the intraocular pressure, using

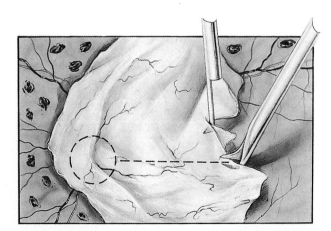

FIG. 9. Membrane segmentation. **A:** An illuminated pick is used to elevate the posterior vitreous surface from the retina while vertical cutting scissors are introduced into this plane to segment the diabetic membranes along the horizontal raphe and around the optic nerve head. **B:** Radial incisions are made in a posterior-to-anterior direction to segment residual fibrovascular tissue and relieve tangential traction.

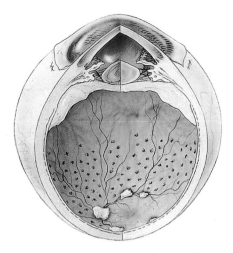

FIG. 10. Membrane segmentation. At the end of membrane segmentation, the anteroposterior and tangential traction has been relieved, but small islands of fibrovascular tissue remain that may obscure retinal breaks or may rebleed in the postoperative period.

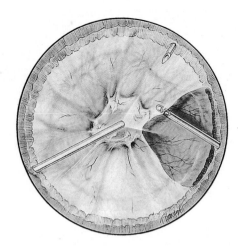

FIG. 12. En bloc excision of diabetic membranes. A small area of the posterior hyaloid between one of the sclerotomies and a posterior vitreoretinal attachment is excised.

bipolar diathermy on the cut edges of fibrovascular tissue, and adding thrombin to the infusion solution.

Membrane segmentation is an effective technique to relieve anteroposterior and tangential traction. However, it leaves islands of fibrovascular tissue that may obscure retinal breaks (that frequently lead to a retinal detachment, because the retinal breaks are under traction) and may rebleed postoperatively (Figs. 10 and 11). Therefore, this technique has largely been abandoned in favor of other techniques that allow for complete removal of the posterior vitreous surface and fibrovascular tissue.

En Bloc Excision of Posterior Hyaloid and Fibrovascular Tissue

This technique leaves the posterior vitreous surface attached to the vitreous base until all posterior attachments have been amputated; therefore, the anteroposterior traction exerted by the vitreous is used to keep the edge of the fibrovascular tissue elevated, thus providing an advantage similar to that of having an additional instrument in the eye. Initially, only enough posterior hyaloid is excised (from the vitreous base to an area of posterior vitreoretinal adhesion) to allow evacuation of the subhyaloid blood and introduction of the horizontal cutting scissors between the posterior hyaloid and the retina (Figs. 12 and 13). An illuminated pick is used as a second instrument to provide illumination and elevate the posterior vitreous surface and fibrovascular tissue, thereby further improving visualization of the fibrovascular epicenters. Using illuminated horizontal cutting scissors, each vascular epicenter is amputated from the retina (Fig. 13). At the time the fibrovascular epicenters are cut, minimal bleeding occurs and it frequently ceases spontaneously. Once the posterior vitreous surface and the fibrovascular tissue have been completely released from the

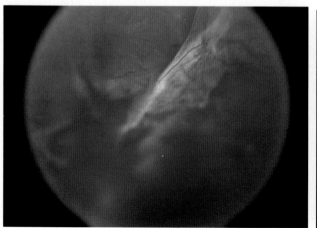

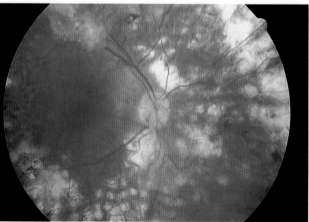

FIG. 11. A: Traction macular detachment and vitreous hemorrhage. **B:** After vitrectomy and membrane segmentation, small islands of fibrovascular tissue remain.

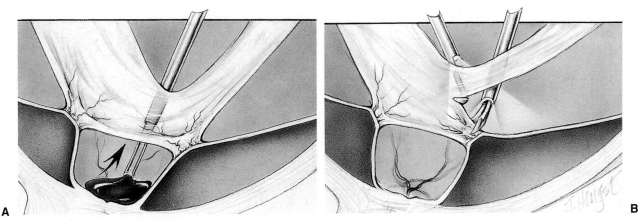

FIG. 13. En bloc excision of diabetic membranes. **A:** An extrusion cannula is introduced through the opening in the posterior hyaloid to evacuate the subhyaloid blood. **B:** While an illuminated pick and the remaining anteroposterior vitreous attachments elevate the posterior hyaloid surface and fibrovascular tissue, an illuminated horizontal scissors is used to amputate the fibrovascular tissue from its retinal epicenter.

retina, the vitrectomy probe is used to remove these tissues (Fig. 14).

The main advantages of this technique include (1) better visualization of fibrovascular epicenters, (2) complete removal of the posterior hyaloid surface and fibrovascular proliferation (Figs. 15 and 16), and (3) minimal intraoperative bleeding. The principal disadvantage is the possibility of causing iatrogenic retinal breaks, which occur in approximately 35% of cases. However, because the traction is completely relieved, the retinal breaks frequently do not lead to a postoperative rhegmatogenous retinal detachment. If retinal breaks occur, they should be treated with photocoagulation, and the eye should be insufflated with gas such as sulfur hexafluoride (SF_6) (Figs. 17 and 18).

Delamination by the Bimanual Technique

This technique is an alternative to en bloc excision of diabetic membranes and is particularly effective in eyes with broad vitreoretinal adhesions. A bimanual approach, with instruments such as the tissue manipulator and scissors, is used to remove the entire posterior vitreous surface and fibrovascular tissue. The tissue manipulator is a multifunction instrument consisting of a 19- or 20-gauge fiberoptic through which a 30-gauge hollow tube protrudes and is used for infusion or aspiration, to pick up or release tissue, and bipolar diathermy. As in membrane segmentation, the initial step consists of excising the partially detached posterior vitreous surface between the vitreous base and the posterior vitreo-

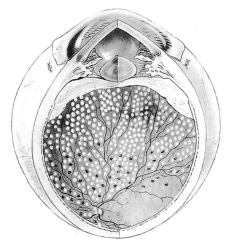

FIG. 14. En bloc excision of diabetic membranes. Complete removal of posterior vitreous surface and fibrovascular tissue exposes a preexisting retinal break located adjacent to a fibrovascular epicenter. The separated vitreous gel and fibrovascular tissue are removed with a vitrectomy probe.

FIG. 15. After en bloc excision or bimanual delamination of diabetic membranes, the retina is completely free of fibrovascular tissue and posterior vitreous surface.

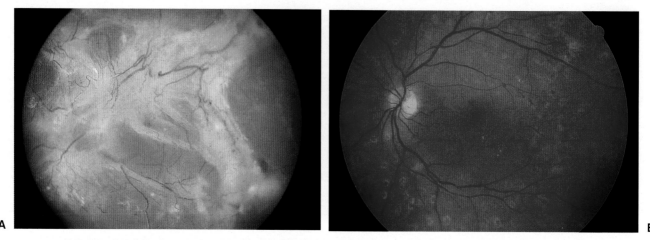

FIG. 16. A: Traction macular detachment. **B:** En bloc excision of diabetic membranes was performed, and the entire posterior surface and fibrovascular tissue were removed.

retinal attachments and thereby releasing anteroposterior traction (see Fig. 8). The dissection is carried from anterior to posterior by using the tissue manipulator to reflect the proliferative tissue or posterior hyaloid and identifying the fibrovascular epicenters that are then amputated from the retina with horizontal or membrane peeler–cutter scissors (Fig. 19). If bleeding occurs, the tissue manipulator can be used to infuse fluid to brush the blood away from the retina and diathermize the bleeding vessel (Fig. 19).

In severe cases, when there are broad areas of vitreoretinal adhesion, a combination of segmentation and delamination is used to accomplish the objectives of surgery. Initially, the fibrovascular membranes are segmented into smaller islands that are then removed by bimanual delamination (Fig. 20).

Independent of the technique used to accomplish the goals of surgery, endophotocoagulation is used at the end of the procedure to treat the retina and all iatrogenic retinal breaks. Placement of a prophylactic scleral buckle is not recommended, and all efforts should be made to release vitreoretinal traction completely. A scleral buckle is only placed if a retinal dialysis occurs intraoperatively.

Results

In expert hands, the results obtained with en bloc excision or bimanual delamination of diabetic membranes for the treatment of traction macular detachments are similar. Long-term retinal reattachment is achieved in 83%–88% of cases, and a visual acuity of 5/200 or better is obtained in 65%–71%. (See also Chapter 15 by S. Charles and B. Wood.)

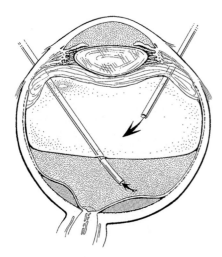

FIG. 17. If preexisting or iatrogenic retinal breaks are present, a fluid–air exchange with internal drainage of subretinal fluid is performed.

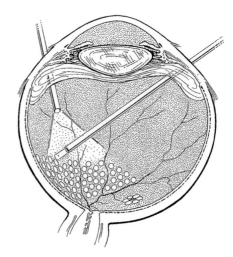

FIG. 18. Endophotocoagulation is applied in a panretinal pattern and is used to treat all retinal breaks.

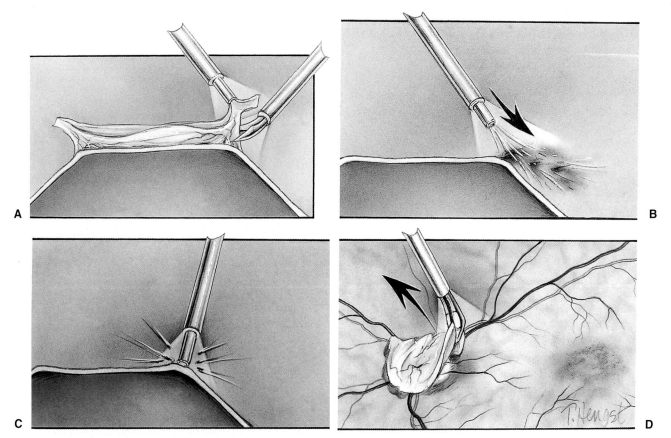

FIG. 19. Bimanual delamination of diabetic membranes. **A:** The tissue manipulator is used to reflect the posterior hyaloid and fibrovascular tissue and to identify vascular epicenters that are cut by illuminated horizontal scissors. **B:** If bleeding occurs, fluid is infused through the tissue manipulator to brush the blood away from the retina and visualize the bleeding vessel. **C:** The diathermy of the tissue manipulator is then used to cauterize the bleeding vessel. **D:** The lighted forceps are used to pull the residual fibrovascular membrane from the optic nerve head.

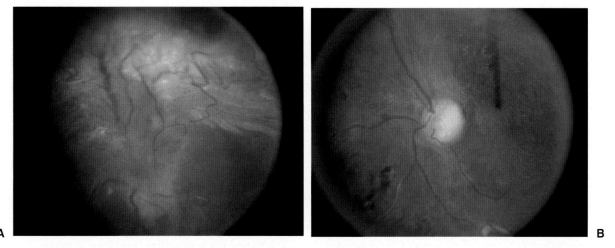

FIG. 20. A: Traction macular detachment. **B:** Fundus photograph following vitreoretinal surgery using bimanual delamination of diabetic membranes.

COMBINED TRACTIONAL AND RHEGMATOGENOUS RETINAL DETACHMENT

Definition

In some diabetic eyes, the traction exerted by the contracted posterior vitreous surface will cause retinal breaks that frequently occur adjacent to fibrovascular epicenters and lead to combined tractional and rhegmatogenous retinal detachments. In contrast to pure tractional retinal detachments, combined detachments tend to be more bullous (although sometimes they have a purely tractional appearance) and may extend into the periphery.

Treatment

In contrast to purely tractional diabetic retinal detachments that are operated only when the macula is detached, combined tractional and rhegmatogenous diabetic retinal detachments are operated on even if the macula is still attached. The rationale for this approach is the high likelihood of progression and macular involvement in combined detachments, and the improved visual results obtained when surgery is performed prior to macular detachment.

The traction is relieved by either en bloc excision or bimanual delamination (Figs. 12–15 and 19). Membrane segmentation is not used because the residual traction keeps the retinal break open and frequently results in a recurrent retinal detachment. Once the traction is released, internal drainage of subretinal fluid is performed (Fig. 17), endophotocoagulation is used to treat retinal breaks and applied in a panretinal pattern (Fig. 18), and the air is exchanged for a nonexpansile concentration of SF_6. Because the retinal breaks are located posteriorly, a scleral buckle is not required.

Results

The anatomic results are similar to the ones obtained in purely tractional macular detachments. The visual results are disappointing, however, with only up to 36% of eyes achieving a visual acuity of 20/200 or better.

DIABETIC MACULAR EDEMA AND TRACTION ASSOCIATED WITH POSTERIOR HYALOIDAL TRACTION

Definition

Some diabetic eyes develop a thickened, taut, and glistening premacular posterior hyaloid that causes traction on the macula and/or contributes to macular edema. In these eyes, the traction is caused by abnormalities of the posterior vitreous surface and not by fibrous proliferation. Angiographically, a characteristic pattern of deep and late retinal fluores-

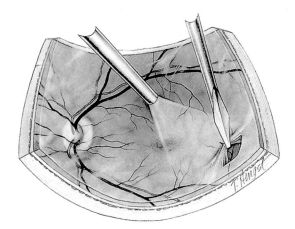

FIG. 21. Vitrectomy for diabetic macular edema and traction associated with posterior hyaloidal traction. The thickened posterior hyaloid is engaged with a bent myringotomy blade.

cence is seen in the macula. Occasionally, focal macular leakage and/or cystoid macular edema can also be present.

Treatment

The diabetic macular edema seen in these eyes does not respond to macular photocoagulation. However, pars plana vitrectomy with separation and removal of the posterior hyaloid is highly effective in causing resolution of the macular edema and traction, and in improving visual acuity. After removing the posterior two-thirds of the vitreous gel, a myringotomy blade is used to engage the posterior hyaloid in an area where it appears to be the thickest (Fig. 21). This maneuver can be easily performed because the posterior vitreous surface is thickened and taut. Then, vitreoretinal forceps are used to separate the posterior hyaloid from the macula, posterior pole, and equatorial retina (Fig. 22).

Results

Results of a pilot study showed that nine of 10 eyes that had been operated on had improvement in visual acuity, with six of them achieving a visual acuity of 20/60 or better. In eight of the 10 cases the macular edema resolved, and in the remaining two cases it decreased. To date, the visual acuity following the surgery has improved in 90% of the patients, and 30% of the eyes achieved a visual acuity of 20/40 or better. Although no intraoperative complications occurred, postoperative complications included a vitreous hemorrhage (one eye), a rhegmatogenous retinal detachment (one eye), and a moderately dense cataract (one eye).

We currently believe that, in addition to the observed macular thickening, the tangential traction exerted by the thickened and taut posterior hyaloid causes a very shallow macular detachment that can explain the angiographic features and the improvement in visual acuity following surgery (Fig. 23).

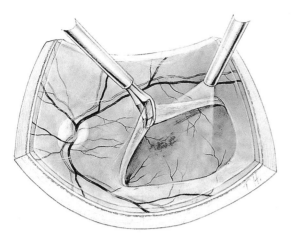

FIG. 22. Vitrectomy for diabetic macular edema and traction associated with posterior hyaloidal traction. Once an opening in the posterior hyaloid is made, intraocular forceps are used to separate the posterior vitreous surface from the retina.

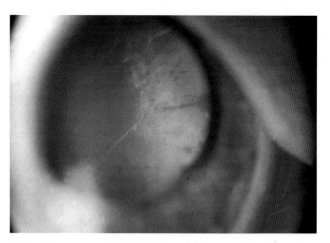

FIG. 24. Anterior hyaloidal fibrovascular proliferation. Neovascularization, hemorrhage, and fibrous proliferation are seen on the posterior lens capsule.

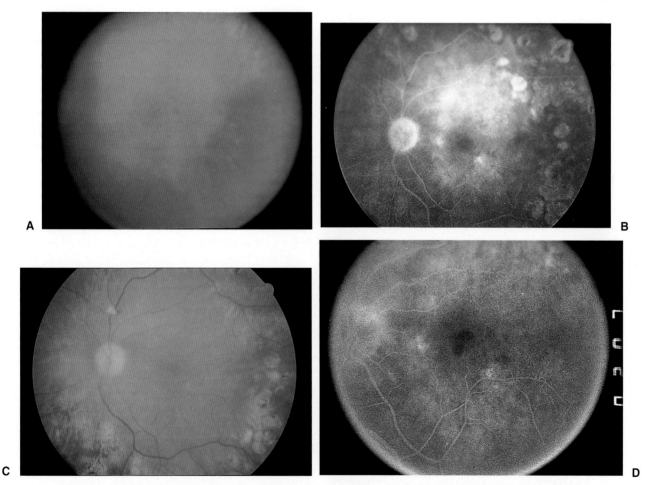

FIG. 23. A: Preoperative color photograph demonstrating opacification of the macular region due to thickening of the posterior hyaloid with parafoveal photocoagulation scars. Contact lens biomicroscopy shows the thickening of the macular and an opacified, thickened, premacular cortical vitreous. Visual acuity is 20/100. **B:** Preoperative fluorescein angiogram demonstrating diffused macular leakage in the late phases. **C:** Postoperative color photograph demonstrating resolution of macular edema. Visual acuity is 20/40. **D:** Postoperative fluorescein angiogram demonstrating resolution of macular edema. 3 months after surgery.

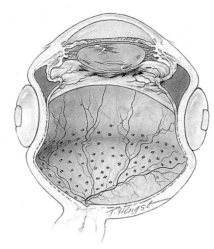

FIG. 25. Anterior hyaloidal fibrovascular proliferation after diabetic vitrectomy. The fibrovascular tissue originates from the anterior retina and grows along the anterior hyaloid to the posterior lens capsule, causing an anterior retinal and ciliary body detachment.

ANTERIOR HYALOIDAL FIBROVASCULAR PROLIFERATION

Definition

This proliferation occurs in phakic and pseudophakic (with posterior capsule) diabetic eyes, and is characterized by the development of neovascularization and fibrous proliferation from the anterior retina extending along the anterior hyaloid to the posterior lens surface. This entity is mostly seen in diabetic eyes that have undergone a previous vitrectomy in which the posterior lens capsule and anterior vitreous are not removed; however, it can also rarely occur in eyes without a previous vitrectomy. Risk factors for the de-

velopment of this complication include (1) young males, (2) type I diabetes mellitus, (3) extensive retinal ischemia, (4) severe retinal neovascularization that does not respond to photocoagulation, (5) traction macular detachment as an indication for surgery, and (6) intraoperative placement of a scleral buckle. This condition frequently occurs within the first 12 weeks after diabetic vitrectomy. Early manifestations include anterior extraretinal vascularization, with the development of vessels on the anterior hyaloid or lens capsule that can be best seen by indirect ophthalmoscopy and scleral depression or by biomicroscopy (Fig. 24). Then, a hemorrhage occurs in between the anterior hyaloid and posterior lens capsule or in the vitreous cavity (Fig. 24). As fibrous proliferation develops, an anterior retinal and ciliary body detachment occurs, causing hypotony, a cyclitic membrane, and eventually atrophy with shrinkage (Fig. 25). Wide-scan echography is useful in making the diagnosis in eyes with a cataract or a vitreous hemorrhage by demonstrating the anterior extraretinal fibrovascular proliferation extending to the posterior lens surface or an anterior retinal or ciliary body detachment.

Treatment

Making an early diagnosis is of utmost importance if the eye is to be saved. This condition should be suspected in all eyes that develop a hemorrhage into the vitreous cavity soon after vitrectomy, particularly if the above risk factors are present. If a diagnosis is made early on, before the development of a cataract, dense vitreous hemorrhage, hypotony, or anterior retinal detachment, the use of extensive panretinal photocoagulation is frequently beneficial. In cases with a cataract, vitreous hemorrhage, and/or retinal or ciliary body traction, a lensectomy with removal of the anterior vitreous

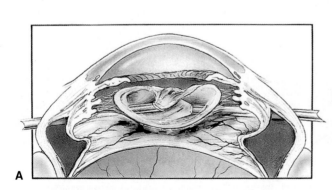
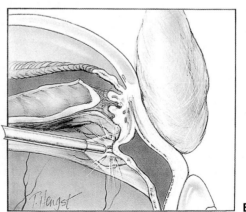

FIG. 26. Anterior hyaloidal fibrovascular proliferation. **A:** Pars plana phacofragmentation is used to remove the lens. **B:** Scleral depression is used to visualize the anterior extraretinal neovascular tissue that is diathermized.

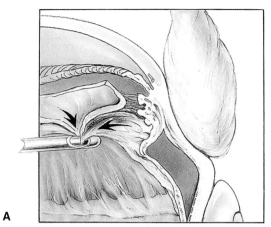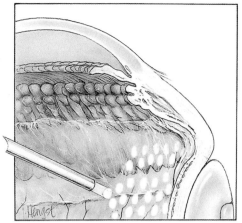

FIG. 27. Anterior hyaloidal fibrovascular proliferation. **A:** Performing scleral depression, the anterior fibrovascular tissue, basal vitreous gel, and lens remnants are removed. **B:** Endophotocoagulation is applied in a panretinal pattern and also over the pars plana.

and fibrovascular proliferation in conjunction with endophotocoagulation should be performed (Figs. 26 and 27). The results are frequently disappointing, however, if the eye has already developed a ciliary body detachment.

Anterior hyaloidal fibrovascular proliferation can be prevented in most cases by performing extensive panretinal photocoagulation before and during vitrectomy, and by removing the clear lens and anterior vitreous in eyes that are at great risk of developing this complication. If the lens is removed during diabetic vitrectomy, extensive endophotocoagulation should be performed to decrease the risk of neovascular glaucoma.

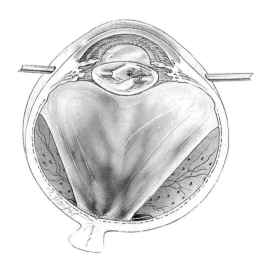

FIG. 28. Implantation of intraocular lens during diabetic vitrectomy. Pars plana lensectomy in eye with cataract and vitreous hemorrhage.

IRIS NEOVASCULARIZATION IN THE PRESENCE OF MEDIA OPACIFICATION

Definition

Eyes that develop iris and/or angle neovascularization and in which transpupillary panretinal photocoagulation cannot be performed because of the presence of a cataract or a vitreous hemorrhage are candidates for vitrectomy.

Treatment

In these circumstances, the media opacities are removed, and extensive endophotocoagulation is performed to induce regression of the iris and/or angle neovascularization and to prevent neovascular glaucoma.

HEMOLYTIC GLAUCOMA

Definition

Intraocular blood can obstruct the angle and trabecular meshwork and lead to hemolytic glaucoma. This complication is more commonly seen in previously vitrectomized and aphakic eyes, but can also occur in diabetic eyes without previous vitreous surgery.

Treatment

If the intraocular pressure is unacceptably elevated, despite antiglaucoma medications, vitreoretinal surgery should be considered. In vitrectomized eyes with residual hemorrhagic basal gel, a vitrectomy with debulking of the basal gel should be performed. If the eye is vitrectomized, however, and most of the blood is in the vitreous cavity, an outpatient fluid–air exchange might be all that is required.

CONTROVERSIAL ISSUES

Removal of Clear Crystalline Lens

Traditionally, the crystalline lens is removed when (1) preexisting lens opacities prevent adequate visualization of the fundus during vitrectomy, (2) if lens opacities will significantly reduce postoperative vision, or (3) when the lens is damaged or opacifies during vitreous surgery. However, removal of a clear crystalline lens might be considered in the following situations:

1. Eyes at high risk for development of anterior hyaloidal fibrovascular proliferation in which removal of the lens and anterior vitreous gel prevents the development of this complication—in these cases, extensive endopanretinal photocoagulation should be performed to decrease the likelihood of developing neovascular glaucoma.

2. Eyes with tractional retinal detachment extending into the periphery—if the clear lens is not removed, adequate membrane dissection cannot be performed, and residual traction remains leading to postoperative retinal detachment. A scleral buckle is not adequate to manage peripheral traction retinal detachments.

Implantation of Intraocular Lens During Diabetic Vitrectomy

Traditionally, intraocular lenses have not been placed during diabetic vitrectomy, because of the risk of developing

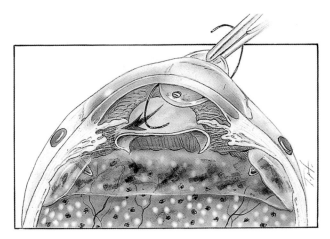

FIG. 30. Implantation of intraocular lens during diabetic vitrectomy. After the vitrectomy, the fundus is examined and if there are no contradictions for intraocular lens implantation, a superior limbal incision is made to insert a preselected intraocular lens anterior to the anterior lens capsule and into the ciliary sulcus.

significant complications if anterior segment neovascularization occurs postoperatively. Because very few aphakic diabetics will wear contact lenses, implantation of an intraocular lens during diabetic vitrectomy might be considered in selected cases such as eyes in which the proliferative disease appears to be inactive (during vitrectomy) and the visual potential is good.

The technique used depends on the surgeon's preference. One possibility is to phacoemulsify the lens through a scleral tunnel, leaving the posterior capsule intact. During the vitrectomy, the posterior capsule is filled with sodium hyaluronidase to improve visualization. After the vitrectomy, the fundus is examined, and if the patient is a candidate for intraocular lens implantation, the scleral wound is enlarged and a posterior chamber intraocular lens is implanted in the bag.

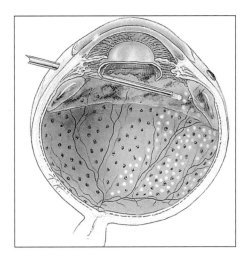

FIG. 29. Implantation of intraocular lens during diabetic vitrectomy. While the anterior lens capsule and zonules remain in place, the vitrectomy is performed.

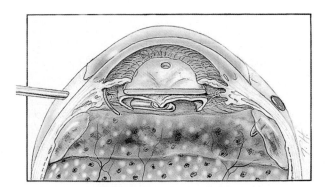

FIG. 31. The vitreous cutter is introduced and the anterior capsule is cut centrally.

An alternative operation if the surgeon has no experience with this technique involves performing a pars plana lensectomy, leaving the anterior lens capsule and zonules intact (Figs. 28 and 29). After performing the vitrectomy and determining that the patient is a candidate for intraocular lens implantation, the superonasal sclerotomy is closed, a superior limbal incision is made, and a preselected intraocular lens is placed above the anterior lens capsule and into the ciliary sulcus (Fig. 30). Then, through the superotemporal sclerotomy, the vitrectomy probe is used either to aspirate the cells from, or to make a central opening in, the anterior lens capsule (Fig. 31).

Both of these techniques offer the advantages of being able to examine the fundus after the vitrectomy and prior to inserting the intraocular lens, preventing corneal edema during vitrectomy, and maintaining corneal transparency during vitreoretinal surgery.

Use of Tissue Plasminogen Activator for Postvitrectomy Fibrin Deposition

Postvitrectomy fibrin deposition is a severe complication of diabetic vitrectomy occurring in approximately 10% of cases. Fibrin deposition can lead to pupillary or cyclitic membranes, pupillary block glaucoma, ciliary body detachment with hypotony, and recurrent tractional retinal detachment. Tissue plasminogen activator is a fibrin-specific thrombolytic agent that has been found to be very useful in the clearance of postvitrectomy fibrin. However, a few cases with severe neovascularization have been reported in which the injection of tissue plasminogen activator has resulted in intraocular bleeding.

Use of Silicone Oil as Intraocular Tamponade

This use of silicone oil in primary diabetic retinal detachments offers no advantages over gas and might have adverse effects if the eye bleeds postoperatively. However, its use might be necessary in patients who cannot maintain a face-down position postoperatively.

BIBLIOGRAPHY

Aaberg TM, Abrams GW. Changing indications and techniques for vitrectomy in the management of complications of diabetic retinopathy. *Ophthalmology* 1987;94:775–779.

Abrams GW, Williams GA. "En bloc" excision of diabetic membranes. *Am J Ophthalmol* 1987;103:302–308.

Blankenship GW. Proliferative diabetic retinopathy: principles and techniques of surgical treatment; vol 3. In: Ryan SJ, ed. *Retina.* St. Louis: CV Mosby, 1989:515–539.

Blankenship GW, Flynn HW, Kokame GT. Posterior chamber intraocular lens insertion during pars plana lensectomy and vitrectomy for complications of diabetic retinopathy. *Am J Ophthalmol* 1989;108:1–5.

Dabbs CK, Aaberg TM, Aguilar HE, Sternberg P, Meredith TA, Ward AR. Complications of tissue plasminogen activator therapy after vitrectomy for diabetes. *Am J Ophthalmol* 1990;110:354–360.

Diabetic Retinopathy Vitrectomy Study Research Group. Early vitrectomy for severe vitreous hemorrhage in diabetic retinopathy—Diabetic Retinopathy Vitrectomy Study Report 2. *Arch Ophthalmol* 1985;103:1644–1651.

Diabetic Retinopathy Vitrectomy Study Research Group. Two-year course of visual acuity in severe proliferative diabetic retinopathy with conventional management—Diabetic Retinopathy Vitrectomy Study Report 1. *Ophthalmology* 1985;92:492–501.

Diabetic Retinopathy Vitrectomy Study Research Group. Early vitrectomy for severe proliferative diabetic retinopathy in eyes with useful vision: results of a randomized trial—Diabetic Retinopathy Vitrectomy Study Report 3. *Ophthalmology* 1988;95:1307–1320.

Diabetic Retinopathy Vitrectomy Study Research Group. Early vitrectomy for severe proliferative diabetic retinopathy in eyes with useful vision: clinical applications of results of a randomized trial—Diabetic Retinopathy Vitrectomy Study Report 4. *Ophthalmology* 1988;95:1321–1334.

Diabetic Retinopathy Vitrectomy Study Research Group. Early vitrectomy for severe vitreous hemorrhage in diabetic retinopathy. Four years results of a randomized trial: Diabetic Retinopathy Vitrectomy Study Report 5. *Arch Ophthalmol* 1990;108:958–964.

Koenig S, Han DP, Mieler WF, Abrams GW, Jaffe GJ, Burton TC. Combined phacoemulsification and pars plana vitrectomy. *Arch Ophthalmol* 1990;108:362–364.

Lewis H, Abrams GW, Williams GA. Anterior hyaloidal fibrovascular proliferation after diabetic vitrectomy. *Am J Ophthalmol* 1987;104:607–613.

Lewis H, Abrams GW, Foos RY. Clinicopathologic findings in anterior hyaloidal fibrovascular proliferation after diabetic vitrectomy. *Am J Ophthalmol* 1987;104:614–618.

Lewis H, Aaberg TM, Abrams GW. Current causes of failure after diabetic vitrectomy. *Invest Ophthalmol Vis Sci* 1988;29:220(abst).

Lewis H, Abrams GW, Blumenkranz MS, Campo R. Vitrectomy for diabetic macular edema and traction associated with posterior hyaloidal traction. *Ophthalmology* 1992;99:753–759.

Michels RG, Wilkinson CP, Rice TA, eds. *Retinal detachment.* St. Louis: CV Mosby, 1990.

Ramsay RC, Knobloch WH, Cantrill HL. Timing of vitrectomy for active diabetic retinopathy. *Ophthalmology* 1986;93:283–289.

Practical Atlas of Retinal Disease and Therapy, Second Edition
edited by William R. Freeman,
Lippincott–Raven Publishers, Philadelphia © 1997.

· 12 ·

Diagnosis and Treatment of Peripheral Retinal Lesions

John S. Lean

Peripheral retinal lesions are common. Only a minority predispose eyes to retinal detachment, and because prophylactic treatment can lead to macular edema or macular pucker, expertise with indirect ophthalmoscopy and scleral depression is needed in order to make an accurate diagnosis and avoid unnecessary surgery. Once a predisposing lesion is identified, appropriate management reflects an assessment of the likely risk of retinal detachment if the lesion is not treated (natural history), as well as the reduction in risk with treatment (likelihood of success), the possibility of retinal detachment despite treatment (likelihood of failure), and how much treatment will need to be applied (likelihood of complications).

In some cases, the decision to treat or not to treat is clearcut; a symptomatic break is always treated, an asymptomatic break is usually not. In other situations, appropriate management is more controversial. Lattice degeneration might be treated if the patient is young, has a family history of retinal detachment, and is going to work for 5 years in a remote area, but not if a posterior vitreous detachment (PVD) is already present and the patient is 75 years old and lives in proximity to a well-trained ophthalmologist.

DIAGNOSIS

The key difference between benign peripheral lesions and those that predispose eyes to tear formation and retinal detachment is the presence of focal vitreoretinal adhesions. These adhesions are best detected by indirect ophthalmoscopy and kinetic scleral depression. As the peripheral retina is rolled over the tip of the scleral depressor, the adhesion is seen in relief as a wispy opaque strand in the vitreous.

Benign Peripheral Lesions

Chorioretinal Degeneration

These lesions range from a mild pigmentary disturbance to multiple large drusen ("cobblestone") to a patch of chorioretinal atrophy ("pavingstone"). At sites of pavingstone degeneration, the retina adheres to the choroid and these areas are never the site of retinal breaks.

Cystoid Degeneration/Retinoschisis

This degeneration is always contiguous with the ora serrata; it frequently extends as far as the equator, more rarely further posteriorly. The retina is slightly opaque and contains tiny cystoid spaces. When peripheral cystoid degeneration becomes more marked and a cavity forms in the retina, it is called retinoschisis. The clinical appearance is of a smooth-domed, thin-walled cyst posterior to the ora that is continuous with less elevated areas of cystoid at the ora. White dots are scattered on the inner surface of the schisis cavity, which has a beaten metal appearance. Sometimes, large holes are seen in the outer leaf (Fig. 1), which may then be elevated ("schisis retinal detachment"). Holes in the inner leaf are round. If holes are present in both leaves of schisis, retinal detachment can occur. However, schisis is very common, and the vast majority of cases are static or extend only very slowly.

Whitening With and Without Pressure

These geographic areas of retinal whitening usually have a linear configuration. They can be seen either with or with-

J. S. Lean, M.D., F.R.C.S.: 23521 Paseo de Valencia, Laguna Hills, CA 92653.

[1] See also discussions in Chapter 15 by S. Charles and B. Wood and in Chapter 17 by G. W. Abrams and L. C. Glazer.

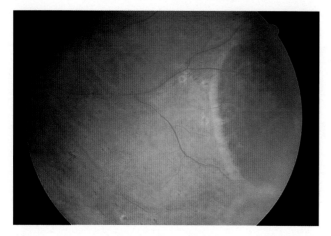

FIG. 1. Retinoschisis: the inner wall of the schisis cavity is shallowly elevated. There is a large peripheral outer leaf break that has a rolled posterior edge.

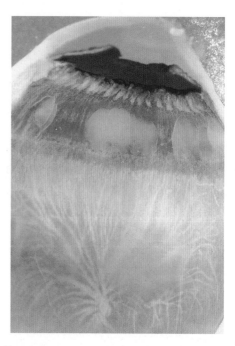

FIG. 2. Pars plana cysts: postmortem specimen showing large pars plana cysts.

out scleral depression. Their explanation is unclear; however, they probably relate to vitreoretinal adhesion and have no ominous significance.

Variants of the Normal Ora Serrata

It is important to be aware of anatomic variants of the ora in order not to confuse these with degenerations predisposing eyes to tears and retinal detachment.

1. *Meridional fold.* The fold is an exaggeration of the normal dentate process. Occasionally, there is a round hole in the base of the fold.
2. *Meridional complex.* This occurs when a ciliary process and meridional fold almost meet. They are commonly seen in the upper nasal quadrant.
3. *Enclosed oral bay.* This is formed by the joining of two adjacent dentate processes. It may look like a hole, but it is distinguished from one by its location anterior to the ora serrata.
4. *Granular tissue.* This tissue appears as tiny white opacities in the vitreous base immediately interior to the retinal surface. These can look like peripheral opercula, but are distinguished by their small size and multiplicity.
5. *Pars plana cysts.* Cysts sometimes form between the nonpigmented and pigmented pars plana epithelium. They may be quite large (Fig. 2).

Lesions That May Predispose Eyes to Retinal Detachment

Lattice Degeneration

The distinguishing features of lattice degeneration are a patch of retinal atrophy with vitreous adhesion at its borders and a pocket of syneretic vitreous overlying the lesion itself (Fig. 3A). Typical lattice lesions are circumferentially oriented oval lesions with thin white (hyalinized) retinal blood vessels (Fig. 3B). However, there is considerable variation. Some lesions are small, and white lines may not be obvious; others are quite heavily pigmented (Fig. 3C). Radially oriented lesions along blood vessels are occasionally found, particularly as one of the ocular manifestations of Stickler's disease. The key distinguishing feature of lattice degeneration is not the "lattice" of white lines, but rather the associated vitreoretinal adhesion at the margin of the lesion.

Atrophic round holes without opercula are often present in lattice lesions, usually toward the ends of an extended patch. The holes may be surrounded by a small cuff of fluid. Following PVD, there is an increased risk of flap tears in eyes with lattice. Saccadic vitreous movement creates dynamic traction on the vitreoretinal adhesions at the posterior edge of the lattice patch; the retina breaks at this point, creating a tear with the lattice lesion in the flap of the tear (Fig. 3D,E). In addition, flap tears in normal retina seem to occur more frequently in eyes with lattice, particularly in aphakic eyes.

Snail Track

Snail track lesions (Fig. 4) are so named because they resemble the track of a snail. They are typically longer than lattice lesions and consist of a fine frosting of white dots on the retinal surface, without white lines. There is overlying vitreous liquefaction, but no obvious vitreoretinal adhesion. Eyes with snail track degeneration are often myopic. Like lattice lesions, atrophic holes without opercula may be present in the patches of degeneration, but, unlike lattice, these holes

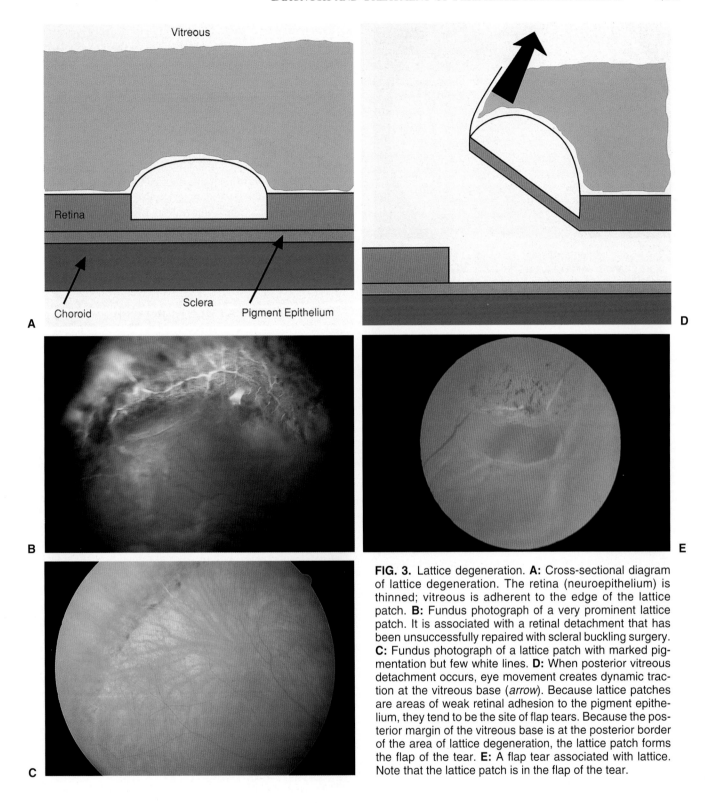

FIG. 3. Lattice degeneration. **A:** Cross-sectional diagram of lattice degeneration. The retina (neuroepithelium) is thinned; vitreous is adherent to the edge of the lattice patch. **B:** Fundus photograph of a very prominent lattice patch. It is associated with a retinal detachment that has been unsuccessfully repaired with scleral buckling surgery. **C:** Fundus photograph of a lattice patch with marked pigmentation but few white lines. **D:** When posterior vitreous detachment occurs, eye movement creates dynamic traction at the vitreous base (*arrow*). Because lattice patches are areas of weak retinal adhesion to the pigment epithelium, they tend to be the site of flap tears. Because the posterior margin of the vitreous base is at the posterior border of the area of lattice degeneration, the lattice patch forms the flap of the tear. **E:** A flap tear associated with lattice. Note that the lattice patch is in the flap of the tear.

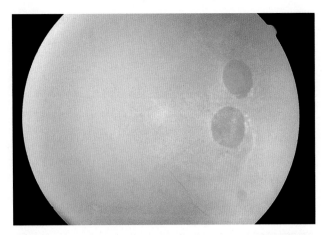

FIG. 4. Snail track degeneration. Multiple tiny white dots are present on the surface of the retina associated with very large retinal holes. As is frequently the case with this degeneration (in contrast to lattice), the holes have led to retinal detachment.

are large and have a strong tendency to cause retinal detachment, whereas flap tears do not occur.

Cystic Tuft

This is a granular tuft of tissue on the surface of the postbasal retina. Cystic tufts frequently occur bilaterally and are usually recognized when retinal detachment due to a cystic tuft has occurred in one eye.

Zonular Traction Tuft

This is a tuft of peripheral retinal tissue directed anterior toward the zonule. Like the cystic tuft, it is usually first detected in the fellow eye of a patient with retinal detachment.

Retinal Breaks

There are three types of postoral peripheral retinal breaks: (1) flap or horseshoe tears, in which the torn retina is attached at the anterior aspect of the tear; (2) operculated (usually round holes), in which the avulsed retina is separated from the retina; and (3) atrophic holes, in which there is normally no overlying operculum. Retinal breaks are usually best detected with the indirect ophthalmoscope and scleral depression. In most cases, the break itself can be seen as a red dehiscence in the pale retina. In some cases, however, the break is revealed only by its attached flap or detached operculum. These are best seen during kinetic examination of the retinal periphery with the scleral depressor. As the retina rolls over the moving depressor, the flap or operculum transiently "pops up" into view. Sometimes the insertion of the posterior hyaloid is visible as an opaque cir-

cumferential line behind the ora; if visible, this is a useful landmark, as the majority of breaks occur at the posterior border of the vitreous base.

Dialysis/Disinsertion

These lesions typically follow contusional injuries. In the superonasal quadrant, they occur as an indirect result of equatorial scleral stretching at the time of a severe injury. In the inferotemporal quadrant, they result from direct, often less severe, contusional damage to the ora; inferotemporal dialyses are sometimes bilateral, and the role of trauma is then less certain. In dialysis, the dentate processes of the retina are pulled away from the pars plana at the ora serrata. In a disinsertion, the retina is pulled away from the ora serrata between the dentate processes.

TREATMENT CRITERIA

Benign lesions require diagnosis but, needless to say, do not require treatment.

Lattice Degeneration

Lattice degeneration is found in approximately 30% of retinal detachment cases. However, the high prevalence of lattice in the general population (5%–10%) and the low incidence of retinal detachment (1:10,000/people/year) means that the risk of lattice degeneration leading to retinal detachment in an individual eye is extremely low. This low statistical probability of retinal detachment has been confirmed by long-term follow-up of asymptomatic eyes with lattice degeneration with or without retinal holes (Table 1). In addition, in eyes that are treated, flap tears are prone to occur at the edge of areas of chorioretinal scars and in previously uninvolved areas of the retina. Therefore, treatment is rarely indicated. I treat lattice degeneration only in the following situations:

TABLE 1. *Natural history of lattice degeneration*

	Percentage of 276 patients with lattice degeneration in nonfellow eyes developing specified changes during long-term follow-up
Symptomatic tears	2%
Subclinical retinal detachment	2%
Retinal detachment[a]	1%

[a] Two patients: atrophic holes in lattice; macula attached. One patient: ∪ tear; macula detached.
Modified from Byer NE. Long term natural history of lattice degeneration of the retina. *Ophthalmology* 1989;96:1396–1401, with permission.

1. *In an eye with retinal detachment.* Lattice patches may be the site of subsequent flap tears that can lead to recurrent retinal detachment. The most vulnerable area for secondary tears appears to be close to the site of the primary tears. Thus, I am particularly concerned to treat lattice in the vicinity of all the original tears. If possible, I use a circumferential buckle to support the lattice on either side of the primary tears. I also generally encircle these eyes, because in eyes with lattice there is a risk of subsequent tears in areas of normal retina. In eyes with multiple large lattice patches, I sometimes delay treatment of remote lattice patches until the postoperative period in order to avoid extensive cryotherapy at the time of initial surgical repair. An alternative strategy, in areas of attached retina, would be to use the laser indirect ophthalmoscope.

2. *In the fellow eye of patients who have had a retinal detachment in one eye.* This is particularly important if the fellow eye has not had a PVD, because flap tears are likely to occur when the vitreous eventually detaches. Under these circumstances, I treat all areas of lattice. In an eye without PVD, in which the other is blind from retinal detachment, I consider 360° treatment in the fellow eye, because of the risk of tears occurring outside visible lattice patches. If a PVD has already occurred and no tears are present, the risk of tears developing subsequently is probably minimal. I generally treat only the patches of lattice that form the "mirror image" of the tears that occurred in the eye with retinal detachment. A recent study has suggested that treatment of lattice in phakic fellow eyes has little impact on the risk of retinal detachment. This may be because, in the majority of cases, treatment was applied in eyes in which PVD had already occurred.

3. *Prior to cataract surgery.* This is a difficult issue. Although eyes with lattice degeneration are at higher risk of retinal detachment following cataract surgery and tears occur in lattice patches, tears are also more likely than in phakic eyes to occur in areas of normal retina. Current cataract surgery, in which the posterior capsule is left intact, also appears to be associated with a lower overall risk of retinal detachment. If posterior capsulotomy is performed, however, the risk of retinal detachment rises. Furthermore, increasing numbers of younger patients (in their 40s and 50s) are undergoing cataract surgery. Premature PVD is induced by the surgery or the subsequent yttrium–aluminum–Garnet capsulotomy. The vitreous in these younger patients is a more solid structure, creating greater dynamic traction on the retina and a correspondingly greater risk of flap tears and retinal detachment. I consider treatment of lattice degeneration prior to cataract surgery in these patients and arbitrarily use 55 years of age as the "cutoff point" below which I usually recommend treatment if a PVD is not present. However, I warn the patient that the treatment may not be successful, that tears may subsequently occur in areas of untreated retina, and that the indications for this treatment are not clear-cut.

4. *In aphakia.* This is similar to the situation prior to cataract surgery; indeed, if the cataract is dense, treatment may have to be applied after the cataract is removed. Again, I consider treatment in younger patients if the vitreous is not already detached. Treatment should be applied as soon as possible, because retinal detachment may occur quite quickly following cataract surgery or posterior capsulotomy.

5. *Lattice and flap tears/round holes.* By itself, this combination does not require treatment. However, if it occurs in the context of the situations previously described, or in high myopia, or with a family history of retinal detachment, I advise treatment.

Snail Track

The large round holes found in this degeneration have a strong tendency to progress to retinal detachment and therefore should always be treated. There appears to be little tendency for new hole formation in other areas, which are often extremely extensive, so these should not be treated.

Cystic Tuft/Zonular Traction Tuft

When these are discovered either incidentally or in the fellow eye of a patient with retinal detachment (the majority), I advise treatment.

Retinal Breaks

Round holes or flap tears are found in about 10% of otherwise normal (asymptomatic) eyes. Their presence generally indicates that PVD has occurred and that subsequent dynamic vitreous traction has been sufficient to create a break but not to lead to retinal detachment. With few exceptions, they are benign, because if a break is to cause retinal detachment, it is likely to do so within the first 6 weeks of its formation and be associated with symptoms (Table 2). However, there is a small group of patients in whom progression to retinal detachment from asymptomatic flap tears occasionally occurs. These high-risk situations occur in cataract surgery (particularly if the eye is myopic), in fellow eyes

TABLE 2. *Natural history of asymptomatic retinal breaks*

	Percentage of 196 patients with asymptomatic breaks in nonfellow eyes developing specified changes during long-term follow-up
New asymptomatic breaks	13%
Subclinical detachment	5%
Retinal detachment	0%

Modified from Byer NE. The natural history of asymptomatic retinal breaks. *Ophthalmology* 1982;89:1033–1039, with permission.

(particularly if the eye is aphakic), and in patients with a family history of retinal detachment. In these cases, I treat asymptomatic flap tears. A more controversial group of patients are those with myopia or preexisting aphakia, but without other high-risk characteristics. Although myopic or aphakic eyes are at increased risk of retinal detachment, this rarely occurs without symptoms. I consider treatment of flap tears in myopic eyes only if the patient is young and has a high degree of myopia, and if long-term observation may be difficult. I treat asymptomatic flap tears in aphakic eyes only if these are definitely new.

A minority of retinal breaks are symptomatic, and the patient complains of flashes of light, floaters, or visual loss from vitreous hemorrhage. The majority of these breaks have an attached flap. Under these circumstances, the risk of progression to retinal detachment is high. All such breaks should be treated. Symptomatic operculated breaks are less likely to lead to retinal detachment than are flap tears, because traction on the break is relieved when the operculum forms. However, residual vitreoretinal traction is sometimes present on the edge of the hole, and holes with this configuration should be treated as flap tears. I also treat operculated holes if they are superiorly located, particularly if associated with much vitreous hemorrhage. Atrophic round holes without traction (for example, in a lattice patch) and a coincidental PVD do not need to be treated. The symptoms of retinal break formation are generally those of the associated PVD. Approximately 15% of patients with a symptomatic PVD will have a retinal tear and in the majority the tear will be found when the patient is first examined. A tear is highly likely if substantial hemorrhage is present or pigment (Shafer's sign) is found in the vitreous. A single tear is most common; multiple tears occur in about 20% of cases.

Following treatment, I routinely reexamine the eye at 1 and 4 weeks, since further tears may rarely occur during this time. Patients with a symptomatic PVD but *without* a retinal tear at the first examination should also be reexamined periodically for several weeks to detect the minority of cases in which a delayed tear occurs. All patients should be reexamined at any time that their symptoms recur, because, although rarely, tears and retinal detachment can sometimes occur months or years after an original PVD.

Retinal Dialysis/Disinsertion

These breaks almost always progress to retinal detachment, which usually develops slowly and may be symptomless until macular retinal detachment occurs. These breaks should therefore always be treated.

Giant Retinal Breaks

A special indication for prophylaxis is the fellow eye of a patient with a retinal detachment due to nontraumatic giant break. The reported risk of bilaterality with giant breaks is as high as 75%. Occasionally, the fellow eye contains extensive areas of lattice; more usually, it appears completely normal. Whatever the findings, I apply 360° prophylaxis.

TECHNIQUE OF TREATMENT

Prophylactic treatment is performed in two contexts: at an office visit or at the time of surgical repair of retinal detachment in the other eye.

In the first situation, laser photocoagulation is preferred. Only topical anesthesia is required. With eye movement and manipulation of the three-mirror lens, it is usually possible to surround the lesion entirely with contiguous 500-μm spots. If available, the laser indirect delivery system may facilitate more anterior treatment.

Occasionally, if there are considerable medial opacities or if very anterior treatment is required, it may be necessary to use cryotherapy. Care must be taken with large breaks to avoid treating the pigment epithelium in the bed of the tear, as this may disperse pigment epithelial cells into the vitreous. To perform this treatment satisfactorily, it is necessary to ensure good anesthesia. For very anterior cryotherapy, a subconjunctival injection of 2% lidocaine in the area of treatment may be sufficient. This allows the patient to rotate the globe in the direction of the tear to allow good visualization. For more posterior treatment, I have found that extensive peribulbar or retrobulbar anesthesia may be required. With inadequate local anesthesia, patients find office cryotherapy extremely uncomfortable, as indentation of the eye is unavoidable, and there is usually some spread of the freeze into the palpebral conjunctiva.

In the operating room, it is generally easier to use cryotherapy. However, if a large amount of treatment is required (for example, in the fellow eye of a giant break), I will apply it in two sessions, using cryotherapy in the operating room and following this up, 6 weeks later, with laser photocoagulation as an office procedure. The aim of these divided treatment sessions is to reduce the risk of subsequent macular pucker or macular edema. An alternative strategy is to use the indirect laser, if this is available in the operating room.

Lattice Degeneration

The entire patch of lattice is treated, but it is important to extend treatment into the normal retina on each side of the patch. The retina is very thin in areas of lattice, and the tensile strength of the chorioretinal adhesion induced by treatment is low; flap tears can still form following PVD. Provided the retina surrounding the lattice has been treated, however, retinal detachment should not develop even if flap tears occur. It is particularly important to apply treatment anterior to the areas of lattice. Although tears occur along the posterior border of lattice patches, vitreous traction is exerted on the surrounding retina at the anterior edge of the lattice and failure of treatment usually occurs because of inadequate treatment in this area (Fig. 5).

Snail Track

Treatment is applied to surround the large round holes completely.

Cystic Tuft/Zonular Traction Tuft

These tufts should be surrounded with chorioretinal reaction.

Retinal Breaks

Symptomatic breaks can be treated with chorioretinal reaction alone, provided they are flat or surrounded by only a narrow cuff of subretinal fluid. If extensive fluid is present, then the break should be buckled (or otherwise treated as a retinal detachment). The cutoff point between these two strategies is somewhat arbitrary. However, if fluid extends more than one optic disc diameter from the breaks, it should be treated as if for a retinal detachment.

It is particularly important to apply generous treatment to the anterior aspect of a flap tear, trying if possible to extend the treatment anteriorly as far as the ora serrata (Fig. 6A). There are several reasons for this. First, dynamic vitreous traction is exerted on the retina at the base of the flap; localized retinal detachment is common at this point and may subsequently extend through the prophylactic treatment and lead to failure if this treatment is inadequate (Fig. 6B). Second, PVD may be incomplete when the tear forms; further

separation of the vitreous toward the ora then tears the flap anteriorly (Fig. 7A,B). Although treatment will probably not prevent the anterior extension of the flap, provided chorioretinal reaction has been applied almost to the ora on either side of the tear, it will remain sealed despite this development (Fig. 7C). Finally, the horns of a flap tear sometimes initially extend almost to the ora; these anterior extensions may be slitlike and hard to visualize. If they are not surrounded by treatment, retinal detachment will develop from the anterior aspect of the break (Fig. 7D).

Following treatment, I examine the patient at 1, 2, and 4 weeks and at 3 months. A small proportion of patients develop new breaks, most of which occur within 3 months of treatment.

Asymptomatic breaks usually require no treatment. Occasionally, however, they are surrounded by subclinical retinal detachment. Subclinical retinal detachment is defined as subretinal fluid extending more than one disc diameter from the break, but not more than two disc diameters, or any fluid extending posterior to the equator. Treatment is indicated in most of these cases. If the extent of retinal detachment is demarcated by a heavy pigment line, then the retinal detachment is almost certainly stationary and may sometimes spontaneously flatten. However, a pigment line confers no protection against further extension and thus retinal detachment of this type needs to be kept under periodic review. Treatment consists of applying a barrier of laser photocoagulation (4–5 rows of contiguous 500-μm spots) in the flat retina beyond the retinal detachment. The treatment is taken out as far anteriorly as possible. If this fails to halt the spread of fluid, then it is treated as if for a retinal detachment. If cataract surgery is planned, the fellow eye has had or develops a retinal detachment, there is a family history of retinal detachment, or regular observation may be difficult, ophthalmologists should treat as if for a clinical retinal detach-

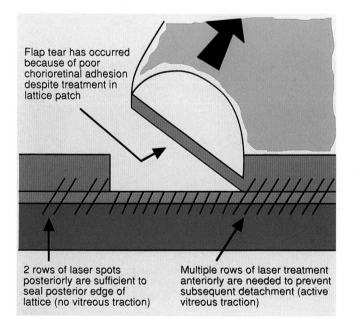

Flap tear has occurred because of poor chorioretinal adhesion despite treatment in lattice patch

2 rows of laser spots posteriorly are sufficient to seal posterior edge of lattice (no vitreous traction)

Multiple rows of laser treatment anteriorly are needed to prevent subsequent detachment (active vitreous traction)

FIG. 5. Prophylactic treatment of lattice degeneration. Cross-sectional diagram of the treatment pattern. It is important to surround the lattice patch completely with laser treatment. Breaks may be present and, because the lattice patch is thin, the chorioretinal adhesion induced by treatment of the lattice itself is weak and flap tears can subsequently occur. Tears form along the posterior border of lattice, so it is important to treat along this edge of the lattice. However, a double row of laser treatment or a single row of cryotherapy applications is sufficient. More extensive treatment should be applied *anteriorly*, because if tears are present or develop, vitreous traction on the attached retina is exerted via this portion of the lattice (*thick arrow*).

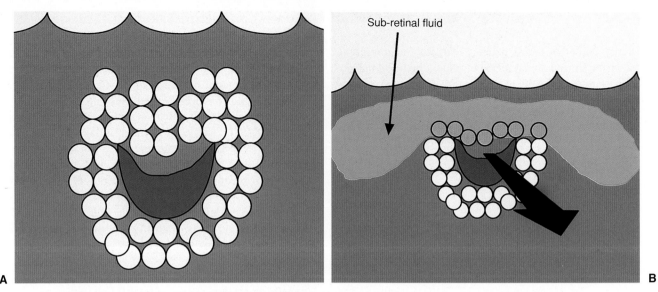

FIG. 6. Prophylactic treatment of flap tear. **A:** A double row of contiguous laser or a single row of applications of contiguous cryotherapy is used to seal the posterior edge of the tear. More extensive treatment is applied anteriorly extending, where possible, to the ora serrata. Inadequate *anterior* treatment is the most usual cause of failure of prophylaxis of flap tears. **B:** Continuing vitreous traction (*thick black arrow*) breaks through insufficient laser photocoagulation at the base of the flap.

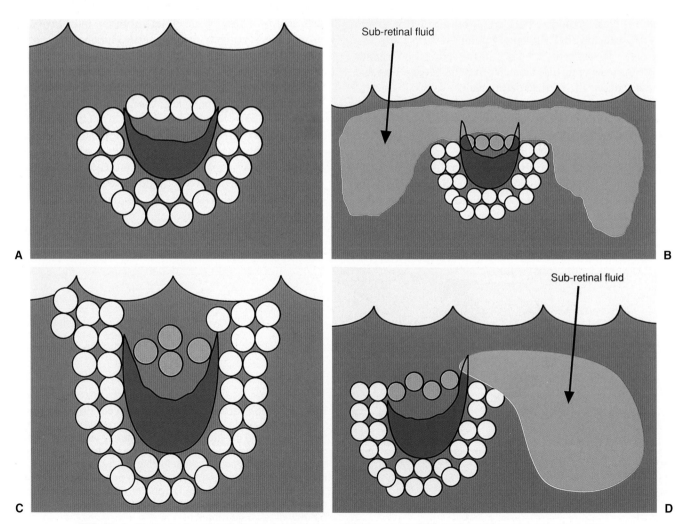

FIG. 7. **A:** Posterior break initially sealed with laser treatment. **B:** With further vitreous separation, the break extends anteriorly through inadequate laser treatment. **C:** Extensive treatment anteriorly prevents failure of prophylaxis. **D:** Failure to surround completely the radial horn of a flap tear anteriorly allows subretinal fluid to leak under this aspect of the break.

238

ment. An argument could be made for treating all of these subclinical asymptomatic detachments as if they were symptomatic detachments. However, retinal detachment surgery is not without complications, some of which can result in profound visual loss, and probably most of these detachments will either not progress or can be halted with laser treatment. Under these circumstances, it seems reasonable to individualize their management.

Dialysis/Disinsertion

These should be treated with confluent reaction along their posterior border. The treatment must be extended to the ora to seal each end of the break; therefore, cryotherapy is usually easier.

Giant Breaks

Prophylactic treatment for giant breaks presents two problems. First, it must be extensive. Second, it needs to be applied at the point in the retina where the break is likely to occur. The first problem is overcome by applying the treatment in two sessions. I usually apply patchy treatment to the fellow eye for 360° at the time of the repair of the giant tear in the first eye. Subsequently, I fill in the treatment with either cryotherapy (if an additional anesthetic is being given, for example, for silicone oil removal) or laser photocoagulation.

I find it is easier to divide the treatment by filling in areas of treatment than to perform two sessions of 180° confluent treatment.

The second problem is more difficult. Giant breaks, like flap tears (of which they are only a very large manifestation), form at the posterior border of the vitreous base after PVD has occurred. Their location therefore depends on the posterior extent of the vitreous base. This is difficult to determine before PVD has occurred. One can use as a guide the anteroposterior location of the giant break in the first eye. If this is equatorial, one should apply treatment from the equator to the ora; if oral, the surgeon should apply treatment just behind the ora of the fellow eye.

BIBLIOGRAPHY

Aaberg TM, Stevens TR. Snail track degeneration of the retina. *Am J Ophthalmol* 1972;73:370–376.

Byer NE. Review: lattice degeneration of the retina. *Surv Ophthalmol* 1979;23:213–248.

Byer NE. The natural history of asymptomatic retinal breaks. *Ophthalmology* 1982;89:1033–1039.

Byer NE. Long term natural history of lattice degeneration of the retina. *Ophthalmology* 1989;96:1396–1401.

Byer NE. Natural history of posterior vitreous detachment with early management as the premier line of defense against retinal detachment. *Ophthalmology* 1994;101:1503–1514.

Chignell AH. *Retinal detachment surgery.* 2nd ed. New York: Springer-Verlag, 1989.

Folk JC, Arrindel EL, Klugman MR. The fellow eye of patients with phakic lattice retinal detachment. *Ophthalmology* 1989;96:72–77.

Practical Atlas of Retinal Disease and Therapy, Second Edition
edited by William R. Freeman,
Lippincott–Raven Publishers, Philadelphia © 1997.

· 13 ·

Management of Rhegmatogenous Retinal Detachment

Harvey A. Lincoff and Ingrid Kreissig

Rhegmatogenous retinal detachment occurs when fluid from the vitreous passes through a break in the retina and dissects retina from pigment epithelium. To reattach the retina, it is necessary to find and close the retinal break. Closing the retinal break is the sole surgical problem. Difficulty increases as the size of the break increases, but it is independent of the extent of the retinal detachment (Fig. 1).

DIAGNOSIS AND PATHOPHYSIOLOGY

Finding the Retinal Break

Finding the break is the task at the preoperative examination. If the break is very small, it can be a laborious task for even the most skilled ophthalmoscopist. The examination benefits from biomicroscopy through a three-mirror contact lens combined with scleral depression. The latter technique, which uses a small-tip stick depressor, is widely practiced in Western Europe but is infrequently applied in the United States.

Finding the break can be made easier by first defining the borders of the detachment (1). A retinal detachment proceeds predictably from the break that causes it; conversely, the eventual shape of the detachment indicates the location of the primary break (the superior break that alone could produce the detachment). Retinal detachments assume three different shapes: (a) lateral detachments that extend into the superotemporal or nasal quadrant, (b) superior detachments that cross the 12:00 o'clock radian and proceed down both sides of the eye to become total detachments, and (c) inferior detachments. The analysis of 1,000 retinal detachments indicated the following:

1. In superior nasal or temporal detachments, the primary break lies within 1½ clock hours of the highest border of the detachment 98% of the time (Fig. 2). (When drawing a detachment for analysis, place the disc and not the macula in the center of the diagram. Detachments rotate around the disc and the rules relating to the 12:00 and 6:00 o'clock radians are valid only if the radians are vertical to the disc.)

2. In superior detachments that cross the 12:00 o'clock radian and total detachments, the primary break lies within a triangle whose apex is at 12:00 o'clock and whose sides intersect the equator 1 hour to either side of 12:00 o'clock 93% of the time. The more posterior the break, the more it can deviate from 12:00 o'clock within the triangle (Fig. 3).

3. For inferior detachments, the highest border of the detachment indicates that side of the 6:00 o'clock radian on which the primary break will be found 95% of the time (Fig. 4).

Inferior detachments caused by inferior breaks are relatively shallow and do not form bullae. An apparent inferior bullous detachment implies a superior break that connects through a shallow lateral sinus (Fig. 5). The sinus and the break can be demonstrated if the patient is examined while he or she is prone with the head turned to one side and then the other. The sinus will fill with fluid and become more evident when the side with the break is dependent (Fig. 6). (*Pitfall:* An inferior detachment that distributes symmetrically to 6:00 o'clock, if rhegmatogenous, is caused by a break on the 6:00 o'clock radian. If a break cannot be found, the detachment is probably exudative from a choroidal tumor or an inflammatory process. If the head of the supine patient is turned to one side and the other, the upper borders of the detachment rise symmetrically.)

H. A. Lincoff, M.D.: Department of Ophthalmology, The New York Hospital–Cornell University Medical College, New York, NY 10021.
I. Kreissig, M.D.: Department of Ophthalmology, University Eye Clinic, 72076 Tübingen, Germany; and Department of Ophthalmology, New York Hospital–Cornell University Medical Center, New York, NY 10016.

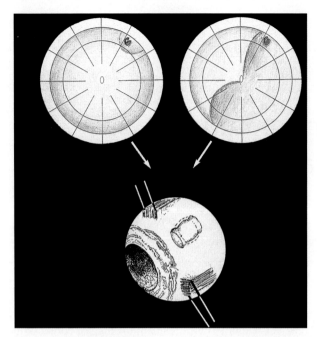

FIG. 1. The small detachment to the *left* and the large detachment to the *right* are caused by horseshoe tears of similar size. Both responded to an identical surgical procedure: a 5-mm radial sponge without drainage.

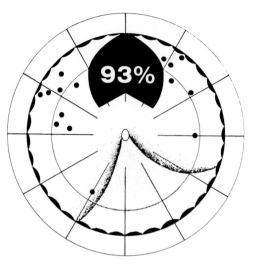

FIG. 3. In superior detachments that cross the 12 o'clock radian (many of which are total), the primary break lies within a triangle whose apex is at 12 o'clock and whose sides intersect the equator 1 hour to either side of 12 o'clock 93% of the time.

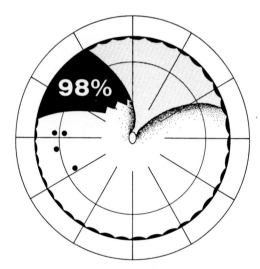

FIG. 2. In superotemporal or nasal detachments, the primary retinal break lies within 1½ hours of the highest border 98% of the time. (Note that the disc is drawn in the center of the diagram).

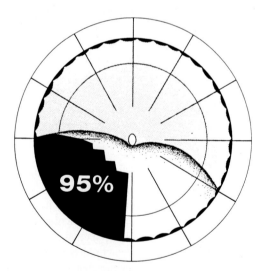

FIG. 4. In inferior detachments, the primary break lies beneath the highest border 95% of the time.

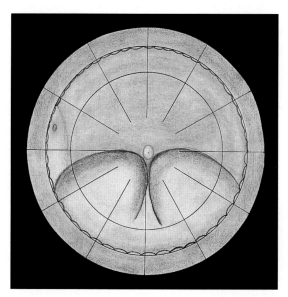

FIG. 5. An apparent inferior bullous detachment is actually a temporal detachment emanating from a barely visible retinal break at 10 o'clock and connecting to the inferior detachment by a shallow peripheral sinus.

More than one break is present in about half of the retinal detachments. The secondary break tends to be located, in order of frequency, (a) adjacent to the primary break, (b) remote from the break but in the same latitude, or (c) elsewhere.

Vitreous Hemorrhage

Vitreous hemorrhage, a consequence of the retina tearing, may obscure the retina and prevent adequate examination. Immobilization and binocular occlusion with the patient's head elevated at least 45° will cause most of the blood to settle to the bottom of the eye and make the retina available for examination often within 6–12 hours (2). This is because initially and, for a few days after a preretinal hemorrhage, most of the blood is in the retrohyaloidal space, an aqueous filled compartment through which red cells will settle if the eye is relatively still (Fig. 7). In a prospective study of vitreous hemorrhage associated with retinal detachment, 38 of 43 eyes in which the hemorrhage was of rhegmatogenous origin cleared with immobilization and binocular occlusion (Table 1) (3). Before the current limits on hospital inpatient days, patients with acute vitreous hemorrhage were hospitalized for immobilization. We still hospitalize those in whom a retinal detachment is perceived or confirmed with ultrasonography. Others are sent home with both eyes covered, asked to rest overnight in a chair or recliner, and return in the morning. If a patient with an acute hemorrhage is examined in the early morning and the retina is obscured, we bandage both eyes, have the patient sit in the waiting room, and reexamine the patient again late in the day. Frequently, the blood will have settled enough to disclose the retinal break.

Preoperative immobilization with binocular occlusion and bed rest are useful adjuncts to therapy quite apart from the presence of vitreous hemorrhage. Immobilization and occlusion will usually curtail progress of the detachment, a consideration that is important when the macula is attached but threatened. Immobilization will frequently reduce the elevation of retinal bullae and make localization of the breaks at operation easier and more accurate. In a few patients, immobilization with occlusion will effect complete reattachment of the retina and enable the repair solely by applying laser or cryopexy to the edges of the break. The earliest sign of settling of the retina is a crinkling effect on the posterior edges of the bullae. If the crinkling sign appears the next day after occlusion and immobilization, it may be worth delaying the operation in expectation of additional flattening.

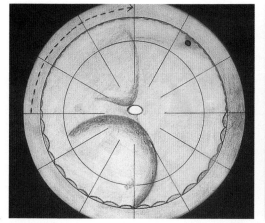
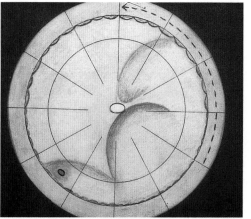

A   B

FIG. 6. When the patient with the detachment in Fig. 5 turns his head so that the side of the break is superior, the lateral sinus becomes less apparent (**A**); when he turns so that the side of the break is dependent, the sinus becomes distended and demonstrates the retinal break (**B**).

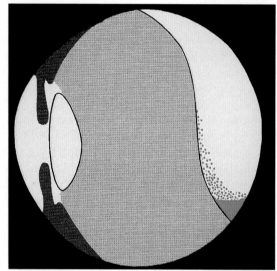

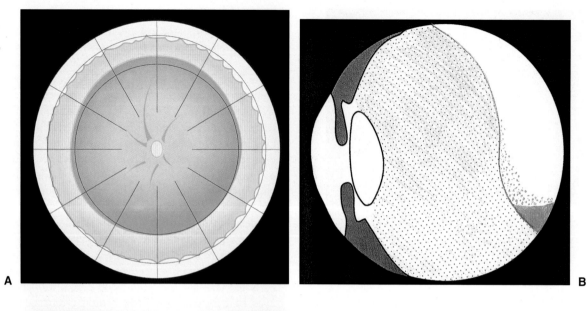

FIG. 7. An acute preretinal hemorrhage that obscures the posterior retina. The anterior retina and the disc are visible, indicating that most of the blood is retrohyaloidal (**A**). Sixteen hours after both eyes were occluded and the patient maintained an elevated posture, the blood settled inferiorly and a retinal tear at 11: 00 o'clock was revealed (**B**). Cross section demonstrates that the blood collected dependently in the retrohyaloidal space (**C**).

TABLE 1. *Prospective study of vitreous hemorrhage associated with retinal detachment*

Etiology	No. of patients	Clearing time (days)		
		1	2–4	5–7
Retinal tears	9	7	2	—
Tears with detachment	16	9	6	1
Bridging vessel on scleral buckle	4	2	1	1
Posterior hyaloidal detachment without tear	9	2	6	1
Total	38	20	15	3

SURGICAL REPAIR WITH SEGMENTAL BUCKLING WITHOUT DRAINAGE OF SUBRETINAL FLUID

Most operations for rhegmatogenous retinal detachments can be completed in less than 2 hours and so can be done under retrobulbar anesthesia. A lid block is not required. An adequate scleral field is made available if the conjunctival incision extends 90° to either side of the break. Localization is obtained by directing a scleral depressor or cryoprobe to the break while the retina is being observed with the indirect ophthalmoscope. The position of the break is marked on the sclera with ink or cautery. The edges of the break may be treated at the same time with transscleral cryopexy or the next day, after the retina is in contact with the buckle, with applications of laser.

The break is closed by compressing an elastic silicone sponge against the overlying sclera, with a mattress suture tied under tension. One mattress suture with long intrascleral limbs (6 mm) is preferable to multiple sutures with short intrascleral passages because the short ones tend to tear out of sclera (Fig. 8). Compression of the sponge causes an abrupt rise in intraocular pressure, and it is necessary to monitor the central retinal artery to ascertain that it has not closed. Momentary closure or a pulsating artery is not infrequent. The artery reopens within minutes if the patient does not have glaucoma. The reopening can be accelerated by digital massage. A paracentesis is rarely required. Mannitol or acetazolamide have little effect and may encourage postoperative choroidal effusion.

The break does not need to be in contact with the buckle at the conclusion of the operation. As the eye decompresses over the next hours, the sponge will expand beneath the break and create a buckle high enough to close it. With the pathway between the vitreous and the subretinal space closed, the fluid beneath the retina is "pumped out" by the

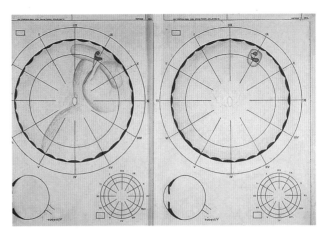

FIG. 9. A horseshoe tear on a circumferential buckle leaked through a fishmouth, and the detachment persisted (*left*). The tear was closed by replacing the circumferential buckle with a radial buckle, and the retina became attached (*right*).

pigment epithelium and cannot be replenished, and the retina reattaches. Reattachment usually occurs within 16–24 hours (4–7).

Radial Versus Circumferential Buckles

Whenever possible, the scleral sponge is oriented with the long axis in a radial direction (8,9). The retina, fixed at the ora and disc, tends to form radial folds when it detaches. A circumferentially oriented buckle preserves and augments the radial folds because it shortens the circumference of the eye, making the circumferential dimension of the retina redundant. Compounding the problem is the tendency for the folds on a circumferential buckle to aggregate and align with the retinal tear that is upon it. The posterior edge of the tear opens like a fish's mouth (called "fishmouthing") and provides a path for vitreous fluid to flow into the subretinal space. Radial buckles fill potential folds and prevent this complication (Fig. 9).

Limits of Radial Buckling

There are limits to the application of radial buckles. Most retinal breaks are smaller than 3 mm (15° or ½ hour at the equator) and can be closed by a 5-mm cylindrical sponge sewn into place on the sclera with an 8-mm mattress suture. The suture indents the half circumference of the sponge to provide a buckle 8 mm wide.

Breaks as large as 5 mm (25°) can be closed by a 7½ × 5-mm oval sponge sewn into place with a 10-mm mattress suture. Breaks as large as 8 mm (40°) can be closed with two 7½-mm overlapping sponges tied into place with a mattress suture with intrascleral limbs that are 14 mm apart (Fig. 10). Two sponges side by side mark the limit of the radial sponge operation. Three or more sponges and a mattress suture

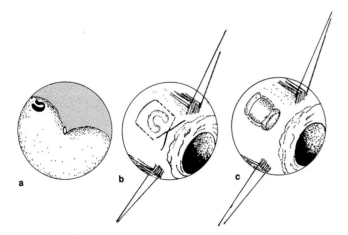

FIG. 8. A temporal detachment with a horseshoe tear at 10 o'clock (*a*). The localization of the break on the sclera is surrounded by one broad mattress suture whose intrascleral limbs are 6 mm long (*b*). The suture is tied under tension to compress a silicone sponge (*c*).

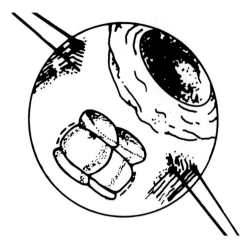

FIG. 10. Two overlapping sponges oriented in a radial direction are compressed by a single mattress suture to treat a retinal tear 8 mm wide.

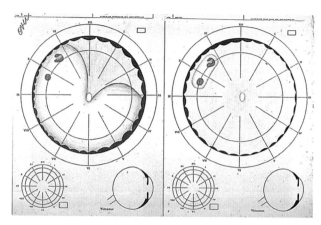

FIG. 12. Two retinal tears close together in a three-quadrant detachment (*left*) are buckled with a short circumferential sponge. The ends of the sponge do not extend beyond the breaks (*right*).

wider than 14 mm have little compression potential and make a poor buckle (10).

The "Half-Thickness" Sponge

It is apparent that shallower buckles may be adequate for shallow detachments and higher buckles are required for breaks in bullous detachments. A 3 × 5-mm oval sponge was designed for anterior breaks in shallow retinal detachments. The 5-mm cylinder, however, is the standard sponge that closes most retinal breaks in bullous detachments. When compressed by an 8-mm mattress suture, it yields a buckle that is 2.5 mm high. An ingenuous idea has been advanced that suggests that because only half of the sponge indents the eye, a half-thickness of sponge would be as effective and eliminate the subconjunctival hump. This idea disregards the principle of compression of an elastic sponge to obtain a

higher buckle (through internal drainage) as the eye decompresses. Half-thickness sponges and solid silicone forms might provide buckles of equivalent height if accompanied by external drainage of subretinal fluid.

Multiple Breaks

Multiple retinal breaks are treated with a radial sponge beneath each break, providing they are separated by at least 2 clock hours (Fig. 11). Multiple breaks separated by less than 2 clock hours are necessarily treated with a circumferentially oriented sponge (radial sutures would overlap). The circumferential buckle is made as short as possible to diminish the likelihood of radial folds (Fig. 12). The geometry of circumferential buckles indicates that buckles shorter than 90° are unlikely to cause folds, because the sloping edges of the buckle compensate for the redundancy of the retina over the middle portion of the buckle (Fig. 13).

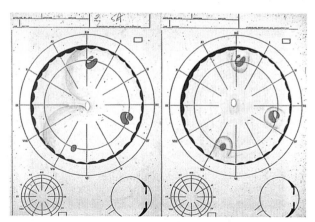

FIG. 11. Three breaks in a three-quadrant detachment (*left*) are buckled with three radial sponges, and the retina has reattached (*right*).

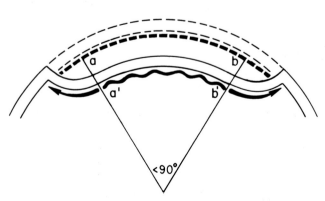

FIG. 13. A circumferential buckle diminishes the circumference of the scleral wall and makes the area of retina (*a,b*) redundant (*a',b'*). The sloping edges (*arrows*) of a buckle that is shorter than 90° can compensate.

Large Tears (40°–70°)

Radial buckling can be done for breaks larger than 8 mm (40° at the equator) and up to 14 mm (70°) by resorting to a scleral pouch operation (Fig. 14). The pouch is made with Dacron-reinforced silicone sheeting cut to a radial shape and sewn over the retinal break with a running suture (Fig. 15). The elastic buckling effect is obtained by stuffing it with silicone sponge pellets (Fig. 16). The pouch operation is time consuming, but works without drainage and has a reattachment rate of 95%, which is as good as that of the sponge operation (11).

COMPLICATIONS OF SEGMENTAL BUCKLING

The extrascleral sponge operation without drainage of subretinal fluid has no significant intraocular complications. There may be a rare choroidal effusion in elderly patients. Uveitis occurs even less frequently. Extraocular complications of segmental buckling are infection of the buckle and diplopia. Since the use of closed cell silicone sponge material and a prophylactic lavage of the operative site with antibiotic at the conclusion of the operation, the incidence of infection has fallen to 0.5% (12). Diplopia occurs if the sponge is sutured anteriorly beneath a rectus tendon. A 5-mm radial sponge beneath a rectus tendon has been observed to erode through the tendon. If a sponge is required anteriorly beneath a muscle, it is advisable to detach and rotate the muscle to one side of the sponge or the other.

TEMPORARY BUCKLES (BALLOONS)

The extraocular complications of buckling (infection and diplopia) can be eliminated by using a temporary balloon instead of a scleral sponge (13–15). There has been one infection in the first 1,000 balloon operations even though antibiotic therapy is limited to topical bacitracin ointment. Balloons are less likely to cause scleral infection or abscess because the catheter acts as a drain to the buckle site and because lysozyme washes the entrance of the catheter through

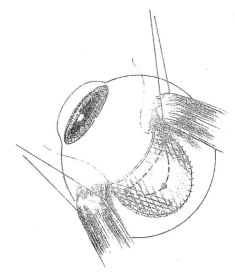

FIG. 15. Transparent Dacron-reinforced silicone sheeting cut to the shape of a radial pouch for the break in Fig. 14. The pouch is fixed over the break with a running suture.

the conjunctiva. The one patient with an infection complained of deep (uveal) pain on postoperative day 3. There was tenderness over the balloon and purulence around the tube. A culture was positive for *Staphylococcus aureus*. The balloon was deflated and removed, and the symptoms and signs resolved rapidly.

Diplopia, the other complication of scleral buckles, does not occur with the balloon. For this reason, it is an operation of choice when the retinal break is beneath a rectus muscle, particularly a vertical rectus. To insert the balloon beneath a rectus, the incision in conjunctiva is made over the tendon. The tendon fibers are separated in a radial direction for about 2 mm. The balloon is inserted through the opening in the tendon, maneuvered posteriorly until it is beneath the retinal break, and then expanded with 1 ml of sterile water. Muscle

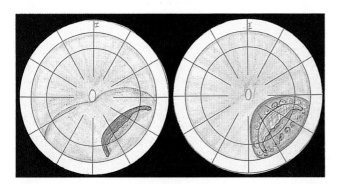

FIG. 14. A retinal detachment caused by a horseshoe tear of 70° (*left*) was buckled with a radial pouch. The retina reattached without drainage of subretinal fluid (*right*).

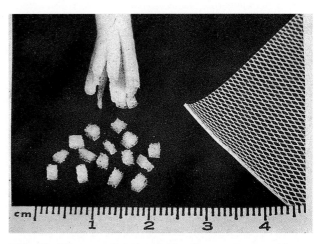

FIG. 16. Silicone pellets for stuffing the pouch are cut from a silicone sponge cylinder. Silicone sheeting is on the *right*.

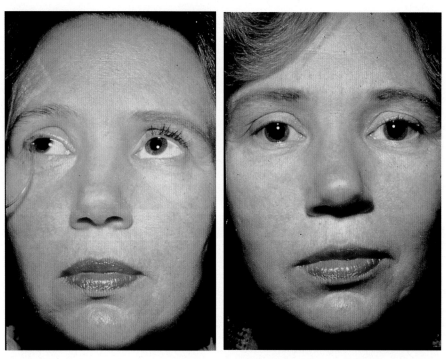

FIG. 17. A patient with a balloon beneath the superior rectus has limited elevation and experiences diplopia (*left*). Ocular rotations are normal 3 hours after the balloon was deflated and withdrawn (*right*).

function is limited, and there is diplopia while the balloon is in place; but, within hours after the balloon is deflated and removed, the muscle function is normal again and diplopia will have disappeared (Fig. 17).

The balloon procedure is suitable for retinal detachments caused by a single break or a group of breaks close together that do not subtend an arc greater than 1 clock hour at the equator (Fig. 18). The break is localized transconjunctivally, and the position of the break and the radian (anteriorly) marked with ink (Fig. 19). The conjunctiva and Tenon's capsule are opened at the anterior mark, and the balloon inserted to the break and expanded with 1–2 ml of distilled water. The balloon buckle looks and acts like a 7.5 × 5-mm scleral sponge (Fig. 20). Initially, the balloon maintains its position because it is compressed between the globe and the wall of the orbit and the intraocular pressure is temporarily increased. As the intraocular pressure decreases over the next hour, the balloon expands and sinks into an indentation in the globe from which it shows no tendency to move when ocular rotations are restored, even though there are no sutures. The increased buckle that is produced by the expanded balloon closes the retinal break and reattaches the retina (Fig. 21). The proximal end of the balloon catheter is taped to the patient's temple. Additional volume can be added to the balloon on subsequent days if a bigger buckle is required. The balloon is deflated and removed after 7 days. Long-term adhesion is obtained by cryopexy around the break prior to inserting the balloon or applications of laser on subsequent days after the retinal break has come into contact with the buckle (Fig. 22). The balloon reattaches 93% of the eyes selected for it after the first procedure and 99% after reoperation; 2%–5% will redetach in the first weeks or months and require a permanent buckle (15). If a second operation is required, the ocular tissues have not been significantly disadvantaged by the balloon insertion.

Pseudophakic Retinal Detachment

The diminished rate of reattachment in pseudophakic eyes is largely due to the difficulty in finding the retinal break. Less effort might be expended to find the breaks because of a misapprehension that the breaks in aphakic and in pseu-

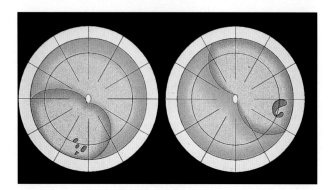

FIG. 18. The parabulbar balloon yields a scleral indentation sufficient to buckle a retinal break (*left*) or a group of breaks close together (*right*) that do not subtend an arc greater than 1 clock hour at the equator.

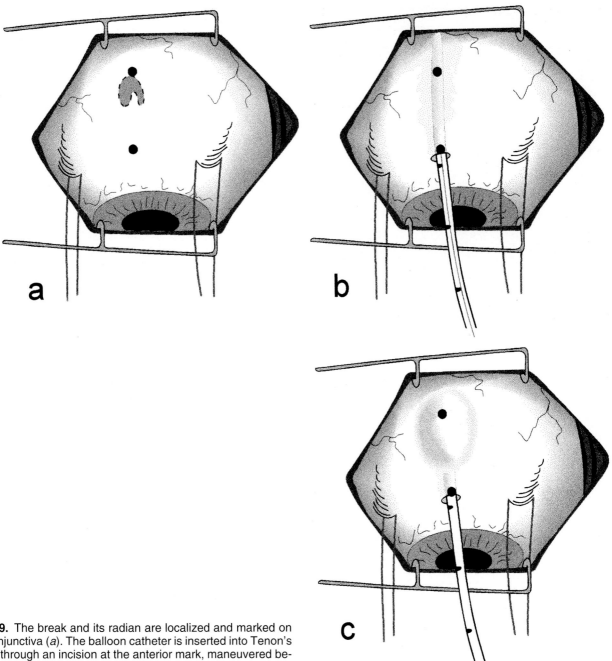

FIG. 19. The break and its radian are localized and marked on the conjunctiva (*a*). The balloon catheter is inserted into Tenon's space through an incision at the anterior mark, maneuvered beneath the break (*b*), and expanded (*c*).

dophakic eyes tend to be so small as to be beyond the resolution of indirect ophthalmoscopy or biomicroscopy and are located so far in the periphery as to be inaccessible for viewing. In our series, 60% of the breaks were horseshoe tears with perceptible flaps, and only one of 45 breaks was not visible by indirect ophthalmoscopy or biomicroscopy. The average distance from the ora serrata was 11.6 mm (9–15 mm), which is only 1.4 mm more anterior than breaks in phakic eyes (16,17).

Contributing to the difficulty of finding the breaks in pseudophakic eyes is the failure of the Goldmann lens to pro-

vide a clear image for biomicroscopy. The image is blurred because of marginal astigmatism induced by the steep angle of view through the edge of the intraocular lens. The view can be further compromised by lens and capsular opacities. Boldrey (18) has succeeded in diminishing the astigmatism by superimposing a −6 diopter cylinder on the 67° mirror of the Goldmann lens.

The wide-field indirect contact lenses of Mainster and Volk, with some tilting and scleral depression, can provide a clear image anterior to the equator in most pseudophakic eyes (17). The indirect optics provide an image around a

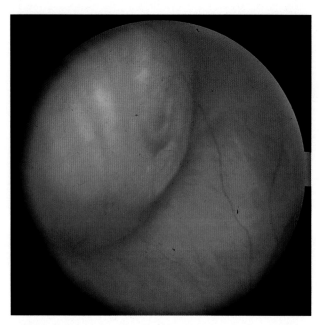

FIG. 20. Photo of a balloon beneath a retinal break. The balloon was expanded with 1 ml of distilled water.

moderate lens opacity and through thin capsular opacities similar to the view obtained with the indirect ophthalmoscope. Given a 5- to 6-mm pupil, the anterior retina and, with depression, the ora serrata can be brought into view in pseudophakic eyes.

Reasons for Encircling and for Not Encircling

The encircling buckle was originally used to confine anterior leaks from horseshoe tears that were incompletely buckled on narrow circumferential elements, such as the polyethylene tube. When larger local elements were adopted to buckle the breaks more completely, encirclement was retained to wall away suspicious areas in the peripheral retina that could not be clearly defined—what one retinal surgeon used to call "porous retina." With the advent of biomicroscopic techniques through the mirrors of the Goldmann lens and the wide-angle indirect contact lenses of Mainster and Volk, suspicious areas in most eyes can be defined as having a retinal break or not. Many retinal surgeons nevertheless retain the encircling band because they believe it supports the anterior vitreous and prevents additional retinal breaks from occurring, particularly in aphakic eyes. We argue against this because we think the prophylactic value of routine encircling is doubtful. It would prevent redetachment in only the small percentage of eyes in which a subsequent break fortuitously lies on the meridian of the band. A break that is anterior to the band and above the horizontal is likely to cause redetachment. If the subsequent break is posterior to the band, it is even more likely to cause redetachment.

There is evidence that a constricting band may be deleterious to function. Dobbie (19) has demonstrated that an encircling band dampens the ocular pulse. Yoshida and et al. (20) have demonstrated that encircling diminishes vascular flow in the posterior eye. Winter and Lipka (21) found it also diminished retinal function. We have observed late pigmentary degeneration of the retina posterior to the buckle and diminished function in some of the eyes that we encircled in the 1950s and 1960s. As a result, we have been cutting the many bands that we placed in those years.

We employ an encircling band solely to provide permanent support for the local buckle that reattached the retina initially, but failed in the weeks or months that followed because the buckle diminished in height. To reestablish the el-

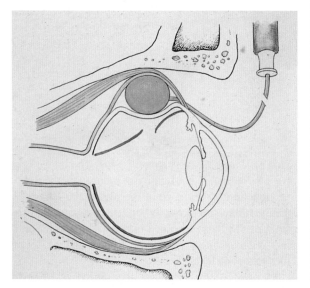
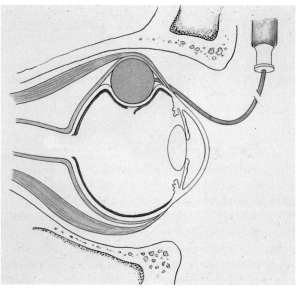

FIG. 21. Initially, the balloon is compressed between the eye, and the bony orbit and the buckle is shallow (*left*). As the eye decompresses, the balloon sinks deeper into the eye and causes a buckle to be high enough to close the retinal break and reattach the retina (*right*).

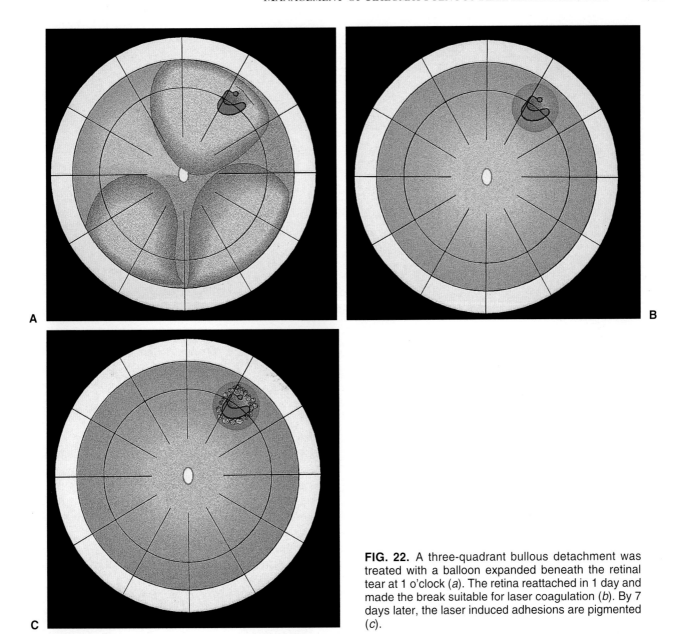

FIG. 22. A three-quadrant bullous detachment was treated with a balloon expanded beneath the retinal tear at 1 o'clock (*a*). The retina reattached in 1 day and made the break suitable for laser coagulation (*b*). By 7 days later, the laser induced adhesions are pigmented (*c*).

evation of the buckle and make it permanent, we place an encircling band over the buckle and constrict it by 10 %–20% of the circumference of the eye (22). This can be done without draining subretinal fluid.

Failure of Nondrainage Operations

At least 90% of retinal detachments are caused by breaks smaller than 70° and are suitable for treatment without drainage of subretinal fluid (23,24). Of these, 4% will fail to attach completely because of another break that was undetected. Providing that the break that was buckled was the superior one, the upper border of the detachment will fall close to the level of the undetected break and help to indicate its location (Fig. 23). If the shape of the detachment is un-

changed after a buckling operation without drainage, it is likely that there is an undetected break above the one that was buckled (Fig. 24). Of the nondrainage procedures, 3% will fail because the buckle was inadequate, either poorly placed (Fig. 25), too narrow (Fig. 26), or rarely not high enough; and 2% will fail because of existing or developing proliferative vitreoretinopathy. Baring an inadvertent perforation by a scleral suture, an iatrogenic complication in a nondrainage operation is unlikely. Because their pigment epithelium and choriocapillaris function poorly, 1% of patients will have delayed absorption.

Patients with another break or an inadequate buckle will respond to a second buckling procedure without drainage of subretinal fluid. Elderly or myopic patients with atrophic pigment epithelium might be considered for drainage if the break is in the inferior retina. If the break is superior, how-

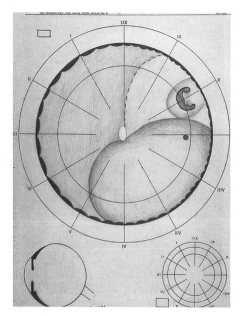

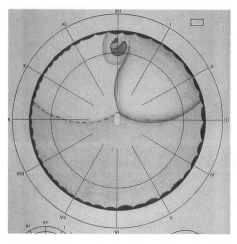

FIG. 23. The horseshoe tear at 2 o'clock was buckled, and the superior margin of the detachment dropped from 12:45 to 3:00, where it remained unchanged because of an undetected break below 3:00. Note that there has been no regression of the inferior margin.

FIG. 25. The buckle at 12 o'clock is not centered beneath the break, and the break continues to maintain the nasal half of a superior detachment.

ever, it will attach on the buckle in 1–2 days, and patients may be left to absorb residual fluid over weeks. Patients are cautioned to sleep with the head elevated to prevent pooling of the fluid into the macula.

Reasons for Draining

Fewer than 5% of retinal detachment patients might be selected for drainage of subretinal fluid. In addition to elderly

patients with inferior breaks, partial drainage might be indicated for an eye with a staphylomatous sclera that might not tolerate the increase in intraocular pressure of a nondrainage procedure. Drainage will be required if the patient has glaucoma, because elevating the intraocular pressure with a compressed sponge could lead to sustained closure of the retinal artery.

Old fluid is not a reason to drain; old subretinal fluid is absorbed as rapidly as recent fluid (Fig. 27). A break in a highly

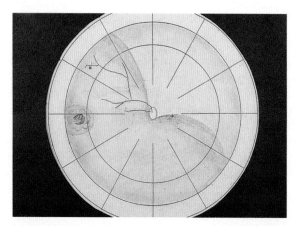

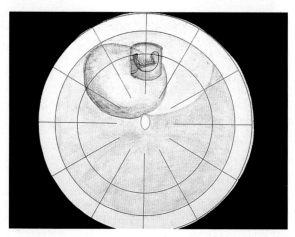

FIG. 24. A break at 9:00 has been buckled, but the margins of the detachment remained unchanged because of another very small break at 10:15 above the buckle that had been overlooked. (*Note:* The break at 9: 00 is more than 1½ hours below the superior margin and had only a 2% chance of being the primary break.)

FIG. 26. The buckle is too small to close this large horseshoe tear, and the temporal edge of the tear continues to leak.

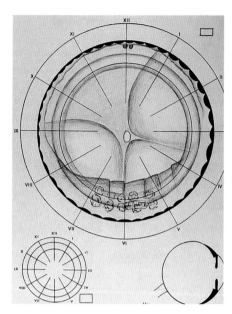

FIG. 27. A total detachment in a 50-year-old man was operated on twice with encircling procedures and coagulation directed at inferior lattice and preretinal proliferation. The detachment that has persisted for 2 years since the last operation was cured with a sponge at 12:00 o'clock that closed two breaks near the ora. The old subretinal fluid completely absorbed in 24 hours.

elevated retina is also not a reason to drain. Even though the break may be widely separated from the buckle at the end of the operation, it will come into contact and close in 1–2 days, providing the sponge was correctly placed. Fewer than 1% of retinal breaks show no tendency to approach the buckle. If another break cannot be found above the buckle, contact can be obtained by raising the buckle with a temporary balloon (Fig. 28). A gas injection is another alternative. Drainage of

subretinal fluid as a secondary procedure is avoided because the choroid is likely to be congested and the perforation of it has an increased risk of subretinal hemorrhage.

Drainage Technique

When drainage for the reasons just listed is planned as part of the primary procedure, it is good practice to get to it within the first hour of the operation. Attempts to drain later are likely to encounter a congested choroid, and the perforation is likely to lead to subretinal hemorrhage.

Drainage of subretinal fluid is the most morbid maneuver in the operation for retinal detachment. Perforating the choroid risks, in addition to subretinal hemorrhage, retinal and vitreous incarceration. The temporary decompression that occurs with drainage may provoke choroidal effusion. To diminish the risk of incarceration, it is good practice to drain 12 mm from the ora serrata in a radian of maximum retinal elevation. To minimize hemorrhage, it is advisable to make a radial incision in the sclera for 3 mm, expose a knuckle of choroid, and transilluminate it to identify vessels or congestion. Choroidal vessels appear as bright red streaks and congestion as a uniform red glow. The perforation is made in a dark area between the vessels with a round needle from a 6-0 suture. The needle should enter the choroid obliquely to minimize the risk of perforating the retina. A bright spot of light at the perforation site and a flow of clear fluid indicates successful drainage. Avoid penetrating congested choroid.

External cautery of the choroid with diathermy or a laser beam has been proposed, but either method is accompanied by a significant incidence of bleeding. If bleeding occurs and is confirmed to be subretinal by ophthalmoscopic examination (it is a streak of red blood flowing toward the posterior pole), one is advised (a) to close the wound with the pre-

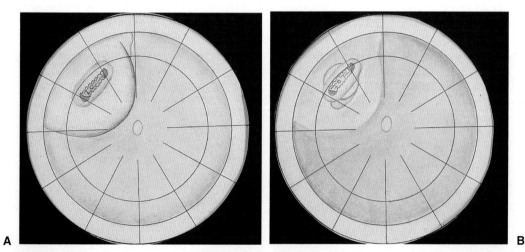

FIG. 28. The detachment caused by two breaks at the edge of a line of lattice degeneration has been buckled with a 5-mm circumferential silicone sponge. The detachment remained unchanged for 4 days (**A**). When a parabulbar balloon was inserted and expanded on top of the buckle, it raised the buckle, and the retina reattached in 16 hours (**B**).

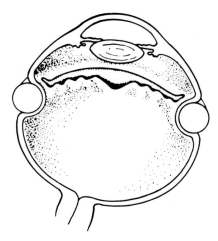

FIG. 29. The retina is compressed by a circumferential buckle. The posterior edge of the large tear is thrown into radial folds, and a large fold (fishmouth) forms in the center.

placed mattress suture, (b) to rotate the head so that the perforation site is dependent, and (c) to raise the intraocular pressure to the level of the central retinal artery pressure by injecting air or Balanced Salt Solution through the pars plana and maintaining ocular ischemia for 3–5 minutes.

Restoration of Volume

Restoration of volume after drainage adds another degree of morbidity to drainage of subretinal fluid. Whatever the substance injected, it will disturb the vitreous structure and stimulate or aggravate proliferative activity. Balanced Salt Solution is least noxious and was preferred for many years. More recently, air or a perfluorocarbon gas is injected because they are less likely to enter the break and cause redetachment. Gas also serves as an internal tamponade to flatten retinal folds. Both air and perfluorocarbon gas provoke a breakdown of the blood retinal barrier. This becomes evident

as a protein and cellular infiltration of the vitreous that appears 24–36 hours after the injection.

Xenon gas is another alternative for restoring volume and tamponading the retina (25). Xenon, which is very soluble, has an intraocular half-life of about 1 hour; 88% is absorbed by 3 hours. Its brief presence and replacement by aqueous minimizes the irritative response that air and other gases cause. The brief intraocular presence of xenon also diminishes the time the patient needs to be in a prone or bent position. Laboratory-grade xenon, like the perfluorocarbons, is available in lecture bottles.

Tears Larger Than 70°

Tears larger than 70° are fortunately infrequent. When encountered, they could only be buckled with a circumferentially oriented sponge (the posterior edge of a radial pouch larger than 70° would intrude on the posterior pole). Circumferential buckling of large tears, however, is prone to cause fishmouthing and to fail (Fig. 29). Large tears are treated instead with intraocular tamponades of air or gas with or without vitrectomy (26).

Oral Disinsertions (Retinal Dialyses)

Long tears at the ora serrata are an exception (Fig. 30) because the posterior edge of a disinsertion, unlike the edge of a horseshoe tear, is not longer than the circumference of the tear. Oral disinsertions as long as 90° reattach upon a circumferential buckle without significant retinal redundancy and rarely fishmouth (27).

Gas without Vitrectomy for Large Tears (>70°)

The perfluorocarbon gases that expand in the eye from two to five times (because of diffusion of the more soluble

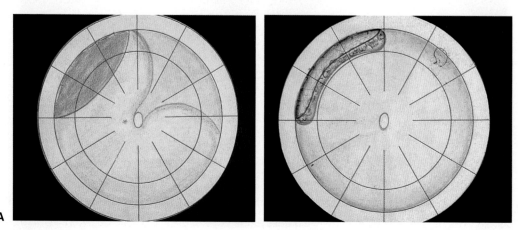

FIG. 30. Retinal detachment caused by an oral disinsertion of less than 90°. The posterior edge is the same length as the anterior edge of the tear (**A**). The retina reattached when the break was buckled with a circumferential sponge without drainage of subretinal fluid (**B**).

blood gases into the bubble) have simplified intraocular gas tamponades (28). The expansion potential of the perfluorocarbons eliminates the need for drainage of subretinal fluid or vitrectomy to make space for an adequate gas bubble (Fig. 31). The normal eye accepts 0.2–0.3 ml of gas, about 5% of its volume, through a combination of choroidal compression and scleral expansion. Larger injections of gas raise intraocular pressure to levels that close the central retinal artery. [*Pitfall:* It is a mistake to expect that larger gas volumes might be accepted because gas is compressible. Injecting gas into the eye is almost equivalent to injecting water: the amount of compression of the bubble in the range of tolerable intraocular pressure is insignificant. For example, an injection of 0.3 ml of air or gas that might increase the intraocular pressure 3 $\times$ (to 60 mm Hg) only compresses the gas bubble by the fraction 780/830 (9%) or 0.027 ml.]

To obtain more space for larger volumes of gas, some surgeons do repeated paracentesis. Others apply a Honan balloon at 30–35 mm Hg to "soften" the eye. More space can be obtained by inserting a parabulbar balloon to the equator in the inferonasal quadrant and expanding it until the central artery is observed to pulsate (29). This triples intraocular pressure and aqueous outflow. When maintained for 1 hour, it provides the intraocular space for the injection of 0.7 ml of gas. If perfluoroethane (C_2F_6) is injected, its expanded volume will be 2.3 ml (3.3 x), enough to fill half of the vitreous space of the average eye and to tamponade tears as long as 160°. If perfluoropropane (C_3F_8) is injected, the expanded amount of gas will be 3.2 ml (4 x). We prefer C_2F_6 because its half-life in the eye is 12 days (30), which is time enough for a secure retinal adhesion, induced by coagulation, to develop (31,32). C_3F_8 has a half-life of 25 days.

The larger volumes of gas for large tears are injected as the parabulbar balloon is deflated to avert hypotension. Patients are supine during the injection, and the gas collects behind the lens. For lateral tears (Fig. 32), patients may be rotated laterally in bed (Fig. 33). For superior or inferior tears, head

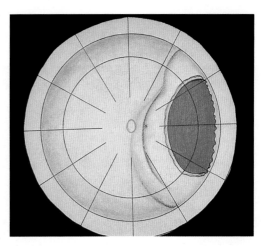

FIG. 32. A large lateral tear with a rolled edge that was treated with rotation across an intraocular gas bubble.

or feet first, a rotating orthopedic frame is useful. It is important to rotate patients initially in the direction that moves the side of the eye that is across from the tear over the gas bubble; rotating the other way invites the bubble to enter the retinal break and become subretinal. The rotation is continued until the bubble approaches the posterior edge of the break. Closure of the edge will occur over the next hours as the bubble expands. When the posterior edge has reattached, it is secured with laser coagulation or cryopexy. The coagulation is carried to the ora serrata at the ends of the tear to seal

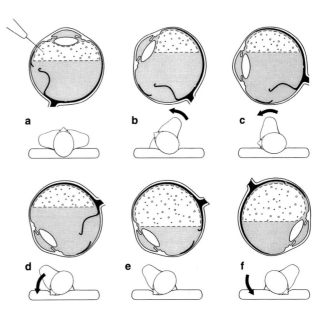

FIG. 33. Rotation of a patient whose eye is depicted in Fig. 32. The gas is injected with the patient supine (*a*); the patient is rotated initially to place the bubble opposite to the tear (*b,c*); then nose oblique down (*d*). Overnight, the bubble of perfluoroethane expands across the retina and flattens the posterior edge of the tear (*e*). The next day, the patient is rotated to optimum tamponade position with the bubble across the tear (*f*).

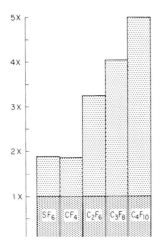

FIG. 31. Graphic display of the intraocular expansion of sulfur hexafluoride and the four straight-chain perfluorocarbon gases.

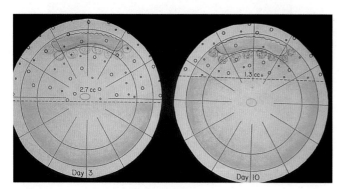

FIG. 34. By day 3, the gas bubble in the eye depicted in Fig. 32 has tripled in volume and tamponades the break. The edges have been cryopexied (*left*). By day 10, the bubble is still large enough to tamponade the break, and the cryo lesions have pigmented (*right*).

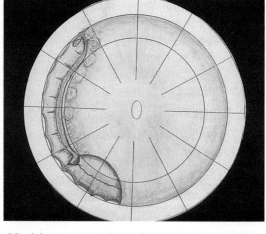

FIG. 36. A long temporal tear that was treated with gas and cryopexy has broken through the inferior cryopexy-induced adhesions and is causing a redetachment.

the edges of the anterior flap of the tear (Fig. 34). The anterior flap is not reattached by a gas tamponade because of vitreous traction. A scleral buckle might attach it but is not required. The posterior edge of a primary tear does not require a buckle because it is not under traction. The curl seen at the posterior edge is a frequent finding in a long retinal tear and does not imply traction. [*Pitfall:* Another source of subretinal gas is from an injection needle that fails to penetrate a transparent membrane that sometimes exists over the pars plana of eyes that have had previous operations or inflammatory episodes (Fig. 35). To avoid this complication, it is necessary to observe the needle tip within the eye by indirect

ophthalmoscopy and ascertain that it is clear of a membrane before injecting. If a membrane is present, it can be perforated by rotating the needle to drill through it. A test bubble should rise to the back of the lens.]

The gas procedure, which is without conjunctival incision, succeeds about 70% of the time (33). It fails when the tear extends through the coagulation line at its ends (Fig. 36) or when preretinal proliferation (induced by the gas) pulls on the posterior edge of the tear and reopens it (Fig. 37). Large tears treated by gas require close follow-up during the days and weeks after reattachment. If a redetachment can be discovered early, before the entire posterior edge of the tear re-

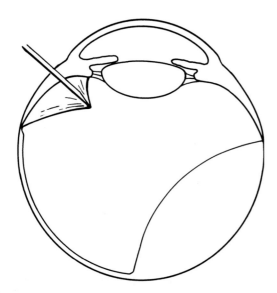

FIG. 35. The needle for gas injection is obstructed by a transparent membrane over the pars plana. If gas is injected, it will enter the subretinal space. The retina on the other side (*right*) is detached.

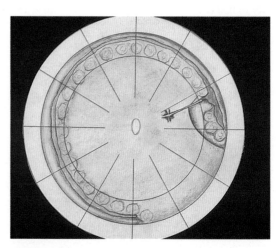

FIG. 37. Preretinal proliferation has developed at 2 o'clock and is redetaching a retina with a 270° tear that was reattached with a gas tamponade 4 weeks before.

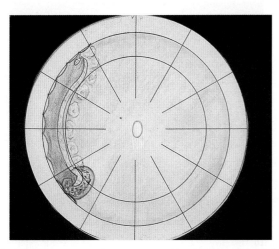

FIG. 38. The small redetachment in Fig. 36 was repaired with a radial buckle at the leaking edge of the long tear.

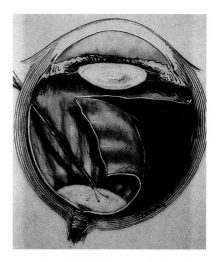

FIG. 40. Perfluorocarbon liquid is injected at the posterior pole to unfold the flap of a giant retinal tear.

opens, it can be repaired with a standard buckle operation (Figs. 38 and 39).

Because of the success of the expanding gases in treating large tears (34), the gas technique has been proposed as a primary outpatient procedure for retinal detachments resulting from less formidable tears (35). The procedure has been called pneumatic retinopexy. However, because intraocular gas may provoke preretinal proliferation, we think small breaks are better managed with an external buckle and without drainage. Pneumatic retinopexy is covered in detail by W.R. Freeman in Chapter 14.

Gas with Vitrectomy for Large Tears (>70°)

The treatment of giant tears has become the province of vitreous surgeons, although a controlled study comparing the

vitrectomy with the gas technique, as outlined in the previous section, has never been done. It is likely, however, that removing the cortical vitreous diminishes the incidence of proliferative vitreoretinopathy after gas injection and for that reason alone might be a better procedure. The use of the perfluorocarbon liquids, which have a specific gravity greater than vitreous, has simplified the problem of unfolding an overhanging posterior edge of a giant tear (36). The liquid is injected at the posterior pole with the patients supine (Fig. 40). It is then replaced by gas, and patients are rotated to optimum tamponade position. (See also Chapter 15 by S. Charles and B. Wood, and Chapter 17 by G.W. Abrams and L.C. Glazer.)

The overhanging flap of a giant tear (Fig. 41) may also be unfolded with gas alone by rotating the flap against a small bubble (less than 1 ml) of expanding gas, for example, C_2F_6 (37). The bubble, which has a thin wafer shape, slides under

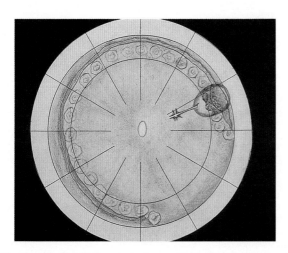

FIG. 39. The beginning detachment in Fig. 37 was treated effectively with a radial sponge at 2 o'clock.

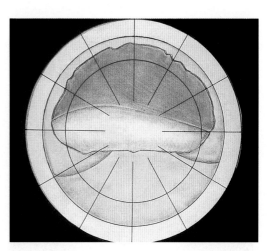

FIG. 41. A large superior tear with an overhanging flap.

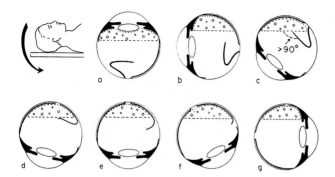

FIG. 42. The flap of the tear in Fig. 41 has been unfolded by rotating it against a wafer-shaped bubble small enough to slide beneath it. The gas is injected with the patient supine on a rotating orthopedic frame (*a*). The patient is rotated so that the bubble approaches the tear from the bottom of the eye (*b,c*). The bubble is small enough (0.75 ml) to slide under the flap (*d*) and unfold it (*e–g*).

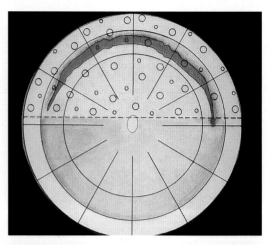

FIG. 44. By day 3, the bubble has tripled in volume and covers the tear when the patient's head is in a vertical position.

the flap and unfolds it (Fig. 42). Initially, the bubble is too small to tamponade the entire tear (Fig. 43). Within a day, however, the bubble will double in size, and in 3 days triple and be large enough to tamponade the entire break when the patient's head is in a vertical position (Fig. 44).

CONCLUSIONS

Segmental buckling with elastic explants will close breaks as large as 70° and reattach the retina in 95% of eyes with detachment. A radial orientation of the explant eliminates leaking radial folds and improves the reattachment rate. Without drainage of subretinal fluid, the operation is without intraocular complications. The extraocular complications are infrequent and reversible. Kreissig et al. (38) have recently demonstrated, from a prospective study of 15 years' duration, that segmental buckling is not deleterious to visual function (38). Tears larger than 70°, except for oral disinsertions, are better managed with an intraocular tamponade of

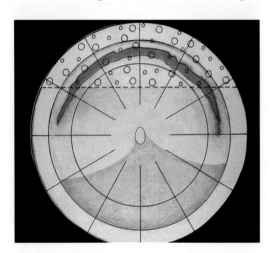

FIG. 43. The bubble in Fig. 42 is initially too small to tamponade the entire extent of the tear.

gas. With the use of expanding gases (the perfluorocarbons), intraocular bubbles of therapeutic volume can be obtained without prior drainage of subretinal fluid. Attachment with the gas operation can be compromised by proliferative vitreoretinopathy that is provoked by the gas. Removing the cortical vitreous by vitrectomy is probably a useful prophylactic measure. However, considering the morbidity of a vitrectomy, a first attempt with gas alone for large tears may be justified.

REFERENCES

1. Lincoff H, Gieser R. Finding the retinal hole. *Mod Probl Ophthalmol* 1972;10:78–87.
2. Lincoff H. Guilty until proved innocent. *Arch Ophthalmol* 1967;78: 271.
3. Lincoff H, Kreissig I. The conservative management of vitreous hemorrhage. *Trans Am Acad Ophthalmol Otolaryngol* 1975;79:858–865.
4. Custodis E. Bedeutet die Plombenaufnähung auf die Sklera einen Fortschritt in der operativen Behandlung der Netzhautablösung? *Berl Dtsch Ophthalmol Ges* 1953;58:102.
5. Lincoff H, Kreissig I. The treatment of retinal detachment without drainage of subretinal fluid. *Trans Am Acad Ophthalmol Otolaryngol* 1972;76:1221–1232.
6. Kreissig I, Rose D, Jost B. Minimized surgery for detachment with segmental buckling and non-drainage with a follow-up of 11 years. *Retina* 1992;12:224–231.
7. Kreissig I. Differential diagnosis of residual detachment after detachment surgery without drainage: a long-term follow-up. *Aktuel Augenheilkd* 1995;20:123.
8. Lincoff H, Kreissig I. Advantages of radial buckling. *Am J Ophthalmol* 1975;79:955–957.
9. Goldbaum MH, Smithline M, Poole TA, Lincoff H. Geometric analysis of radial buckling. *Am J Ophthalmol* 1975;79:958–965.
10. Lincoff H, McLean JM. Modifications to the Custodis procedure. II. A new silicone implant for large tears. *Am J Ophthalmol* 1967;64:877–879.
11. Lincoff H, Kreissig I, Hahn YS. Elastic pouch operation for large retinal tears. *Arch Ophthalmol* 1979;97:708–710.
12. Kreissig I, Lincoff H. A comparative study of sponge infections. *Mod Probl Ophthalmol* 1979;20:154–156.
13. Lincoff H, Kreissig I, Hahn YS. A temporary balloon buckle for the treatment of small retinal detachments. *Ophthalmology* 1979;86: 586–592.
14. Kreissig I: Ten years experience with the balloon operation. *Klin Monatsbl Augenheilkd* 1989;194:145–151.

15. Kreissig I, Failer J, Lincoff H, Ferrari F. Results of a temporary balloon buckle in the treatment of 500 retinal detachments and a comparison with pneumatic retinopexy. *Am J Ophthalmol* 1989;107:381–389.
16. Lincoff H, Kreissig I, Farber M. The results of 100 aphakic detachments treated with a temporary balloon buckle: a case against routine encircling operations. *Br J Ophthalmol* 1985;69:798–804.
17. Lincoff H, Kreissig I. Finding the retinal hole in the pseudophakic eye with detachment. *Am J Ophthalmol* 1994;117:442–446.
18. Boldrey EE. A modified contact lens for peripheral retinal evaluation in pseudophakes. *Ophthalmology* 1988;95(Suppl):16–17.
19. Dobbie C. Circulation changes in the eye associated with retinal detachment and its repair. *Trans Am Ophthalmol Soc* 1980;78:504–566.
20. Yoshida A, Feke G, Green GJ, et al. Retinal circulatory changes after scleral buckling operations. *Am J Ophthalmol* 1983;95:182–188.
21. Winter W, Lipka P. Untersuchungen der Lichtunterschiedsempfindlichkeit nach Operationen von Netzhaut-Ablösungen. *Folia Ophthalmol (Leipz)* 1987;12:315.
22. Lincoff H, Kreissig I, Parver LP. Limits of constriction in the treatment of retinal detachment. *Arch Ophthalmol* 1976;94:1473–1477.
23. Lincoff H, Kreissig I, Goldbaum M. Reasons for failure in nondrainage operations. *Mod Probl Ophthalmol* 1974;12:40–48.
24. Lincoff H, Kreissig I, Goldbaum M. Selection of patients for nondrainage operations. In: Pruett C, Regan DJ, eds. *Retina Congress.* New York: Appleton-Century-Crofts, 1974;397–411.
25. Lincoff H, Kreissig I. Application of xenon gas to clinical retinal detachment. *Arch Ophthalmol* 1982;100:1083–1085.
26. Kreissig I, Stanowsky A, Lincoff H, Richard G. The treatment of difficult detachments with an expanding gas bubble without vitrectomy. *Graefes Arch Clin Exp Ophthalmol* 1986;224:51–54.
27. Nadel A, Gieser R, Lincoff H. Inferior retinal detachments in young patients. *Ann Ophthalmol* 1971;3:1311.
28. Lincoff H, Haft D, Liggett P, Reifer C. Intravitreal expansion of perfluorocarbon bubbles. *Arch Ophthalmol* 1980;98:1646–1647.
29. Kreissig I. The balloon–gas procedure: another move towards minimum surgery. *Dev Ophthalmol* 1987;13:99.
30. Lincoff H, Mardirossian J, Lincoff A, Liggett P, Iwamoto T, Jakobiec F. Intravitreal longevity of three perfluorocarbon gases. *Arch Ophthalmol* 1980;98:1610–1611.
31. Lincoff H, O'Connor P, Bloch D, Nadel A, Kreissig I, Grinberg M. The cryosurgical adhesion. II. *Trans Am Acad Ophthalmol Otolaryngol* 1970;74:98–107.
32. Kreissig I, Lincoff H. Mechanism of retinal attachment after cryosurgery. *Trans Ophthalmol Soc UK* 1975;95:148–157.
33. Lincoff H, Kreissig I, LaFranco F. Mechanisms of failure in the repair of large retinal tears. *Am J Ophthalmol* 1977;84:501–507.
34. Kreissig I. Bisherige Erfahrungen mit SF$_6$-Gas in der Ablatio-Chirurgie. *Berl Dtsch Ophthalmol Ges* 1979;76:553.
35. Hilton GF, Grizzard WS. Pneumatic retinopexy: a two-step outpatient operation without conjunctival incision. *Ophthalmology* 1986;93:626–641.
36. Chang S, Lincoff H, Zimmerman NJ, Fuchs W. Giant retinal tears: surgical techniques and results using perfluorocarbon liquids. *Arch Ophthalmol* 1989;107:761–766.
37. Lincoff H. A small bubble technique for manipulating giant retinal tears. *Ann Ophthalmol* 1981;2:241–245.
38. Kreissig I, Simader E, Fahle M, Lincoff H. Visual acuity after segmental buckling and nondrainage: a 15-year follow-up. *Eur J Ophthalmol* 1995;5:240–246.

Practical Atlas of Retinal Disease and Therapy, Second Edition
edited by William R. Freeman,
Lippincott–Raven Publishers, Philadelphia © 1997.

· 14 ·

Pneumatic Retinopexy for Retinal Reattachment

William R. Freeman

Pneumatic retinopexy was developed independently by Kreissig in Europe and by Hilton in the United States as an in-office operation for the repair of retinal detachments uncomplicated by significant vitreous hemorrhage, proliferative vitreoretinopathy (PVR), or multiple retinal breaks. The procedure is generally limited to retinal detachments caused by breaks located in the superior 8 clock hours (Fig. 1). The standard pneumatic retinopexy procedure consists of cryotherapy of retinal breaks, followed by long-acting gas injection through the pars plana. Patients are positioned so that the expanding gas bubble internally tamponades the retinal break, subretinal fluid is reabsorbed by the retinal pigment epithelium, and a thermal adhesion develops around the break. An alternative approach is to use laser in lieu of cryopexy as a thermal adhesion. In this method, laser is applied through or around the gas bubble after the retina reattaches or is applied prior to gas injections in conjunction with scleral depression if the retina and pigment epithelium can be juxtaposed. The success rate is probably 5%–15% lower than with scleral buckling, particularly in aphakic cases.

Numerous problems associated with pneumatic retinopexy have been reported, including glaucoma, PVR formation, new retinal breaks, subretinal gas, persistent subretinal fluid, endophthalmitis, and potential problems after retrobulbar anesthesia. In addition, surgeons face a confusing variety of choices with regard to surgical technique. Patient selection, the choice and amount of gas, gas injection sites and techniques, utilization of immediate or delayed thermal retinopexy, laser versus cryotherapy for retinal adhesion, and the management of failure to reattach remain important issues for surgeons choosing to perform pneumatic retinopexy. A variety of techniques have evolved to address the these issues and to avoid complications wherever possible.

TECHNIQUE

An often overlooked issue in pneumatic retinopexy is patient selection. Patients chosen for pneumatic retinopexy must have a retinal detachment suitable for repair by this modality. Particularly for beginning pneumatic retinopexy surgeons, the retinal detachment should be characterized by breaks located at or above the horizontal meridian and retinal breaks ideally should be within 1 clock hour of each other with no evidence of PVR, vitreous hemorrhage, or difficulties with visualization. Scleral depression should be able to be performed on patients easily. Patients should have the procedure explained in detail and the ability of patients to maintain appropriate head position should be tested preoperatively. All patients should be given a choice between pneumatic retinopexy and the alternatives of scleral buckling and/or pars plana vitrectomy. Patients should participate in the choice of surgical techniques (this will ensure better postoperative compliance) and should understand that pneumatic retinopexy depends on patient compliance much more so than does scleral buckling or vitrectomy. Obviously, air or mountain travel cannot take place until the intraocular gas is nearly completely absorbed.

Prior to performing pneumatic retinopexy, a second 360° careful scleral depressed retinal examination should be performed. This examination is the equivalent of the "second look" that retinal surgeons typically have available in the operating room if scleral buckling were to be performed. Surgical preparation is important in preventing endophthalmitis. The periorbital skin and conjunctiva should be prepped separately with providone iodine. Subconjunctival lidocaine anesthesia relieves most discomfort associated with cryotherapy and gas injection but allows a patient to move the eye in the direction of the retinal break (Fig. 2). Cryotherapy is placed to surround all retinal breaks. Many surgeons ap-

W. R. Freeman, M.D.: Department of Ophthalmology, University of California–San Diego, Shiley Eye Center, La Jolla, CA 92093-0946.

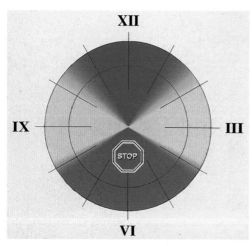

FIG. 1. Favorable and unfavorable locations of retinal breaks in retinal detachments to be considered for pneumatic retinopexy. In the superior 3 clock hours (*green zone*), patients are easily positioned, and the results are most favorable. In the horizontal areas (*yellow zones*), caution is advised because patient positioning is more critical. For retinal detachments associated with the causative break in the inferior 4 clock hours (*red zone*), patient positioning is extremely difficult, and the success rate is much lower.

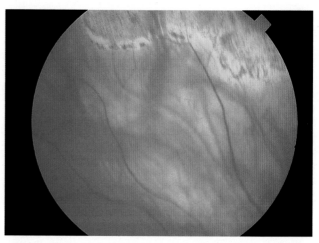

FIG. 3. A relatively broad band of retinal adhesion (in this case, cryopexy) is placed around the causative retinal break during pneumatic retinopexy. A good adhesion is particularly important when the retinal break is not supported by a scleral buckle.

ply a broader band of cryotherapy in pneumatic retinopexy than would be utilized in scleral buckling surgery because traction is not relieved by pneumatic retinopexy (Fig. 3). Laser therapy at the slit lamp or utilizing an indirect ophthalmoscopic delivery system can be performed in lieu of cryotherapy, but often must be delayed until the retina surrounding the retinal break is apposed to the pigment epithe-

lium (Fig. 4). In shallow retinal detachments, scleral depression may close the retinal break and allow laser treatment prior to gas injection.

Numerous problems associated with injection of gas into the vitreous cavity have been described. Slow injection with the needle just beyond the pars plana, while visualizing the tip of the needle, has been advocated to prevent fish-egg formation. Unfortunately, this technique may result in inadver-

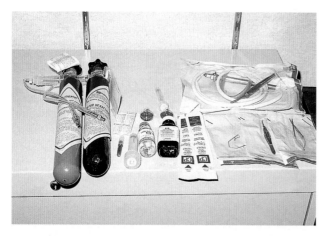

FIG. 2. Materials used in pneumatic retinopexy. An expanding gas (sulfur hexafluoride or perfluoropropane, 0.2–0.4 ml) is injected after sterilizing through a Millipore filter. Subconjunctival anesthesia is adequate and enables the patient to move the eye. A sterile forceps may be useful for stabilizing the globe during the gas injection, and scissors are required in cases where the retinal break is relatively posterior so that the conjunctiva and Tenon's capsule can be opened to allow the cryoprobe to be introduced.

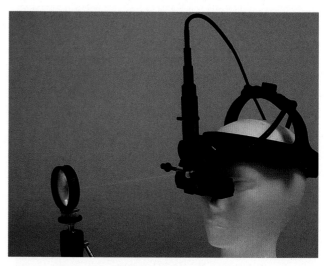

FIG. 4. As an alternative to cryotherapy, surgeons may use laser to form an adhesion around the break. This can be performed in conjunction with scleral depression with the use of the indirect ophthalmoscopic laser delivery system. In relatively shallow detachments, the retina can be placed in apposition to the pigment epithelium with a scleral depressor and the laser can be delivered prior to gas injection. If this is not possible, the laser may be delivered after the retina has reattached; however, the view through the gas bubble can be difficult.

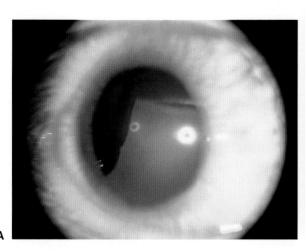
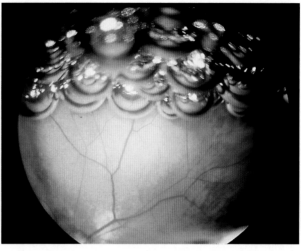

A   **B**

FIG. 5. A: Expanding gas used for pneumatic retinopexy inadvertently injected into prehyaloid space. **B:** Injection of gas into midvitreous cavity may result in multiple small bubbles that can pass through retinal breaks. (Courtesy of H. Richard McDonald, M.D.)

tent subretinal gas injection or gas in the retrolenticular (prehyaloid) space (Fig. 5a). Alternatively, gas can be injected into the midvitreous cavity under direct visualization with the indirect ophthalmoscope. If done briskly, small fish-egg formation can be minimized (Fig. 5b). If patients are supine, the gas will rise to the anterior most vitreous behind the lens and will not be in a position to go through a break. Any small bubbles can be coalesced by tapping on the anesthetized globe with a cotton applicator (Fig. 6). Typically, 0.2–0.4 ml of sulfur hexafluoride (SF_6) or perfluoropropane (C_3F_8) gas is injected after sterilizing the gas through a Millipore filter. Other gases may also be used; perfluoroethane (C_2F_6) has been advocated by some because it has properties intermedi-

ate between SF_6 and C_3F_8. Large breaks are not a contraindication to pneumatic retinopexy, with the exception of giant retinal tears over 3 clock hours. In the presence of large retinal breaks, there is a greater likelihood of small gas bubbles passing into the subretinal space, and therefore when large breaks are present, particular care is required to avoid this complication (Figs. 7 and 8).

Management of subretinal gas may be difficult. The gas may rise into the area anterior to the retinal break, particularly if the break is superior, and keep the break open; this may lead to failure of the treatment (Fig. 9A). Techniques have been described to withdraw this gas via a needle placed through the choroid into the subretinal space (Fig. 9b); bleeding is a potential complication and, if blood accumulates in the subretinal space in the macular area, permanent

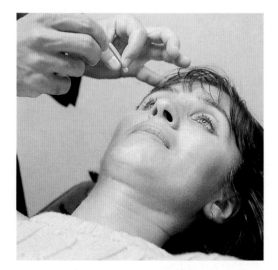

FIG. 6. After gas injection, small bubbles may be present in addition to the larger bubble. If patients remain supine, these bubbles will be unable to pass through the retinal break. Tapping on the anesthetized globe is an effective way of causing the small bubbles to coalesce.

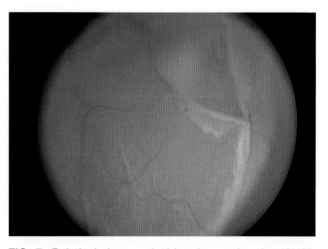

FIG. 7. Relatively large retinal breaks can be closed with pneumatic retinopexy. Care must be taken so that the gas bubble does not pass through the break.

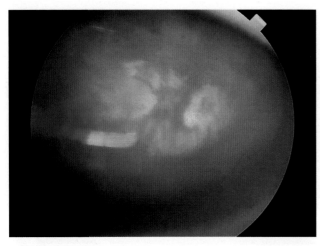

FIG. 8. After gas injection and expansion, the patient with a relatively large and gaping retinal break was rotated into position so that the break was tamponaded. The subretinal fluid reabsorbed in 2 days.

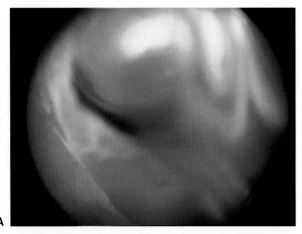

A

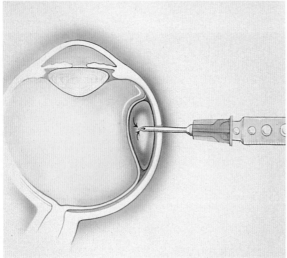

B

FIG. 9. A: Inadvertent injection of subretinal gas keeping retinal break open. **B:** External approach (transscleral) to removal of subretinal gas. (Courtesy of H. Richard McDonald, M.D.)

vision loss may result. Removal of gas via the open break is also a difficult maneuver. If pars plana vitrectomy is performed, gas can be removed in a more controlled manner; however, manipulations in this area are difficult, particularly in the phakic eye.

The intraocular pressure can be allowed to normalize with patients supine, and the perfusion of the optic nerve can be easily monitored. The tonopen can be used to document the intraocular pressure relatively accurately, even in gas-filled eyes. If patients are then rolled over to a face-down position (Fig. 10), the gas bubble will be positioned over the macula and will either reattach it or prevent fluid from detaching the macula.

Postoperative management of retinal detachments repaired by pneumatic retinopexy can be more difficult and is more critical than after scleral buckling. The view may be extremely difficult because of gas bubbles. In addition, the higher incidence of new retinal breaks makes careful scleral depression on each postoperative visit very important. New breaks, if detected, must be treated by thermal adhesion and appropriate positioning.

The issues just discussed are important complications of pneumatic retinopexy. Fortunately, cataract formation does not appear to be a complication despite the injection of intraocular gas. In a recent study by Mougharbel and associ-

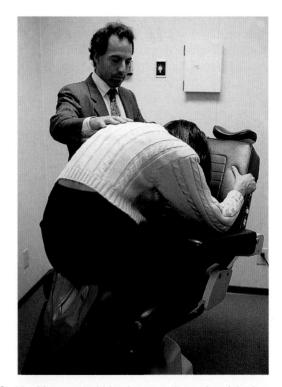

FIG. 10. After gas bubbles have coalesced and the intraocular pressure has normalized, patients may be rotated into the face-down position. This will protect the macula from becoming detached by displaced fluid. If the macula is detached, it will appose it to the pigment epithelium more rapidly. After 24 hours, the gas bubble will have enlarged, and patients can be positioned so that the bubble will tamponade the break.

ates, careful lens examination and photography even 2 years after pneumatic retinopexy showed no evidence of lens opacification.

CAUSES OF PNEUMATIC RETINOPEXY FAILURE

There have been several published case series that have reviewed the initial success rate and causes of failure. In general, most larger case series report a success rate (initially, that is, after the first procedure) in the 70%–80% range. Failures tend to occur within the first 1 month after the procedure, and it has been noted that failures are rare if the retina is attached for 6 months after the pneumatic retinopexy. The major causes of failure include new or missed breaks, reopened initial breaks and, in some cases, breaks that could never be closed. The latter may be the case when vitreous retraction is prominent, even without evidence of PVR. Aphakic or pseudophakic eyes, as discussed below, have a lower success rate as well. Strikingly, more extensive retinal detachments or total retinal detachments seem to have a worse prognosis in most series. The reason for this is unclear, but peripheral retinal examination and the chance to miss breaks would be expected to be greater in eyes in which there is more extensive detachment, particularly if it is bullous. The finding that poor initial vision is also a factor in failure may be explained by more extensive retinal detachment.

APHAKIC EYES

The reason for a lower success rate in aphakes (and pseudophakes) can be understood by considering the two major problems existing in aphakic eyes with retinal detachment: the potential to miss retinal breaks and more significant vitreous traction (Table 1) (see also Chapter 7 by A. Irvine and Chapter 13 by H. Lincoff and I. Kreissig). Aphakic eyes may have more visualization problems than phakic eyes. Aphakic retinal breaks may be very small, round, and located further anteriorly, making visualization difficult. In addition, the "second look" that surgeons have available in operating rooms is often unavailable in offices. The difficulties of visualizing the far periphery in some aphakic eyes further compounds the problem. Data from several groups suggest that the treatment of aphakic eyes with open posterior capsules may be particularly prone to failure (Fig. 11).

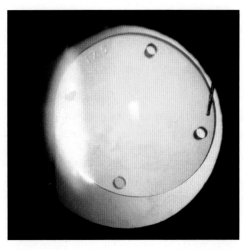

FIG. 11. The aphakic success rate of pneumatic retinopexy is lower in aphakic or pseudophakic eyes. This is particularly true in eyes that have undergone posterior capsulotomy or intracapsular cataract extraction.

Aphakic eyes probably have more vitreous traction on retinal breaks than do phakic eyes. This may relate to liquefaction and collapse of the vitreous, which is more pronounced in aphakes, as well as to the anterior displacement of the vitreous after lens extraction. In some cases, aphakic breaks would be expected to be under more traction and therefore be more difficult to close. Many surgeons include an encircling element as part of scleral buckling surgery in aphakic eyes. Encirclement has been noted by some to improve the success rate in aphakic eyes, possibly because the element will close small difficult-to-see retinal breaks and help to relieve the prominent vitreous traction seen in many such eyes. Thus, encirclement procedures may provide a safety net that does not exist when performing pneumatic retinopexy (Fig. 12). These considerations may help to ex-

TABLE 1. *Pneumatic retinopexy*[a]

Phakic vs. aphakic eyes	Success rate (101 patients)
Aphakic/pseudophakic eyes open or absent posterior capsule	56%
Phakic or intact posterior capsule	85%

[a] From Ambler JS, et al. Reoperations and visual results after failed pneumatic retinopexy. *Ophthalmology* 1990;97: 786–790, with permission.

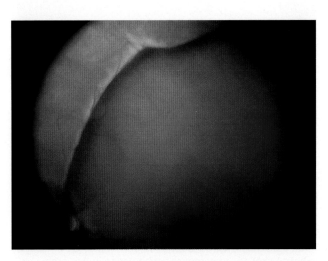

FIG. 12. An encircling buckle is commonly used in aphakic eyes. This allows closure of multiple breaks and tamponades the very tiny breaks that can be present in aphakic eyes. Pneumatic retinopexy cannot provide such a safety net.

plain the apparently lower success rate in aphakic versus phakic eyes.

NEW BREAKS

A second major problem associated with pneumatic retinopexy is the formation of new retinal breaks. New retinal breaks do appear to be more common after pneumatic retinopexy than after scleral buckling procedures. Several groups have speculated that such new or sequential breaks might actually represent missed breaks. Given the difficulties of examining patients in the office and the lost opportunity for a careful second look in the operating room (with patients often under general anesthesia), missed peripheral retinal breaks might be expected to occur more frequently in patients after pneumatic retinopexy. We have documented patients with new posterior retinal breaks after pneumatic retinopexy. In all cases, these breaks were well posterior to the equator and were flap tractional tears and not present preoperatively (Fig. 13). Other possible etiologies of new retinal breaks include motion of gas after pneumatic retinopexy and gas-induced inflammation. It is interesting to speculate that incomplete posterior vitreous detachment may be present in some eyes with retinal detachment and that injection of gas into the subhyaloid space may force a rapid completion of vitreous detachment with an accompanying retinal tear. Because of these considerations, it may be useful to examine eyes with retinal detachment by careful biomicroscopy to document the extent of vitreous detachment.

In summary, pneumatic retinopexy is a recently popularized procedure that may enable successful repair of retinal detachment in the office. Because of the higher incidence of new retinal breaks postoperatively, as well as difficulties in visualizing the retina through a gas bubble, pneumatic retinopexy may be quite difficult. There is no good evidence that pneumatic retinopexy is significantly superior to scleral buckling procedures, and retinal surgeons should feel under no compulsion to use pneumatic retinopexy. Indeed, scleral buckling still remains the "gold standard" in the repair of rhegmatogenous retinal detachment. The lower incidence of discomfort after pneumatic retinopexy and the lower incidence of refractive errors (due to encirclement) or strabismus are potential advantages of the procedure. Clearly, retinal reattachment is the primary concern in choosing an operation, and surgeons should use whatever procedure they feel most comfortable with in that regard. It is suggested that patients be carefully selected for pneumatic retinopexy and that this procedure should be avoided for poorly compliant patients, those who live alone, or those who will have difficulty with positioning. Similarly, retinal detachments characterized by multiple breaks that cannot be simultaneously tamponaded by a single gas bubble or that are complicated by any significant degree of PVR should be repaired with other techniques. There appears to be a consensus that, for "pneumatic retinopexy-eligible eyes," scleral buckling may offer a somewhat higher initial success rate; however, it remains controversial whether visual outcome is statistically worse after pneumatic retinopexy, because most failures can be successfully reattached.

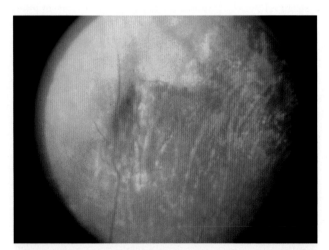

FIG. 13. Secondary breaks after pneumatic retinopexy are probably much more common than after scleral buckling. In this unusual case, a secondary posterior break occurred that was repaired by vitrectomy. This photograph shows the breaks after repair. The break probably occurred secondary to an incomplete vitreous detachment. The force of the gas injection probably caused vitreous traction in this area.

BIBLIOGRAPHY

Ambler JS, Meyers SM, Aegerra H, Paranadi L. Reoperations and visual results after failed pneumatic retinopexy. *Ophthalmology* 1990;97: 786–790.

Bochow TW, Olk RJ, Hershey JM. Pneumatic retinopexy perfluoroethane (C_2F_6) in the treatment of rhegmatogenous retinal detachment. *Arch Ophthalmol* 1992;110:1723–1724.

Boker T, Schmitt C, Mougharbel M. Results and prognostic factors in pneumatic retinopexy. *German J Ophthalmol* 1994:3;73–78.

Coden DJ, Freeman WR, Weinreb RN. Intraocular pressure response after pneumatic retinopexy. *Ophthalmic Surg* 1988;19:667–669.

Freeman WR, Lipson B, Morgan CM, Liggett PE. New posterior retinal breaks in pneumatic retinopexy. *Ophthalmology* 1988;95:14–18.

Grizzard WS, Hilton GF, Hammer ME, Taren D, Brinton DA. Pneumatic retinopexy failures: cause, prevention, timing and management. *Ophthalmology* 1995;102:929–935.

Kreissig I, Failer J, Lincoff H, Ferrari F. Results of a temporary balloon buckle in the treatment of 500. *Ophthalmology* 1986;93:626–641.

Mougharbel M, Koch FH, Boker T, Spitznas M. No cataract two years after pneumatic retinopexy. *Ophthalmology* 1994;101:1191–1194.

O'Malley P, Swearingen K. Scleral buckle with diathermy for simple retinal detachments: 100 pneumatic retinopexy eligible eyes. *Ophthalmology* 1992;99:269–277

Tornambe PE, Hilton GF, Brinton DA, et al. Pneumatic retinopexy: a two year follow up study of the multicenter clinical trial comparing pneumatic retinopexy with scleral buckling. *Ophthalmology* 1991;98: 1115–1123.

Practical Atlas of Retinal Disease and Therapy, Second Edition
edited by William R. Freeman,
Lippincott–Raven Publishers, Philadelphia © 1997.

· 15 ·

Vitreoretinal Surgical Techniques

Steve Charles and Byron Wood

Vitreoretinal surgery requires knowledge of a broad range of diseases, techniques, technologies, and complex surgical anatomy. This knowledge base must be combined with real-time clinical decision making, excellent dexterity, and the ability to manage a team. To be performed at the highest level, vitreoretinal surgery demands a combination of coolness under pressure, resourcefulness, rapid and efficient action, patience and perseverance, compassion, and, most importantly, ethics. This chapter provides an introduction to a system of thinking that is the basis of leading-edge vitreoretinal surgery and a compendium of selected indications and methods.

PATHOANATOMY

An understanding of pathoanatomy is essential to the performance of effective vitreoretinal surgery. Pathoanatomy evolves from normal anatomy as a limited set of interactions that occur between cells and the extracellular matrix. The vitreous is composed of a three-dimensional matrix of collagen fibers suspended in a hyaluronic acid gel. The outer portion of this volume (cortex) is adherent to the retinal surface in varying degrees (Fig. 1). The vitreoretinal adherence is greatest in the preequatorial region known as the vitreous base. Adherence is somewhat less at the macula, retinal vessels, and optic nerve. Intervening regions usually separate first when a posterior vitreous separation occurs. The vitreous develops areas of liquefaction or lacuna in an aging process known as synersis. It was originally thought that vitreous collapse caused by this liquefaction initiated separation. It is now believed that the vitreous cortex loses adherence to the retinal surface. Marked angular acceleration of the vitreous that occurs during a saccade contributes to vitreous separation.

It is crucial to understand the difference between static and dynamic traction. Static traction occurs whether the eye is at rest or in rapid saccadic motion (Fig. 2). Dynamic traction is a result of rapid eye motion (Fig. 3). Classic retinal drawing evolved, in part, to describe retinal breaks and what was thought to be traction. The nearly equal success rate of pneumatic retinopexy and scleral buckling in phakic primary rhegmatogenous retinal detachment repair suggests that buckling static traction is a highly overemphasized paradigm.

Saccadically induced dynamic traction can result in tissue fragments being torn away from the retina. These defects can be full or partial thickness. If full thickness, they can give rise to rhegmatogenous retinal detachment. Full and partial thickness retinal defects allow retinal glial cells and retinal pigment epithelium (RPE) cells to migrate.

PATHOBIOLOGY

The past decade has seen a great revolution in our understanding of pathobiology. In the previous era, tissue-level descriptive concepts derived from histology drove the typical mechanistic, memorized management approach. The application of experimental models, cellular biology, molecular biology techniques, computational fluid mechanics, biomechanics, and electron microscopy has enabled a much greater understanding of the pathogenesis of vitreoretinal disease. This greater understanding brings with it a greater complexity in management options and a more cognitive approach.

Tissue damage is the inciting event in the repair process that results in most vitreoretinal pathoanatomy situations. Damaged cells release growth factors that cause other cells to take action. One of the critical components of the vitreoretinal disease process is the locomotion–contraction process. When stimulated by growth factors, cells utilize coated pits lined with fibronectin to adhere to the extracellular matrix. The extracellular matrix consists of new and old colla-

S. Charles, M.D.: Department of Ophthalmology, University of Tennessee; and Charles Retina Institute, Memphis, TN 38119
B. Wood: Charles Retina Institute, Memphis, TN 38119

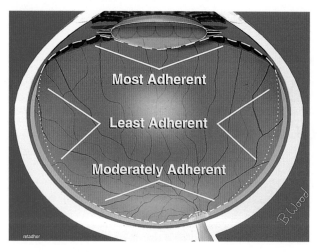

FIG. 1. Zones of retinal adherence.

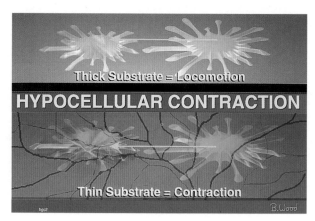

FIG. 4. Hypocellular gel contraction.

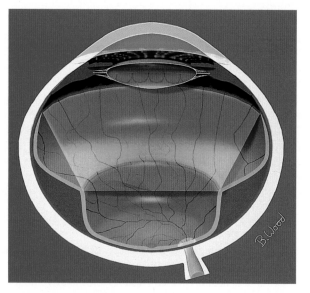

FIG. 2. Static traction.

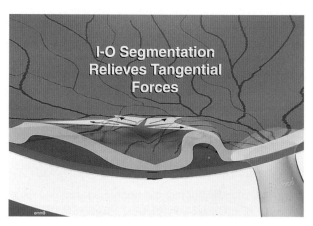

FIG. 5. Tangential traction.

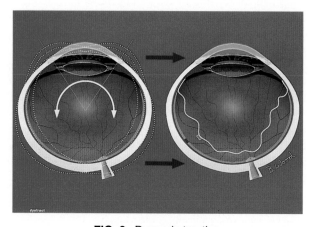

FIG. 3. Dynamic traction.

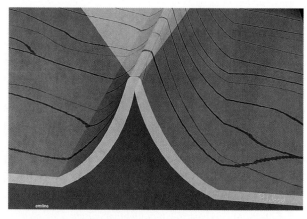

FIG. 6. Linear epiretinal membrane configuration.

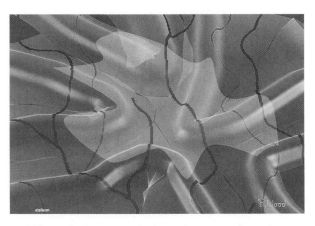

FIG. 7. Stellate epiretinal membrane configuration.

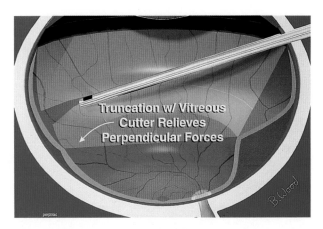

FIG. 9. Perpendicular vitreoretinal traction.

gen, fibrin, and elastin. Fibronectin has specific receptors for each of these structures of the extracellular matrix. As the cytoplasm undergoes shortening through the contraction of microtubules, the cells either migrate or create traction on the extracellular matrix. This process can create vitreous contraction or retinal surface contraction (Fig. 4). In more severe cases, it results in phthisis bulbi. Aberrant repair results in many of the problems seen in all forms of ocular and other surgery. Excellent examples include fibrosis of filtering blebs, retrocorneal membranes, pupillary membranes, and postoperative fibrosis of the extraocular muscle sheaths or lacrimal system.

Retinal static traction can be divided into two nonexclusive types: (1) tangential and (2) perpendicular. Tangential traction on the retina is caused by epiretinal or subretinal membranes (Fig. 5). These membranes can be glial or RPE in origin, although they usually contain a polyclonal milieu of cells. On occasion, residual posterior vitreous cortex (PVC) that remains adherent to the retina contracts in a process known as hypocellular gel contraction. Epiretinal membranes (ERMs) may be linear, stellate, or placoid in configuration. Linear ERMs create a ridgelike retinal geometry (Fig. 6), whereas stellate membranes create a starfold as in classic proliferative vitreoretinopathy (PVR) (Fig. 7). Pla-

coid membranes create a plateaulike configuration typical for epimacular membrane (EMM) and proliferative diabetic retinopathy (PDR) (Fig. 8). Many cases have a combination of these configurations.

Perpendicular vitreoretinal traction creates a geometry that is dependent on the shape and extent of vitreoretinal adherence. A large placoid area of vitreoretinal adherence in combination with hypocellular gel contraction of PVC (perpendicular component) creates a large plateaulike traction retinal detachment (TRD) (Fig. 9). A small, punctate zone of vitreoretinal adherence creates a small, conical TRD. The shape of the posterior vitreous cortex in the region of an associated TRD is a mirror image of the shape of the TRD surface. A TRD means that the retinal elevation from the RPE has occurred because the combined perpendicular and tangential forces on the retina exceed the force generated by the transretinal pressure gradient. The transretinal pressure gradient is generated by an RPE pump and by a difference in osmotic pressure between the vitreous cavity and the choriocapillaris. A TRD has a concave shape in areas between traction apices (Fig 10). A rhegmatogenous retinal detach-

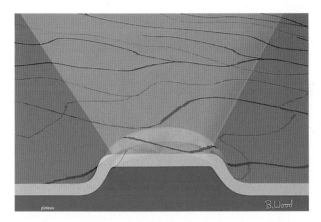

FIG. 8. Placoid epiretinal membrane configuration.

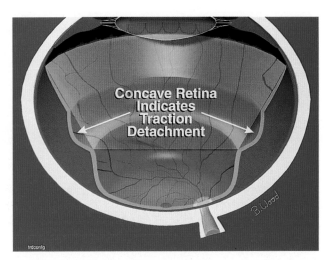

FIG. 10. Traction retinal detachment configuration.

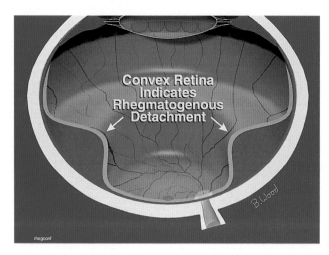

FIG. 11. Rhegmatogenous retinal detachment configuration.

ment occurs because the retinal break and vitreous viscosity factors allow sufficient flow of fluid through the break to overcome attachment forces. Rhegmatogenous retinal detachments have a convex retinal contour (Fig. 11). A TRD with a retinal break with a concave contour does not have hydraulically significant fluid flow through the break. A convex retinal detachment has an exudative or rhegmatogenous component even if the retinal break is not apparent and there is the appearance of traction. Higher-viscosity vitreous fluids (for example, hyaluronic acid) create a higher transretinal pressure gradient because of frictional losses as they move through the retinal break. A scleral buckle works in rhegmatogenous retinal detachment repair largely by bringing the RPE closer to the retina. The narrowing of the retinal–RPE gap acts as a circular venturi or shear zone plate, thus increasing the transretinal pressure gradient. Gas and silicone work, not by buoyancy (except superiorly in the seated patient), but by their interfacial (surface) tension ef-

fects (Fig. 12). Oil or gas in contact with retinal breaks restores the transretinal pressure gradient. An equilibrium is ultimately reached between traction forces on the retina and strength of any retinopexy lesions, balanced against the force of the interfacial tension.

MECHANICS OF VITREOUS SURGERY

The unique mechanical properties of the vitreous coupled with the wide variety of materials to be cut in vitreoretinal surgery present a formidable challenge to the cutting system. High cutter velocity (inertial cutting), shear effect, and sharpness are the three physical principles by which tissue cutting can be accomplished. Vitreous cutters are never sharp and work mostly by shear effects. Ultrasonic mechanical effects will liquefy hyaluronic acid gel but will not cut collagen fibers. Vitreous or ERM cutting with a laser is not practical because it produces a propagating pressure wave, bubbles, and photic damage to the retina. Lasers with very high spatial (10 μm) and temporal (femtoseconds) coherence create minimal remote effects, but have a very low bulk tissue removal rate.

Vitreous cutters should always be operated at the highest possible velocity and frequency. Vitreous cutters, like shavers and lawn mowers, cut best at the highest possible velocity. Velocities cannot exceed the speed of sound or acoustic effects will occur. All vitreous cutter designs are inclusive shears because they have parallel blades and no tendency to squeeze tissue out as the blades close. Scissors are exclusive shears and create a force vector bisecting the blades as the cutting region moves outward with blade closure. The blades are not sharp because sharpening would reduce the structural strength that is needed to create shearing force. Sharpness is defined as minimal thickness and leads to high pressure per unit area of cutting. Sharpness is not a characteristic of vitreous cutters or scissors, as they both use shear effects only.

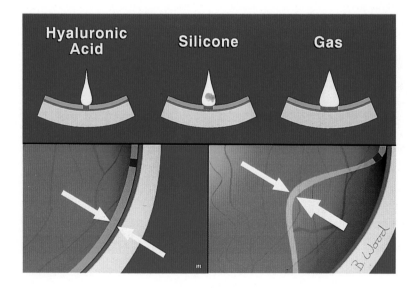

FIG. 12. Interfacial tension restores transretinal pressure gradient.

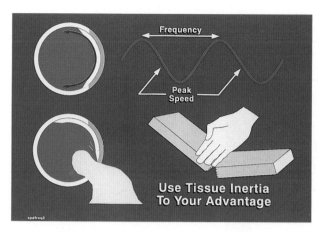

FIG. 13. Cutter speed versus frequency.

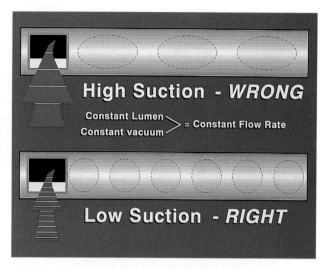

FIG. 15. Vitreous cutter suction.

Vitreous cutters operate at a rate referred to as cutting frequency. This is different than the cutter velocity concept discussed previously (Fig. 13). Vitreous fibers entering the port may be connected to the retina, which points to the need for minimal force during vitreous cutting. High cutting frequency causes the vitreous fibers to be transsected with minimal travel, thereby reducing traction on the retina (Fig. 14). The port should be open the maximum amount of time, with frequent high-velocity cutting action temporarily closing the port. A maximum open duty cycle, high frequency, and reciprocating rotary cutters eliminate pulsatile suction and undesirable traction. Longitudinal cutters pump fluid in and out of the port with each stroke of the inner needle. Reciprocating, rotary cutters (Innovit, Charles, or Alcon) do not exhibit this pulsatile force. Vitreous enters the port because of a pressure gradient across the port (Fig. 15). This transorifice pressure, rather than flow rate, should be the controlled and independent variable in the surgical suction system. The suction should be foot pedal controlled, with its level proportional to the extent that the foot pedal is depressed (linear or proportional suction). It is preferable to have tactile feedback

to indicate the normal and higher-than-normal levels of suction as commanded by foot-pedal position. It is essential that the vacuum levels respond very rapidly, preferably within 100 ms, of any command from the foot pedal. This is particularly true as one rapidly decreases vacuum command from the foot pedal.

The concept that "passive" suction is safer than "active" suction is nonsense. "Passive" suction is due to the difference between intraocular pressure created by the infusion system and the atmospheric pressure. Resistance to flow in the infusion tubing and cannula limits intraocular pressure unless there is no flow. The fingertip on the flute needle port is an imprecise way to modulate the outflow resistance of the "extrusion" needle and any attached tubing.

FLUIDICS

Maintenance of correct intraocular pressure (IOP) during vitreous surgery requires an understanding of the fluid dynamics. Pressure, not flow rate, should be the controlled (independent) variable in the infusion system. Whether air pressure or gravity provides the infusion pressure (IP), the key is to understand the relationship between IP and IOP. This relationship is determined by the resistance (frictional) losses in the infusion tubing between the infusion source and the interior of the eye. In static situations (no outflow), the IOP is equal to the IP. In high-outflow scenarios (high suction or wound leak), there is a large difference between IP and IOP.

INSTRUMENT HANDLES

Surgical dexterity is, in part, a function of the design of hand-held instruments. Lighter instruments are always better, as taught by the Weber–Fechner law of neurophysiology, because they minimize load on the muscle spindles and fibers (Fig. 16). Instruments should be held at their center of

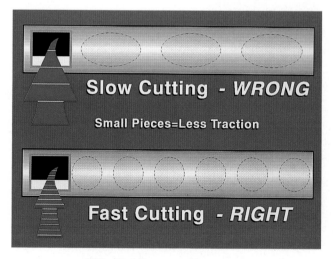

FIG. 14. Vitreous cutter speed.

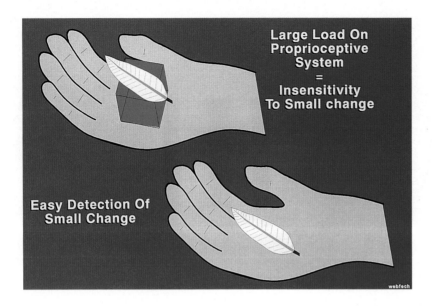

FIG. 16. Weber–Fechner law.

gravity to reduce torque. Shorter handles prevent force from the tubing, fiber, or wires from causing torque on the surgeon's hand (Fig. 17). The handles should be contoured to avoid the need to hold tightly to prevent slipping and dropping. Writinglike motions are the easiest for the human hand. Compound motions, such as actuation of the flute needle or scissors, are the most difficult. Rotation is quite demanding of the surgeon's dexterity, and extension is moderately difficult.

GENERAL VITRECTOMY METHODS

Conjunctival Incisions

The conjunctiva should always be opened parallel to, and about 1 mm from, the limbus. This flap prevents bleeding under the fundus contact lens and enables better closure. If no buckle is planned, a 1 hour of the clock incision should be made just above the 3 or 9 o'clock position for the endoilluminator and a 2 hour of the clock incision should be made extending just above and below the 3 or 9 o'clock position for the infusion cannula and the surgical instruments. No rectus muscle traction sutures are ever to be used for vitrectomy.

If a buckle is planned, the appropriate quadrants are opened, again with a 1- to 2-mm limbus-based flap, and 2-0 silk traction sutures are placed under the appropriate rectus muscle with a fenestrated muscle hook. Minimal cautery, a single area incision through Tenon's capsule and the conjunctiva, and avoidance of cotton-tipped applicators and cellular sponges help to reduce postoperative discomfort, symblepharon, ptosis, strabismus, and ill-fitting contact lenses.

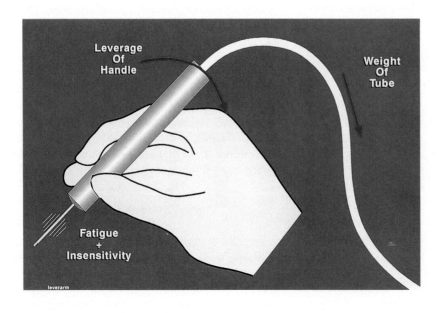

FIG. 17. Handle forces.

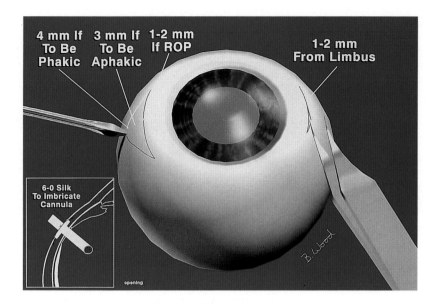

FIG. 18. Openings for vitrectomy.

Sclerotomies

The infusion cannula should be placed, inspected with the operating microscope, and turned on before the other incisions are made. The correct use of the infusion cannula is a critical part of the procedure and requires strict attention to detail. Sclerotomies are made 3 mm from the limbus if the eyes are to be aphakic or pseudophakic at the end of the procedure (Fig. 18). These incisions are made 4 mm from the limbus if the eyes are to remain phakic. Smaller eyes, such as those with persistent hyperplastic primary vitreous or retinopathy of prematurity (ROP), eyes with equatorial retina pulled anteriorly, and eyes with choroidal hemorrhage or detachment require incisions at the posterior edge of the iris (usually 1–2 mm from the limbus). A micro-vitreoretinal (MVR) blade (20-gauge shank, 1.4-mm blade width, and lancet tip) is used for all incisions (Fig. 19). No needle, stiletto, or other instrument is used for the sclerotomy preparation. The MVR blade should be very sharp (single use) to make a full-width opening in the choroid. The infusion cannula sclerotomy is placed just at the inferior border of the lateral rectus. It should be placed in other locations to avoid large vessels, large choroidals, or anterior displacement of the retina.

After the limbus parallel incision is made, a 6-0 silk suture is placed to imbricate the cannula into the surface of the sclera. The first pass should be directed inferiorly (backhand), with the second limbus parallel pass directed superiorly. The bites must be deep in the sclera and far enough apart to imbricate the cannula into the sclera when the sutures are tied up. This suture should not be used to close the sclerotomy. A 4-mm infusion cannula should be used in all cases. The cannula tip should be inspected through the operating microscope and/or the indirect ophthalmoscope after the suture has been tied. Inspecting the tip without magnification is dangerous. If there is any tissue over the cannula, it should be incised with an MVR blade from the superonasal incision if the eye is to be aphakic or pseudophakic at the end of the case (Fig. 20). If the lens is to be retained, the superotemporal sclerotomy should be used for the MVR blade access to incise the tissue over the cannula. The MVR blade should be directed toward the center of the eye when making all three sclerotomies.

It is advisable to observe without utilizing the microscope to check handle orientation at the inception of the sclerotomies. In most instances, the superonasal sclerotomy is used for the endoilluminator, and the superotemporal incision is used for the fragmentor, vitreous cutter, scissors, and similar tools. A three-port, all-20-gauge system allows for the most flexibility, reduces wound leakage, and allows entry of dissection or other instruments from the temporal or the nasal side. High-quality vitreous surgery requires interchangeable use of the surgeon's right and left hands for all tasks.

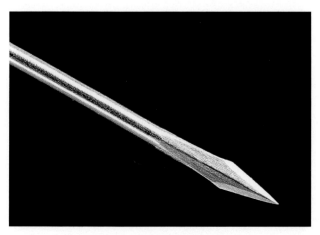

FIG. 19. A micro-vitreoretinal blade.

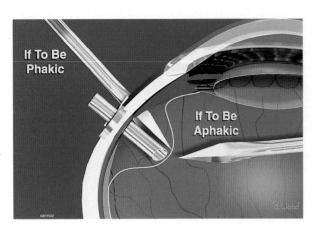

FIG. 20. Incising tissue over the infusion cannula.

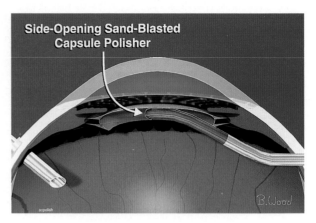

FIG. 22. Polish the anterior capsule.

Lensectomy

In most cases of PVR, giant break, ROP, and trauma, and in many diabetic cases, it is necessary to remove the lens. The fragmentor is basically a 20-gauge phacoemulsifier without the coaxial infusion sleeve. The method of lensectomy is very similar to modern endocapsular phacoemusification except that the nucleus should not be rotated. After placing the infusion cannula, the endoilluminator is inserted through the superonasal incision to retroilluminate the lens and help position the eye.

The author has developed a technique that uses a circular, posterior capsulorhexis rather than equatorial capsular entry. The fragmentor is then introduced through the superotemporal incision and advanced to the back of the lens. The power is usually left at maximum. It is essential to use continuous and simultaneous sonification and aspiration. Pulsation or alteration between suction and ultrasonification is unnecessary and leads to scleral burns and wasted time. If lens "milk" appears, ultrasonic power should be stopped immediately, and the fragmentor backflushed outside the eye with sonification activated to clear the handpiece.

The capsulorrhexis is made by grasping the capsule with angulated, diamond-coated, 20-gauge, Grieshaber, end-opening forceps. The circular tear is made midway between the equator and the posterior pole of the lens. If a radial tear begins, the capsule must be released and grasped again so that the tear can be completed from the opposite direction. Sculpting is initiated centrally to avoid capturing the capsule with the fragmentor. The Alcon 20-gauge titanium fragmentor with a special angulated needle is used to sculpt the nucleus, epinucleus, and finally the cortex (Fig. 21). The anterior cortex is avoided to prevent damaging the anterior capsule.

If the anterior capsule ruptures, decrease suction to allow the anterior chamber to reform through the capsular defect. If the lens material is lost posteriorly, do an anterior vitrectomy, complete the removal of the lens material within the capsule, and then proceed with vitrectomy. When the vitrectomy is complete, the fragmentor suction-only mode can be used to first pick up and then fragment posterior lens material without causing vitreoretinal traction or retinal damage. The anterior lens capsule can be retained to allow placement of a posterior chamber lens in front of the anterior lens cap-

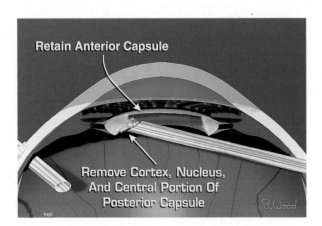

FIG. 21. Removal of lens material.

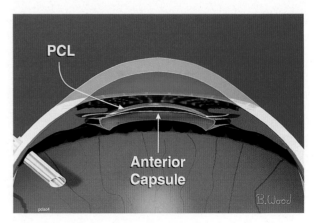

FIG. 23. Insert the intraocular lens in front of the anterior capsule.

sule through the a scleral tunnel after the vitrectomy (Fig. 22). The capsule should be polished with a diamond-dusted or sandblasted capsule polisher (Fig. 23). A primary capsulotomy is not necessary. The Acrysof lens can be placed through a 3.1-mm incision.

Vitrectomy

The initial vitrectomy steps depend significantly on the disease process and resultant pathoanatomy. The specific steps are discussed later, but certain principles should be kept in mind in all vitrectomies.

The essential concept is to cut vitreous in its original position to avoid force on the retina. It follows that the port should be placed directly on the vitreous surface to be removed. After an initial opening in the anterior vitreous cortex (AVC) or PVC has been achieved, the port must be placed on the edge of this opening. It is unsafe and time consuming to jump around to different parts of the vitreous cavity during vitrectomy. It is critical to realize that, in most cases, the surgeon is sectioning the vitreous surface, not removing a volume of vitreous, as in so-called core vitrectomy. Only in young patients with very recent disease is the vitreous *body* present in the volumetric sense. The vitreous cutter port should be moved toward the vitreous to be removed (Fig. 24), not pulled away while cutting. Pulling the probe away adds significant vitreoretinal force to the force produced by the suction effect (Fig. 25).

An orderly approach is essential to resecting the AVC if it is opaque or producing traction, followed by removing enough vitreous opacity to identify the PVC. The PVC can then be entered, and PVC resection can be completed in all cases.

Removal of Free Blood Products

After the PVC has been opened, it is frequently necessary to remove free blood products from behind the PVC to view the dissection plane better. This is done by using a straight 20-gauge cannula connected to the foot-pedal controlled suction system (Fig. 26). This method was previously incor-

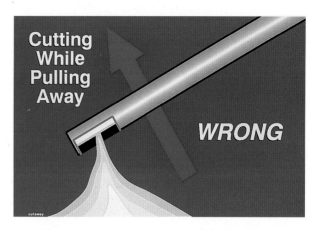

FIG. 25. Pulling away increases traction forces.

rectly called vacuum cleaning or extrusion. The flute needle originally used for this has been obsolete for over a decade. This nonpulsatile source of end-opening, precisely controlled low vacuum will remove all free blood products without turbulence and dispersion of the material. This same method is used to remove blood products from the retinal surface.

Management of Epiretinal Membranes

The goal of ERM dissection must be in concert with those of the plastic surgeon, not the cancer surgeon. Our *biologic* goal is to solve the mechanical problems causing retinal detachment, while causing the least damage and therefore the least likelihood of recurrence. A keloid prevention paradigm (minimize damage) is better than a cancer surgeon paradigm (get it all out and it will not come back).

In PVR, our goals can be achieved with scissors segmentation of ERM without removal. In contrast, our goals in PDR and ROP are usually complete removal by delamination.

Membrane removal methods can be divided into three categories:

1. Membrane peeling by tangential force (Fig. 27).

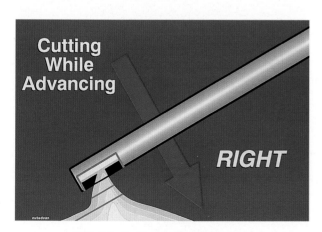

FIG. 24. Cutting while advancing.

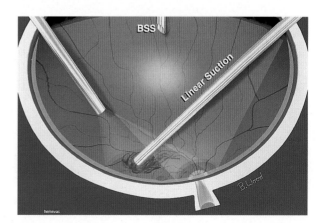

FIG. 26. Removal of blood products in the sub-PVD space.

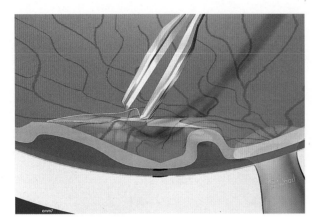
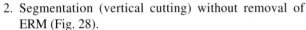

FIG. 27. Membrane peeling.

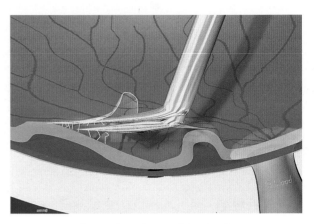

FIG. 29. Membrane delamination.

2. Segmentation (vertical cutting) without removal of ERM (Fig. 28).

3. Delamination (horizontal cutting) with complete removal of ERM without perpendicular or tangential force (Fig. 29).

Membrane peeling is used for low-adherence situations, such as EMM and PVR. Segmentation can be used for more adherent PVR membranes. Delamination is mostly used for PDR and ROP.

Membrane peeling was initially performed with bent needles and picks. The author never uses needles or picks. All membrane peeling is performed with end-opening, microtipped, diamond-coated, 20-gauge forceps (Fig. 30). In most cases, it is best to present the force tangentially to the retina and pull outward with respect to the optic nerve. This method reduces the chance of retinal breaks.

Scissors segmentation of ERM was initially developed by the author for eliminating tangential traction in PDR/TRD and ROP. In the past decade, there has been a much-needed swing toward complete removal of ERM in these cases by using the author's method of scissors delamination. In delamination methodology, the so-called horizontal scissors (Fig. 31) dissect into the potential space between the ERM and the retina. A shear that is under development by the author will eliminate the exclusive shearing (push-out force) problems associated with scissors. There are many reasons that forceps peeling, scissors segmentation, and delamination should be performed in an inside-out manner (starting centrally and progressing toward the periphery). The retina is stronger and thicker centrally. The membrane is thicker and easier to identify centrally. Frequently, no "edge" is visible, and the retina is more redundant centrally. The view is better as well.

Internal Drainage of Subretinal Fluid

If a retinal break or retinotomy is present, a tapered, bent 20-gauge cannula with a 25- or 27-gauge tip (Fig. 32) should be used to drain subretinal fluid (SRF) *through* the break (Fig. 33). This step should precede fluid–air or air–gas exchange. The foot-pedal-controlled suction, not the obsolete flute needle, should be used. The silicone rubber tubing or brush methods are not recommended because they can avulse retina and RPE. The bent, tapered suction cannula

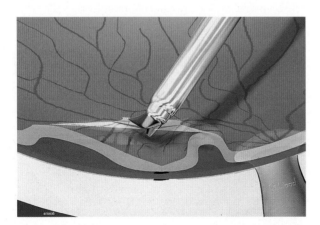

FIG. 28. Membrane segmentation.

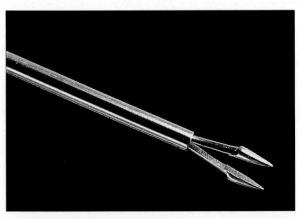

FIG. 30. Diamond-coated, end-opening forceps.

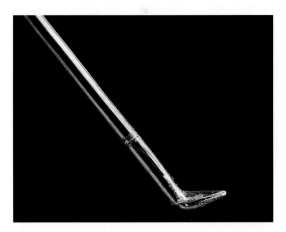

FIG. 31. 70° scissors.

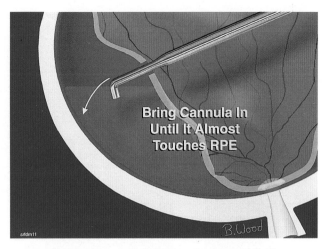

FIG. 33. Internal drainage of subretinal fluid.

should be placed through the break, away from the retina to a position near, but not touching, the RPE. The thick, posterior SRF can then be removed even through a peripheral retinal break. Once the retinal contour stops becoming more concave, fluid–air exchange should be initiated while internal drainage of SRF is continued. When the surface tension of the air "seals" the retinal breaks, the remaining SRF can be removed (Fig. 34).

Fluid–Air Exchange

Fluid–air exchange is performed to allow complete drainage of SRF and reattach the retina, to see through diffusing blood products, to stabilize mobile retina, and as a preparatory step for air–gas or air–silicone exchange (Fig. 35).

A continuous air pump should be connected to the infusion cannula at the inception of fluid–air exchange. The tapered, bent suction cannula should then be placed near the optic nerve and suction initiated with the foot pedal. The fluid meniscus will then proceed posteriorly, and the bubbles will coalesce to provide a single bubble. Occasionally, bub-

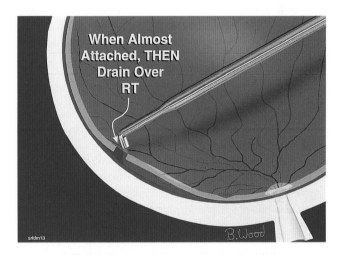

FIG. 34. Repeat drainage of subretinal fluid.

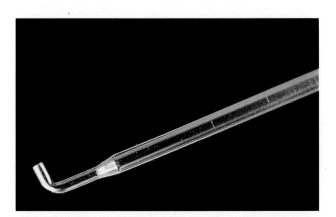

FIG. 32. Tapered, bent suction cannula.

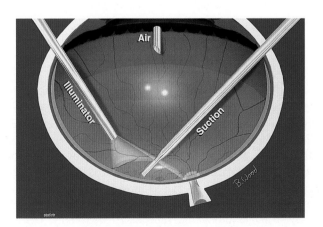

FIG. 35. Fluid–air exchange.

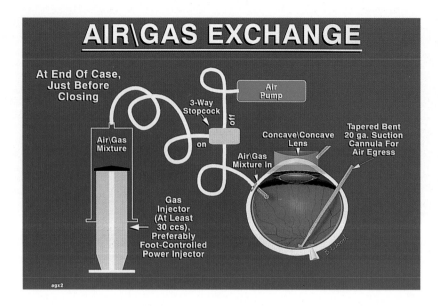

FIG. 36. Air–gas exchange.

bles must be removed from the anterior chamber. If internal drainage of SRF has preceded this step, it should be continued to allow complete removal of SRF and laser endophotocoagulation.

Air–Gas Exchange

Fluid–air exchange provides a complete fill, making use of an expanding concentration of gas unnecessary and dangerous. The usual concentration of sulfur hexafluoride (SF_6) is 25% and perfluoropropane is 15%. At the end of a procedure using fluid–air exchange and internal drainage of SRF, a decision must be made whether to use gas or silicone tamponade. Silicone is reserved for advanced PVR, giant breaks, or occasional trauma cases. The last step before wound closure is air–gas or air–silicone exchange. A power or manually driven syringe containing 50 ml or more of filtered gas mixture is connected to the infusion cannula and at least 30 ml injected while the tapered, bent suction cannula is placed in the middle of the eye to remove the air (Fig. 36). This method ensures a complete fill of the appropriate concentration.

Air–Silicone Exchange

If silicone is selected, a 6 o'clock peripheral iridectomy should be performed in aphakic or anterior chamber lens eyes to allow aqueous humor access to the corneal endothelium and to reduce pupillary block. The initial placement of silicone is best achieved by using a power injector (Grieshaber) and a short, blunt, thin-walled, 16- to 20-gauge cannula (Fig. 37). This is placed through the superotemporal sclerotomy, whereas air is aspirated with a tapered, bent 20-gauge cannula through the superonasal sclerotomy. The air pump is set at 20 mm Hg to maintain the IOP if problems occur with the silicone injection. Silicone is brought to the

pupillary plane, the infusion cannula is clamped, and the incisions are closed. A small amount of Balanced Salt Solution should be used to deepen the chamber should a flat chamber occur. This is accomplished by injecting with a small cannula through the pars plana sclerotomy at the pupillary border. Viscoelastic, air, and iris manipulation should not be used for chamber deepening.

Perfluorocarbon Fluids

Perfluoro-n-octane, perfluorophenanthrene, and perflubron—which are now available and are heavier than water vitreous substitutes—can be used in lieu of air in a fluid–perfluorocarbon exchange to drain fluid through peripheral retinal breaks (reattaching the posterior retina before the anterior retina), enabling the avoidance of posterior retinotomy. In addition, they are particularly helpful in repair of giant retinal tears because they allow the surgeon to unfold the tear by unrolling it in a posterior-to-anterior direction. After intraocular manipulation is completed, the perfluorocarbon is removed via air–perfluorocarbon exchange; to prevent pos-

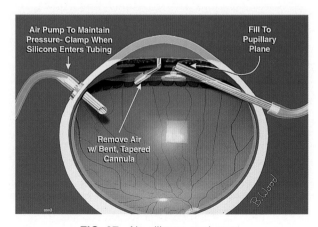

FIG. 37. Air–silicone exchange.

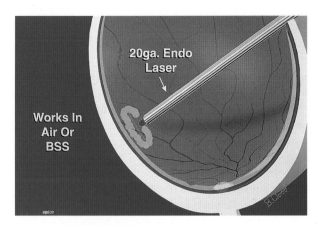

FIG. 38. Endophotocoagulation.

terior slippage of the giant retinal tear, care is taken to avoid any fluid in the eye.

Endophotocoagulation

Argon ion lasers provide an ideal wavelength to coagulate vessels as well as to produce retinopexy, even with lightly pigmented fundi.

The infrared diode lasers are small and more reliable, require no water cooling, and require less power, but will not coagulate bleeding vessels as well or work well with lightly pigmented fundi.

Frequency-doubled diode pumped lasers (532 nm) are the best choice for endophotocoagulation. If the eye is air filled or gas filled, less thermal energy is required than in the fluid-filled eye (Fig. 38). It is recommended that retinal breaks or retinectomies be surrounded with a contiguous treatment by moving the probe rather than by using a pattern of spots. The surgeon and assistant must be protected by appropriate filters.

Endocoagulation

Although 13.56-MHz radio frequency energy (diathermy) can be used for endocoagulation, 1 MHz requires no coaxial cable and is easier to use. The 1-MHz system is usually referred to as bipolar cautery or bipolar diathermy. A single-purpose, 20-gauge probe is very useful, but a 20-gauge multipurpose probe with illumination and irrigation is more versatile. As in all thermal cautery systems, the power should be raised gradually to avoid overtreatment; moderate energy of longer duration provides better control and penetration.

Endocoagulation should usually be utilized after delamination of ERMs (Fig. 39). The goal is to delaminate ERM (as in PDR), immediately recognize bleeding, elevate IOP immediately to stop bleeding, wait briefly, and then proceed. If bleeding recurs, this process should be repeated. If, after two attempts, bleeding cannot be controlled with elevation of IOP, endocoagulation should be utilized. Large retinal vessels that must be resected in retinectomy situations should be pretreated. In no case should ERMs be pretreated. This avoids undue tissue destruction, retinal necrosis, and time delay in surgery.

Wound Closure

The sclerotomies are closed with running three-bite 8-0 nylon monofilament sutures. Absorbable sutures leak during reoperations and can lead to filtering blebs. The nylon ends must be trimmed on the knot with the knot set tangentially to the sclera (Fig. 40). In this way, protrusion of the suture into the conjunctiva is prevented.

The sclera behind the sclerotomies and the buckle, if present, should be irrigated copiously with an antibiotic solution. The conjunctiva and Tenon's capsule should then be closed in a single layer by using a running 6-0 plain gut suture. To reduce ptosis, strabismus, and "buttonholing" on reoperations, Tenon's capsule should not be tacked to the episclera or muscle insertions.

Triamcinolone acetonide (Kenalog) or betamethasone (Celestone) and antibiotics are injected subconjunctivally at the end of the procedure. The repository steroid is injected at the inferior fornix so that it can be removed if steroid glaucoma occurs. Its use is avoided if the patient has a personal or family history of glaucoma.

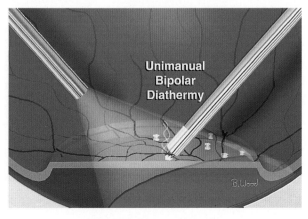

FIG. 39. Endocoagulation.

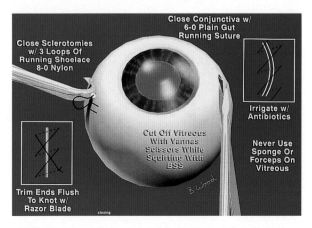

FIG. 40. Wound closure. BSS, Balanced Salt Solution.

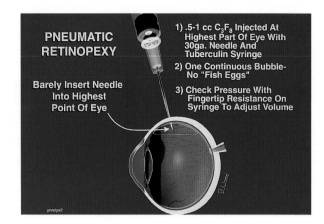

FIG. 41. Pneumoretinopexy.

VITRECTOMY FOR RHEGMATOGENOUS RETINAL DETACHMENT

Management options for repair of rhegmatogenous retinal detachment include scleral buckling, temporary scleral balloon, pneumoretinopexy, and vitrectomy with gas and retinopexy. As a trend, scleral buckling is decreasing in use, and pneumoretinopexy use is on the rise for treatment of straightforward rhegmatogenous retinal detachment (Figs. 41 and 42). Pneumoretinopexy may give equal final anatomic success rates as scleral buckling in selected cases with better final vision, less pain, less refractive error, less strabismus, less cost, and no extrusion or intrusion.

Vitrectomy with gas and retinopexy can be used to treat more difficult rhegmatogenous retinal detachment without retinal foreshortening. Retinal foreshortening of a mild-to-moderate nature can be managed by combining scleral buckling with vitrectomy. If more extensive, direct dissection of ERMs is required.

If vitrectomy, gas, and retinopexy are selected, it is best to perform laser endophotocoagulation after reattachment has been achieved by internal drainage of SRF, fluid–air ex-change, and repeat internal drainage of SRF. In this way, excessive retinopexy and dispersion of RPE cells is avoided.

PROLIFERATIVE VITREORETINOPATHY

PVR is the most common cause of failure of rhegmatogenous retinal detachment surgery. The PVR process is caused by excessive repair after an initial insult. The initial tissue damage could be large retinal breaks, many retinal breaks, membrane peeling, bleeding, or retinopexy, or could involve gas or silicone, which increase PVR by sequestering cells and factors at the retinal surface (Fig. 43). Glial and RPE cells, fibronectin, hemorrhage, and inflammation all play a role in the proliferative process. Although this process is referred to as a proliferative process, it is not characterized by a high rate of mitosis and is better thought of as an excessive repair effort. Just as gas and silicone can sequester the cells and factors of the PVR process at the retinal interface, the lens or intraocular lens (IOL) can increase the concentration of these substances in the vitreous cavity by maintaining a two-compartment eye.

In all except the least severe cases, it is better to remove the lens or IOL in the initial phase of PVR or giant break vitrectomy. In many cases, removal of the lens or IOL will lead to a better result because of decompartmentalization.

Frontal Plane Traction

In PVR, it is typical for there to be a complete posterior vitreous detachment (PVD). The PVC comes forward and fuses with the AVC. This resultant frontal plane structure, (AVC and PVC) must be removed with the vitreous cutter to eliminate traction on the equatorial retina.

Anterior Loop Traction

In most PVR cases, anterior loop traction (anterior PVR) is present. This traction results from hypocellular gel con-

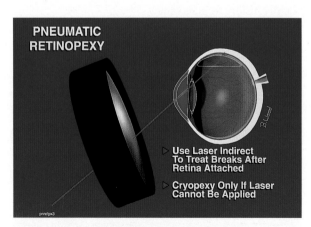

FIG. 42. Application of indirect laser.

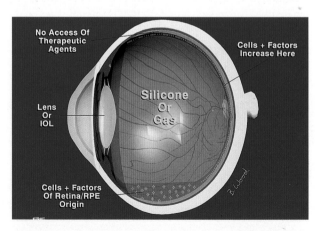

FIG. 43. Compartmentalization with the use of gas or silicone.

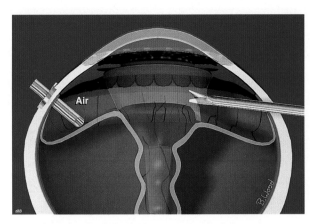

FIG. 44. Segmentation of anterior loop traction.

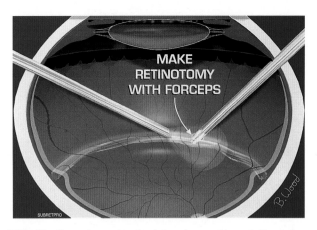

FIG. 46. Grasping subretinal membrane through the retina.

traction of the preequatorial cortex in an anterior–posterior direction. It is not a membrane and must be segmented circumferentially and not peeled (Fig. 44). Retention of the lens or IOL usually results in failure to dissect anterior loop traction properly. Anterior loop traction causes the equatorial retina to be pulled anteriorly, which can result in iridoretinal adherence with concave iris in aphakic cases.

Starfold Dissection

Starfolds are created by a stellate ERM in the epicenter of the starfold. Not infrequently, a thinner extension of the ERM may connect separate starfolds (epicenters). The best method to dissect these folds is to use an inside-out, end-opening, diamond-coated forceps membrane-peeling concept (Fig. 45). Picks, bent needles, viscodissection, liquid perfluorocarbons, and silicone dissection tools are not necessary or advisable for this approach. The epicenter of the ERM in the center of the starfold is grasped perpendicularly by the end-opening, diamond-coated, 20-gauge forceps. It can then be peeled toward the periphery and finally removed.

If it is noted to be highly adherent, inside-out segmentation of the ERM and inside-out delamination can be used.

Subretinal Proliferation

If dendritic, annular, or placoid subretinal membranes (SRMs) are present, an assessment must be made of their role in the retinal detachment. This role can be determined before or after internal drainage by noting their effect on retinal contour. Usually SRMs can be removed in a few pieces by using diamond-coated, 20-gauge, end opening forceps (Figs. 46 and 47). These forceps can be used through a preexisting retinal break, or a small retinotomy without removal of retina can be created for this purpose.

The Reattachment Experiment

After removal of frontal plane traction, ERMs, and any SRMs, an attempt should be made to reattach the retina by internal drainage of SRF, fluid–air exchange, and repeat in-

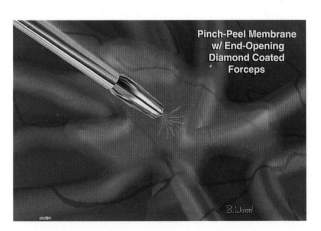

FIG. 45. Inside-out forceps membrane peeling.

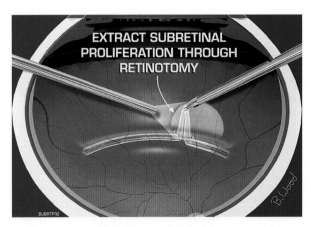

FIG. 47. Removing subretinal membrane in one or two pieces.

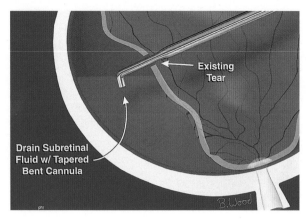

FIG. 48. Pneumohydraulic reattachment of the retina.

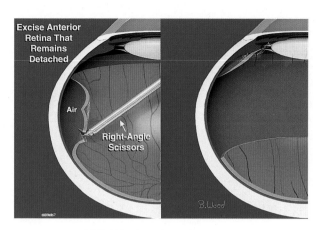

FIG. 51. Anterior retinectomy.

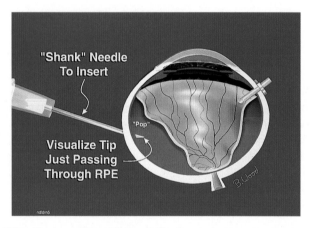

FIG. 49. Insertion of the needle for drainage of subretinal fluid.

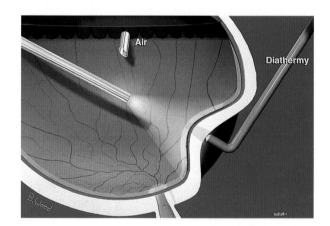

FIG. 52. Transscleral diathermy.

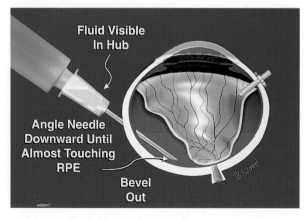

FIG. 50. External needle drainage of subretinal fluid.

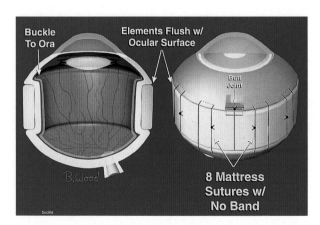

FIG. 53. Scleral buckling in proliferative retinopathy.

ternal drainage of SRF (Fig. 48). This should be done slowly with a low-magnification view of a large area of the retina. If subretinal air appears, the process should be stopped and its initial site inspected. A careful search for residual vitreoretinal traction, ERM, and SRM should be made at this point. Any of these conditions that are detected can usually be dissected under air. No identifiable cause for the subretinal air, this indicates retinal foreshortening and a need for retinectomy.

Retinotomies should not be made for internal drainage of SRF, because these sites can be a source of PVR recurrence. Needle external drainage of SRF is utilized if no retinal breaks or retinectomies are present (Figs. 49 and 50).

Retinectomy

If peripheral retina cannot be made completely flat, it should be excised along with any ERM or adherent vitreous (Fig. 51). All retina anterior to the circumferential so-called relaxing retinotomy should be removed—thus the term retinectomy. This method gives much better results and briefer operating times than tedious bimanual dissection of the so-called anterior PVR membranes.

Retinopexy

Retinopexy should be performed after the retina has been reattached by internal drainage of SRF, fluid–air exchange, and further internal drainage of SRF (Fig. 52). Laser retinopexy is preferable to cryopexy or diathermy because it avoids the need for scleral exposure and scleral damage. Laser and diathermy are probably less likely to cause PVR recurrence than is cryopexy, and certainly have less impact on the blood aqueous barrier. The author has not used cryopexy for over a decade in vitreous surgery cases.

Scleral Buckling

A moderate-height, broad silicone exoplant should be used in most initial PVR management (Fig. 53). In most cases, it is better to encircle with this rather than think of this as a regional disease. Scleral dissection and sponges should be avoided. If an encircling buckle of any type is present, it is usually better to leave it in place and reattach the retina by vitreoretinal methodology.

Tamponade

Gas tamponade should be used for mild-to-moderate PVR, especially in the first vitrectomy situation. Patients with previous vitrectomies for PVR should probably have air–silicone exchange. It is essential to use highly purified, 5,000-centistoke silicone (Adatomed or Richard James) to

TABLE 1. *Silicone complications*

	1,000 centistoke	Adatomed 5,000 centistoke
Silicone keratopathy	39%	20%
Glaucoma	22%	2%
Emulsification	4%	0%

Average number of previous surgeries = 3.9.

reduce emulsification, glaucoma, and corneal problems (Table 1). Silicone is left in place indefinitely if there is residual or recurrent retinal elevation, or if retinal breaks cannot be completely walled off with laser retinopexy. Perfluoropropane gas lasts about 3 weeks, whereas SF_6 gas lasts 1 week. Longer-term gas certainly increases proliferation at the retinal surface while offering longer-term tamponade.

PROLIFERATIVE DIABETIC RETINOPATHY

Vitreous surgery is commonly indicated for vitreous hemorrhage and TRD, complicating PDR. The decision-making process is very complex in the treatment of these patients. Whereas duration of vitreous hemorrhage is an important aspect of the decision-making process, it is not the only concern.

Knowledge of the pathobiology of neovascularization leads to better management decisions in diabetic vitrectomy cases. Hyperglycemia results in serum protein-induced platelet aggregation and capillary damage. Hyperglycemia has a direct effect on metalloproteinases implicated in neovascularization. Leakage, hemorrhage, and ischemia result in turn from the capillary occlusive process. Ischemia causes retinal cells to release vasoproliferative factor (VPF), which then diffuses to target endothelial cells, causing endothelial cell mitosis. The PVC, AVC, lens, and trabecular meshwork act as barriers to the diffusion of VPF. The presence of a barrier allows concentration of VPF to be higher on the retinal

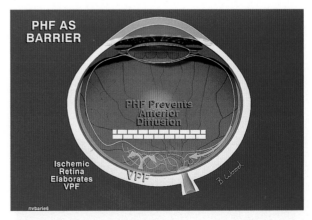

FIG. 54. Posterior hyaloid face (PHF) as a barrier to vasoproliferative factors (VPF).

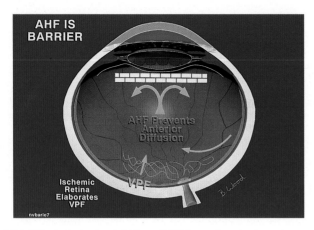

FIG. 55. Anterior hyaloid face (AHF) as a barrier to vasoproliferative factors (VPF).

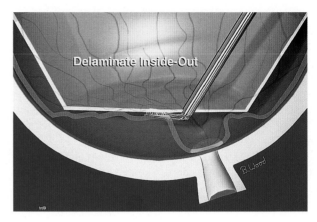

FIG. 57. Delamination of the epiretinal membrane–posterior vitreous cortex complex.

side of the barrier and lower on the anterior side. Proliferating endothelial cells release a factor that causes replication of glial cells; thus, the typical fibrovascular proliferation that occurs on each of these barriers/substrate structures.

Neovascularization extends from the retina onto the PVC, but does not penetrate the vitreous cavity. Both the retina and the PVC act as a substrate for neovascularization (Fig. 54). Anterior vitreous fibrovascular proliferation (retrolenticular neovascularization) is the most common cause of failure in phakic diabetic vitrectomy. Neovascularization starts on the peripheral retinal and cellular body and goes across the anterior hyaloid face behind the lens (Fig. 55). As glial proliferation accompanies this process, ringlike equatorial TRD, total traction detachment, and then phthisis ensue. If the lens, PVC, and AVC are removed, there is a tremendous increase in trabecular meshwork and iris neovascularization (Fig. 56). There is even an increase in neovascular glaucoma after yttrium–aluminum–Garnet laser capsulotomy in PDR patients.

Panretinal photocoagulation is the only method by which neovascularization of the retina and elsewhere can be managed. Incremental panretinal photocoagulation (titration)

must be continued until retinal, retrolental, and iris trabecular meshwork neovascularization become inactive. Panretinal photocoagulation should be used before cataract or vitrectomy surgery, if possible; during vitrectomy; and after surgery if neovascularization or recurrent hemorrhage is noted. Panretinal photocoagulation works by decreasing the production of VPF, releasing an inhibitor of neovascularization, and increasing the ability of the choroid to provide retinal oxygenation. Intraoperative panretinal photocoagulation should not be applied to retina that has been detached before surgery, or overtreatment and fibrin syndrome will ensue.

Indications for Vitrectomy

If a patient has a hemorrhage in the better eye and has marked visual loss in the other eye, vitrectomy should be performed very soon unless the hemorrhage appears to be clearing rapidly. If hemorrhage occurs in a legally blind eye, ultrasound reveals no detachment, and the other eye has useful vision, vitrectomy could be postponed indefinitely.

If an extramacular traction detachment is present and stable, frequent follow-up and self-checking of vision should be used instead of immediate vitrectomy. In general, every effort must be made to consider the patient's visual needs, health, status of the other eye, clinical course if not operated upon, and likely outcome of surgery.

Vitrectomy

AVC that is opaque or semiopaque must be carefully removed by using temporal and nasal instrument entry to avoid bumping the lens. This should be done without the fundus contact lens to better judge the location of the posterior lens capsule. The AVC should be allowed to fall back to avoid the lens as it is removed. Only enough central vitreous hemorrhage should be removed (core vitrectomy) to identify the PVC. An opening should then be made in the PVC in an area thought to have a PVD. Any free blood products can then be

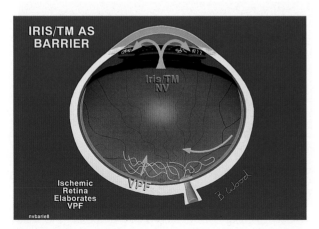

FIG. 56. Trabecular meshwork (TM) as a barrier to vasoproliferative factors (VPF).

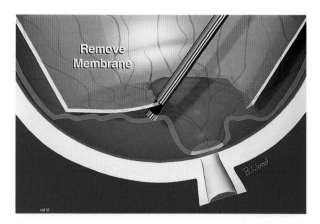

FIG. 58. Removal of the epiretinal membrane–posterior vitreous cortex complex.

removed by the straight suction cannula method through this opening. The PVC should then be truncated circumferentially to eliminate all anteroposterior traction. If TRD is present, inside-out delamination starting near the optic nerve should precede truncation of the posterior vitreous cortex (Fig. 57). In this way, retinal breaks secondary to vitreous cutter-induced vitreoretinal traction can be avoided. Inside-out delamination with a few inside-out segmentation cuts to gain access should be used in all TRDs. Membrane picks and peeling should never be used in PDR with TRD. The ERM–PVC complex can be removed in one or more pieces with the vitreous cutter after the delamination process is complete (Fig. 58). This is not to be confused with the somewhat dangerous en bloc method in which the direction of dissection is outside-in and the vitreous is used to pull on the ERM–retinal interface.

Endocoagulation

Endocoagulation should not be applied prior to delamination. Endocoagulation should be used on the vascular attachment points on the retina after two attempts have been made to control bleeding by transient elevation of the IOP. In no case should endocoagulation be used on or contiguous to the optic nerve.

Fluid–Air Exchange

There is no evidence that air reduces bleeding, and it is *never* required if there is no retinal break. Air or gas has no effect on a strictly TRD. Fluid–air exchange, internal drainage of SRF, and air–gas exchange are used only if a retinal break is present after the dissection has been completed.

Endophotocoagulation

Endophotocoagulation is primarily used for treating any retinal breaks and for initial panretinal photocoagulation or panretinal photocoagulation fill-in. Occasionally, it is used to treat abnormal retinal vessels not treated with endocoagulation. A panretinal photocoagulation fill-in or initial treatment should be used in any case with retinal, anterior vitreous cortex, iris, or trabecular meshwork neovascularization. Most diabetic vitrectomies require additional panretinal photocoagulation at the time of surgery, even if a "complete" panretinal photocoagulation is present.

Scleral Buckling

The author no longer uses routine scleral buckling in most diabetic vitrectomies. Vitreous cutters, fluidics, and techniques have improved to the point that this is an unnecessary step.

TRAUMA

Vitrectomy has radically improved the success rate in the management of corneoscleral lacerations, penetrating injuries, and intraocular foreign bodies (IOFBs). The retinal detachments in trauma cases are almost always traction induced rather than secondary to a retinal laceration. The prognosis in trauma cases depends on many factors spaced out over a few weeks after injury. Obviously, initial optic nerve or macular injury can render the eye legally blind even if the eye is not lost because of endophthalmitis or retinal detachment. Initial management should be oriented toward avoiding loss of intraocular contents and prevention of endophthalmitis.

The single most important management goal of the next few weeks following the injury is the prevention of PVR, which is secondary to hypocellular gel contraction of the vitreous and fibrous proliferation on the retinal surface. Rhegmatogenous retinal detachment from retinal injury is quite rare because the sites are usually self-sealing.

Corneoscleral Laceration

It is essential to close the wounds in such a manner as to avoid loss of intraocular contents, while establishing a watertight closure to permit subsequent vitrectomy. Running 8-0 or 9-0 monofilament nylon suture is elastic and will reclose the wound if undue pressure causes a wound leak. Absorbable sutures and silk have no place in the repair of corneoscleral lacerations. Whereas 10-0 sutures can be used in the cornea, they have much less tensile strength than 9-0 and frequently lead to wound leaks during subsequent vitrectomy. Running sutures reduce astigmatism, irritating suture ends, and operating time in most instances. Viscoelastics can be used to a great advantage to reposition tissue and maintain the anterior chamber while repairing the laceration. Viscoelastics should not be used if the use of silicone is planned, asviscoelastics increase emulsification of silicone.

Most traumatic cataracts in corneoscleral laceration cases have defects in the peripheral and posterior lens capsule, even if these are not identified. Pharcoemulsification and planned extracapsular cataract extraction have no place in most of these cases because of undue vitreous force and potential loss of lens material posteriorly. It is far better to close the wound and give the cornea a few days to slide endothelial cells into the wound, leading to deturgescence of the cornea. With delayed lensectomy, the surgeon encounters less bleeding and miosis, and is prepared to proceed with vitrectomy.

Scleral wounds should be closed without *any* pressure on the eye. It is unnecessary to remove muscles or explore the entire globe. One should close what is visible before exposing any more of the laceration. Retinopexy should *never* be applied to corneoscleral lacerations. It should be recalled that the detachments that occur are secondary to proliferation from tissue damage and are not rhegmatogenous in nature. Cellulose sponges should *never* be applied to the vitreous in a trauma wound or the anterior chamber. It is far better to irrigate the vitreous with Balanced Salt Solution while trimming it flush with the surface of the sclera with the Vannas scissors.

It is now well known that the phenomenon of fibrovascular ingrowth occurs rarely, if at all. All layers of the eye (including the retina, RPE, choroid, sclera, and episclera) and Tenon's capsule are susceptible to excessive repair. An obsession with exploring the globe frequently leads to unnecessary tissue prolapse, just as cellulose sponges to clean the wound lead to vitreoretinal traction and detachment.

Cryopexy to the wounds leads to excessive proliferation. Lensectomy is preferable to phacoemulsification and, in most cases, is easily combined with vitrectomy. If the vitreous shows decreased motility from hypocellular gel contraction or has a significant vitreous hemorrhage, the surgeon should proceed with vitrectomy. In most cases, it is better to perform vitrectomy 5–14 days after the injury.

Double-Penetrating Injury

Double-penetrating injury can occur from screwdrivers, knives, shotguns, nails, ice picks, explosions, and high-velocity industrial accidents. In most cases, it is unnecessary and inadvisable to close the posterior exit wound (Fig. 59). The entry wound must be closed immediately to avoid endophthalmitis and tissue prolapse. The exit wounds are invariably self-sealing and require no retinopexy. Vitrectomy should be performed when decreased vitreous mobility is noted during saccadic motion using real-time, ultrasound imaging, or ophthalmoscopy. This is typically 5–14 days after injury. It is extremely difficult to perform the essential removal of the PVC if no PVD is present. Young trauma patients typically do not develop a PVD until 7 days after injury. It is far easier and safer to do the vitrectomy after PVD has occurred. Vitreous stuck in a posterior wound should be left in place to avoid hemorrhage, wound leaks, and retinal damage. Endophotocoagulation should not be used around exit wounds.

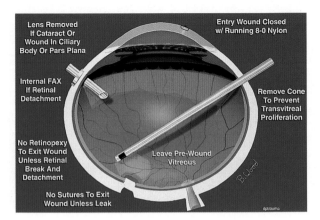

FIG. 59. Double-penetrating injury.

All anterior loop traction and lens capsule should be removed to reduce the incidence of late detachment, epiciliary membranes, and phthisis.

Intraocular Foreign Bodies

The vitrectomy approach should be used for essentially all IOFBs. If there is a small magnetic IOFB in the vitreous cavity but no hemorrhage, cataract, or retinal damage, the magnet can be used. The author has not used a magnet in 20 years. The vitrectomy approach allows safe and controlled removal of organisms, management of vitreous hemorrhage and cataract, and removal of the matrix for late proliferation.

The entry wound should be closed immediately and subconjunctival antibiotics administered if the referral process creates a long delay prior to vitrectomy. To reduce endophthalmitis risks and retinal tissue damage if ferrous or caustic materials are near the macula, most foreign bodies should be operated on immediately rather than postponing the operation to the next day. Steel, copper, chemical, and biologic material indicate immediate vitrectomy. Glass and plastic can be observed indefinitely. Shotgun wounds usually are double-penetrating injuries and should be managed by delayed vitrectomy. Intraocular lead can be observed for a few days to wait for a PVD to develop.

Small-to-Medium IOFBs

The typical 1- to 3-mm foreign body should be removed by first closing the entrance wound as previously described. The lensectomy is performed if there is a cataract in the pupillary axis or extensive cataract. Small, localized cataracts can be observed. A complete vitrectomy is performed *before* removing an IOFB. The foreign body should then be grasped with diamond-coated IOFB forceps and moved to near the center of the eye, and the size compared with that of the sclerotomy. If the IOFB is no larger than 1.4 mm (sclerotomy size), a 20-gauge, cross-sectional area can be removed without enlarging the wound. If the wound re-

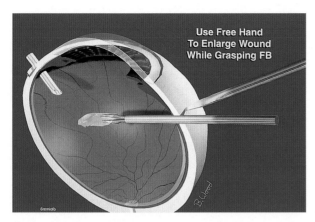

FIG. 60. Wound enlargement for removal of an intraocular foreign body smaller than 6 mm.

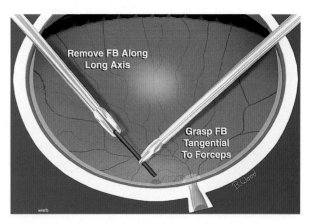

FIG. 62. Removal of a cylindrical intraocular foreign body.

quires enlarging, it should be accomplished after the IOFB is moved to the center of the eye by using the forceps shaft to stabilize one end of the wound and using a sharp blade to cut sclera and choroid to the desired size (Fig. 60). Some surgeons use a 20-gauge rare-earth magnet to initially pick up the IOFB, but the author has not found this necessary. Others use liquid perfluorocarbons to float the IOFB anteriorly, but, again, the author believes this is unnecessary in most instances. Endo or pre-op laser photocoagulation should not be used at the IOFB contact site because it will lead to excessive scarring. Scleral buckling is usually not required.

Large IOFBs

Very large IOFBs should be removed through the limbus after vitrectomy and lensectomy have been performed (Fig. 61). The IOFB can then be grasped with the forceps and the limbal wound made with the other hand. Liquid perfluorocarbons can offer an advantage in some of these cases.

Cylindrical IOFBs

A long, wire IOFB is usually grasped with its long axis perpendicular to the forceps (Fig. 62). Using coaxial illumi-

nation, a second pair of forceps through the opposite pars plana sclerotomy can then be used to position the IOFB to make it colinear with the removing forceps, allowing it to be grasped on the end. This eliminates the need for wound extension.

Retained IOFBs

Encapsulated, retained IOFBs should be removed if evidence of siderosis or chalcosis is present (Fig. 63). The capsule should be incised with scissors and the IOFB completely mobilized within the capsule before the diamond-tipped forceps are used for removal. Extreme care should be taken to avoid retinal breaks in the area surrounding the encapsulated site. All metallic particles and oxidized materials should be removed from the capsule after the IOFB is removed. The capsule can be left in place.

Subretinal IOFBs

Subretinal IOFBs should be removed transretinally, usually through the original retinal wound (Fig. 64). The diamond forceps can be passed for great distances underneath the retina to remove an IOFB, or a retinotomy away from the

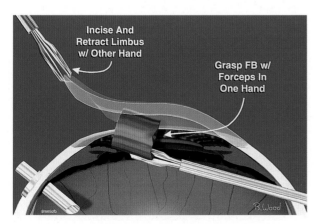

FIG. 61. Translimbal removal of IOFB < 6mm.

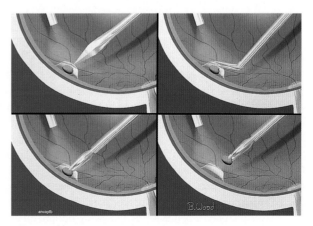

FIG. 63. Removal of an encapsulated IOFB.

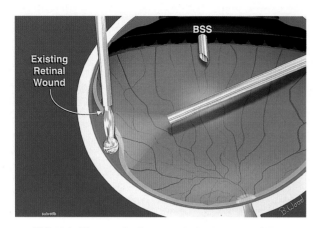

FIG. 64. Transretinal removal of subretinal IOFB..

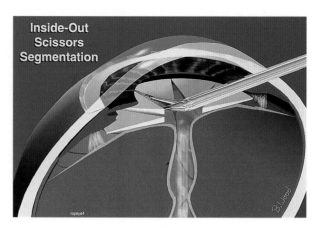

FIG. 65. Inside-out segmentation of the anterior hyaloid face–posterior hyaloid face.

macula can be made for this purpose. Transscleral removal causes retinal prolapse, bleeding, and more scarring.

Opaque Cornea with Retinal Detachment

Occasionally, trauma cases present with a bloodstained, but otherwise relatively normal cornea, vitreous hemorrhage, and a retinal detachment. These cases can be managed by using the temporary epikeratoprosthesis. After placement of the epikeratoprosthesis, lensectomy and vitrectomy, and gas or silicone, are used, and the patient's cornea replaced. The author usually prefers trephination of the opaque cornea, open sky vitrectomy with better visualization, removal of epiciliary tissue and iris, silicone injection, and then placement of a donor button.

RETINOPATHY OF PREMATURITY

ROP, as with all diseases, is best managed with prevention. Stage III patients treated with the laser have a 15% chance of progression to stage IV or V, necessitating vitrectomy. The usual prognosis in vitrectomy for stage V is poor. Over 95% can be operated on successfully, but recurrent proliferation in the first 2 months reduces the anatomic success rate to 30%–35%. Late proliferation reduces the anatomic success rate to 15%–20%. Essentially none of the patients have better than ambulatory vision, and only about 10%–15% of the stage V patients end up with useful vision.

The lens must be removed in all vitrectomies for ROP stage V and most stage IV cases. The sclerotomies are made at the iris root, 1.0–1.5 mm posterior to the limbus. A sector iridectomy is made with the vitreous cutter at both sclerotomy sites unless the pupil is large. Two-port vitrectomy is the best approach for ROP, and viscoelastics and sew-in infusion cannulas should not be used. The infusion is provided by a blunt, 20-gauge bent infusion cannula that usually is placed superonasally. The fragmentor is used to remove the lens because it does a better job of removing peripheral lens material and takes less operating time. The capsule can be removed with the end-opening, 20-gauge forceps without trac-

tion on the thin, preequatorial retina. If the capsule and zonules are tough, they are best removed by scissors delamination from the ciliary processes or by using the vitreous cutter.

There is essentially no core vitreous in the ROP cases. All vessels seen behind the lens are retinal vessels in the stage V case. The PVC is markedly adherent to the retinal surface in most areas, and the AVC and PVC are in contact in most areas.

As in diabetic TRDs, starfolds in PVR, and EMMs, the dissection begins centrally and progresses toward the periphery (Fig. 65). The initial cuts of segmentation are to the AVC and PVC in a single cut. This then exposes the retinal surface. As in all situations, the membrane (PVC and AVC) is matte finish and white, whereas the retina is shiny and pale yellow. The cuts are extended over the equatorial ridge and past the preequatorial "trough" until the cut visibly separates. These triangular pieces are then delaminated away from the retinal surface with horizontal scissors (Fig. 66). No pics or membrane peeling of any kind can be utilized in ROP cases. These delaminated triangular pieces are then amputated from the ciliary body by dividing the anterior loop traction by circumferential scissors segmentation. Gas or silicone is not used, because there is no rhegmatogenous component.

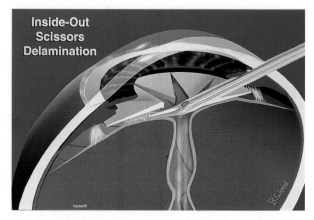

FIG. 66. Inside-out delamination of the anterior hyaloid face–posterior hyaloid face.

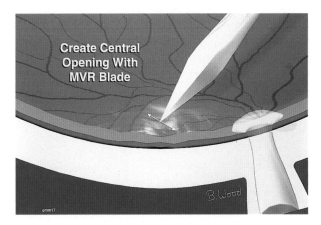

FIG. 67. Micro-vitreoretinal entry into epimacular membrane.

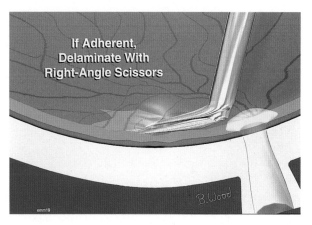

FIG. 69. Scissors delamination of epimacular membrane.

Bleeding is controlled by transient elevation of IOP. Endocoagulation is used very rarely. Scleral buckling is not used in these cases, because it can lead to brachycardia or cardiac arrest and late intrusion of the buckle.

EPIMACULAR MEMBRANES

EMMs have been called macular pucker, premacular fibrosis, cellophane maculopathy, surface-wrinkling retinopathy, and epimacular proliferation. These membranes are usually of mixed glial and RPE origin. As is typical for other conditions described, EMMs have a hypocellular nature and are caused by interaction of cells and internal limiting lamina, residual posterior vitreous cortex, or new collagen.

Many surgeons look for a peripheral "edge" to the membrane. This is not the best method and is not possible in many cases. As in all other conditions discussed, the dissection should begin by looking for the thickest portion of EMM (the epicenter). This may be foveal or extrafoveal in location. The MVR blade is then used to make a slit in the EMM at that point (Fig. 67). This creates a central "edge." This central edge is grasped by the end-opening, 20-gauge, diamond-coated forceps (Fig. 68). The membrane is removed in 1–3 pieces circumlinearly with traction being applied outward

and tangential to the retinal surface. The fovea is observed carefully during this process to prevent tearing. If strong adhesion, especially to the fovea is noted, delamination is substituted for peeling (Fig. 69).

Vitrectomy is utilized only if the vitreous has condensation or hypocellular gel contraction. Normal vitreous can be left in place to reduce the incidence of cataract and postoperative retinal detachment. Approximately 2% of these membranes recur, and the vast majority of those can be successfully reoperated on.

Progression of nuclear sclerotic cataract, presumably from heating the nucleus and ultraviolet exposure from the operating microscope, occurs in 10%–50% of the cases. If a substantial nuclear sclerotic cataract is present, it is suggested that the lensectomy approach of leaving the anterior capsule and placing a posterior chamber lens in front of the anterior lens capsule at the end of the case be utilized. Cooling the infusion fluid and infrared and ultraviolet filters in the microscope may be ways to reduce nuclear sclerosis progression.

SUMMARY

Vitreoretinal pathobiology, biotechnology, and electromechanical knowledge are rapidly evolving crafts. General ophthalmologists managing vitreoretinal patients, as well as vitreoretinal surgeons, must have an understanding of the pathobiology and pathoanatomy to make the best management decisions. Retinal disease and surgery are certainly the most challenging, exciting, and rewarding ophthalmic subspecialties, and require continued study.

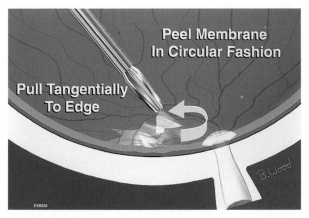

FIG. 68. Forceps peeling of epimacular membranes.

BIBLIOGRAPHY

Charles S. *Vitreous microsurgery.* 2nd ed. Baltimore: Williams and Wilkins, 1987.

Machemer R, Aaberg T. *Vitrectomy.* 2nd ed. New York: Grune and Stratton, 1979.

Michels R. *Vitreous surgery.* St. Louis: CV Mosby, 1981.

Peyman G, Schulman J. *Intravitreal surgery: principles and practice.* Norwalk, CT: Appleton-Century-Crofts, 1986.

Ryan S. *Retina.* St. Louis: CV Mosby, 1989.

Practical Atlas of Retinal Disease and Therapy, Second Edition
edited by William R. Freeman,
Lippincott–Raven Publishers, Philadelphia © 1997.

· 16 ·

Posterior Penetrating Trauma

H. Michael Lambert

Posterior penetrating trauma is one of the most complex and emergent problems to face ophthalmologists. The approach to patients with a possible ruptured globe begins with the suspicion that there may have been a global rupture and the realization that even the most trivial appearing lid or periocular injury may be associated with a penetration of the globe (Fig. 1). (*Pitfall:* Failure to suspect a rupture of the globe when a minor periocular injury is present.)

DIAGNOSIS

History

A complete history is very important. The ophthalmologist must determine the circumstances of the injury and its cause. The mechanism of the damage and the causative agent (blow with bare fist versus pounding metal on metal) may suggest a different course of workup and evaluation. Specific questions, such as these, should be asked: Was the patient pounding metal on metal? Was the patient near an explosion? Was the patient working under a car? Was there possible trauma by organic matter (higher incidence of infection)? Was the injury of a blunt (crush injury) or a cutting nature (with injuries from glass and debris)? Of what is the offending material made (radiopaque versus radiolucent)? Is the offending material available for examination (to determine the nature of the piece missing and nature of material)? This information may be necessary to direct the examination and treatment. In unconscious patients, similar information from witnesses may be vital. (*Pitfall:* Failure simply to ask the patient and witnesses the circumstances of the injury.)

The patient's past ocular history is also important. Does the patient have a history of decreased vision from previous trauma, amblyopia, glaucoma, hereditary disorder, or other cause (Fig. 2)? Has the patient undergone previous ocular surgery? (Rupture may be at the site of previous penetrating keratoplasty, cataract wound, and so on.) Is the patient tak-

ing any medications? Does the patient have a history of allergies to antibiotics? When did the patient last receive tetanus toxoid?

Examination

General Principles

1. *Do not apply pressure to the eye in any way.* Be sure to admonish anyone referring a patient to you to cover the eye with a protective device, be it a Fox shield, a cut Dixie cup, or a similar contrivance (Fig. 3). (*Pitfall:* Failure to cover the eye during radiologic or other exams allowing further damage by uninformed personnel.)

2. In a child or an uncooperative or inebriated patient, or if an open eye is predetermined, you may consider proceeding directly to the operating room to avoid possible examination damage to the eye.

3. Consider the whole patient. Occasionally, a patient may arrive with eye trauma that may have more urgent systemic or head complications requiring treatment before you proceed with eye repair. (*Pitfall:* That clear fluid coming from the patient's nose could be cerebrospinal fluid.)

4. Consider a lid block in the patient with severe blepharospasm or in whom general anesthesia may be contraindicated.

5. Remember the classic signs of perforation: lid edema, chemosis, perilimbal hyperemia, lacrimation, deep or flat anterior chamber (corresponding to posterior or anterior perforation), peaked pupil, and persistent hypotony. (*Pitfall:* Failure to realize that an eye with normal pressure may have been perforated.)

Vision

An accurate assessment of visual acuity should be obtained as early as possible in the examination process. Post-

H. M. Lambert, M.D., F.A.C.S.: Retina and Vitreous of Texas, PLLC, 6500 Fannin Suite 1100, Houston, TX 77030; and Uniformed Services University of Health Sciences, Bethesda, MD 20841.

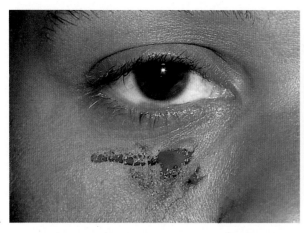
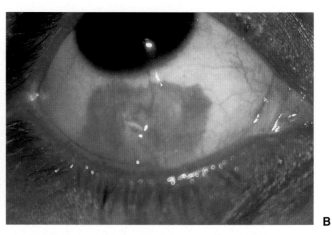

FIG. 1. **A:** Inferior lid puncture referred to an ophthalmologist for repair. **B:** Ocular penetration missed by a referring emergency-room physician. The eye had obvious conjunctival laceration and subconjunctival hemorrhage and, despite clear vitreous, had a ruptured globe. (Courtesy of William R. Burks, M.D., Margate, FL.)

traumatic visual function is the best indicator of final vision in damaged eyes. No light perception immediately after the trauma, although prognostically bad, does not necessarily rule out later visual recovery. The best vision possible should be determined whether by wall chart, hand card, reading newsprint, counting fingers, hand motion, or light perception. To open swollen lids, be sure to retract by applying pressure over the brow, not over the globe. The use of a lid speculum or fashioning retractors from paper clips may prove helpful (Fig. 4). (*Pitfall:* Pressure on the globe during examination.)

External Examination

Note lid swelling, lacerations, and penetrations. Minor brow and lid damage by narrow, sharp objects (information obtained from the history) such as darts, knives, scissors, and wire may be accompanied by ocular damage despite little or no evidence of the classic signs of penetration. Look for chemosis, subconjunctival hemorrhage (penetration may underlie hemorrhage), evidence of lacerations, and abnormal substances under the conjunctiva. Consider transparent substances to be vitreous, black substances to be uvea, gray substances to be retina, and others to be foreign bodies until proven otherwise (Fig. 5).

Motility

Check motility as in a complete ophthalmologic examination. Look for muscle damage, pain on ocular motion, or limited motion, particularly in upgaze that might suggest a blow-out fracture (Fig. 6). Decreased sensation in the in-

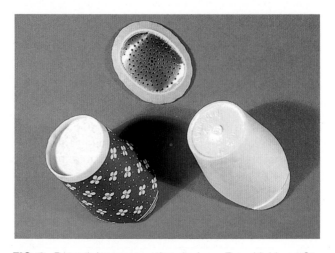

FIG. 2. The history of this patient referred with possible ruptured globe and markedly decreased visual acuity to the finger-counting level included poor vision from previous trauma and a macular hole.

FIG. 3. Potential eye protection devices: Fox shield, cut Styrofoam cup, and cut Dixie cup.

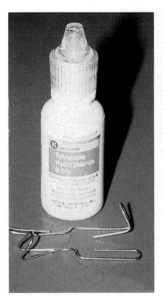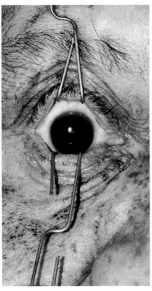

A   B

FIG. 4. A,B: Paper clips bent and used as a retractor lid speculum that affords minimal pressure on the globe.

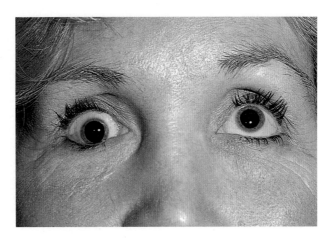

FIG. 6. Patient with a blow-out fracture.

fraorbital area also would indicate a blow-out fracture. (*Pitfall:* Failure to examine for a blow-out fracture because there appears to be only minor trauma.)

Visual Fields

Finger-counting visual fields, if possible to perform, might suggest areas of retinal damage or intraocular hemorrhage.

Pupils

Determine pupillary reactivity. Reaction may not be present and/or the pupil may appear irregular due to the trauma.

Look for a Marcus Gunn or a reverse Marcus Gunn pupil to help in your determination of retinal/nerve damage versus traumatic immobility. Look for a peaking of the pupil that will point toward a corneal or scleral wound (Fig. 5).

Slit-Lamp Examination

1. *External:* Look for small areas of perforation of the lids and conjunctiva that might indicate penetration off the globe.

2. *Conjunctiva:* Carefully look for conjunctival lacerations, through hemorrhage for scleral ruptures, and for small embedded foreign bodies that may extend into the globe (Fig. 7).

3. *Cornea:* Look for small penetrations, foreign bodies (Fig. 8A), and lacerations. Many shelved lacerations self-seal and are overlooked. These may not require suturing, but a gentle examination using fluorescein will show the patency of the wound (Fig. 8B). Look carefully in the limbal region for ruptures.

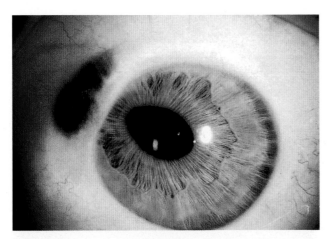

FIG. 5. Exposed uvea underlying the conjunctiva in a traumatized patient. The iris is peaked toward the scleral laceration site and is plugging the perforation site.

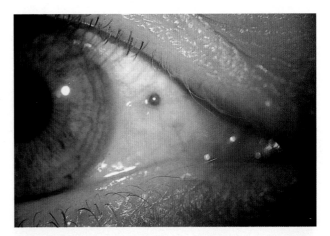

FIG. 7. Patient with a mildly irritated eye who, after inquiry, admitted to pounding metal on metal. The metallic fragment extended into the globe.

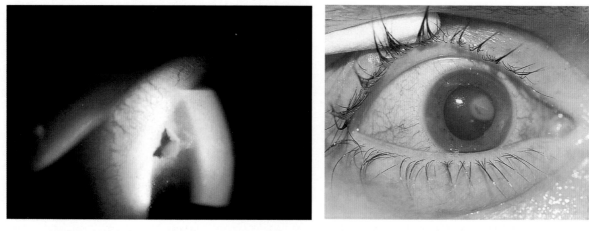

FIG. 8. A: Metallic transcorneal foreign body in a patient who was near a grenade blast in the invasion of Panama. **B:** Self-sealing corneal wound in a second patient from shrapnel in the Panama conflict.

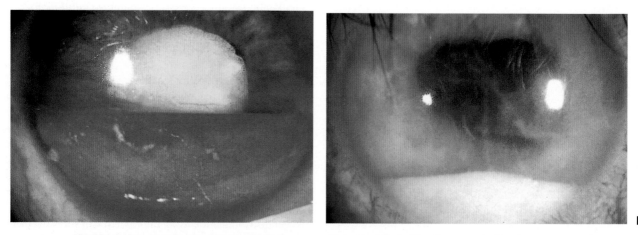

FIG. 9. A: Hyphema after trauma. **B:** Hypopyon with endophthalmitis after penetrating trauma.

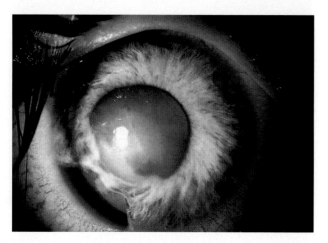

FIG. 10. Traumatic iris tear.

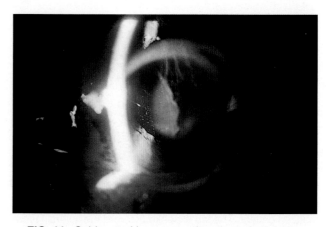

FIG. 11. Subluxated lens secondary to ocular trauma.

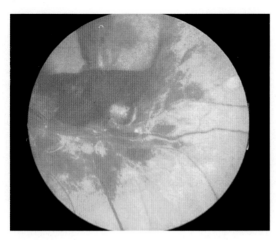

FIG. 12. Metallic intraocular foreign body with vitreous hemorrhage in the posterior pole.

4. *Anterior chamber:* Look for hyphema, hypopyon, inflammatory reaction, and foreign bodies (Fig. 9A,B).

5. *Iris:* Look for peaking (iris "points" toward rupture), tears (Fig. 10), small holes (if present, an intraocular foreign body should be assumed), and dialysis.

6. *Lens:* Look for traumatic subluxation or true luxation (Fig. 11). Determine whether the lens exited the globe at the time of the trauma. Determine whether there is evidence of a foreign body passage through the lens. Determine whether a Vossius ring (ring of pigment from the iris margin on the lens from trauma to the eye) is present.

7. *Vitreous:* Examine for clarity and to determine whether pigment (from iris anteriorly or from retinal tear), hemorrhage, or stranding (will point to scleral laceration) is present. (*Pitfall:* Failure to recognize vitreous stranding pointing to a posterior penetration site.)

8. *Macula/disc:* A noncontact method (60, 78, or 90 diopter lens or Hruby lens) may afford a view of the posterior pole to allow macular and disc examinations (Fig. 12). Examine early because hemorrhage, cataract, and inflammatory reaction may quickly obscure the view. Avoid pressure on the globe.

Supplementary Testing

For any supplementary tests, ensure that the eye is well protected and that ancillary personnel understand that the eye is open and pressure cannot be placed on or near the eye.

1. *Computed tomographic (CT) scanning* is probably the best single test for an intraocular foreign body if direct visualization is not possible. A good rule to follow is that if examination cannot definitely rule out a foreign body, a CT should be performed. The CT is less reliable when foreign bodies are extremely small or nonmetallic. Stranding of hemorrhage and vitreous, which may point to a posterior rupture or penetration, and foreign bodies in the orbit can occasionally be seen (Fig. 13).

2. *Ultrasound* is complementary to the CT scan. The ultrasound carefully performed can determine vitreous stranding, foreign body tracks through the vitreous, radiolucent foreign bodies, choroidal (Fig. 14) and retinal detachments, lens rupture, absence, dislocation, localization of small foreign bodies in fibrous tissue, and perforations of the globe.

3. *Orbital x-rays* are rarely used since the advent of the CT scan. Anteroposterior and lateral x-rays can be used in localizing a foreign body.

4. *Bone-free x-rays* can be useful in geographic locations not near a CT scanner or without ultrasound, but with dental

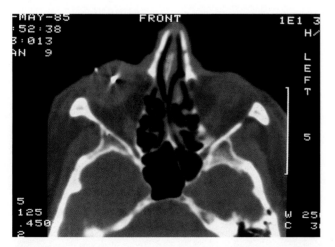

FIG. 13. Computed tomographic scan localization of an intraocular metallic foreign body with scatter from the foreign body. (Courtesy of Paul Sternberg, Jr., M.D., Emory University Eye Center, Atlanta, GA.)

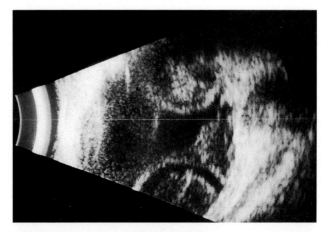

FIG. 14. Ultrasound of choroidal detachments in a posttraumatic patient. (Courtesy of Paul Sternberg, Jr., M.D., Emory University Eye Center, Atlanta, GA.)

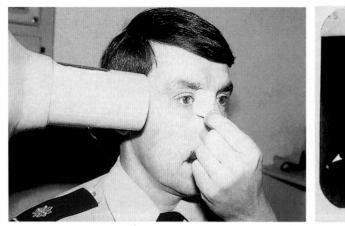
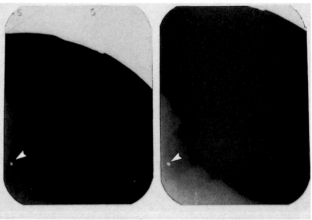

FIG. 15. A: Technique of using a dental x-ray to locate an anterior foreign body. **B:** Conjunctival metallic foreign body (*arrow*) on dental x-ray.

x-ray equipment available. This technique can be useful in the localization of anterior foreign bodies (Fig. 15).

TREATMENT

The general principles of treatment apply to all ruptured globes. When there is any doubt of penetration, explore the globe. Classic teaching is to avoid anesthetic depolarizing agents (succinylcholine) during induction to avoid the initial muscle contraction and possible resultant expulsion of intraocular contents. A review of a large number of patients, however, failed to corroborate this assumption, and a recent animal trial showed no expulsion on induction with succinylcholine. Perhaps the best course of action is to allow the anesthesiologist to make the decision based on the best induction agent for the patient. The goals of initial operation

should include finding and closing all lacerations and repositing any herniated tissues, if possible. If tissue is removed, it should be sent to the pathology department for histologic evaluation. Pathologic diagnosis may be helpful in considering and planning for future therapy. Incarcerated tissue should never be left in the wound. After these steps, surgeons should restore the intraocular pressure and visual axis, and provide prophylaxis against tetanus and infective endophthalmitis, if needed. The patients should be immediately referred to a vitreoretinal surgeon after initial repair if further therapy is necessary.

Exploration of a ruptured globe should proceed in a similar manner to the opening of a scleral buckle procedure. The surgeon must avoid any pressure on the globe: the conjunctiva should be opened with a 360° peritomy, even if the laceration is quite evident (Fig. 16). Damage remote from an obvious perforation may not be readily apparent or may be hidden under a muscle. The surgeon should use either a wire

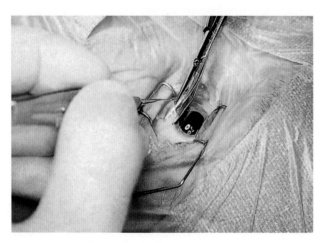

FIG. 16. Open conjunctiva similar to scleral buckle. Start 180° from obvious lacerations. Avoid pressure on the globe.

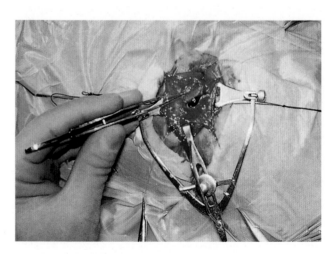

FIG. 17. Conjunctiva "filleted" away from the globe by 6-0 plain traction sutures on mosquito forceps.

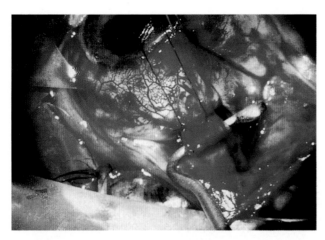

FIG. 18. Rectus muscle hooked with a Jameson muscle hook.

speculum (that allows more maneuverability) or a mechanical speculum, depending on swelling and circumstances. The surgeon should consider lid sutures for maximal exposure, especially in very swollen lids (4-0 silk through tarsus). "Fillet" the conjunctiva away from the globe with conjunctival traction sutures to maximize exposure (Fig. 17). Clean each quadrant with curved Stevens scissors, looking for damage other than the obvious. Gently hook each of the four major rectus muscles with a traction suture (I prefer 2-0 silk) (Fig. 18). Each muscle is picked up with large toothed forceps to avoid pressure on the globe, and a Jameson muscle hook is placed under the elevated muscle. This is important because of the high likelihood of hidden scleral ruptures under the rectus muscles.

At this point, the surgeon should explore all quadrants as far posteriorly as possible. The most common sites for rupture: the limbus, parallel to the equator between the limbus and the equator (usually superior); under the rectus muscles

(perpendicular to the limbus); and, rarely, in the posterior pole and the cornea.

The surgeon should repair all lacerations with nonabsorbable suture (nylon or mersilene). We use 8-0 for the sclera, 8-0 or 9-0 for the limbus, and 10-0 for the cornea. Many patients will require further surgery later, so it should be assumed that reoperation will be necessary. Nonabsorbable sutures ensure a strong lasting closure and one less likely to open during later intraocular surgery.

Lacerations crossing the limbus are closed first at the limbal junction to allow proper alignment. A stab incision is performed into the anterior chamber before beginning the closure to aid in globe reformation (access site) after all wounds are closed. The surgeon should close all lacerations with interrupted stitches. Interrupted sutures allow maximal closure with minimal problems, even if one stitch ruptures postoperatively (Fig. 19). During closure, the lips of the wound can be lifted by the assistant to allow tissue to be reposited without inclusion in the wound. For stellate or angular lacerations, the angle is closed first. A purse-string suture (Fig. 20) is used for large stellate closures to ensure closure of the center of the wound. The surgeon should avoid placing sutures through the points of the stellate portion, as these will tear, complicating the closure. The stellate wound's legs are closed last with interrupted stitches.

For lacerations that leak despite good closure with interrupted sutures, consider oversewing the wound with a baseball stitch (interrupteds left in place) (Fig. 21). If the laceration still leaks despite the use of the previously described techniques, consider the use of cyanoacrylate glue. The wound is dried thoroughly and the glue is applied directly over the sutured wound (Fig. 22). If the wound still leaks, consider sewing a scleral patch graft over the wound or gluing a scleral buckle over the leaking site (used especially when a buckle will be applied anyway) (Fig. 23). If the laceration extends to a muscle insertion, disinsert the muscle to

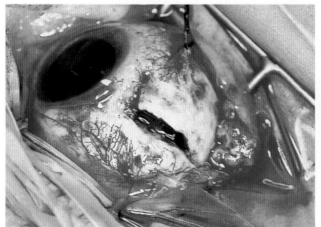
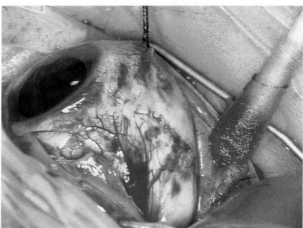

A   B

FIG. 19. A: L-shaped scleral laceration caused by blunt trauma at the time of a motor vehicle accident. **B:** Closure with interrupted 8-0 nylon sutures. The angle was closed first to ensure proper alignment.

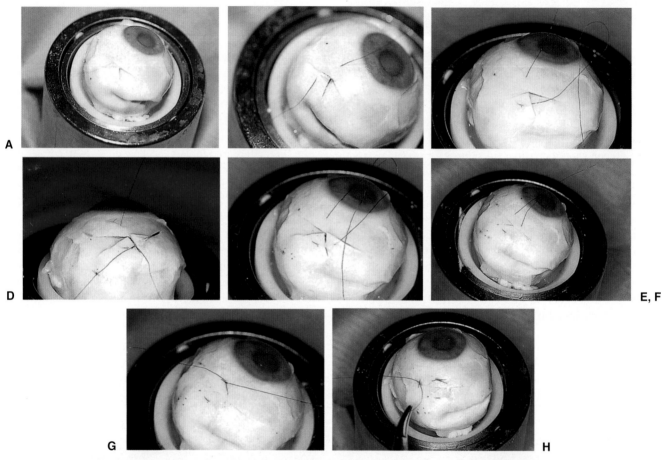

FIG. 20. Stellate lacerations. Stellate scleral laceration in a cadaver eye. **A:** Initial stitch from external to half-depth sclera and exiting a wound edge. **B:** Stitch enters the second edge, exits in midflap, reenters at midflap (to half-scleral depth), and exits at the wound edge. **C:** Repeated in the second flap. **D:** Third flap with demonstration of the needle at midflap. **E:** Stitch reenters at midflap and exits at the final wound stage. **F:** Stitch enters last the wound edge and is angled toward the initial entry site. **G:** Closure of the wound and the tight stellate wound. **H:** Legs of the wound are closed with interrupted sutures.

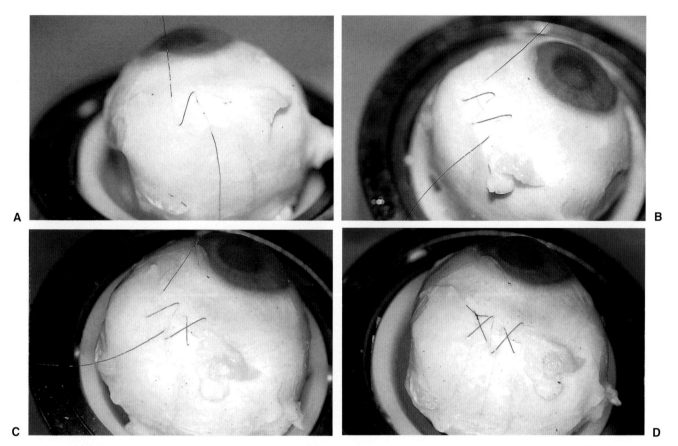

FIG. 21. Baseball stitch for leaking despite adequate interrupted suture closure. **A:** Linear laceration (for clarity, interrupted sutures are not shown) with suture entering externally to half-depth sclera across the wound edge and out with an external angular cross-stitch and a similar intrascleral stitch. **B:** Continuation with the last intrascleral stitch near the end of laceration. **C:** External cross-stitch with reentry (all intrascleral stitches are perpendicular to the wound margin). **D:** Final external cross-stitch tied to the initial suture.

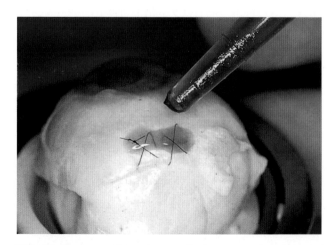

FIG. 22. Cyanoacrylate glue applied over a sutured wound after the area has been dried.

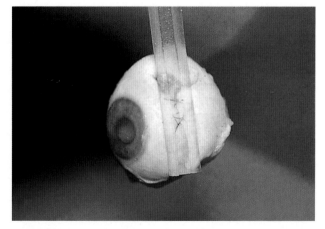

FIG. 23. Silicone scleral buckling material glued to the globe to close a leaking wound.

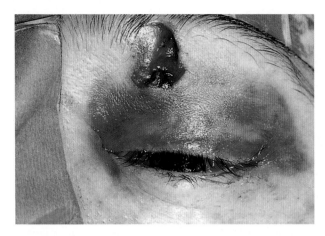

FIG. 24. Lid laceration in a 30-year-old ammunitions plant worker.

complete repair. Never assume that a laceration ends at a muscle insertion, as it will not. Reform the globe via the stab incision after all lacerations are repaired. If any tissue is removed, send it to pathology for evaluation. If a foreign body is removed, culture it. We do not routinely use intraocular antibiotics in trauma cases unless the eye has obvious intraocular vegetable matter or has a grossly dirty wound. If used, we prefer intraocular amikacin (400 μg in 0.1 ml) and vancomycin (1 mg in 0.1 ml).

The role of vitrectomy is still undergoing evaluation in patients with ruptured globes. Most vitreous surgeons would perform a vitrectomy, when necessary, as a secondary procedure. Primary vitrectomy would be considered (assuming the proper equipment and trained personnel are available) in cases with obvious endophthalmitis, if vitreous has prolapsed into an anterior segment wound, or when removal of a reactive foreign body is necessary.

Secondary vitrectomy is indicated in cases with retained reactive intraocular foreign bodies, retinal detachment and vitreous hemorrhage, admixed lens and vitreous, double-perforating injuries with vitreous hemorrhage, and vitreous incarcerated in an anterior wound (see also Chapter 15 by S. Charles and B. Wood, and Chapter 17 by G.W. Abrams and L.C. Glazer). The timing of vitrectomy remains controversial, with one group advocating vitrectomy in the first 72 hours and the second at 7–14 days after the injury. The group advocating early surgery feels that the risk of intraocular proliferation is minimized, that the eye is rehabilitated more quickly, and that the risk of a second anesthesia is eliminated. The group advocating later surgery feels that the risk of secondary hemorrhage is reduced, the cornea is allowed to clear, the vitrectomy is inherently easier because of detachment of the posterior vitreous, and the procedure is safer after resolution of choroidal and ciliary detachments. We usually defer secondary vitrectomy to the later period, but will do early vitrectomy in certain instances. We rec-

ommend referral to a vitreoretinal surgeon when possible after primary closure to allow the surgeon to make the timing decision.

Further details of vitreoretinal surgical techniques in trauma, including timing and the role of scleral buckling, are in Chapter 15 on vitreoretinal surgical techniques by Steve Charles and Byron Wood.

The use of prophylactic antibiotics in penetrating trauma is controversial, with advocates both for and against the use of intraocular antibiosis. The "for" group justifies the use of intraocular antibiotics based on the seriousness of endophthalmitis after penetrating trauma. These patients, when endophthalmitis occurs, have a higher incidence of loss due to "bad actors" such as *Bacillus*. The "con" group points out that infection occurs in a minority of cases and that many uninfected patients would be treated with the potential toxicity of intraocular injection. My approach is to use intraocular antibiosis only if there are indications of infection (hypopyon, aqueous or vitreous inflammatory cells, and so on). I do not use intravenous antibiotics unless there are extraocular indications for their use. The Endophthalmitis Vitrectomy Study (although performed in postcataract not posttraumatic endophthalmitis) showed that intravenous antibiotics were not efficacious in the treatment of postcataract endophthalmitis. I currently use intraocular vancomycin (1 mg) and amikacin (400 μg) and periocular vancomycin (25 mg) and ceftazidime (100 mg) in indicated cases.

Enucleation should not be considered as a primary procedure unless restoration and closure of the globe is completely impossible. Some eyes that are NLP immediately following trauma may regain vision, and modern vitreoretinal techniques can now save many eyes previously lost. Never enucleate with bilateral trauma unless there is no alternative—the eye regaining the best vision is usually impossible to determine based on the initial assessment.

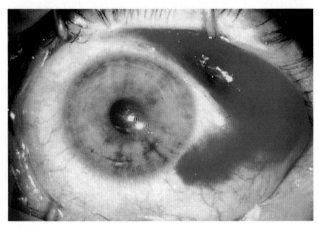

FIG. 25. External globe appearance (the same patient as Fig. 24.)

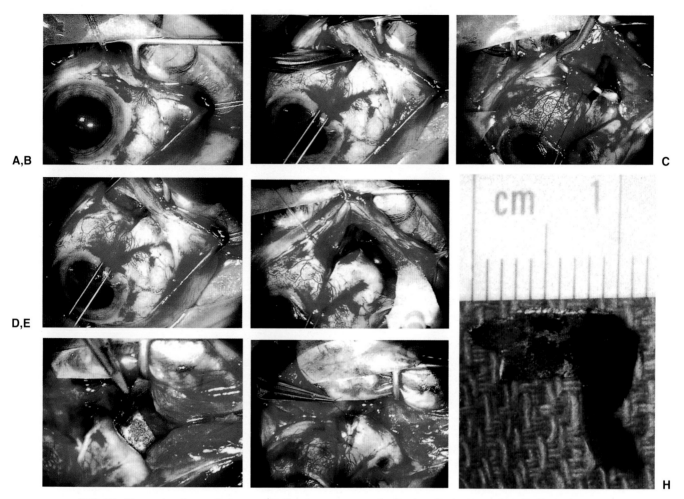

FIG. 26. Example of a posterior penetrating trauma case. **A:** Conjunctival preparation. **B:** Tenon's capsule dissection. **C:** Muscle disinsertion. **D,E:** Exploration of the laceration. **F:** Removal of foreign body. **G:** Closure of the opening. **H:** The removed foreign body. See the text for details.

SAMPLE CASE

A 30-year-old ammunition factory worker presented after an explosion occurred in his plant. His history indicated that a shell casing had exploded while it was being stamped, and he immediately felt pain in his left upper lid and the loss of vision in his left eye. He had previously been 20/20 in this eye, had no family history of eye disease, had no medical illnesses, and had not had a tetanus shot for approximately 8 years. He was not allergic to antibiotics. Examination at the scene by the plant physician revealed light perception vision. He was instructed to cover the eye carefully with a shield and send the patient to us. (He had no other injuries and was stable.) On arrival, a brief exam revealed an upper lid laceration (Fig. 24). Gentle lid opening revealed a collapsed globe with a superior subconjunctival hemorrhage (Fig. 25). The eye was immediately covered with a Fox shield, the patient was given tetanus toxoid, a CT of the head and orbits was performed (which showed a large metallic foreign body equivocally intraocular), and the patient was taken to the operat-

ing room. Anesthetic induction was uneventful, and the anesthesiologist did not use succinylcholine for induction.

After achievement of full anesthesia, the patient was prepped and draped and a lid speculum placed. A 360° conjunctival peritomy was performed. Conjunctival traction sutures were placed, and the conjunctiva was "filleted" away from the globe (Fig. 26A). A traction suture was placed at the limbus to provide global mobility, and blunt Wescott scissors were used to clean Tenon's capsule carefully from the laceration (Fig. 26B). Care was taken to avoid cutting any extruded intraocular tissue. The superior rectus muscle, through which the laceration extended, was hooked with a Jameson muscle hook, and 7-0 Vicryl suture placed through its tendon insertion and tied to each edge of the muscle (Fig. 26C), and the muscle was disinserted, exposing the posterior extent of the laceration (Fig. 26D). Further conjunctival traction sutures were used to fillet the conjunctiva away from the globe, and the hint of a large copper-colored foreign body was seen (Fig. 26E). Tenon's capsule was gently cleaned along the laceration and posterior globe, and the foreign body was further delineated. The copper shell casing was grasped with a needle holder, and the foreign body (anchor shaped, with extensions in three planes) was rotated away and out of the globe (Fig. 26F) and finally out of the orbit. The laceration was progressively closed from anterior to posterior with interrupted 8-0 nylon suture (Fig. 26G,H), and the conjunctiva was closed after exploration of all quadrants for further damage. The rectus muscle was reinserted, and the conjunctiva was closed with 6-0 plain suture. No antibi-otics other than the usual postoperative subconjunctival gen-tamicin were used in this case. Vitrectomy, endolaser, and gas tamponade 10 days later restored vision to 20/40.

ACKNOWLEDGMENTS

Many thanks to William R. Burks, M.D., Paul Sternberg, Jr., M.D., Donald K. Lowd, Jim Gilman, and Ray Swords for their efforts in the compilation of this chapter.

Practical Atlas of Retinal Disease and Therapy, Second Edition
edited by William R. Freeman,
Lippincott–Raven Publishers, Philadelphia © 1997.

· 17 ·

Proliferative Vitreoretinopathy

Gary W. Abrams and Louis C. Glazer

PATHOPHYSIOLOGY

Proliferative vitreoretinopathy (PVR) remains a leading cause of failure in retinal detachment surgery, occurring in approximately 7% of all retinal detachments. During the past 2 decades, major advances have been made in both the understanding of the pathogenesis of PVR and in the surgical treatment of the disease.

Massive preretinal retraction and massive periretinal proliferation were the terms used in the past to describe the fixed folds in the retina and formation of membranes on the surface of the retina in eyes that had long-standing retinal detachments or redetachments after retinal detachment surgery. Opacification and retraction of the vitreous body that occur with long-standing detachment have been called massive vitreous retraction. A committee of the Retina Society renamed this condition proliferative vitreoretinopathy.

Using an experimental model of retinal detachment in the owl monkey, Machemer and coworkers identified the cellular basis of PVR that they called massive periretinal proliferation. A single layer of cells resembling retinal pigment epithelial (RPE) cells was found on the retinal surface after long-standing detachment. These cells were also present in the vitreous body. The cells that proliferated along the retinal surface were identical to normal RPE cells based on light-microscopy and electron-microscopy techniques. These investigators found that some RPE cells liberated after a retinal detachment assumed characteristics of fibroblasts, whereas other RPE cells underwent metaplastic differentiation into a macrophage-like cell with phagocytic activity. Proof of this hypothesis came when pigment epithelial cells isolated from one eye were injected into the vitreous of the contralateral eye. The RPE cells underwent transformation into both fibrocytes, with the ability to produce collagen, and macrophages.

Proliferating retinal glial cells, probably derived from Müller cells, have also been identified along the retinal surface after a detachment. The glial cells could apparently grow through the internal or external limiting membrane, forming retroretinal membranes on the outer surface of the retina or epiretinal membranes on the inner surface of the retina. Autoradiography demonstrated the proliferative activity of these cells. The earliest glial cell proliferation occurred 3 weeks after retinal detachment.

Once RPE cells gain access to the vitreous, proliferative myofibroblast-like cells, which extend pseudopods, can pull and contract a strand of collagen in a "hand-over-hand" manner and cause retraction of the vitreous body. Only a small number of cells are required to create a great deal of vitreous contraction, a phenomenon termed *hypocellular gel contraction*. Thus, vitreous contraction and the formation of contractile membranes on the retinal surface are both caused by the proliferation of RPE and glial cells (Fig. 1).

More recent immunohistochemical studies have further defined the nature of preretinal membranes found in PVR. Jerdan and colleagues demonstrated that the extracellular matrix of PVR membranes contained type 1, type 2, and type 3 collagen. RPE cells expressed the class 2 histocompatibility antigen HLA-DR.

Baudouin and colleagues also found the expression of human leukocyte antigens HLA-DR and HLA-DQ on pigment epithelial cells, in vitro, and on epiretinal membranes and cellular components of vitreous and subretinal fluid in PVR. These investigators found linear deposits of immunoglobulin and complement in the pars plana. The expression of class 2 antigens and the presence of immunoglobulin in the pars plana suggest a role for the immune system in the pathogenesis of PVR.

PVR can occur in a number of clinical situations. The most common form of PVR follows previous retinal reattachment surgery. This type of PVR may follow either a scleral buckling procedure, pneumatic retinopexy, or vitrectomy. No previous retinal surgery is required, however, and PVR can occur in a long-standing retinal detachment. Cases

G. W. Abrams, M.D., and L. C. Glazer, M.D.: Kresge Eye Institute, Wayne State University, 4717 St. Antoine, Detroit, MI 48201.

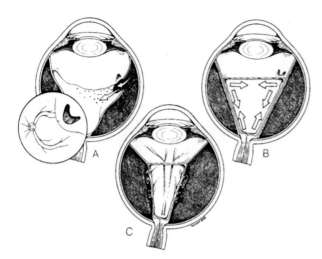

FIG. 1. A: Migration of pigment epithelial and other cells into the vitreous cavity and the subretinal space. **B:** Proliferation and contraction of cells on the retinal and vitreous interfaces. **C:** Fixed folds due to contraction of cellular membranes. (Courtesy of Churchill-Livingstone, from Abrams GW, Aaberg TM. Posterior segment vitrectomy. In: Waltman SR, ed. *Surgery of the eye.* New York: Churchill-Livingstone, 1988: 903–1012, with permission.)

of PVR, which follows vitrectomy, have features that are different from cases that have not had a vitrectomy, with a greater percentage of cases after vitrectomy exhibiting anterior forms of retinal contraction. Severe PVR can sometimes be found associated with penetrating ocular injuries and following proliferative vascular retinopathies, such as diabetic retinopathy. Pathophysiology of the retinal detachment and proliferation in the latter two conditions are different from the pathophysiology found associated with rhegmatogenous retinal detachment with PVR and are not considered in this chapter.

DIAGNOSIS AND CLASSIFICATION

The major clinical findings in eyes with PVR are fixed retinal folds. PVR is classified according to the severity and extent of retinal folding. The current classification of PVR (the updated Retina Society classification) subdivides PVR into three grades with progressive severity (Table 1). This classification is a modification of the earlier Retina Society classification of PVR and the classification used by the Silicone Study Group. Grade A PVR is the earliest phase and includes vitreous haze, vitreous pigment clumps, and pigment clusters on the inferior retina. Grade B PVR has wrinkling of the inner retinal surface, without full-thickness folds. The retina stiffens, with tortuosity of the vessels. Retinal breaks may have rolled and irregular edges, and there is decreased mobility of the vitreous on eye movement. Grade C PVR has full-thickness retinal folding and is

subdivided into anterior and posterior varieties. Although some eyes will have posterior PVR only, most eyes with anterior PVR will also have posterior PVR. Posterior PVR includes proliferation and contraction posterior to the equator, whereas anterior PVR encompasses proliferation and contraction anterior to the equator. Several types of contraction are present (Table 2). The most common form of contraction is the starfold, which is caused by contraction of an epicenter of proliferation on the retinal surface (Fig. 2). A focal contraction is a starfold less than four disc areas in size. Clinically, the retinal folds radiate away from the epicenters; thus, the starfold configuration. A diffuse contraction contains starfolds more than four disc areas in size, with confluent epicenters of proliferation (Fig. 2). The multiple confluent epicenters create irregular folds in the retina. In addition, subretinal proliferation can create membranes beneath the retina. These can present as an annular construction of the retina anterior to the optic disc ("napkin ring") (Fig. 3) or as a linear fold ("clothesline") (Fig. 4), or as a diffuse membrane with moth-eaten–appearing sheets (Fig. 5). In the updated Retina Society classification, the extent of contraction is graded according to the number of clock hours encompassed by the proliferation (1–12 clock hours). For example, a posterior area of diffuse proliferation involving 4 clock hours would be classified as grade C P 4 PVR, whereas if 8 clock hours were involved, the classification would be grade C P 8 PVR.

The two major forms of retinal contraction found in anterior PVR are anterior circumferential contraction and anterior retinal displacement (Table 1). In anterior PVR, retinal folds can be caused by epiretinal membranes, vitreous con-

TABLE 1. *Proliferative vitreoretinopathy described by grade*

Grade	Features
A	Vitreous haze Vitreous pigment clumps Pigment clusters on inferior retina
B	Wrinkling of inner retinal surface Retinal stiffness Vessel tortuosity Rolled and irregular edges of retinal break Decreased mobility of vitreous
CP1–12[a]	Posterior to equator Focal, diffuse, or circumferential full-thickness folds Subretinal strands
CA1–12	Anterior to equator Focal, diffuse, or circumferential full-thickness folds Anterior displacement Subretinal strands Condensed vitreous with strands

[a] Expressed in the number of clock hours involved.

TABLE 2. *Grade C proliferative vitreoretinopathy described by contraction type*

Type	Location	Features
Focal	Posterior	Starfold posterior to vitreous base
Diffuse	Posterior	Confluent starfolds posterior to vitreous base Optic disc may not be visible
Subretinal	Posterior/anterior	Proliferations under retina "Napkin ring" around disc "Clothesline" Moth-eaten–appearing sheets
Circumferential	Anterior	Contraction along posterior edge of vitreous base with central displacement of the retina Peripheral retina stretched Posterior retina in radial folds
Anterior displacement	Anterior	Vitreous base pulled anteriorly by proliferative tissue Peripheral retinal trough Ciliary processes may be stretched or may be covered by membrane Iris may be retracted

traction or, less commonly, by subretinal membranes. Focal or diffuse contraction just posterior to the vitreous base tends to cause circumferential contraction of the retina (Fig. 6). The circumferential contraction, in effect, shortens the circumference of the retina and produces a vector force that pulls the retina toward the central vitreous cavity (Fig. 7). Radial folds extend posteriorly from the plane of contraction, whereas the retina anterior to the plane of contraction appears smooth as it is stretched centrally. A similar picture can be seen due to contraction of the posterior hyaloid that can pull the posterior aspect of the vitreous base centrally. In addition, following vitrectomy, the residual frill of the pos-

terior hyaloid can contract circumferentially to create a similar picture. Anterior displacement of the retina is found most commonly in eyes that have undergone a previous pars plana vitrectomy. Membranes may form on the remaining posterior hyaloid, over the vitreous base area, and on the remaining anterior hyaloid (Fig. 8). These membranes can transmit vector forces of contraction in both anterior–posterior and circumferential directions. The anterior retina at the posterior aspect of the vitreous base is displaced anteriorly, variably toward the pars plana, ciliary processes, or the iris (Fig. 9). A trough of peripheral retina is created peripheral to the displaced retina in advanced cases. The ciliary processes may be stretched, possibly creating hypotony. In advanced cases, the iris is retracted. Anterior PVR is classified by the extent of involvement (Table 1). For example, if there is anterior displacement or anterior circumferential contraction involving 6 clock hours, the classification in either case would be grade C A 6 PVR.

The retina is characteristically contracted into a funnel-shaped configuration. The funnel configuration that was included in the original Retina Society classification was dropped from the updated Retina Society classification.

The Silicone Study evaluated the prognostic utility of the Silicone Study classification and the original Retina Society classification systems, which include most components of the revised Retina Society classification system. In general, the more extensively the PVR was classified, the worse was the visual outcome. Eyes with both anterior and posterior PVR had worse visual acuity and more hypotony than did eyes with posterior PVR only. For eyes with both anterior and posterior PVR, there was a decreasing trend in successful visual acuity outcome, with increasing severity of PVR as measured by extent of retina involved.

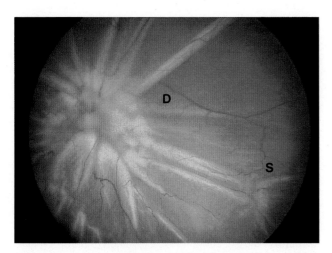

FIG. 2. Posterior proliferative vitreoretinopathy: S, starfold (posterior type 1); D, diffuse contraction (posterior type 2). Classification is C P 12. (Courtesy of Churchill-Livingstone, from Abrams GW, Aaberg TM. Posterior segment vitrectomy. In: Waltman SR, ed. *Surgery of the eye.* New York: Churchill-Livingstone, 1988:903–1012, with permission.)

Text continues on p 308.

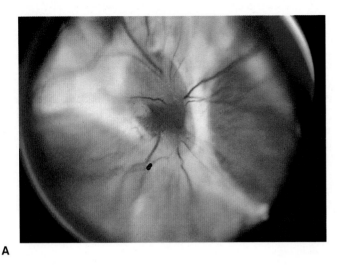

A

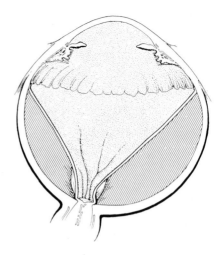

B

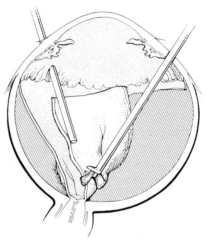

C

FIG. 3. A,B: Subretinal "napkin ring" membrane (posterior type 3). **C:** Membrane sectioned and removed through peripheral retinotomy. (A: courtesy of Hilel Lewis, M.D., Cleveland Clinic Foundation, Cleveland, OH; B and C: courtesy of CV Mosby, from Abrams GW. Retinotomies and retinectomies. In: Ryan SJ, ed. *Retina;* vol 3. St. Louis: CV Mosby, 1989:317–346, with permission.)

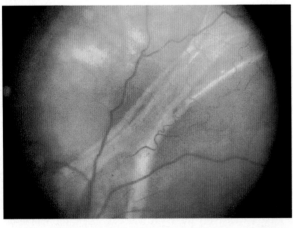

A

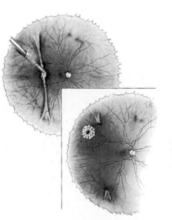

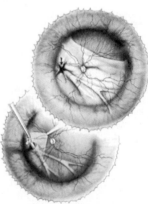

B, C

FIG. 4. A: Branching subretinal strand. **B:** Sectioning of subretinal strand through peripheral retinotomy. **C:** Extraction of subretinal strand through retinotomy. (A: courtesy of Hilel Lewis, M.D., Cleveland Clinic Foundation, Cleveland, OH; B and C: courtesy of CV Mosby, from Abrams GW. Retinotomies and retinectomies. In: Ryan SJ, ed. *Retina;* vol 3. St. Louis: CV Mosby, 1989:317–346, with permission.)

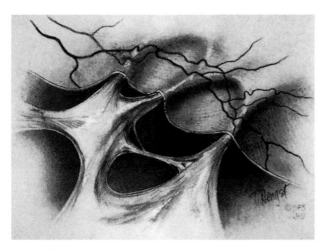

FIG. 5. Moth-eaten–appearing sheets of subretinal membranes. (Courtesy of Ophthalmic Communications Society, Inc., from Michels RG. Surgery of retinal detachment with proliferative vitreoretinopathy. *Retina* 1984;4:63–83, with permission.)

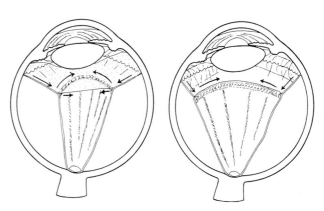

FIG. 7. Proliferative vitreoretinopathy grade C. Type 4, circumferential contraction with proliferation immediately behind insertion of the posterior hyaloid pulling the retina centrally, stretching the retina anterior to it, and creating radial folds posteriorly. Schematic drawing of situation in nonvitrectomized eye (*left*) and vitrectomized eye (*right*). *Arrows* show the direction of pull. (Courtesy of Ophthalmic Publishing Company, from Machemer R, Aaberg TM, Freeman HM, Irvine AR, Lean JS, Michels RM. An updated classification of retinal detachment with proliferative vitreoretinopathy. *Am J Ophthalmol* 1991;112:159–165, with permission.)

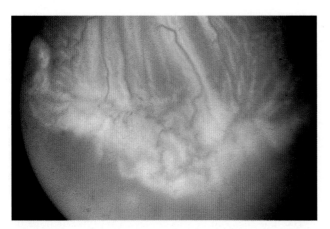

FIG. 6. Contraction along the posterior edge of the vitreous base with central displacement of retina. Peripheral retina stretched; posterior retina in radial folds (anterior type 4). (Courtesy of Ophthalmic Publishing Company, from Machemer R, Aaberg TM, Freeman HM, Irvine AR, Lean JS, Michels RM. An updated classification of retinal detachment with proliferative vitreoretinopathy. *Am J Ophthalmol* 1991; 112:159–165, with permission.)

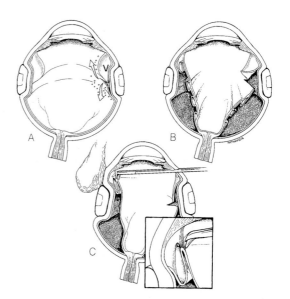

FIG. 8. Anterior retinal displacement in proliferative vitreoretinopathy. **A:** Proliferation of cells on the vitreous base and the retina following vitrectomy and scleral buckle. **B:** Contraction of cellular membranes pulls the retina at the posterior vitreous base anteriorly. **C:** Vitreous base depressed into view. Membrane exerting anterior–posterior traction is sectioned with vertically cutting scissors. (Courtesy of Churchill-Livingstone, from Abrams GW, Aaberg TM. Posterior segment vitrectomy. In: Waltman SR, ed. *Surgery of the eye.* New York: Churchill-Livingstone, 1988;903–1012, with permission.)

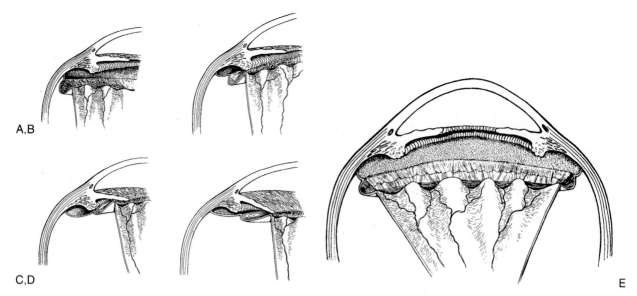

FIG. 9. Anterior proliferative vitreoretinopathy: anterior retinal displacement. Retina at the posterior aspect of the vitreous base drawn to the anterior vitreous base (**A**), to the ciliary processes (**B**), to the posterior iris (**C**), and to the pupil with iris retraction (**D**). **E:** Posterior insertion of the vitreous base drawn anteriorly, creating a retinal trough. Folds that radiate posteriorly are caused by circumferential contraction. (Courtesy of Ophthalmic Publishing Company, from Lewis H, Aaberg TM. Anterior proliferative vitreoretinopathy. *Am J Ophthalmol* 1988;105:277, with permission.)

SURGICAL TECHNIQUES

Vitrectomy is seldom indicated in grade A and grade B PVR. Those eyes and some eyes with limited grade C PVR may be managed with a scleral buckle (see also Chapter 13 by H. Lincoff and I. Kreissig). Nearly all eyes with PVR involving more than 6 clock hours and many eyes with lesser grades of PVR will require vitrectomy. Vitrectomy is indicated when it is not anticipated that a scleral buckle will adequately relieve traction to reattach the retina.

When a vitrectomy is done for an eye with PVR, if no scleral buckle is present, we recommend encircling the eye with a scleral buckle to support the vitreous base and the retina just posterior to the vitreous base. In most cases, we use a 4.5-mm-wide encircling band to create a moderately high buckle. If the eye already has an encircling scleral buckle, we usually do not revise or replace that element. Sometimes it is necessary to supplement an existing scleral buckle, especially inferiorly, if there is not adequate inferior support of the vitreous base. If the eye has previously had only a radial scleral buckle, the radial element is usually removed and an encircling scleral buckle placed. We often place the sutures for the scleral buckle prior to vitrectomy. At this time, the eye is firmer and it is easier to place the sutures. We usually wait until after the vitrectomy is completed to place the buckling element around the eye.

For vitrectomy, we use a three-port vitrectomy system. Sclerotomy sites are usually made 3 mm posterior to the limbus through the anterior pars plana, unless the retina is pulled anteriorly by anterior PVR, in which case we make the sclerotomy sites more anteriorly through the ciliary processes. We use the 4-mm infusion port, and the tip is visualized prior to starting infusion to make sure that the tip has penetrated the pars plana pigmented and nonpigmented epithelium in order to prevent subretinal or choroidal infusion.

If the pupil will not dilate adequately, we dilate the pupil by mechanical pupillary stretching (Fig. 10). Our preferred pupillary stretching devices are small plastic hooks placed through the limbus in four quadrants (Flexible Iris Retractors; Grieshaber, Kennesaw, GA, U.S.A.). We lyse synechiae and remove residual capsular material as much as possible prior to placing the stretching hooks in order to minimize iris trauma. Limbal openings are made parallel with and just anterior to the iris plane with a Ziegler-type blade. The small hooks are secured externally with a small locking device at the limbus.

The lens ring can be placed following placement of the pupillary stretching devices. We suture a lens ring in place and utilize several lenses as necessary to visualize the posterior and peripheral retina. We peel most posterior membranes by using a planoconcave lens, while prism lenses are used in the periphery. A wide-angle lens system with image inverter is also used in selected situations. The wide-angle lens is especially useful if there is a constricted view due to a posterior chamber lens with opacified peripheral capsule.

Removal of the lens is necessary in almost all phakic eyes, even if the lens is clear. One of the most important parts of the vitrectomy procedure for PVR is removal of anterior vit-

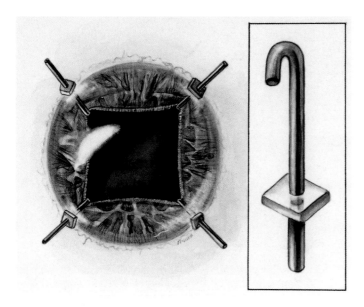

FIG. 10. Pupillary stretching using flexible iris retractors (Grieshaber, Inc., Kennesaw, GA.)

reous and membranes. In the phakic eye, an adequate vitreous base dissection is not possible. In addition, with prolonged gas tamponade, the lens will almost always develop a cataract. Management in the postoperative period, including the ability to do a fluid–gas exchange and to administer postoperative laser photocoagulation, is facilitated by removing the lens.

The lens is removed through the pars plana, except in cases with extremely hard nuclei, in which case the nucleus is removed through the limbus. Following fragmentation of the nucleus and removal of the cortical material, the vitrectomy instrument is used to make an opening in the anterior capsule. One can then grasp the peripheral capsule with vitreous forceps and exert enough traction to expose the zonules in the pupil. While retracting the capsule, the

zonules can then be cut with the membrane peeler–cutter (MPC, Grieshaber, Inc., Kennesaw, GA.) placed through the opposite sclerotomy site. We feel that complete removal of the lens capsule will reduce the likelihood of recurrent anterior PVR that can sometimes present with membranes adherent to the peripheral lens capsule. In addition, removal of the capsule will prevent synechiae of the iris to the lens capsule, which can leave a distorted, retracted, fixed pupil.

We do not always remove posterior chamber intraocular lenses (IOLs). An adequate vitreous base dissection in the presence of a posterior chamber lens may be possible in many cases. If significant membranes appear to adhere to the peripheral lens capsule, or if the posterior chamber IOL is unstable, we remove the IOL through the limbus. We remove unstable anterior chamber IOLs. An unstable anterior chamber lens may damage the cornea if it is pushed forward by the gas bubble postoperatively.

We remove the central vitreous with the vitreous cutting instrument and then remove gross peripheral vitreous. We delay extensive shaving of the vitreous base and peripheral membrane dissection until after posterior membranes have been removed. We begin epiretinal membrane dissection at the posterior pole. The preferred instruments for bimanual epiretinal membrane removal are an illuminated pick (Fig. 11) and vitreous forceps (Fig. 12). There are several types of forceps that can be used to grasp membranes. The membrane is elevated with the illuminated pick initially and then grasped with the forceps for stripping. Membranes can usu-

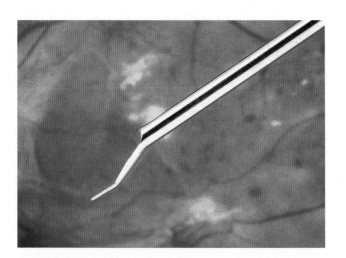

FIG. 11. Illuminated pick. Bending shaft of the pick 30° away from the light axis gives a broader field of illumination and reduces the shadow cast by the pick.

FIG. 12. De Juan pick–forceps. (Grieshaber, Inc., Kennesaw, GA.)

ally be easily seen, but sometimes with extensive confluent membranes, no edges can be identified. Signs of these type membranes include obscuration of portions of retinal vessels by the membrane and a stiff, smooth, grey appearance of the retina. Large retinal folds can be obscured by the membranes. In this situation, the pick is placed in a fold and gently pulled toward the center of the fold in order to engage the membrane (Fig. 13). Once the membrane is engaged and the edge elevated, it is grasped with the forceps for stripping (Fig. 14). We utilize a bimanual technique to strip the membrane. As the membrane is pulled by the forceps, the blunt portion of the pick is placed against the retina to fixate the retina during the stripping process (Fig. 15). During removal of peripheral membranes, the membrane is often pulled centrally with the forceps, and the blunt edge of the pick is placed between the membrane and the peripheral retina. As the membrane is pulled centrally, the blunt edge of the pick separates the membrane from the retina (Fig. 16). All membranes that can be located are meticulously stripped from the retinal surface. Some tightly adherent membranes can be more easily engaged with a sharp-barbed blade such as the microvitreoretinal blade. Immature membranes will fragment, and it is important to separate all of the fragments from the retina. Sometimes, immature membranes cannot be adequately grasped for removal. A helpful technique for elevating very immature membranes is to stroke them with a silicone "brush" found on the tip of the backflush brush. Zivojnovic has found the "membrane scratcher" useful for this technique.

The posterior hyaloid is often adherent to peripheral membranes posterior to the vitreous base. This probably occurs because of incorporation of the posterior hyaloid into membranes formed at the junction of the separated posterior vit-

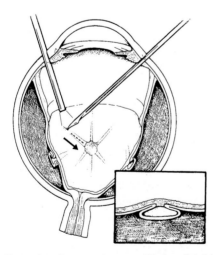

FIG. 13. Engaging the membrane with the pick by stripping toward the center of the starfold in the radiating fold. Note the redundant retina obscured within the fold beneath the membrane. (Courtesy of Churchill-Livingstone, from Abrams GW, Aaberg TM. Posterior segment vitrectomy. In: Waltman SR, ed. *Surgery of the eye.* New York: Churchill-Livingstone, 1988:903–1012, with permission.)

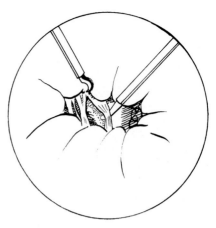

FIG. 14. Bimanual membrane removal. Membrane engaged by the pick is grasped with the forceps. (Courtesy of Churchill-Livingstone, from Abrams GW. Posterior segment vitrectomy. In: Packer AJ, ed. *Manual of retinal surgery.* New York: Churchill-Livingstone, 1989, with permission.)

reous and the vitreous base. With increasing and more posterior membrane formation, we suspect that the vitreous is gradually pulled in by the contracting membranes to give a relatively posterior adherence of the posterior hyaloid, well posterior to the vitreous base. It is important to strip the posterior hyaloid anteriorly to its insertion into the vitreous base. We have found it useful to grasp the edge of the posterior hyaloid with the vitreous forceps, place the blunt portion of the illuminated pick at the junction between the hyaloid and the peripheral retina, and pull the hyaloid centrally to allow the pick to separate the hyaloid from the retina (similar to the method described in Fig. 16). This technique also identifies the point of permanent adherence of the hyaloid to the posterior border of the vitreous base. Once the peripheral hyaloid is separated to the vitreous base, it is excised with the vitrectomy instrument.

Once the posterior and peripheral membranes have been removed, the retina becomes quite mobile. The pars plana is often detached, and any remaining vitreous is easily incarcerated in the sclerotomy sites. There is risk of peripheral retina incarceration in the sclerotomy sites. The retina can be stabilized and further peripheral vitreous removal and membrane dissection can be facilitated by the use of a perfluorocarbon liquid (PFCL) (Fig. 17). An initially small volume of PFCL (usually approximately 1 ml) is injected over the optic nerve. We usually wait until posterior membranes have been completely removed before injecting the PFCL. While a small posterior retinal break is not a contraindication to the use of PFCL, we usually do not use PFCL in the presence of large breaks. Excessive traction on the retina in the presence of even a small retinal break may also cause PFCL to go through the break. It is important not to inject the PFCL directly over a break, because the stream of PFCL will go beneath the retina. Initially, only enough PFCL is injected to stabilize the posterior retina and improve the ability to re-

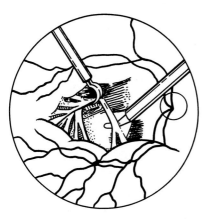

FIG. 15. Bimanual membrane removal. Retina is held back with blunt edge of pick as membrane is peeled with the forceps. (Courtesy of Churchill-Livingstone, from Abrams GW. Posterior segment vitrectomy. In: Packer AJ, ed. Manual of retinal surgery. New York: Churchill-Livingstone, 1989, with permission.)

move peripheral vitreous and membranes. Injection of too much PFCL may cover and compress the remaining vitreous. Additional PFCL can be injected to flatten the retina further as the dissection is carried anteriorly.

The vitreous base should be shaved to the surface of the peripheral retina and pars plana. The PFCL will stabilize the retina and prevent overly mobile peripheral retina from being pulled into the vitreous cutter during the shaving of the vitreous base. The vitreous base can be visualized with standard lens systems (either hand held or with a sutured lens ring) by using scleral depression, or by using a wide-angle system without scleral depression. Using a standard lens system, we perform anterior vitrectomy by two methods. In the first method, the vitreous cutter and the fiberoptic endoillu-

mination probe are both placed in the eye. An assistant depresses the peripheral retina and vitreous base into view as the vitreous is excised. This method is especially useful for removing vitreous in the inferior 140° and the superior 100°. Using this method, it is difficult to excise all of the peripheral vitreous in the horizontal meridians. The second method, especially useful in the horizontal meridians, utilizes external illumination. The vitrectomy cutter is placed through a sclerotomy site. A plug is placed in the opposite sclerotomy site, and the surgeon depresses the retina and vitreous base in the area 180° from where the vitreous cutter has entered the eye. An assistant holds the fiberoptic light probe in contact with the contact lens, directing the light toward the area to be cut (Fig. 18). Because the light probe actually touches the contact lens, there is no light reflection, and the visualization is similar to that seen with endoillumination. We have found this method superior to that in which the microscope light is used for peripheral visualization.

Scleral depression is not always required to visualize and shave the vitreous base when using the 125°-wide angle lens with an image inversion system. A "bullet" light probe is used to disperse the light over a broad area when using the wide-angle lens system. The vitreous structure is more easily seen when using a standard light probe held close to the vitreous, so we have found the standard lens system with scleral depression most useful for PVR.

If anterior PVR is present, peripheral membranes must be dissected. Membranes may be focal, diffuse, or subretinal. Focal and diffuse membranes are peeled in a fashion similar to posterior membrane peeling, although vitreous is often adherent to the membranes. Subretinal membranes may not be apparent until after epiretinal membranes have been removed. The most difficult form of anterior PVR to manage is anterior retinal displacement, in which the retina at the posterior vitreous base or even more posteriorly is pulled an-

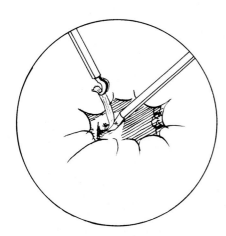

FIG. 16. Bimanual membrane removal. Blunt portion of membrane pick held at junction of membrane and retina as membrane is pulled centrally. (Courtesy of Churchill-Livingstone, from Abrams GW. Posterior segment vitrectomy. In: Packer AJ, ed. *Manual of retinal surgery.* New York: Churchill-Livingstone, 1989, with permission.)

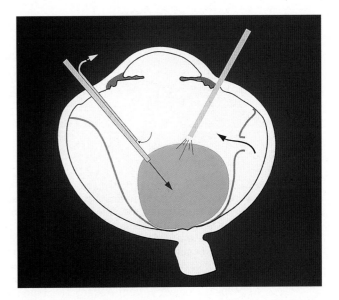

FIG. 17. Stabilization of the posterior retina with a perfluorocarbon bubble facilitates anterior membrane removal.

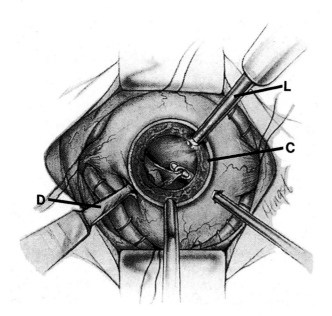

FIG. 18. Lightpipe (L) held in contact with the contact lens (C) illuminates the vitreous base pushed into view by the scleral depressor (D). (Courtesy of the American Medical Association, Chicago, IL, from Murray TG, Boldt HC, Lewis H, Abrams GW, Mieler WF, Han DP. A technique for facilitated visualization of the vitreous base, pars plana, and pars plicata. *Arch Ophthalmol* 1991;109:1458–1459, with permission.)

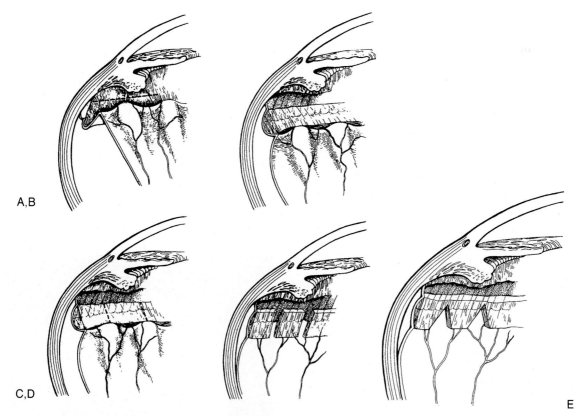

FIG. 19. A: An incision (*dotted line*) is made by a sharp blade or scissors in the anterior and posterior hyaloid vitreous surface remnant adhesions to the ciliary body processes or posterior iris. **B:** The meridional distance between the anterior and posterior vitreous base insertions is markedly reduced by the anteroposterior contraction within the vitreous base. **C:** The circumferentially contracted vitreous base is relaxed by multiple transecting incisions through the posterior and anterior insertions (*dotted lines*). **D:** When the circumferential vitreous base traction has been adequately relieved, the meridional retinal pleatlike folds disappear. **E:** Circumferential vitreous base traction is eradicated by multiple incisions of the posterior insertion without full-width radial transection of the vitreous base. (Courtesy of Ophthalmic Publishing Company, from Aaberg TM. Management of anterior and posterior proliferative vitreoretinopathy [45th Edward Jackson Memorial Lecture]. *Am J Ophthalmol* 1988;106:519–532, with permission.)

teriorly by contracting anterior vitreous and membranes. A circumferential "trough" of variable depth and area may be present at the vitreous base formed between the anteriorly displaced retina and the anterior retina and pars plana. Initially, the type of anterior PVR must be identified. Sometimes, in advanced forms of anterior PVR, a peripheral trough is difficult to see, and the surgeon might erroneously think no anterior retinal displacement is present. The only sign of anterior retinal displacement may be obscuration of the ora serrata and the finding of a fibrous circumferential membrane adherent to the pars plana or ciliary processes. Usually, however, a peripheral trough can be seen peripheral to a circumferential fold of anteriorly displaced retina (Figs. 8 and 9). The membrane that bridges from the anteriorly displaced retina toward the anterior structures must be cut (Fig. 8). It is often easiest to open this membrane initially with the sharp tip of the microvitreoretinal blade (Fig. 19). Then, vertically cutting vitreoretinal scissors can be inserted to section the membrane circumferentially. The membrane should be circumferentially sectioned throughout the extent of anterior displacement of the retina. When the membrane is sectioned, the anterior–posterior element of traction is relieved, and the anteriorly displaced retina will fall posteriorly. Remnants of the membrane can exert circumferential traction and sometimes can be excised with the vitrectomy instrument. If membrane remnants are tightly adherent, then a bimanual technique is used in which the membrane is fixated with an illuminated pick or illuminated forceps as it is cut with the vertically cutting scissors. If possible, the whole extent of the membrane should be eliminated, but if this is not possible, remnants should be sectioned vertically in multiple areas along its circumference in order to eliminate circumferential traction (Fig. 19). Vitreous in the trough should be trimmed back to the surface of the pars plana and peripheral retina with the vitreous cutter. Retinal breaks are sometimes created during the dissection process. Breaks should be identified, and all traction relieved around the area of these breaks. In some cases, anterior contraction cannot be relieved adequately with dissection, so a peripheral retinectomy is necessary. Because removing posterior and peripheral membranes is difficult after an extensive retinectomy, we wait until all of the posterior and peripheral membranes have been removed before proceeding with retinectomy.

After all of the membranes have been removed and the retina is mobile, the retina is reattached with injection of further PFCL or, if PFCL was not used, a fluid–air exchange (Fig. 20). In the PFCL technique, we inject enough PFCL to reattach the anterior and posterior retina. This usually means bringing the PFCL to the level of the vitreous base. Try to avoid immersing the tip of the infusion port in the PFCL because multiple bubbles of PFCL are created by the fluid flow. We usually perform laser photocoagulation with PFCL in the eye. We treat retinal breaks with confluent treatment around the breaks (Fig. 21), then do 360° scatter photocoagulation in two or three rows on the scleral buckle (Fig. 22). At least 1 burn width should be left between laser burns dur-

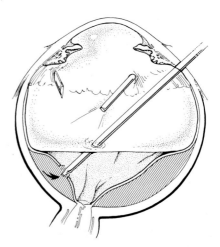

FIG. 20. Fluid–air exchange. Subretinal fluid is aspirated through the posterior retinal break as the eye is simultaneously filled with air pumped by the air pump. (Courtesy of CV Mosby, from Abrams GW. Retinotomies and retinectomies. In: Ryan SJ, ed. *Retina;* vol 3. St. Louis: CV Mosby, 1989: 317–346, with permission.)

ing scatter photocoagulation (Fig. 23). Treatment intensity should be moderate. We usually start at low power, with burns of $^1/_2$-second duration. Power is increased until a moderately white burn is obtained. Confluence of the peripheral scatter treatment should be avoided because excessive treatment may cause stasis of venous return from the ciliary body to the vortex system (Fig. 24). We treat any posterior retinal breaks with laser, but do not perform scatter treatment posterior to the scleral buckle.

PFCL is removed with a soft-tipped needle during fluid–air exchange. We initially remove any subretinal fluid that may remain anterior to the PFCL meniscus. We do this

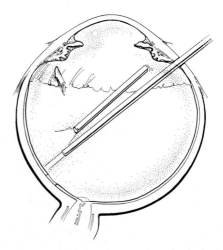

FIG. 21. Laser endophotocoagulation. Treated retinal breaks with one or two rows of confluent laser. (Courtesy of CV Mosby, from Abrams GW. Retinotomies and retinectomies. In: Ryan SJ, ed. *Retina;* vol 3. St. Louis: CV Mosby, 1989: 317–346, with permission.)

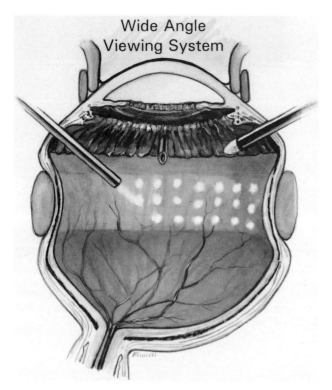

FIG. 22. Laser endophotocoagulation using a wide-angle system. The wide-angle view enables visualization of the peripheral retina during endophotocoagulation. Treatment is applied using a scatter technique on the retina supported by the scleral buckle. The bullet light probe is used with the wide-angle viewing system to give wide-field illumination.

by aspirating with a soft-tipped needle through anterior retinal breaks during the initial portion of the fluid–air exchange. The anterior breaks are best visualized by using the wide-angle system or via indirect ophthalmoscopy. Once any anterior subretinal fluid is removed, the remainder of the PFCL is aspirated posteriorly during the fluid–air exchange. Perfluoro-*n*-octane is easily seen and removed, and any remaining small bubbles will evaporate in air at body temper-

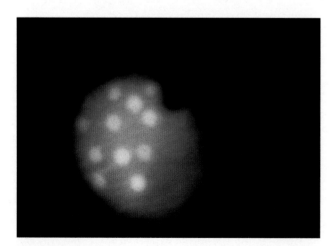

FIG. 23. Leave 1 burn width between laser applications during scatter treatment.

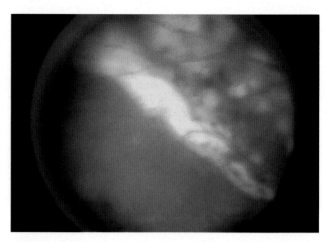

FIG. 24. Excessive laser treatment to peripheral retina on scleral buckle.

ature. However, perfluorodecalin and perfluorophenanthrene, two other commonly used PFCLs, are less easily seen and will not evaporate in air, so we recommend flushing the eye with approximately 0.5 ml saline injected over the posterior retina to identify any remaining PFCL to facilitate identification and removal.

If PFCL is not used, we reattach the retina with a fluid–air exchange. Air is supplied by the air pump, and fluid is usually removed with a soft silicone-tipped needle. We usually use active suction from the vitrectomy console, although an extrusion device, such as a Charles needle or backflush brush, can be utilized. A posterior or peripheral retinal break is usually available for removal of subretinal fluid. If a posterior break is present, it is used for subretinal fluid drainage (Figs. 20 and 25). If no posterior break is present, we do not usually make a posterior drainage retinotomy. Drainage through a peripheral break is facilitated by the use of the extendable cannulated extrusion needle in which the soft silicone tube can be extended through the peripheral break into the subretinal space posteriorly (Fig. 26). In most cases, a simple nonextendable, soft-tipped cannula will suffice for the same purpose. If there is no accessible break for drainage, we usually make a drainage retinotomy with the endodiathermy probe in the peripheral retina in an area to be supported by the scleral buckle.

All retinal breaks should be marked with endodiathermy prior to fluid–air exchange so they can be seen and treated through the air bubble (Fig. 25). We do laser treatment in a manner similar to that just described in the PFCL technique (Figs. 21–23).

Following laser treatment, two sclerotomy sites are closed, usually with no. 7-0 polyglycolic acid sutures. At least 25 ml of a nonexpansile mixture of perfluoropropane (C_3F_8) gas (12%–15%) is flushed through the eye. We have shown experimentally that a predictable gas concentration can be obtained by using this method. The gas mixture is insufflated through the infusion port and allowed to egress through a 27-gauge, $^1/_2$-inch-long needle inserted through the pars plana and vented to atmosphere. A tuberculin sy-

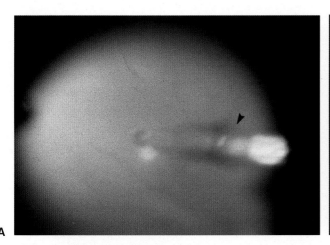

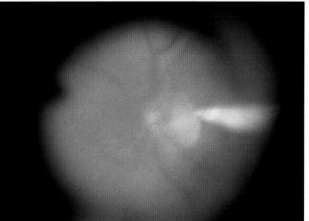

A

B

FIG. 25. A: Fluid–air exchange. Tip of the suction needle held just anterior to the break. Note the fluid meniscus (*arrow*) on the shaft of the drainage needle. **B:** Removing the final bit of fluid over the optic nerve. The needle tip is repeatedly "dipped" into the fluid at the retinal break and over the optic disc. A light reflex is seen as the needle tip contacts the fluid meniscus. (Courtesy of Churchill-Livingstone, from Abrams GW, Aaberg TM. Posterior segment vitrectomy. In: Waltman SR, ed. *Surgery of the eye.* New York: Churchill-Livingstone, 1988:903–1012, with permission.)

ringe with the plunger removed can be used as a handle for the needle. Following the gas flush, the needle is removed, then the infusion port is removed, and that site closed. We then reform the eye to a normal pressure with the gas mixture via a 30-gauge needle through the limbus or the pars plana.

Retinotomy and Retinectomy

In the management of PVR, retinotomies and retinectomies are indicated when anterior contraction cannot be adequately relieved by membrane dissection. This most commonly occurs with severe anterior displacement of the retina in eyes that have had previous vitrectomy. After all other membranes have been removed, diathermy is applied posterior to the area of contraction (Fig. 27). It is important to diathermize all vessels to prevent hemorrhage. The actual retinotomy is usually made with vertically cutting vitreous scissors. The retinotomy should be extended beyond the area of contraction into uninvolved retina on each end of the area of contraction. The retinotomy is made circumferentially and after cutting behind the area of contraction; the retinotomy is angled anteriorly to the ora serrata or, if the pars plana is detached, to the posterior edge of the ciliary processes. The contracted retina and other detached, devitalized retina anterior to the retinotomy should be excised with the vitrectomy instrument (Fig. 28). The anterior excision is performed to prevent anterior contraction of this devitalized retina that can contract circumferentially and exert traction on the ciliary body. Radial retinotomies are rarely indicated. Radial retinotomies tend to extend posteriorly into the posterior pole and often inadequately relieve traction. Retinotomies in the posterior pole, which involve more functionally important retina, should also be avoided.

A retinotomy greater than 90° in circumference creates the problem of management of a giant retinal tear. The best method for reattaching the retina in the presence of a giant tear is the use of a PFCL. PFCLs have the advantage of ease of use and do not require manipulation of the flap under gas

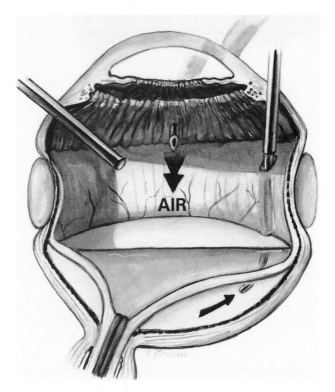

FIG. 26. Fluid–air exchange by using a peripheral retinal break. Drainage retinotomy created anteriorly over the scleral buckle. Extendable soft silicone tubing of the cannulated extrusion needle passed through retinotomy into the posterior subretinal space for fluid–air exchange.

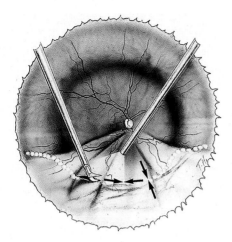

FIG. 27. Inferior relaxing retinotomy to relieve traction in the contracted retina. Diathermize the retina to be cut, primarily diathermizing the blood vessels. Extend into the normal retina on each end of the contracted retina. Make the cut with vertically cutting scissors along the posterior edge of the contracted retina. (Courtesy of CV Mosby, from Abrams GW. Retinotomies and retinectomies. In: Ryan SJ, ed. *Retina;* vol 3. St. Louis: CV Mosby, 1989:317–346, with permission.)

or silicone oil. Care must be taken prior to injection of the PFCL that all traction be relieved from the retina. In the presence of persistent traction, which prevents retinal flattening, the PFCL will run through elevated breaks and go beneath the retina. The heavier-than-water PFCL is slowly injected over the posterior pole. The enlarging bubble of PFCL reattaches the retina from posteriorly to anteriorly, forcing the subretinal fluid anteriorly (Fig. 29A). During injection, fluid is allowed to escape from the sclerotomy site. The eye is filled with PFCL to the posterior edge of the giant tear. Fol-

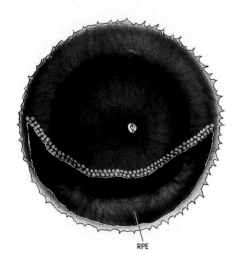

FIG. 28. Retina reattached following the relaxing retinotomy in Fig. 24. Retinotomy extended anteriorly to the ora serrata or the ciliary body (if pars plana is involved). Anterior retina excised. (Courtesy of CV Mosby, from Abrams GW. Retinotomies and retinectomies. In: Ryan SJ, ed. *Retina;* vol 3. St. Louis: CV Mosby, 1989:317–346, with permission.)

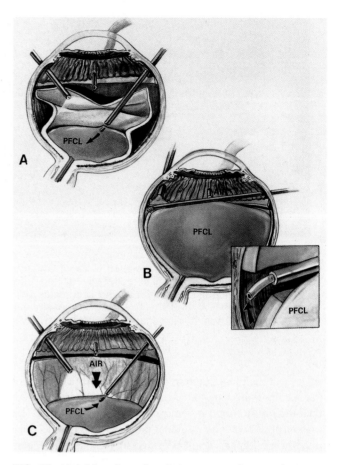

FIG. 29. Unfolding flap of a giant tear or a large retinotomy with perfluorocarbon liquid (PFCL). **A:** PFCL is injected over the posterior pole to unfold the flap of the giant tear. With the retina stabilized with PFCL, removal of the anterior vitreous and the anterior dissection are made easier. PFCL can be injected to the level of the anterior edge of the giant tear after all membranes are removed. **B:** PFCL–air exchange. The space anterior to the PFCL is filled with air. The edge of the tear is "dried" to prevent slippage. Fluid behind the edge is aspirated with the soft-tip needle until the edge is completely flat. **C:** PFCL–air exchange is completed. All PFCL is removed with the soft-tip needle.

lowing laser treatment, the PFCL is exchanged with air (followed by gas) or silicone oil. In the presence of a giant retinotomy (usually 180° or more), there is a risk of retinal slippage during the exchange for air. This can be prevented by adequate "drying" of the edge of the retinotomy during the air exchange. This is accomplished by filling the vitreous cavity with air anterior to the flap of the giant retinotomy and then aspirating fluid from beneath the anterior edge of the retinotomy before removing the PFCL (Fig. 29B). The anterior edge of the retina can be visualized during fluid–air exchange with a wide-angle viewing system or, alternatively, with an indirect ophthalmoscope. If fluid is left behind the edge of the retinotomy, as PFCL–air exchange proceeds, fluid forced posteriorly during the exchange will allow posterior slippage of the edge of the tear. If PFCL goes beneath the retina, it must be removed. This may require refilling the eye with fluid. Once fluid is removed from behind the anterior edge of the retina, PFCL–air exchange is completed and all PFCL is removed from the eye (Fig. 29C).

Silicone Oil in Proliferative Vitreoretinopathy

The Silicone Study found that visual and anatomic results in eyes with PVR were similar in most analyses regardless of whether silicone oil or C_3F_8 gas was used as the intraocular tamponade, and both modalities were superior to sulfur hexafluoride (SF_6) gas. While the surgeon and patient will jointly decide on the tamponade to use in most cases, some factors will contribute to the decision. Gas may be preferred over silicone oil if it is likely that silicone oil will herniate into the anterior chamber and contact the cornea, such as when the iris diaphragm is not intact or when an IOL is present without an intact iris–capsular–IOL diaphragm. Oil may be preferred for patients, such as children or mentally or physically impaired patients, who are unable to maintain prone positioning. Silicone oil may be preferred in the face of a giant tear or retinotomy, which might more likely have hypotony postoperatively. Silicone oil is preferred if the pa-

tient must travel by air or if the patient must travel to a higher elevation. Gas is preferred over silicone oil in the presence of residual vitreous, choroidal, or large subretinal hemorrhage.

When silicone oil is to be used, an inferior iridectomy should be created in the aphakic eye (Fig. 30). If the retina has been reattached with air, then silicone oil can be infused into the air-filled eye at the end of the case. Alternatively, a fluid–silicone exchange or PFCL–silicone oil exchange can be performed. When infusing silicone oil into the air-filled eye, the 5,000-centistoke oil that is most commonly used has high viscosity and requires high-pressure tubing if injected through the infusion port. We usually inject silicone oil into the air-filled eye in the following manner. With the infusion port in place and the air pump engaged to the infusion port tubing, we close one sclerotomy site and preplace a suture in the other site. We inject the silicone oil through an 18- or 20-gauge catheter (Angiocath, Becton Dickinson Infusion Therapy Systems, Sandy, Utah) that has been trimmed to approximately 15 mm in length. As the silicone oil is injected, the pressure is adjusted and maintained at the preset pressure by the air pump. The silicone oil is injected to the plane of the iris, which may require tilting the infusion port anteriorly in the latter portion of the silicone oil infusion. The anterior chamber is left at normal depth. If the anterior chamber shal-

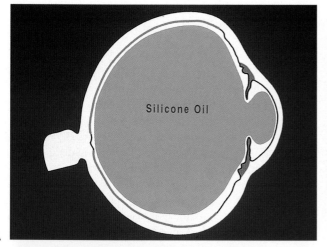

A

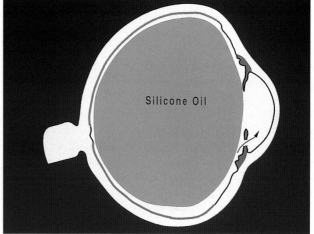

B

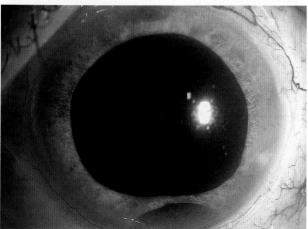

C

FIG. 30. Inferior iridectomy. **A:** Without inferior iridectomy, silicone oil herniates into the anterior chamber due to pupillary block mechanism. **B:** Inferior iridectomy allows access of aqueous into the anterior chamber, relieving pupillary block so aqueous no longer forces silicone oil into the anterior chamber. **C:** Inferior iridectomy.

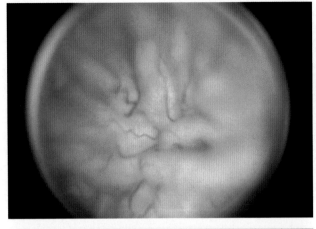

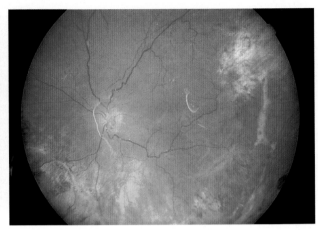

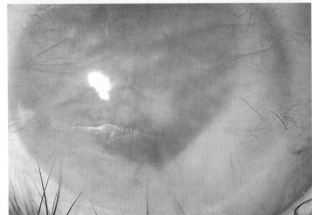

FIG. 31. Atrophia bulbi following silicone oil removal in an eye with reduced intraocular pressure. **A:** Preoperative photograph shows severe proliferative vitreoretinopathy. **B:** Four months postoperatively with silicone oil in eye. Large inferior retinotomy. Visual acuity is 20/400, and intraocular pressure is 5 mm Hg. **C:** Atrophy, hypotony, and visual acuity of only hand motions 4 months after removal of silicone oil and poor follow-up.

lows, a small amount of oil is removed and the anterior chamber is reformed with air injected through the limbus. It is important that the intraocular pressure (IOP) be left at the low end of normal level so as not to inadvertently overfill or underfill the eye with silicone oil.

If a posterior chamber IOL is present with an intact iris–capsular–IOL diaphragm, we do not make an inferior iridectomy. If the diaphragm is not intact and/or silicone oil herniates around the IOL into the anterior chamber, an inferior iridectomy will sometimes keep the silicone oil out of the anterior chamber; sometimes, however, the oil will go into the anterior chamber in spite of the iridectomy. Residual capsular material can obstruct an iridectomy, so patency should be confirmed at surgery. If the iridectomy is open and oil has gone into the anterior chamber, the oil can be pushed posteriorly with viscoelastic material injected into the anterior chamber. If the eye is making adequate aqueous, it may be necessary to remove the IOL and capsule and reopen the iridectomy in order to keep the silicone oil out of the anterior chamber. A stable anterior chamber lens can be left in place if an adequate inferior iridectomy is made. Unstable anterior chamber lenses should be removed.

If the IO is within a normal range and the retina is stable, the silicone oil can be removed 2 months or more following surgery. Recurrent epiretinal membranes can often be removed at the time of silicone oil removal. The Silicone

Study found that approximately 20% of retinas detach following silicone oil removal.

In the presence of hypotony, it is probably best to leave the silicone oil in the eye. Hypotonus eyes usually end up with corneal decompensation in the presence of silicone oil, because the silicone oil herniates forward and touches the corneal endothelium. Unfortunately, with silicone oil removal, these eyes often become phthisical (Fig. 31). Whereas the visual prognosis is poor in either situation, the eye will probably remain more stable with silicone oil remaining in the eye than otherwise.

POSTOPERATIVE MANAGEMENT

Postoperative management is critical to a successful outcome in an eye with PVR. The initial portion of the postoperative management is directed toward (1) careful control of the IOP, (2) adequate retinal tamponade, (3) control of inflammation, (4) elimination of hemorrhage and fibrin, and (5) early detection and management of recurrent retinal detachment.

IOP is commonly elevated following vitrectomy, and 36% of patients reported by Han and colleagues developed an IOP of 30 mm Hg or more. Patients undergoing surgery for PVR are at particular risk for pressure elevation because they have a scleral buckle, often undergo lensectomy, are treated with scatter endophotocoagulation, and often develop a fibrin pupillary membrane postoperatively, all risk factors for postoperative pressure elevation. Pressure should be monitored carefully in the postoperative period. Pressure should be normalized at the end of the case, then rechecked approximately 2–4 hours following surgery, and then rechecked as needed. Elevated pressure is treated medically in most cases, but extreme elevation of pressure that may cause vascular occlusion is usually treated with paracentesis of fluid or gas. In patients with temporary loss of light perception due to elevated IOP after vitrectomy, we have sometimes seen recovery of excellent visual acuity following prompt reduction of IOP.

Adequate and prolonged postoperative retinal tamponade is necessary. This is most important in the presence of inferior retinal breaks. We prefer to have the eye at least 80% filled with gas in the postoperative period. If, as sometimes occurs, the gas bubble is inadequate postoperatively, we do a fluid–gas exchange to "top up" the gas bubble. For fluid–gas exchange in the aphakic eye, we prepare the eye with 5% Betadine (povidone–iodine) solution to the lids and the conjunctival cul-de-sac. A limbal incision is made with a disposable Ziegler-type blade and then, with the patient prone, gas is injected into the eye through a 30-gauge needle inserted through the limbal keratotomy. As gas is injected, fluid will run out around the shaft of the needle through the limbal keratotomy. Once the eye is filled with gas and the fluid has drained out of the eye, the needle is removed. The limbal keratotomy is self-sealing and usually leaves a relatively normal IOP. We usually use a 15% mixture of C_3F_8 for the postoperative fluid–gas exchange.

In phakic eyes or in eyes with a posterior chamber im-

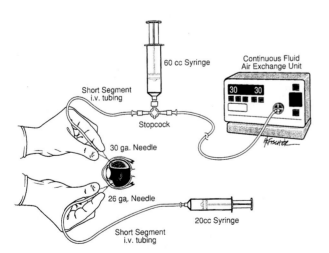

FIG. 32. Fluid–gas exchange with two needles. (Courtesy of Ophthalmic Communications Society, Inc., from Han DP, Murphy ML, Mieler WF, Abrams GW. Outpatient fluid–air exchange for severe postvitrectomy diabetic vitreous hemorrhage: long-term results and complications. *Retina* 1991; 11:309–314, with permission.)

plant, the fluid–gas exchange is performed through the pars plana. We use a two-needle technique and the air pump during the fluid–air exchange (Fig. 32). With the patient placed on his or her side, a 30-gauge needle attached to the air pump is placed in the most superior position through the pars plana into the vitreous cavity. A second 30-gauge needle attached to a syringe is placed through the pars plana at the most dependent position. Usually, the needle for air insufflation is placed nasally (which is now superior), while the needle for fluid aspiration is placed temporally (which is now dependent, inferiorly). With the air pump insufflating air at approximately 30 mm Hg, fluid is aspirated from the dependent position. The eye simultaneously fills with air as the fluid is aspirated. As more fluid is aspirated and the eye fills with air, the head is turned toward a more prone position so further fluid can be aspirated. Aspiration is performed as the needle is slowly withdrawn to remove as much fluid as possible. After fluid is aspirated, the eye is flushed with at least 25 ml of a nonexpansile gas mixture (12%–15% C_3F_8). The flush procedure is facilitated by having a three-way valve on the gas insufflation tubing. Then, it is easy to turn the valve from the air pump to the gas syringe when desired. During the flush procedure, the dependent needle is usually vented to atmosphere.

If an air pump is not available, the exchange can be completed by using a 25-ml or larger syringe filled with 15% C_3F_8 gas. It is important to equalize sequentially the volume of fluid aspirated through the dependent aspirating syringe with the amount of gas injected through the filling syringe. We usually sequentially aspirate 0.5 ml of fluid and then inject 0.5 ml of gas until the fluid is replaced with gas.

To control inflammation, we give preoperative topical steroids and, at the conclusion of the case, we give subconjunctival Decadron (dexamethasone, 5–10 mg). We also treat with frequent topical corticosteroids postoperatively. We usually administer the topical corticosteroids every hour while the patient is awake in the postoperative period for the first few days. We usually do not administer systemic corticosteroids, because of the potential systemic risks involved and because the benefit has not been clearly demonstrated. There is experimental evidence that preoperatively administered corticosteroids suppress postoperative inflammation better than do postoperatively applied corticosteroids. In preoperative eyes with significant inflammation, suppression of inflammation with preoperative systemic corticosteroids might be of benefit.

If significant postoperative fibrin formation causes pupillary block, interferes with postoperative fluid–gas exchange, or interferes with the view to the extent that it complicates postoperative evaluation and management, we treat the fibrin with tissue plasminogen activator (tPA). To minimize the possibility of intraocular hemorrhage, we usually wait 48–72 hours following surgery to inject the tPA. We currently recommend a dose of 3 μg in 0.1 ml, usually injected via a 30-gauge needle through the limbus. In the presence of severe fibrin and/or hemorrhage, we usually do a fluid–gas exchange to clear the fibrin products and/or hemorrhage after lysis with the tPA.

Patients are monitored closely for the development of recurrent retinal detachment. Retinal detachment is most easily seen when looking around, not through, a gas bubble. We usually examine the patients every 1–2 weeks until the gas bubble has resolved. If retinal detachment is detected, we look for its cause. Usually retinal detachment will indicate the presence of an untreated retinal break and/or excessive retinal traction. The most common cause of recurrent retinal detachment is residual anterior traction that opens an anterior break. However, recurrent retinal detachment may result from residual posterior epiretinal membranes, usually manifest by residual posterior retinal folds. In the presence of residual posterior membranes and folding, fluid–gas exchange is contraindicated and reoperation is usually necessary. If the eye is filled with gas and there is then further contraction of posterior epiretinal membranes, the retina can spontaneously tear to relax the traction. However, eyes with anterior contraction can sometimes be successfully reattached with a repeat fluid–gas exchange. After the retina is flattened, laser treatment is applied in several rows to the retina over the scleral buckle and sometimes just posterior to the scleral buckle 360°. We have found that postoperative laser photocoagulation in the air-filled eye is most easily administered by using a laser with a long wavelength, such as krypton red or diode laser and a panfunduscopic contact lens. Whereas some degree of retinal detachment anterior to the scleral buckle may remain, often fluid can be demarcated and the posterior retina will remain attached. This is compatible with long-term stability and recovery of functional visual acuity in some cases; however, some cases with anterior retinal detachment will become hypotonus.

PROGNOSIS AND RESULTS OF TREATMENT OF PROLIFERATIVE VITREORETINOPATHY

There have been rapid advances in the surgical management of PVR in the past 20 years. Grizzard and Hilton, who used a high encircling scleral buckle technique, reported a 35% retinal reattachment rate in eyes with the equivalent of C1 to D2 PVR by the Retina Society classification. Machemer and Norton were the first to use vitrectomy techniques in the management of PVR. In their initial series of 28 eyes treated with vitrectomy and scleral buckling techniques, none were treated successfully. However, Machemer and Laqua combined membrane-peeling techniques with vitrectomy, and their retinal reattachment rate at 6 months increased to 36%.

Early surgical techniques of vitrectomy and membrane peeling were effective in managing posterior membranes in PVR. The major cause of failure was anterior retinal proliferation and contraction. Charles first described anterior displacement of the retina in PVR. Lewis and Aaberg have described the pathoanatomy, and Elner and associates have shown the histopathology of anterior PVR. Aaberg correlated the chronology of surgical advances and understanding of the pathoanatomy of PVR with improvement in results and management of PVR.

There has been continued improvement in both anatomic and visual results in management of PVR. Lewis, Aaberg, and Abrams reported the results of vitrectomy for cases of PVR that had not had a previous vitrectomy. All cases had posterior PVR, whereas 22% also had anterior PVR. Of 81 eyes with C3 to D3 PVR followed for 6–62 months (median, 19 months), 73 retinas (90%) were completely reattached and 76 (94%) were attached posterior to the scleral buckle at the last follow-up. With one operation, 66 retinas (81%) remained completely attached. Visual acuity of 5/200 or better was obtained in 62 (85%) of 73 eyes in which retinas were completely reattached. In eyes in which the retina redetached, cellular reproliferation and traction were the cause of failure, with associated anterior PVR in half of the failed cases.

The results of surgery for cases with previous vitrectomy for PVR were not as good as those for cases without previous vitrectomy. Lewis and Aaberg reported their surgical results in 37 eyes with PVR that had undergone a previous vitrectomy. All of the cases had posterior PVR, whereas 32 (86%) of 37 cases also had anterior PVR. Of 37 cases, the retinas in 27 (73%) were completely reattached at the last follow-up, whereas the retinas in 32 (86%) of 37 cases were reattached posterior to the scleral buckle. Final visual acuity was 5/200 or better in 18 (67%) of 27 retinas that were completely attached, whereas none of the eyes with anterior retinal detachment had ambulatory vision at the last follow-up. The IOP was less than 5 mm Hg in four of five cases with anterior retinal detachment. The cause of failure was cellular reproliferation and traction, with anterior PVR present in nine of 12 cases that developed a recurrent retinal detachment.

The Silicone Study was a multicenter, randomized, controlled clinical trial funded by the National Eye Institute comparing silicone oil and gases in the management of PVR. The Silicone Study included many surgeons from many academic and private centers throughout the United States. The results of the study included all patients entered into the study, and all cases were followed prospectively, so the study probably best demonstrates the level of results to be expected in the treatment of PVR by the typical vitreoretinal surgeon. Recent improvements such as PFCLs and wide-angle viewing were not available for the Silicone Study, so these advances might have improved results further. The surgical method included vitrectomy, removal of posterior membranes, dissection for anterior PVR if present, and reattachment of the retina with air, followed by randomization to 1,000-centistoke silicone oil or gas. An inferior iridectomy was created in silicone oil eyes. There were two groups of eyes: group 1 eyes had not had a previous vitrectomy, whereas group 2 eyes had had a previously unsuccessful vitrectomy with gas for retinal detachment.

Eyes were randomized to silicone oil or 20% SF_6 gas in the initial portion of the study and to silicone oil or 14% C_3F_8 gas in the major portion of the study. Although results with silicone oil were superior to SF_6, there was little difference between silicone oil and C_3F_8 gas. Both silicone oil and C_3F_8 gas produced better results than SF_6 gas.

Of 101 eyes in group 1, silicone oil was superior to SF_6 in most analyses: silicone oil eyes were more likely than SF_6 eyes to obtain a visual acuity of 5/200 or better (50%–60% silicone oil eyes versus 30%–40% SF_6 eyes, p < 0.05). Macular attachment was also more frequent in silicone oil eyes than in SF_6 eyes (80% vs 60%, p < 0.05). Hypotony was more prevalent in eyes with detached maculae (40%–50% for SF_6 eyes versus 25%–30% for silicone oil eyes) when compared with those with attached maculae (<5% for either modality).

In the latter, major portion of the study, 14% C_3F_8 gas was used instead of SF_6. There were 131 eyes in group 1 and 134 eyes in group 2. In contrast to the results comparing silicone oil and SF_6 gas, at 24 months most analyses showed no difference between C_3F_8 gas and silicone oil. The visual acuity was 5/200 or better in 43% of gas eyes versus 45% of silicone oil eyes in group 1, and in 38% of gas eyes versus 33% of silicone oil eyes in group 2. There was complete posterior retinal reattachment in 73% of gas eyes versus 64% of silicone oil eyes in group 1, and in 73% of gas eyes versus 61% of silicone oil eyes in group 2. For group 1 eyes with more than 18 months of follow-up, there was an advantage favoring C_3F_8 gas over silicone oil eyes in achieving complete posterior retinal reattachment (83% vs 60% at 36 months, p = 0.045).

There was no difference in retinal reattachment or visual acuity between group 1 eyes (no previous vitrectomy) and group 2 eyes (at least one unsuccessful vitrectomy with gas tamponade prior to entry into the study). Though uncommon, elevated IOP (>25 mm Hg) was more common in silicone oil eyes (8%) than in C_3F_8 eyes (2%) (p < 0.05). Chronic hypotony (IOP < 5 mm Hg) was (1) more prevalent in eyes randomized to C_3F_8 gas than in those randomized to silicone oil (31% vs 18%, p < 0.05); (2) more prevalent in eyes with anatomic failure (48% vs 16%, p < 0.01); and (3) correlated with poor postoperative vision (p < 0.001) and retinal detachment (p < 0.001). Diffuse contraction of the retina anterior to the equator was an independent factor prognostic of chronic hypotony.

Relaxing retinotomies were more commonly done in group 2 eyes (42%) than in group 1 eyes (20%) (p < 0.0001). The incidence of hypotony (IOP < 5 mm Hg) was greater in gas eyes than in silicone oil eyes undergoing relaxing retinotomies. There were more relaxing retinotomies in group 2 eyes than group 1 eyes. Relaxing retinotomies were done more commonly in eyes with anterior PVR than in eyes without anterior PVR. Visual acuity was better and the retinal reattachment rate was better in eyes without relaxing retinotomies than in eyes with relaxing retinotomies.

Silicone oil was removed from 45% of 222 eyes that re-ceived silicone oil in the study. At the time of silicone oil removal, eyes with oil removed were more likely to have attached retinas (85% vs 40%), have a visual acuity of 5/200 or better (63% vs 35%), and not be hypotonous (5% vs 22%). In a matched-pairs analysis, eyes with silicone oil removed were more likely (1) to experience improvement in visual acuity and (2) to experience retinal detachment than were eyes with silicone oil retained. In eyes with attached maculae, the incidence of corneal abnormalities at 24 months was 27% and did not differ significantly between silicone oil and gas groups. Corneal abnormalities were correlated with poor visual acuity and hypotony. Factors predictive of corneal abnormalities were iris neovascularization, aphakia or pseudophakia, postoperative aqueous flare, and reoperations.

The overall prevalence of macular pucker among eyes with attached maculae was 15%. There was no difference in the prevalence of postoperative macular pucker between eyes randomized to gas versus silicone oil or between group 1 and group 2 eyes. Postoperative macular pucker was three times as likely to develop in eyes that were preoperatively aphakic or in pseudophakic eyes than in eyes that were preoperatively phakic.

Additional follow-up (to 36 months) of eyes randomized to C3F8 gas or silicone oil has shown no change from the initially reported results. In addition, there has been little change in the results with further follow-up (up to 72 months) of gas and silicone oil eyes that had attached retinas at 36 months. Eyes in which oil was removed had the best overall result in comparison to eyes in which oil was retained or eyes that had been randomized to gas. Compared to oil-retained eyes, oil-removed eyes had higher rates of complete posterior attachment and of a visual acuity of 5/200 or better and less keratopathy. Compared with oil-removed eyes, gas-treated eyes had a worse visual acuity outcome and more hypotony.

PHARMACOLOGIC ADJUVANTS IN PROLIFERATIVE VITREORETINOPATHY

In spite of the excellent surgical results in PVR, many problems with recurrent proliferation remain. Whereas an improved percentage of retinas in PVR cases can be reattached with surgery, inhibition of reproliferation with pharmacologic agents to prevent subsequent retinal detachment has been sought by many investigators for over 20 years. The three major areas of investigation into reducing cellular proliferation in PVR are anti-inflammatory therapy, direct inhibition of cellular proliferation, and prevention of attachment of proliferating cells to collagen.

Corticosteroids may reduce reproliferation by both reducing the inflammatory response of tissues and by inhibiting the mitotic activity of cells. Work by Machemer and colleagues suggests that corticosteroids may help to reduce intraocular reproliferation. Pretreatment with corticosteroids prior to surgery may induce synthesis of proteins that inhibit the inflammatory cascade. This may help stabilize the blood–ocular barrier and reduce the leakage of mitogenic serum components from tissue. Triamcinolone acetonide injected into the vitreous cavity in a depot form has been shown experimentally to inhibit cellular proliferation and neovascularization in rabbits. This inhibition is probably due to a reduction in inflammation and a direct inhibition of the mitotic activity of cells. Nonsteroidal anti-inflammatory drugs also cause a reduction in proliferation in vitro, although their potency is much lower than corticosteroids such as triamcinolone or dexamethasone.

Since cellular proliferation and contraction of the extracellular matrix are central to the development of PVR, it is not surprising that many investigators have used a wide variety of cytotoxic agents to arrest vitreoretinal scarring. The fluoropyrimidines were the first family of agents studied because of their potent inhibition of RPE cell proliferation and lack of toxicity in the vitreous cavity. Subsequent investigators have studied anthracyclines (such as daunorubicin), retinoic acid, immunotoxins, and anticontractile agents (such as colchicine). Some of the difficulties in using cytotoxic drugs include their possible ocular toxicity along with the lack of availability of a slow-release or depot form. Several new delivery systems are currently being investigated to lengthen the time that the pharmacologic agent remains in the eye.

Another approach in the pharmacologic therapy of PVR involves the prevention of attachment of proliferating cells to collagen. Fibronectin is a protein secreted from fibroblasts that participates in cell attachment to collagen. Several different pharmacologic agents have been designed that interfere with the attachment of fibronectin to various ligands. RGDS, a tetrapeptide that blocks fibronectin attachment to cells, has been shown in vitro to inhibit RPE cell contraction. Heparin also binds to fibronectin, but possesses numerous other properties that may be useful in treating PVR, including prevention of fibrin formation, decreasing collagen polymerization, and direct antiproliferative action on RPE cells.

One problem with many of the aforementioned agents is that they act on only one phase within the cell cycle. An agent such as heparin may be more amenable to infusion therapy or a single injection, since its multiple biochemical actions affect several different phases in the cell cycle. Low molecular weight heparin, a heparin fragment with decreased hemorrhagic potential, has recently been shown to decrease fibrin formation and traction retinal detachment in an animal model of PVR.

Another form of pharmacologic therapy now used clinically is fibrinolytic therapy using tPA. Fibrin formation is frequently encountered following vitrectomy for PVR and probably results from surgically induced breakdown of the blood–ocular barrier. Fibrin is most commonly observed at the pupil on the surface of a gas or silicone oil bubble, but fibrin can be deposited on the posterior iris, ciliary body, vitreous base, retina, and the vitreous cavity. The most clinically apparent problems induced by fibrin are pupillary-block glaucoma, adhesion of iris to cornea, and reduced view of the posterior segment that complicates postoperative care. Fibrin may also stimulate cellular reproliferation and act as a scaffold for proliferating cells. Fibrin is normally lysed by plasmin, which is derived from plasminogen, and tPA is one of several plasminogen activators that convert plasminogen to plasmin. Recombinant tPA was developed to treat acute coronary artery thrombosis, and tPA stimulates formation of plasmin within a fibrin clot to cause rapid fibrinolysis. Whereas large doses of tPA are used systemically to treat coronary artery thrombosis, low doses of tPA, as low as 3 μg injected intracamerally, are effective in lysing postvitrectomy fibrin. While retinal toxicity and increased potential for hemorrhage may occur with doses greater the 25 μg, lower doses appear to be safe. The tPA is prepared for intraocular use by initially preparing the commercially available product as recommended by the manufacturer. These vials, which contain 20 or 50 mg, are then diluted with sterile physiologic saline to a concentration of 3–6 μg per 0.1 ml. Studies have shown that aliquots prepared under sterile conditions and frozen at $-70°C$ maintain activity and sterility for at least 1 year.

ACKNOWLEDGMENT

This study was supported in part by an unrestricted grant from Research to Prevent Blindness, Inc.

BIBLIOGRAPHY

Aaberg TM. Management of anterior and posterior proliferative vitreoretinopathy [45th Edward Jackson Memorial Lecture]. *Am J Ophthalmol* 1988;106:519–532.

Abrams GW. Retinotomies and retinectomies. In: Ryan SJ, ed. *Retina;* vol 3. St. Louis: CV Mosby, 1989:317–346.

Abrams GW. Posterior segment vitrectomy. In: Packer AJ, ed. *Manual of retinal surgery.* New York: Churchill-Livingstone, 1989:71–105.

Abrams GW, Aaberg TM. Posterior segment vitrectomy. In: Waltman SR, ed. *Surgery of the eye.* New York: Churchill-Livingstone, 1988: 903–1012.

Abrams GW, Azen SP, Barr CC, et al., and the Silicone Study Group. The incidence of corneal abnormalities in the Silicone Study: Silicone Study report #7. *Arch Ophthalmol* 1995;113:764–769.

Abrams GW, Azen SP, McCuen BW II, Flynn HW, Jr., Lai MY, Ryan ST, Silicone Study Group. Vitrectomy with silicone oil or long-acting gas in eyes with severe proliferative vitreoretinopathy: Results of additional and long-term follow-up: Silicone Study Report #11. *Arch Ophthalmol* 1997;115:335–344.

Barr CC, Lai MY, Lean JS, et al., and the Silicone Study Group. Postoperative intraocular pressure abnormalities in the Silicone Study: Silicone Study report #4. *Ophthalmology* 1993;100:1629–1635.

Baudouin C, Brignole F, Bayle J, Fredj-Reygrobellet D, Lapalus P, Gastaud P. Class II histocompatibility antigen expression by cellular components of vitreous and subretinal fluid in proliferative vitreoretinopathy. *Invest Ophthalmol Vis Sci* 1991;32:2065–2072.

Blumenkranz MS, Azen SP, Aaberg TM, et al., and the Silicone study group. Relaxing retinotomy with silicone oil or long-acting gas in eyes with severe proliferative vitreoretinopathy: Silicone Study report #5. *Am J Ophthalmol* 1993;116:557–564.

Chang S, Ozmert E, Zimmerman NJ. Intraoperative perfluorocarbon liquids in the management of proliferative vitreoretinopathy. *Am J Ophthalmol* 1988;106:668–674.

Charles S. *Vitreous microsurgery.* 2nd ed. Baltimore: Williams and Wilkins, 1987:137–138.

Cox MS, Azen SP, Barr CC, et al., and the Silicone Study Group. Macular pucker after successful surgery for proliferative vitreoretinopathy: Silicone Study report #8. *Ophthalmology* 1995;102:1884–1891.

Elner SG, Elner VM, Diaz-Rohena R, Freeman HM, Tolentino FI, Albert DM. Anterior proliferative vitreoretinopathy: clinicopathologic, light microscopic and ultrastructural findings. *Ophthalmology* 1988;95:1349–1357.

Fekrat S, de Juan E, Campochiaro R. The effect of oral 13 *cis* retinoic acid on retinal redetachment after surgical repair in eyes with proliferative vitreoretinopathy. *Ophthalmology* 1995;102:412–418.

Grizzard WS, Hilton GF. Scleral buckling for retinal detachment complicated by periretinal proliferation. *Arch Ophthalmol* 1982;100:419–422.

Han DP, Lewis H, Lambrou FH Jr, Mieler WF, Hartz A. Mechanisms of intraocular pressure elevation after pars plana vitrectomy. *Ophthalmology* 1989;96:1357–1362.

Han DP, Murphy ML, Mieler WF, Abrams GW. Outpatient fluid–air exchange for severe postvitrectomy diabetic vitreous hemorrhage: long-term results and complications. *Retina* 1991;11:309–314.

Heath TD, Lopez NG, Lewis GP, Stern WH. Fluoropyrimidine treatment of ocular cicatricial disease. *Invest Ophthalmol Vis Sci* 1986;27:940–945.

Hutton WL, Azen SP, Blumenkranz MS, et al., and the Silicone Study Group. The effects of silicone oil removal: Silicone Study report #6. *Arch Ophthalmol* 1994;112:778–785.

Innocenzi R, Glazer L, Stec L, Hartzer M, Iverson D, Blumenkranz M. Treatment of experimental PVR in the rabbit with low molecular weight heparin. *Invest Ophthalmol Vis Sci* 1993;34:950.

Jaffe GJ, Green GDJ, Abrams GW. Stability of recombinant tissue plasminogen activator. *Am J Ophthalmol* 1989;108:90–91.

Jerdan J, Pepose J, Michels RG, et al. Proliferative vitreoretinopathy membranes: an immunohistochemical study. *Ophthalmology* 1989;96:801–810.

Kangas TA, Bennett SR, Flynn HW Jr, et al. Reversible loss of light perception after vitreoretinal surgery. *Am J Ophthalmol* 1995;120:751–756.

Laqua H, Machemer R. Glial cell proliferation in retinal detachment (massive periretinal proliferation). *Am J Ophthalmol* 1975;80:602–618.

Lean JS, Stern WA, Irvine AR, Azen SP, and the Silicone Study Group. Classification of proliferative vitreoretinopathy used in the Silicone Study. *Ophthalmology* 1989;96:765–771.

Leaver PK, Cooling RJ, Feretis EB, Lean JS, McLeod D. Vitrectomy and fluid/silicone–oil exchange for giant retinal tears: results at six months. *Br J Ophthalmol* 1984;68:432–438.

Lewis H, Aaberg TM. Anterior proliferative vitreoretinopathy. *Am J Ophthalmol* 1988;105:277–284.

Lopez R, Chang S. Long-term results of vitrectomy and perfluorocarbon gas for the treatment of severe proliferative vitreoretinopathy. *Am J Ophthalmol* 1992;15:424–428.

Machemer R, Laqua H. Pigment epithelial proliferation in retinal detachment (massive periretinal proliferation). *Am J Ophthalmol* 1975;80:1–23.

Machemer R, Laqua H. A logical approach to the treatment of massive periretinal proliferation. *Ophthalmology* 1978;85:584–593.

Machemer R, McCuen BW, de Juan E. Relaxing retinotomies and retinectomies. *Am J Ophthalmol* 1986;102:7–12.

Machemer R, Norton EW. A new concept for vitreous surgery. 3. Indications and results. *Am J Ophthalmol* 1972;74:1034–1056.

Machemer R, Aaberg TM, Freeman HM, Irvine AR, Lean JS, Michels RM. An updated classification of retinal detachment with proliferative vitreoretinopathy. *Am J Ophthalmol* 1991;112:159–165.

McCuen BW II, Azen SP, Stern W, et al., and the Silicone Study Group. Vitrectomy with silicone oil or perfluoropropane gas in eyes with severe proliferative vitreoretinopathy: Silicone Study report #3. *Retina* 1993;13:279–284.

Michels RG. Surgery of retinal detachment with proliferative vitreoretinopathy. *Retina* 1984;4:63–83.

Murray TG, Boldt HC, Lewis H, Abrams GW, Mieler WF, Han DP. A technique for facilitated visualization of the vitreous base, pars plana, and pars plicata. *Arch Ophthalmol* 1991;109:1458–1459.

Silicone Study Group. Vitrectomy with silicone oil or sulfur hexafluoride gas in eyes with severe proliferative vitreoretinopathy: results of a randomized clinical trial—Silicone Study report #1. *Arch Ophthalmol* 1992;110:770–779.

Silicone Study Group. Vitrectomy with silicone oil or perfluoropropane gas in eyes with severe proliferative vitreoretinopathy: results of a randomized clinical trial—Silicone Study report #2. *Arch Ophthalmol* 1992;110:780–792.

Wiedemann P, Sorgente N, Bekhor C, Patterson R, Tran T, Ryan SJ. Daunomycin in the treatment of experimental proliferative vitreoretinopathy: effective doses in vitro and in vivo. *Invest Ophthalmol Vis Sci* 1985;26:719–725.

Williams DF, Peters MA, Abrams GW, Han DP, Mieler WF. A two-stage technique for intraoperative fluid–gas exchange following pars plana vitrectomy. *Arch Ophthalmol* 1990;108:1484–1486.

Živojnovíc R: Silicone oil in vitreoretinal surgery: Dordrecht, The Netherlands, Martinus Nijhoff/Dr. W. Junk Publishers 1987:32.

Practical Atlas of Retinal Disease and Therapy, Second Edition
edited by William R. Freeman,
Lippincott–Raven Publishers, Philadelphia © 1997.

· 18 ·

Retinopathy of Prematurity

Eugene de Juan, Jr., and Anat Loewenstein

Retinopathy of prematurity (ROP), which is the major cause of blindness in infants (Fig. 1), is characterized by a fibrous gliovascular proliferation arising from the inner retina. This gliovascular proliferation is unique to premature, developing retinas and is associated with very low birth weights (under 1,000 g) with gestational ages of less than 32 weeks.

PATHOPHYSIOLOGY AND DIAGNOSIS

History

ROP was first described in 1942 by Theodore Terry (Terry, 1942), a pathologist and ophthalmologist from Texas, while he was at the Massachusetts Eye and Ear Infirmary. He termed the disease retrolental fibroplasia because of its end-stage appearance showing a vascularized fibrous membrane behind a clear lens (Fig. 2). It was 8 years later, in 1951, that the high concentrations of oxygen routinely used in incubators at the time was first suggested by Kate Campbell (Campbell, 1951) in Melbourne, Australia, to be associated with the development of ROP. She observed that there was a higher incidence of ROP in the hospitals where oxygen use was more prevalent than in poorer hospitals where oxygen was considered too expensive to use without clear need. However, it was Arnall Patz (Patz, 1957) in a landmark study who clearly demonstrated the causal effect of high oxygen administration on the development of ROP. This represented one of the first prospective and controlled trials performed in ophthalmology. These findings and similar ones later proved the association of high oxygen administration with the development of ROP in premature infants.

Following these studies, a worldwide recommendation was made to decrease incubator oxygen levels to no greater than 30%. This rapidly reversed the worldwide epidemic of ROP, and the disease nearly disappeared. However, as neonatal intensive care units became more successful at saving the lives of very premature infants (under 1,000 g), a new epidemic of ROP occurred. It has recently been estimated that ROP leads to blindness in approximately 500 infants per year (Gibson et al., 1990). Hopefully, with the advent of new therapies, including cyrotherapy to the peripheral avascular retina and laser photocoagulation, this number will be greatly reduced.

Pathoanatomy

Normal Retinal Development

In normal retinal development, the retina begins to be vascularized in the second trimester of gestation. This vascularization of the retina occurs in concert with the normal differentiation of the retinal architecture. Preceding this normal retinal vascularization is a well-developed hyaloid vascular system (Fig. 3) that courses along the retinal surface, into the vitreous, and along the lens, forming the tunica vasculosa lentis. The hyaloid vascular architecture is potentially important in defining the vitreoretinal anatomy in the later stages of ROP. In premature infants, the tunica vasculosa lentis is often still visible as spindly vessels encroaching on the surface of the lens when the pupil has been dilated (Fig. 4).

Risk Factors

A child born prematurely (weighing less than 1,000 g) is very likely to develop some degree of ROP. The vast majority of the children that lose vision from ROP are represented in this very low birth weight group. Oxygen therapy is no longer the greatest risk factor for the development of ROP. Additional risk factors that have been shown to be independent and have a potentially greater correlation with the development of ROP include the following:

E. de Juan, Jr., M.D., and A. Loewenstein, M.D.: Wilmer Ophthalmological Institute, Johns Hopkins Hospital, Baltimore, MD 21287.

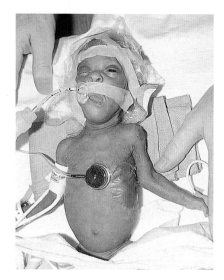

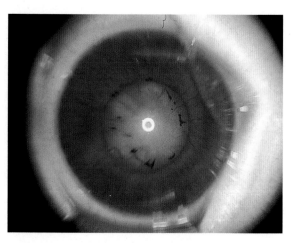

FIG. 1. A 2½-lb infant being prepared for cryosurgery because of severe retinopathy of prematurity.

FIG. 2. Typical appearance of end-stage retinopathy of prematurity, known as retrolental fibroplasia, as described by Terry (Terry et al., 1942) in the early 1940s.

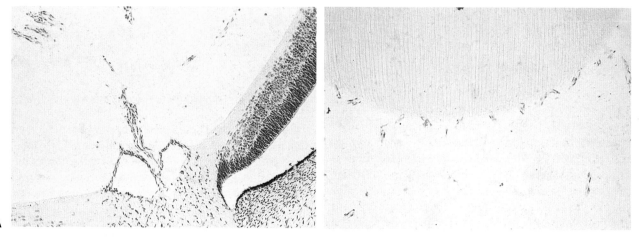

A   B

FIG. 3. A: Histologic sections of hyaloidal vessels in a 16-week fetus eye. (Note the immaturity of the retina and no vascularization of the retina proper.) The hyaloidal system appears to arise from the optic disc and extends to a capillary border around the posterior aspect of the lens (**B**).

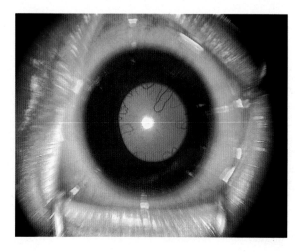

FIG. 4. Persistent lacy vessels on the anterior surface of the lens in active retinopathy of prematurity. Some have mistaken these for rubeotic vessels, but they represent a persistence of the tunica vasculosa lentis.

1. Low birth weight, particularly under 1,000 g.
2. Early gestational age, particularly less than 28 weeks of gestation.
3. Oxygen administration and prolonged intubation.
4. Associated intracranial hemorrhage and the requirement for multiple transfusions.
5. Correlation of light exposure in the nursery with the severity of the ROP (Fielder et al., 1992; Seiberth et al., 1994).
6. Multiple gestation.

Etiology

The exact cause of ROP has not been determined. Previously, a widely held belief was that the avascular retina is ischemic or hypoxic, presumably because no retinal vessels are in this area. Histologic studies show, however, that the avascular retina is poorly developed, particularly with regard to photoreceptors, indicating that the oxygen consumption might be low. In addition, the premature avascular retina is less than 120 μm thick, which indicates that the choroid might supply adequate oxygen and prevent hypoxia in avascular retinas. Vaso-occlusion has not been well documented in this disease.

ROP is highly dependent on the developmental stage and age of the infant: it rarely occurs before 32 weeks of gestational age and rarely progresses in an active form past 40 weeks of gestational age. Thus, in 8 weeks, from a vascular standpoint, the disease will appear and burn out in the vast majority of cases. The retinal detachment can progress because of fibrous contraction. This is discussed later in the *Retinal Detachment* section.

Diagnosis, Clinical Course, and Stages

The earliest clinical change noticed in ROP is the cessation of normal retinal vascularization. Usually, this is a temporary slowing of vascular development. This can then proceed to a more clearly defined demarcation line that represents a clear demarcation between the capillary development (the rear guard) and the location of a visibly apparent collection of spindle cells (the vanguard). In the early stage, known as stage I, no thickening in the retina can be appreciated clinically. At this stage and the next (stage II), where the capillary proliferation within the retina becomes more prominent, a ridge separating the more normal vascularized retinal area and the avascular peripheral retinal area is visible (Figs. 5 and 6). Histopathologically, the thickened ridge is the result of intraretinal capillary proliferation (Fig. 7). Anterior to this capillary proliferation are the spindle cells, the exact origin and nature of which remain unclear. These cells are glycogen rich and are thought to be in some way precursors to vascular development.

In stage III, the capillary plexus exits the retina proper and extends through the internal limiting membrane, reaching

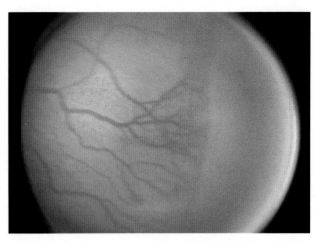

FIG. 5. Early stage II retinopathy of prematurity. (Note an elevated ridge but no intravitreal neovascularization at the ridge.) Some intravitreal proliferations (popcorn lesions) posterior to the ridge are not considered in the classification (stages).

into the vitreous gel. This is apparent ophthalmoscopically as a fine brush border of vessels extending into the vitreous cavity (Fig. 8). Clinically, only the blood-filled channels are seen. Ultrasonographically, however, a more diffuse involvement of the vitreous can be seen. This proliferation often grows toward the back of the lens, probably because of the proliferation's relation to the vitreous anatomy (Fig. 9).

Histopathologically, this proliferation is quite active mitotically and extends in a veil-like fashion to the lens anteriorly, but also progresses posteriorly along the retinal surface (Figs. 10 and 11). In the more limited cases of ROP, this proliferation is confined to the temporal retina. The temporal and nasal retinal regions are characteristically more involved than the superior and inferior retinal areas, presumably be-

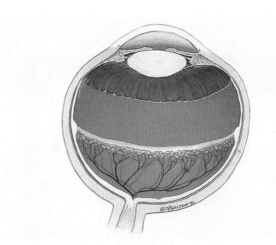

FIG. 6. Artist's drawing of stage II retinopathy of prematurity with no extraretinal neovascular proliferation. (From Machemer R. Description and pathogenesis of late stages of retinopathy of prematurity. *Ophthalmology* 1985;92: 1000–1004, with permission.)

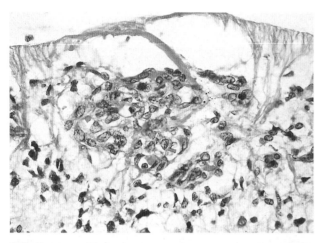

FIG. 7. Histopathologic section showing detail of intraretinal capillary proliferation corresponding to the ridge. Spindle cells are peripheral to the ridge.

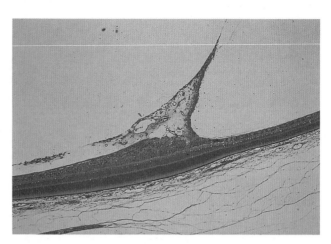

FIG. 10. Histopathologic view of stage III retinopathy of prematurity. Proliferation is very active and nearly purely vascular, extending in a veil-like fashion to behind the lens. A preretinal component (*left*) is also extending posteriorly. (Courtesy of Richard Green, M.D., Johns Hopkins Hospital, Baltimore, MD.)

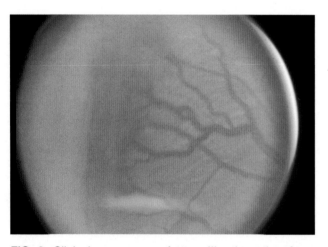

FIG. 8. Clinical appearance of stage III retinopathy of prematurity. Note the intravitreal proliferation and the tortuosity of the vessels.

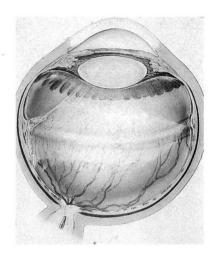

FIG. 11. Artist's conception of stage III retinopathy of prematurity demonstrating vitreous membranes that are often transparent on clinical examination.

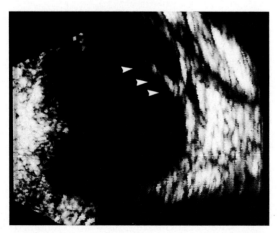

FIG. 9. Ultrasound appearance of intravitreal proliferation that can be seen to be exiting the retina (*arrows*) and growing toward the lens.

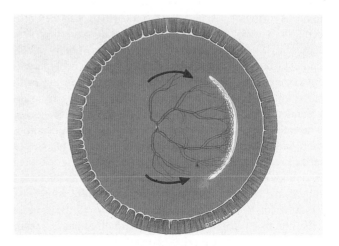

FIG. 12. Artist's conception showing contraction of the temporal ridge, causing early dragging of retinal vessels. (From Machemer R. Description and pathogenesis of late stages of retinopathy of prematurity. *Ophthalmology* 1985;92: 1000–1004, with permission.)

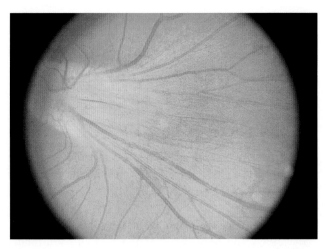

FIG. 13. Clinical appearance of dragged disc and vessels caused by peripheral contraction of the fibrovascular proliferation.

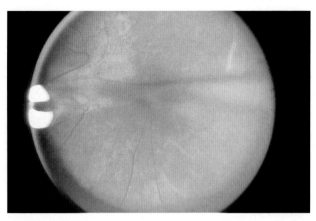

FIG. 15. Fundus photograph showing the clinical picture of a retinal fold caused by temporal contraction of the peripheral ridge. (Courtesy of John Flynn, M.D., Bascom Palmer Eye Institute, Miami, FL.)

cause of the increased light exposure of the temporal and nasal retinal areas compared with the superior and inferior aspects. Because the retinal vascularization extends radially from the optic disc, usually the temporal area has the longest path and is therefore more frequently involved in the more severe stages of ROP. Once the vascularization regresses and the cicatricial stages begin, the vessels contract and are dragged temporally, giving the appearance of the so-called dragged disc (Figs. 12 and 13). In the most severe cases of this temporal dragging, these proliferations can cause retinal folds or temporal retinal detachment (Figs. 14 and 15).

Pathoanatomy of Cicatricial Retinopathy of Prematurity

Sometimes, cicatricial vitreous veils can be identified as they course toward the back of the lens (Fig. 16). Ultrastruc-

turally, these membranes are composed of glial cells that directly invade the vitreous, as well as neovascular vessels that also directly invade the vitreous cavity (Figs. 17 and 18). This is different from other types of neovascular proliferation, for example, in diabetic retinopathy where the gliovascular proliferation develops on the posterior surface of the vitreous, not invading it directly. Presumably, this is because the immature endothelial and glial cells that invade the vitreous do not have the same matrix requirements as more mature adult tissues might. Embryologically, the vitreous is more firmly attached in the area behind the lens. The vitreous collagen is normally present in a loose matrix. The invasion of the cells, however, causes the vitreous to become stretched and oriented, increasing the tension and secondarily increasing the proliferation in a mechanism of development not unlike tendon development in muscles (Fig. 19). Why there is a more firm adherence of the vitreous behind the lens is not clear, but it may be related to the vitreous and

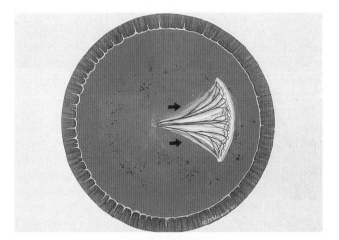

FIG. 14. Artist's conception of more prominent dragging of retinal vessels causing a retinal fold and a nearly avascular retina elsewhere due to severe and focal temporal dragging. (From Machemer R. *Ophthalmology* 1985;92:1000–1004, with permission.)

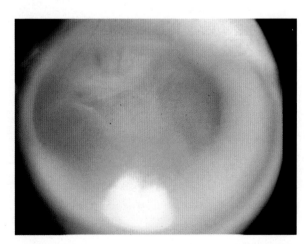

FIG. 16. Fundus photograph showing a peripheral retinal fold (caused by intravitreal veil formation and contraction).

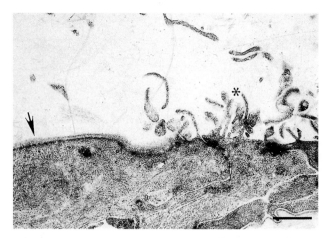

FIG. 17. Electron micrograph showing glial tissue projecting microvillous projections (*arrow*) into the overly vitreous cavity.

lens development associated with the tunica vasculosa lentis. These contracting cells lead to an anterior and inward pulling of the peripheral retina toward the lens. This process can sometimes occur over a period of days. Figure 20 shows the ultrasound photographs from a patient with a progressive traction detachment. The series starts with intravitreal proliferation (Fig. 20A) that progresses to a peripheral traction detachment [stage IV (Fig. 20B)], then to a total open-funnel retinal detachment (Fig. 20C), and finally to a posteriorly closed-funnel detachment (Fig. 20D).

The clinical appearance of the retinal configuration is best understood with reference to the histopathology. Often, in these eyes, there is a bright red reflex. The retina is still relatively transparent, making the clinical diagnosis of detachment more difficult because the choroidal pattern is easily visible. This is particularly true because infants are often difficult to examine, and poor pupillary dilation and/or scarring is often associated with ROP. Figures 21 and 22 show the appearance of a large peripheral trough and a narrow

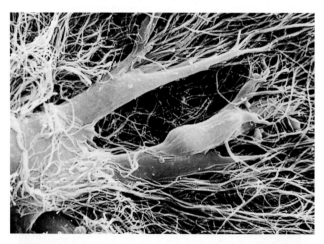

FIG. 18. Scanning electron micrograph of a human retinal glial cell interacting with the collagen matrix. Note the cell extending pseudopods in the direction of and orienting the fibrils of the collagen gel.

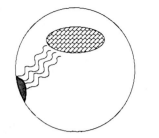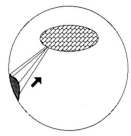

FIG. 19. Artist's drawing showing orientation and contraction of vitreous collagen fibers caused by cells exiting the ridge.

vascularized funnel being pulled up toward the disc. Clinically, this would have the appearance of an open-funnel type of detachment, as is evident in Fig. 23. In this instance, a typical nonvascular glial proliferation arising from the disc leads to an anterior–posterior traction, with much of the disc substance drawn into the eye (Fig. 24). The peripheral traction gives rise to the clinical appearance of a trough in the periphery, a consistent feature of eyes with severe ROP (Fig. 25). The trough forms as the retina is pulled up in a ringlike fashion by the proliferation, and against the retinal pigment epithelium and choroidal suction forces trying to keep the retina attached. This leads to a stretching of the peripheral avascular retina, with the development of a peripheral trench or trough. Surgically, the trough is important to identify and open in order to release the anterior traction (Figs. 25 and 26).

In certain cases, the proliferation not only pulls on the peripheral retina, but the ciliary body epithelium as well. This can sometimes be seen clinically (Fig. 27), where the pars plana and ciliary body epithelium have been pulled into the eye. The sub–pars plana space communicates directly with the subretinal space and is adjacent to the lens, as is shown in the histopathologic section in Fig. 28.

Sometimes the view of a bright red reflex can be misleading because the peripheral troughs can be so large as to lead to the impression of attached retina (Fig. 29). The retinal periphery must be inspected carefully. Rarely, a total detachment of the vascularized retina occurs in a narrow-funnel configuration, leaving only the peripheral troughs that are apparent. This unusual ultrasound and histopathologic appearance is shown in Fig. 30.

The process of retinal and vitreous contraction usually leads to a total closed-funnel appearance, drawing the retina into many folds and causing a retinal degeneration with severe photoreceptor atrophy and proliferative changes in the retina resulting in a disruption of normal retinal architecture (Figs. 31 and 32). When this process is very advanced and begins very posteriorly, all that may be evident is a posterior fibrous scar (Fig. 33). These eyes are difficult to approach surgically, because there is essentially no viable retina remaining (Fig. 34).

Text continues on p 334.

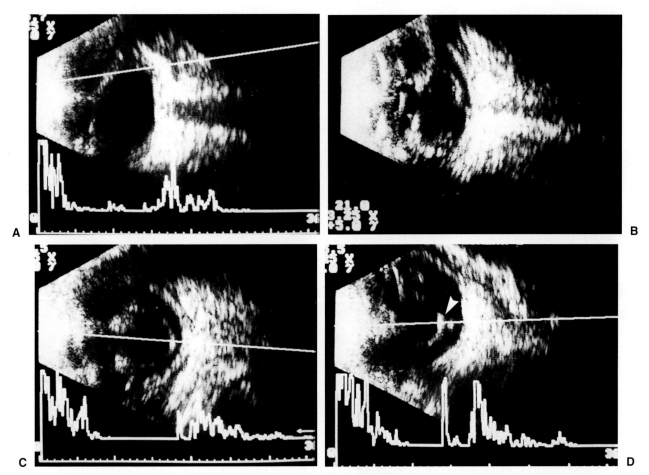

FIG. 20. A series of ultrasound photographs showing the rapid progression of retinal detachment. **A:** Intravitreal proliferation. **B:** Partial peripheral traction detachment stage IV. **C:** Total retinal detachment, although open funnel both anteriorly and posteriorly. **D:** The funnel is beginning to close posteriorly (*arrow*). This process occurred over a 1-week period. (From de Juan E, et al. The role of ultrasound in the management of retinopathy of prematurity. *Ophthalmology* 1988;95:884–888, with permission.)

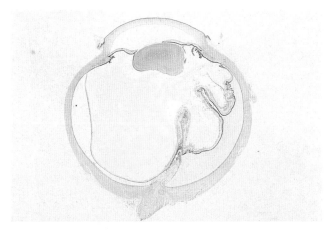

FIG. 21. Histopathologic section of an entire eye showing a large peripheral trough to the left and intravitreal proliferation pulling the retina toward the lens centrally.

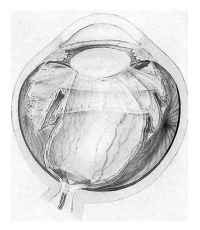

FIG. 22. Artist's conception of the process shown in the preceding figure: an open-funnel type of detachment.

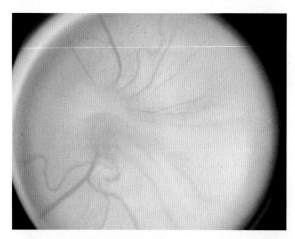

FIG. 23. Fundus photograph showing an avascular glial remnant exiting the optic disc, causing traction and pulling of the optic disc into the eye. (From Noorily S, et al. Scleral buckling surgery for Stage 4B retinopathy of prematurity. *Ophthalmology* 1992;99:263–268, with permission.)

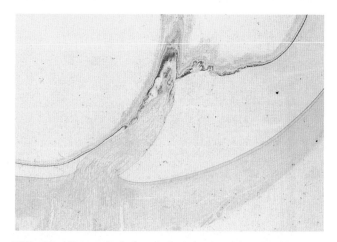

FIG. 24. Histopathologic section emphasizing the dragged disc and pulling of disc tissue into the vitreous cavity.

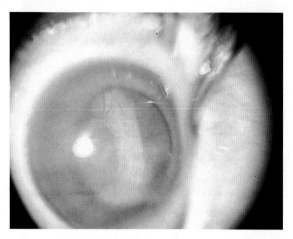

FIG. 25. Fundus photograph showing to the *left* the open-funnel appearance in the center of the pupil. A whitish area or ridge is evident, and an additional reddish reflex is evident to the *right* of the whitish ridge that is a peripheral trough. The trough is filled with vitreous and vessels that arise from the retina.

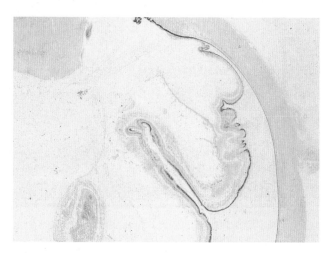

FIG. 26. Histopathologic section showing the detail of the retinal folding and vessels that are present in the peripheral trough.

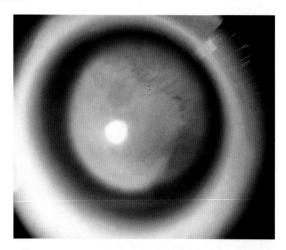

FIG. 27. Fundus photograph of severe anterior traction detaching the pars plana and ciliary body epithelium, pulling it in toward the lens. The space beneath the pars plana epithelium communicates with the subretinal space. Surgically, it is important to recognize this, because any tears that occur in this area are often very difficult to repair.

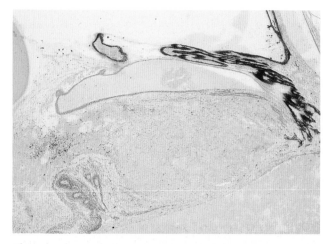

FIG. 28. Histopathologic appearance of detached pars plana epithelium showing the one- to two-cell-layer-thick epithelium just behind the dragged ciliary body processes that are pigmented. These are pulled in toward the lens.

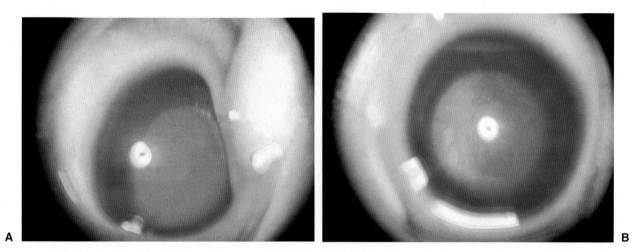

FIG. 29. A: Bright red reflex in infant eye. **B:** When viewed at another angle, however, the retrolental fibrovascular tissue can be seen.

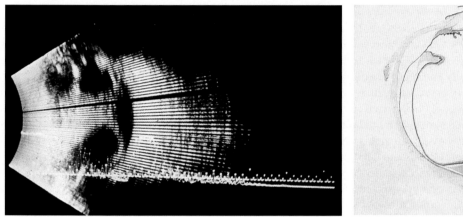

FIG. 30. A: Ultrasound appearance an eye such as in the preceding figure, with large peripheral troughs and a closed central funnel. Such an eye might have the appearance histopathologically of **B** or of Fig. 21, where a large peripheral trough is attached, but the retina proper is totally detached.

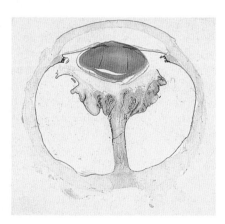

FIG. 31. Histopathologic view of a typical narrow anterior/narrow posterior funnel configuration showing total retinal detachment, retinal folds, and severe retinal degeneration. (Courtesy of Alec Graner, M.D., Moorfields Hospital, England.)

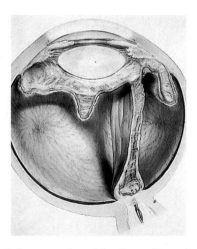

FIG. 32. Artist's conception of the three-dimensional character of the view in the preceding figure. Such cases have an extremely poor prognosis surgically.

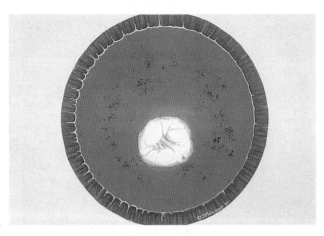

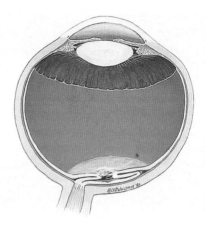

A

B

FIG. 33. A: Artist's conception of proliferation starting very posteriorly, leaving the retina fully attached in a large peripheral trough, but only a nubbin of fibrous tissue occurring posteriorly. **B:** No viable retinal tissue is present posteriorly. (From Machemer R. *Ophthalmology* 1985;92:1000–1004, with permission.)

Differential Diagnosis

The differential diagnosis of ROP includes essentially all other causes of retinal detachment or vitreous fibrosis in infants. These include Coats' disease (Fig. 35), which fortunately is very rare in infants, is usually unilateral, occurs predominantly in males, and is usually not associated with prematurity. Given the appearance of a vascularized retrolental mass, though, in this case retina often with lipid-containing subretinal fluid, infantile Coats' can mimic the whitish pupil of severe ROP. Familial exudative vitreoretinopathy is a bilateral autosomal dominant disorder of peripheral retinal vascular development often associated with retinal traction, with abrupt termination of temporal retinal vasculature and dragging of the macula, disc, and retinal vessels, which can have an appearance similar to ROP (Fig. 36). Other types of infantile retinal degeneration, including Norrie's disease (Fig. 37), which is a progressive neural degeneration associated with mental retardation, deafness, and a fi-

brous vitreoretinal dysplasia, can mimic ROP. Incontinentia pigmenti is a bilateral, asymmetric X-linked dominant or sporadic disorder of pigmentary skin abnormalities. Ocular involvement includes pigmentary changes of the retinal pigment epithelium and peripheral vascular abnormalities associated with an avascular zone, peripheral fibrovascular proliferation, and tractional retinal detachment that can mimic ROP (Fig. 38). Persistent hyperplastic primary vitreous (PHPV), particularly that with posterior involvement, can also give the appearance of ROP. In fact, Reese (Reese, 1951) felt that ROP was an abnormal development of the primary vitreous, and he associated the disease with PHPV. Retinal dysplasia usually occurs unilaterally. In addition, other diseases, such as Snead's syndrome, are associated with retinal vascular hypoplasia, although not usually retinal detachment. Finally, there are a series of cases that are essentially indistinguishable from ROP in the late cicatricial phases, although there is no history of ROP. These cases are probably best defined as vitreous fibrosis in the infant. Other

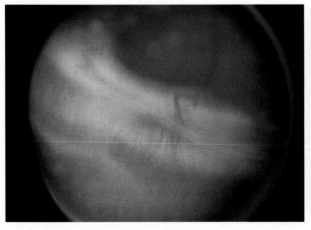

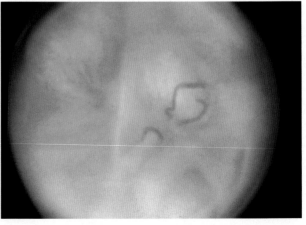

A

B

FIG. 34. A: Posterior proliferation in such a case as that in the preceding figure. [Note that the ridge is extremely posterior, causing the neovascular proliferation to contract and roll on itself toward the optic disc (**B**).] Surgical attempts at opening these folds are often unsuccessful.

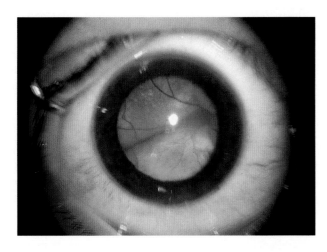

FIG. 35. Fundus photograph of a patient with Coats' disease showing the retrolental presence of an elevated bullous retina and subretinal lipid-containing material. Coats' disease is in the differential diagnosis of severe retinopathy of prematurity as it can occur in infants. However, usually it is unilateral and present in males typically with no history of prematurity.

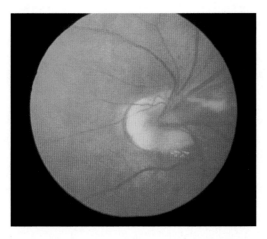

FIG. 36. Fundus photograph showing the clinical picture of dragged blood vessels in familial exudative vitreoretinopathy. (Courtesy of Irene Maumenee, M.D., Wilmer Eye Institute, Baltimore, MD.)

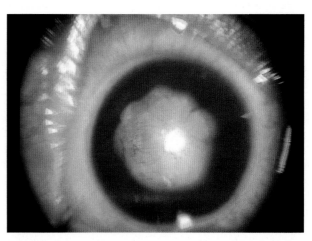

FIG. 37. Fundus photograph of a patient with Norrie's disease. This was a bilateral condition. Notice the retrolental fibrous membrane that is partially vascularized, giving an appearance not unlike retinopathy of prematurity. The child had no history of prematurity and was subsequently developmentally delayed, leading to the diagnosis of Norrie's.

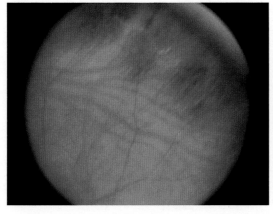

A

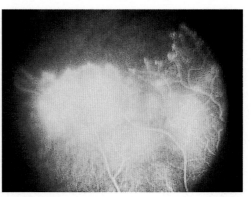

B

FIG. 38. Fundus photograph and fluorescein angiography showing the retinal pigment epithelial changes (A) and peripheral vascular abnormalities (B) in incontinentia pigmenti. (Courtesy of Morton Goldberg, M.D., Wilmer Eye Institute, Baltimore, MD.)

causes of leukokoria include cataract, retinoblastoma, and coloboma. However, all of these diseases are typically not associated with prematurity and do not have a progressive onset from the time of birth.

CURRENT RECOMMENDATIONS FOR EXAMINATION AND TREATMENT

The key to successful treatment of ROP is diligent and careful screening in the neonatal nursery. Because it is quite unusual for ROP to develop before 4 weeks of age or 32 weeks of gestational age, screenings are usually delayed until this time. This screen is done with indirect ophthalmoscopy and scleral depression. A small lens loop or forceps is often helpful in this regard after topical anesthesia. Once the retina fully vascularizes, no further examinations are needed until the infant is 3 months old. The reason for these late examinations is because of a higher incidence of myopia, strabismus, and amblyopia.

If there is incomplete vascularization, even with no evidence of ROP, examinations should be performed every 2 weeks until the retina is vascularized. If ROP is present, weekly follow-up is indicated. A recent report from the Cryo-ROP Cooperative Group confirmed that the degree of early retinal vessel development is a significant predictor of outcome in ROP. In addition, iris vessel dilatation was found to be associated with increased risk for developing threshold retinopathy and is an important indication for greater vigilance in following up the cases of these infants (Kivlin et al. 1996).

Cryotherapy

The study by the Cryotherapy for ROP Cooperative Group has shown a beneficial effect of cryotherapy on eyes with threshold ROP, which has been defined as 5 contiguous or 8 cumulative clock hours of stage III ROP in zone I or II (Cryotherapy for ROP Cooperative Group 1988, 1990a and b, 1993; Committee for the Classification of ROP 1984). Specifically, for the 234 children examined $5^1/_2$ years after randomization, fundus structure showed a reduction in unfavorable outcomes [stage IVB (partial retinal detachment, retinoschisis, or fold with foveal involvement) and stage V (total retinal detachment, retinoschisis, or retrolental membrane); view of the posterior pole and near periphery is blocked owing to total cataract or total corneal opacity, or enucleation] in treated (26.9%) versus control eyes (45.4%) (p < 0.001) (Cryotherapy for ROP Cooperative Group 1996). Detailed analysis of visual acuity outcomes for all eyes, however, revealed that although fewer treated eyes (31.5%) than control eyes (48%) were blind (p < 0.001), there was a slight trend toward fewer eyes with a visual acuity of 20/40 or better in the treated (13%) versus control (17%) groups (p = 0.19) (Quinn et al. 1996a). Thus, these long-term results support the long-term efficacy and safety of cryotherapy in the treatment of severe ROP, but show evidence of a possible adverse effect of this treatment on visual acuity. It was also recently demonstrated that eyes that have retinal structure and acuity preserved by cryotherapy for severe acute-phase ROP have slightly smaller visual fields than do untreated eyes with severe acute-phase ROP that had vision preserved (Quinn et al. 1996b).

Cryotherapy in infants is a difficult procedure, particularly for those not experienced with performing it in infants (Fig. 39). We typically use a cataract probe with either topical or general anesthesia, dilating the eyes with 0.5% Cyclogyl (cyclopentolate) or, if this is not sufficient, we add a single drop of 2.5% phenylephrine and close the tear duct to block systemic absorption. The indirect laser ophthalmoscope delivery system can be used to deliver laser photocoagulation to the avascular retina in conjunction with scleral depression (Fig. 40). Eyes with stage III (extraretinal proliferation) plus disease (posterior vascular tortuosity) with 5 or more contiguous or 8 total clock hours of involvement and no retinal detachment should be treated with cryotherapy. The cryotherapy is placed to ablate the avascular retina totally. A silicone-sleeved cataract probe has been found to be the most useful. Usually, it is not necessary to incise the conjunctiva, but the conjunctiva may be focally opened in the area of the probe by applying slight pressure and breaking through Tenon's capsule with the blunt tip of the probe. This allows easy access to the midperipheral retina. Although there is usually no attempt to administer cryotherapy to the ridge, freezing the total avascular retina will often result in freezes to the ridge. No particular adverse or beneficial outcomes have been associated with cryotherapy of the ridge.

Figure 41 shows a series of eyes that received cryotherapy during a randomized cryotherapy trial. The left eye received cryotherapy. As can be seen, there was marked plus disease (Fig. 41A) and 360° of extraretinal (stage III) vascular proliferation. Cryotherapy was placed with the cataract probe in a contiguous fashion, as shown in Fig. 41B. Nine days after the cryotherapy, the untreated right eye (Fig. 41C) had pro-

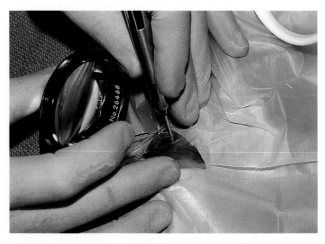

FIG. 39. Cryotherapy being placed to an infant eye to treat retinopathy of prematurity under sterile conditions because of the necessity of posterior placement. A silicone-sleeved cataract probe is being used.

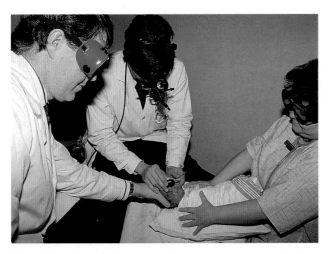

FIG. 40. In cases where a cryotherapy probe is not available or thought to be too traumatic because of extensive posterior proliferation, laser therapy can be used.

gressive marked fibrovascular proliferation (Fig. 41E). However, the disease in the treated left eye had totally regressed, with resolution of the plus disease (Fig. 41D) and involution of the peripheral neovascularization (Fig. 41F). This response is consistent and dramatic, and reduces vascular tortuosity and causes involution of the vessels quickly. In certain cases, however, particularly those with more severe degrees of ROP, an avascular fibrous component may cause retinal traction even though the vascularization regresses.

The few complications reported from cryotherapy include late retinal detachment with tears, particularly at the posterior edge of cryotherapy scars. Failure of cryotherapy will most often result in traction retinal detachments. In addition, cryotherapy itself can cause an exudative detachment, particularly when traction is already present. This type of early traction detachment can be quite mild and difficult to detect.

Figure 42 shows a traction detachment of the macula (stage IVB) that would have been very easy to miss if not for the appearance of subretinal blood delineating the extent of the detachment as it progressed toward the fovea. The eye of this patient was successfully treated with scleral buckling. In these cases, we use a small band placed around the eye and typically have not had to drain subretinal fluid, but rather prefer an anterior chamber paracentesis to allow tightening of the band.

Laser Treatment

Although cryotherapy has been shown to be en effective means of treating infants with threshold ROP, the introduction of laser indirect ophthalmoscopy has made laser photocoagulation an increasingly popular means of therapy for these infants. Successful treatment of acute ROP with both the argon laser and the diode laser has been reported (Benner et al. 1993, Capone et al. 1993, Fleming et al. 1992, Goggin and O'Keefe 1993, Hunter and Repka 1993, Iverson et al. 1991, Landers et al. 1990 and 1992, McNamara et al. 1991

and 1992, Preslan 1993, Laser ROP Study Group 1994, Margolis et al. 1994, Tasman 1992). The incidence of unfavorable outcome varied in most of these studies from 0 to 10%, and only two studies reported a higher failure rate, which was similar to those of the Cryo-ROP Cooperative Group study (Landers et al. 1990, Margolis et al. 1994). Several controlled studies have compared the efficacy of laser photocoagulation and cryotherapy (Goggin and O'Keefe 1993, Hunter and Repka 1993, Landers et al. 1990 and 1992), a meta-analysis of which suggests that laser therapy is better tolerated and as effective as cryotherapy for treating most cases of threshold ROP (Laser ROP Study Group 1994, Tasman 1992). The retinal and preretinal hemorrhage that occurred in 22% of the Cryo-ROP Cooperative Group study eyes was rarely reported to occur with the laser treatment probably because the pressure of scleral depression during laser photocoagulation on the globe is minimal compared with the pressure on the globe created by the cryotherapy probe. With the indirect laser, it is not necessary to open the conjunctiva even when treatment is applied to posterior zone 2 or zone 1 whereas, in cryotherapy, the conjunctiva has to be opened to reach the posterior retina with the probe. Usually the laser treatment causes minimal conjunctival trauma and less postoperative chemosis and eyelid edema than does cryotherapy. The major drawback to the use of the laser indirect ophthalmoscope is the need for relatively optically clear media. Thus, significant corneal haze or vitreous hemorrhage may preclude its use or require the use of adjunctive cryotherapy.

Both argon laser and diode laser have been proved equal to cryotherapy in the aforementioned studies. However, the blue–green argon laser light (wavelengths, 488 and 514 nm) has several disadvantages when compared with the semiconductor diode laser (wavelength, 810 nm). The argon laser is well absorbed by reduced hemoglobin and oxyhemoglobin. Thus, it may be less optimal for treating eyes that have a prominent anterior tunica vasculosa lentis as compared with the diode laser, which is minimally absorbed by hemoglobin. Indeed, after argon laser treatment of ROP, transient lenticular opacities and cataract formation were noticed in single cases (Drack et al. 1992, Pogrebniak et al. 1994). These were not reported to occur with use of the diode laser (Seiberth et al. 1995a). Additionally, the diode laser is portable, making curb-side treatment with topical anesthesia possible. Theoretically, the fact that the diode laser does not cause a significant direct damage to the inner retinal layers might be a disadvantage: it might not damage the spindle cells, which are precursors of capillary endothelial cells in the immature retina and may contribute to ROP development. It has therefore been proposed that the laser intensity be adjusted in an attempt to extend damage into the inner retinal layers, thereby destroying all retinal layers, including the spindle cells (Seiberth et al. 1995b).

When applying laser and using scleral depression, it should be remembered that spots are more intense in indented areas when the same laser energy is used. The duration of laser treatment is similar to that of cryotherapy.

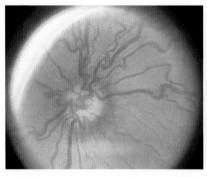 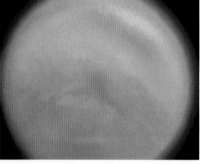 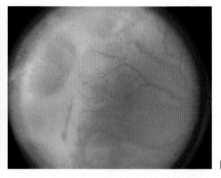

A,B   **C**

The patient had bilateral severe plus disease (**A**) with peripheral neovascularization.

B: Cryotherapy placed in a contiguous fashion in the left eye (note the ridge treatment).

C: Plus disease of the right eye.

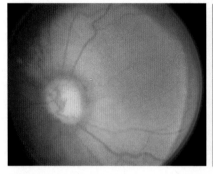 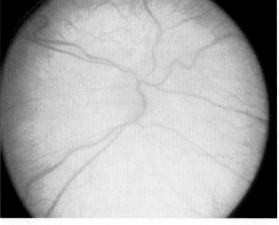

D,E   **F**

D,E: Postoperative appearance 9 days later, following cryotherapy. (Note the resolution of plus disease in the left eye.) The right eye showed progression of the peripheral neovascularization and early retinal detachment (**E**).

F: Peripheral resolution of the neovascularization in the left eye with placement of the cryotherapy

FIG. 41. A patient treated in the Cryo-ROP Cooperative Group study.

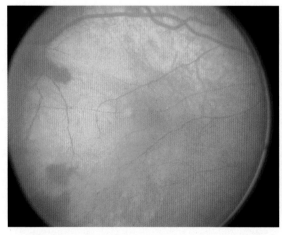 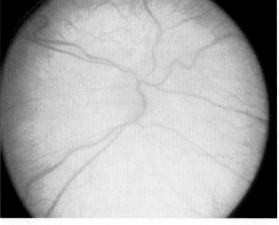

A   **B**

FIG. 42. A,B: Fundus photographs of stage IVB retinal detachment. The transparent retina allows the choroidal pattern to be seen despite retinal elevation. On cursory examination, posterior retinal detachment can be quite difficult to detect. In this patient, the detachment is easier to detect because of the presence of subretinal hemorrhage.

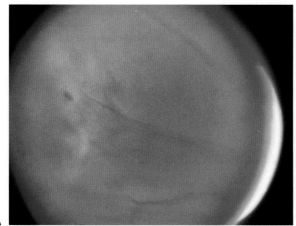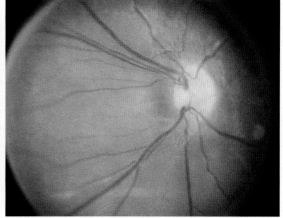

A   B

FIG. 43. A,B: Fundus photographs showing peripheral and posterior views of rhegmatogenous retinal detachment. The patient was a product of a twin birth with no evidence of detachment after retinopathy of prematurity had regressed from stage II. After some weeks, however, the mother noticed that the child had decreased vision and, on examination, a rhegmatogenous retinal detachment was diagnosed.

Placement of laser spots close to the ridge was found to be associated with an increased risk of small retinal or preretinal bleeding that appears immediately after the spot application but stops spontaneously (Seiberth et al. 1995b).

Retinal Detachment

Rhegmatogenous detachment is extremely rare in ROP, but does occur (Fig. 43) and can be successfully treated with scleral buckling and cryotherapy in certain instances.

Most cases that progress to retinal detachment will proceed to total retinal detachment (stage V). The international classification now recognizes four types of total retinal detachment. These are broken down by description of the shape of the retinal configuration, that is, whether the anterior half of the retina has an expanded or a narrow-funnel appearance, and likewise for the posterior portion of the retina (Fig. 44). These are known as narrow/narrow, wide/wide, and so on. The best diagnoses of these configurations are made ultrasonographically.

The treatment of stage V ROP is in flux. Instrumentation has had to change dramatically to accommodate the small eyes of infants. In Fig. 45, a small 27-gauge pick–forceps (Storz Ophthalmic Products, St. Louis, MO, U.S.A.) is shown passing through the eye of a needle. Figure 46 shows a 0.5-mm scissors and a new instrument known as a vitreous dissector, which is a vitreous cutter with a small scoop at the tip (Storz). This instrument is also 25 gauge and enables delicate removal of the proliferations in ROP. Our preferred approach is anteriorly through the corneal limbus (Fig. 47). We can achieve excellent dilation with the use of small iris retractors that are made of flexible materials (Grieshaber, Bern, Switzerland). We place an anterior chamber angled infusion cannula especially designed for pediatric use to provide infusion (Fig. 47A) (Grieshaber). The anterior chamber

infusion cannula tends to protect the cornea, as well as the underlying pars plana epithelium and ciliary epithelium that can be detached, and directly communicates with the subretinal space. The lens is removed by a combination of cutting and aspiration with the standard 20-gauge vitreous cutter (Fig. 47D). We use Balanced Salt Solution infusion without addition for infusion fluid and keep the infusion pressure low to promote good retinal perfusion. A bimanual technique is used to delaminate the membranes from the retinal surface. In these cases, we place the pick–forceps and membrane peeler–cutter into the eye to facilitate the delamination (Fig. 48A,B). Scleral depression is used to expose the peripheral trough that can be opened with the membrane peeler–cutter (Fig. 48C,D). (See also Chapter 15 by S. Charles and B. Wood.)

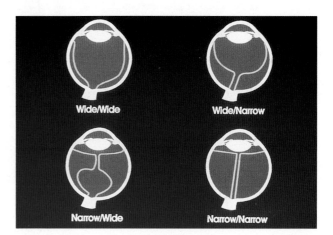

FIG. 44. International classification of total retinal detachment (stage V) showing anatomic configurations of wide/wide and narrow/narrow. The most uncommon of these presentations is the narrow-anterior/wide-posterior configuration. Usually, the configurations are much more complex than is shown in these photos, and these photos do not emphasize the peripheral architecture adequately.

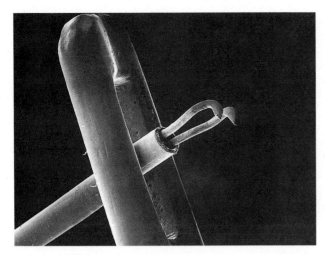

FIG. 45. Scanning electron micrograph of a tiny 30-gauge pick–forceps being passed through the eye of a needle.

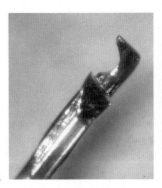
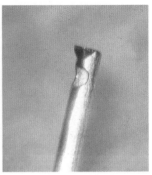

FIG. 46. Small scissors (**A**) and membrane dissector (**B**), 25-gauge (0.5 mm). Note the small tip at the end for engaging tissue.

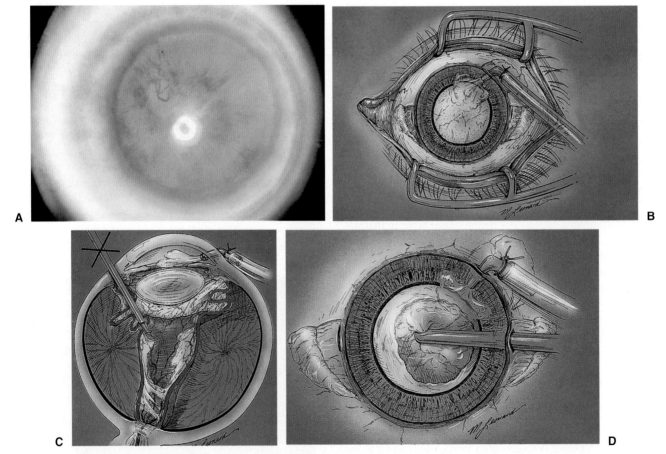

FIG. 47. Current vitreous surgical approach used by the authors. **A:** Typical appearance of stage V retinopathy of prematurity requiring vitreous surgery. **B:** An infusion cannula into the anterior chamber that is angled and sutured with a single suture through the limbus. Small, limited conjunctival peritomies are made at the 3 and 9 o'clock positions to gain access to the 12 and 6 o'clock positions equally. **C:** Demonstrated is why the pars plana or pars plicata approach is not recommended in certain cases where there is severe peripheral traction with folding of the retina. Often there can be detached ciliary body epithelium that communicates with the subretinal space that can easily be torn when entering posterior to the iris (see Figs. 27 and 28). Although anterior iris entry can be difficult because of poor pupillary dilation, new iris retractors have facilitated this approach. **D:** The lens being removed by a combination of aspiration and irrigation. (From de Juan E, Machemer R. *Retina* 1987;7:63–69, with permission.)

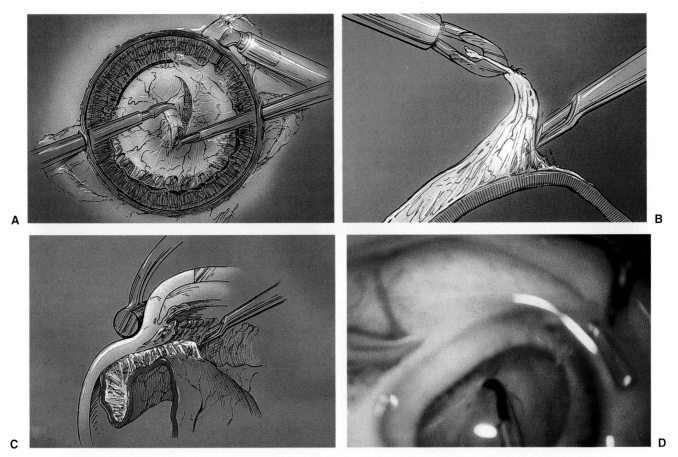

FIG. 48. Once the lens has been removed, the bimanual technique is used to grasp the preretinal tissue, and scissors are used to delaminate the membranes from the retinal surface (**A**). **B:** Artist's conception of bimanual surgery showing delamination of anterior membrane. **C:** Drawing demonstrating peripheral scleral depression allowing access to the trough. (Note that the trough is filled with vitreous and fibrous tissues.) **D:** Surgical microscope photograph showing the use of scleral depression to expose the peripheral trough for opening with the scissors. (From de Juan E, Machemer R. *Retina* 1987;7:63–69, with permission.)

Surgical success can be achieved. The postoperative anatomic success is highly dependent on the preoperative anatomy, and open-funnel detachments have the best chance for success (Fig. 49). Once the traction is released, the retina can settle into place, but the retinal vessels often become atrophic, and typically any lipid beneath the retina gradually resorbs over a period of a year or so. Most cases do not develop total retinal reattachment, but have either peripheral or posterior retinal detachment evident. In those cases where the funnel can be expanded but not fully reattached, vision typically does not return, although exceptions exist. Failures are usually due to fibrous proliferation, in addition to inadequate primary removal of tissue. Secondary causes of failure, such as creating retinal breaks, are disastrous in ROP surgery.

As stated previously, the surgical success rate is highly dependent on the preoperative configuration (Figs. 50 and 51). Surgery in eyes with active disease often leads to failure (Fig. 52). The Cryo-ROP Cooperative Group study recently reported on the long-term results of the structural status and visual function at $5^1/_2$ years of age for 128 eyes of 98 infants who participated in the multicenter clinical trial in whom total retinal detachment developed from ROP by the 3-month study examination. The group found that at least partial retinal attachment was present at $5^1/_2$ years in 21% compared with 28% at 1 year of age (difference not significant). All except one of the eyes tested at $5^1/_2$ years had vision limited to light perception or had no light perception, regardless of whether a vitrectomy had been performed. Only one eye that underwent vitrectomy had minimal pattern vision. This poor visual outcome suggests that the emphasis should be placed on prevention of retinal detachment in premature infants (Quinn et al. 1996c). According to our experience, approximately 11% of our patients with total retinal detachment will develop hand-motion or better vision (Fig. 53). This visual improvement correlates highly with the presence of retinal attachment, although there are some so-called visual successes even when the retina is detached. Similarly, patients who lose light perception after the operation are much more likely to have retinas that are detached than attached. Those infant eyes with both wide/anterior and wide/posterior retinal detachments (shallow detachments) have a much better

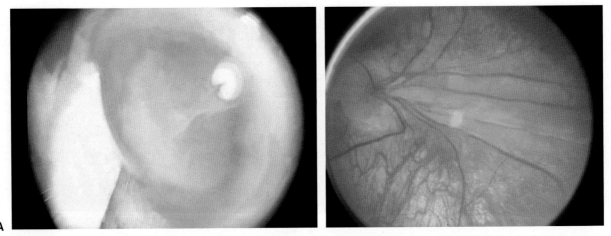

FIG. 49. Preoperative (**A**) and postoperative (**B**) views of a patient with open-funnel detachment and a good postoperative result.

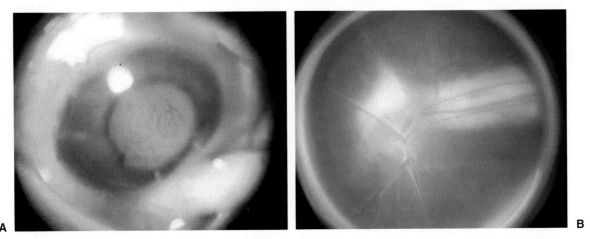

FIG. 50. A,B: A patient with more severe anterior scarring, with a reasonable postoperative result. (Note the atrophy of the retinal vessels and the presence of subretinal lipid.) Subretinal lipid will resorb over a period of months.

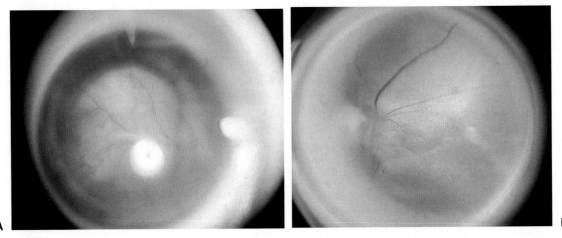

FIG. 51. Preoperative (**A**) and postoperative (**B**) views of patients with open-funnel retinal detachment with inadequate release of traction leading to an expanded posterior funnel appearance with improved configuration, but not yet retinal attachment.

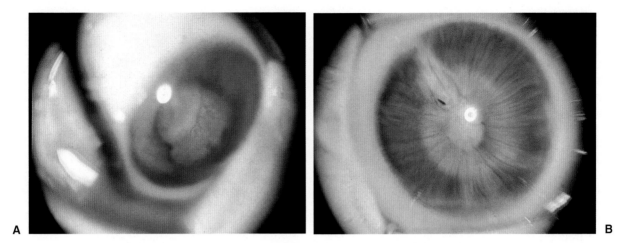

FIG. 52. A: Preoperative appearance of a patient with active disease. (Note the rather prominent neo-vascularization behind the lens and some hemorrhage.) **B:** The postoperative result was complicated by severe scarring leading to failure.

prognosis, with approximately 50% of these eyes achieving some posterior attachment (Fig. 54). This success decreases anatomically, so that narrow/narrow configurations result in retinal reattachment in fewer than 20% of the cases. The visual results are also better in these wide-open funnel configurations.

At present, we do not have great enthusiasm for vitreous surgery of closed-funnel detachments, particularly those with flat anterior chambers with glaucoma, the presence of subretinal blood, or failed vitreous surgery (Fig. 54). Because these eyes have such a poor prognosis, usually no therapy is recommended. Similarly, if one eye has full resolution of its ROP and the other eye has a partial retinal detachment, we will often recommend scleral buckling. However, if the eye progresses to a very narrow funnel configuration such that the success rate is low and the necessary aphakia results in another visual handicap, we will often not recommend any surgery. We believe correction of the aphakia is of

paramount importance to allow the rapidly developing visual system to develop. Intensive contact lens therapy appears to be the mode of operation that is most preferred by our pediatric ophthalmology staff, although epikeratophakia can result in excellent results as well. Postoperative glaucoma is rare, probably occurring in fewer than 5% of the cases. Although it has been suggested to be a cause of visual loss, we have not seen it often with our approach.

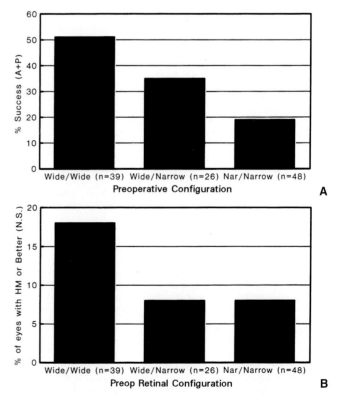

FIG. 54. With regard to anatomic success (*vertical axis*), a wide/wide-funnel configuration is much more likely to lead to postoperative success (**A**), as well as visual success (**B**), than is a narrow/narrow-funnel configuration (p = 0.02).

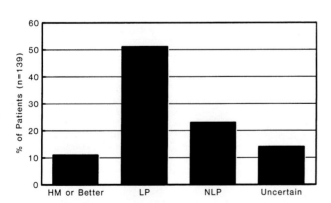

FIG. 53. Graphical representation of surgical results for stage V retinopathy of prematurity. (Data from Jack Zillis, M.D., Devers Eye Institute; and Eugene de Juan, Jr., M.D., and Robert Machemer, M.D.) We are able to obtain visual results of hand motions (HM) or better in approximately 11% of patients. LP, light perception; NLP, no light perception.

It should be noted that the major reason for failure in treatment of infants with ROP is noncompliance with the screening and follow-up needed. The infants who suffer from ROP nowadays are smaller and sicker than ever before. Nonocular medical problems, however, should be no means delay the screening examination and the treatment needed, which can easily be accomplished since the treatment nowadays can be performed with topical anesthesia only and as a curb-side procedure. This is of paramount importance, because timely screening and treatment of ROP is necessary to prevent the dreadful results of this blinding disease, and incomplete and delayed treatment might not have optimal results in preventing an unfavorable outcome. Another important pitfall is many infants are lost for follow-up upon discharge from the nursery. It is still not clear who is responsible for the continued follow-up of the infants upon discharge from the nursery. It has been suggested to include an order for an eye examination on the standard admission order form, to use computerized data, such as an admission summary noting the need for ROP screening in infants that meet the standard criteria, and to include a screening eye examination as a requirement on the discharge checklist in the nurseries (Trainor et al. 1988 and 1989). In addition, we recommend that ophthalmologists screening infants and scheduling a follow-up examination document in writing the responsibility of the nursery for keeping up the appointment.

REFERENCES

Benner JD, Morse LS, Hay A, Landers MB III. A comparison of argon and diode photocoagulation combined with supplemental oxygen for the treatment of retinopathy of prematurity. *Retina* 1993;13:222–229.

Campbell K. Intensive oxygen therapy as a possible cause of retrolental fibroplasia: a clinical approach. *Med J Aust* 1951;2:48–50.

Capone A, Diaz-Rohena R, Sternberg P, Mandell B, Lambert M, Lopez PF. Diode-laser photocoagulation for zone 1 threshold retinopathy of prematurity. *Am J Ophthalmol* 1993;116:444–450.

Committee for the Classification of Retinopathy of Prematurity. The international classification of retinopathy of prematurity. *Arch Ophthalmol* 1984;102:1130–1134.

Cryotherapy for Retinopathy of Prematurity Cooperative Group. Multicenter trial of cryotherapy for retinopathy of prematurity: preliminary results. *Arch Ophthalmol* 1988;106:471–479.

Cryotherapy for Retinopathy of Prematurity Cooperative Group. Multicenter trial of cryotherapy for retinopathy of prematurity: 3-month outcome. *Arch Ophthalmol* 1990a;108:195–204.

Cryotherapy for Retinopathy of Prematurity Cooperative Group. Multicenter trial of cryotherapy for retinopathy of prematurity: 1-year outcome—structure and function. *Arch Ophthalmol* 1990b;108:1408–1416.

Cryotherapy for Retinopathy of Prematurity Cooperative Group. Multicenter trial of cryotherapy for retinopathy of prematurity: $3^1/_2$-year outcome—structure and function. *Arch Ophthalmol* 1993;111:339–344.

Cryotherapy for Retinopathy of Prematurity Cooperative Group. Multicenter trial of cryotherapy for retinopathy of prematurity: Snellen visual acuity and structural outcome at $5^1/_2$ years after randomization. *Arch Ophthalmol* 1996;114:417–424.

de Juan E Jr., Machemer R. Retinopathy of prematurity. Surgical technique. *Retina* 1987; 7:63–69.

de Juan E Jr., Shields S, Machemer R. The role of ultrasound in the management of retinopathy of prematurity. *Ophthalmology* 1988;95:884–888.

Drack AV, Burke JP, Pulido JS, Keech RV. Transient punctate lenticular opacities as a complication of argon laser photocoagulation in an infant with retinopathy of prematurity. *Am J Ophthalmol* 1992;113:583–584.

Fielder AR, Robinson J, Shaw DE, Ng YK, Moseley MJ. Light and retinopathy of prematurity: does retinal location offer a clue? *Pediatrics* 1992;89:648–653.

Fleming TN, Ringe PE, Charles ST. Diode laser photocoagulation for prethreshold, posterior retinopathy of prematurity. *Am J Ophthalmol* 1992;114:589–592.

Gibson DL, Sheps SB, Hong Uh S, Schechter MT, McCormick AQ. Retinopathy of prematurity-induced blindness: birth weight-specific survival and the new epidemic. *Pediatrics* 1990;86:405–412.

Goggin M, O'Keefe M. Diode laser for retinopathy of prematurity: early outcome. *Br J Ophthalmol* 1993;77:559–562.

Hunter DG, Repka MX. Diode laser photocoagulation for threshold retinopathy of prematurity: a randomized study. *Ophthalmology* 1993;100:238–244.

Iverson DA, Trese MT, Orgel IK, Willimans GA. Laser photocoagulation for threshold retinopathy of prematurity [Letter]. *Arch Ophthalmol* 1991;109:1342–1343.

Kivlin JD, Biglan AW, Gordon RA, et al. Early retinal vessel development and iris vessel dilatation as factors in retinopathy of prematurity. Cryotherapy for Retinopathy of Prematurity (CRYO-ROP) Cooperative Group. *Arch Ophthalmol* 1996;114:150–154.

Landers MB III, Semple HC, Ruben JB, Serdahl C. Argon laser photocoagulation for advanced retinopathy of prematurity. *Am J Ophthalmol* 1990;110:429–430.

Landers MB III, Tooth CA, Semple HC, Morse L. Treatment of retinopathy of prematurity with argon laser photocoagulation. *Arch Ophthalmol* 1992;110:44–47.

Laser ROP Study Group. Laser therapy for retinopathy of prematurity. *Arch Ophthalmol* 1994;112:154–156.

Machemer R. Description and pathogenesis of late stages of retinopathy of prematurity. *Ophthalmology* 1985;92:1000–1004.

Margolis TI, Duker JS, Reichel E, Puliafito CA. Indirect diode laser photocoagulation for threshold and posterior prethreshold retinopathy of prematurity. *Invest Ophthalmol Vis Sci* 1994;35(Suppl):1443(ARVO abst).

McNamara JA, Tasman W, Brown GC, Federman JL. Laser photocoagulation for stage 3+ retinopathy of prematurity. *Ophthalmology* 1991;98:576–580.

McNamara JA, Tasman W, Vander JF, Brown GC. Diode laser photocoagulation for retinopathy of prematurity: preliminary results. *Arch Ophthalmol* 1992;110:1714–1716.

Noorily S, et al. *Ophthalmology* 1992;99:263–268.

Patz A. The role of oxygen in retrolental fibroplasia. *Pediatrics* 1957;19:504–524.

Preslan MW. Laser therapy for retinopathy of prematurity. *J Pediatr Ophthalmol Strabismus* 1993;30:80–83.

Pogrebniak AE, Bolling JP, Stewart MW. Argon laser-induced cataract in an infant with retinopathy of prematurity. *Am J Ophthalmol* 1994;117:261–262.

Quinn GE, Dobson V, Barr CC, et al., on behalf of the Cryotherapy for Retinopathy of Prematurity Cooperative Group. Visual acuity of eyes after vitrectomy for retinopathy of prematurity: follow-up at $5^1/_2$ years. *Ophthalmology* 1996a;103:595–600.

Quinn GE, Miller DL, Evans JA, Tasman WE, McNamara JA, Schaffer DB. Measurement of Goldman visual fields in older children who received cryotherapy as infants for threshold retinopathy of prematurity. *Arch Ophthalmol* 1996b;114:425–428.

Quinn GE, Dobson V, Barr CC, et al., on behalf of the Cryotherapy for Retinopathy. Visual acuity of eyes after vitrectomy for retinopathy of prematurity: follow-up at $5^1/_2$ years. *Ophthalmology* 1996c;103:595–600.

Reese AB, Blodi F. Retrolental fibroplasia. *Am J Ophthalmol* 1951;34:1–24.

Seiberth V, Linderkamp O, Knorz MC, Liesenhoff H. A controlled clinical trial of light and retinopathy of prematurity. *Am J Ophthalmol* 1994;118:492–495.

Seiberth V, Linderkamp O, Vardarli I, Knorz MC, Liesenhoff H. Diode laser photocoagulation of threshold retinopathy of prematurity in eyes with tunica vasculosa lentis. *Am J Ophthalmol* 1995a;119:748–751.

Seiberth V, Linderkamp O, Vardarli I, Knorz MC, Liesenhoff H. Diode laser photocoagulation for stage 3+ retinopathy of prematurity of Prematurity Cooperative Group. *Graefes Arch Clin Exp Ophthalmol* 1995b;233:489–494.

Tasman W. Threshold retinopathy of prematurity revisited [Editorial]. *Arch Ophthalmol* 1992;110:623–633.

Terry TL. Extreme prematurity and fibroblastic overgrowth of persistent vascular sheath behind each crystalline lens. I. Preliminary report. *Am J Ophthalmol* 1942;25:203–204.

Trainor S, White GL, Trunnell E, Kivlin JD. Compliance with a standard of care for retinopathy of prematurity in one neonatal intensive care unit. *J Pediatr Ophthalmol Strabismus* 1988;25:237–239.

Trainor S, White GL, Kivlin FD, Thiese SM, Trunnell E. Follow up retrospective study of compliance with a standard of care for retinopathy of prematurity in one neonatal intensive care unit. *J Pediatr Ophthalmol Strabismus* 1989;26;285–287.

Practical Atlas of Retinal Disease and Therapy, Second Edition
edited by William R. Freeman,
Lippincott–Raven Publishers, Philadelphia © 1997.

· 19 ·

Retinal Arterial Obstructive Disease

Gary C. Brown

Arterial obstructive diseases affecting the circulation in the retina are discussed in descending order in this chapter, from the large arterial vessels emanating from the aorta to the terminal retinal arterioles. The subcategories include

1. Ocular ischemic syndrome
2. Ophthalmic artery obstruction
3. Central retinal artery obstruction
4. Central retinal artery–vein obstruction
5. Branch retinal artery obstruction
6. Cotton-wool spots

OCULAR ISCHEMIC SYNDROME

In 1963, Kearns and Hollenhorst described "venous stasis retinopathy," the posterior segment manifestations seen with severe carotid artery obstructive disease. They noted this abnormality in approximately 5% of their patients with carotid artery obstructive disease. Other authors have since used the term "venous stasis retinopathy" to signify mild (nonischemic) central retinal vein obstruction. Because of this confusion in the literature, the term preferred by the Retina Vascular Unit at Wills Eye Hospital for the ocular symptoms and signs occurring secondary to severe carotid artery obstruction is the *ocular ischemic syndrome.*

The ocular ischemic syndrome is most often caused by carotid artery obstruction, although chronic ophthalmic artery, and rarely central retinal artery, obstructions can also cause a similar clinical picture. Atherosclerosis is the most common etiology, although giant cell arteritis and other inflammatory diseases causing arteritis can also be responsible. Eisenmenger's syndrome has also been implicated, indicating that diffuse systemic ischemia can also play an etiologic role.

Flow within an artery is not usually substantially affected unless there is at least a 70% obstruction. With most cases of the ocular ischemic syndrome, there is at least a 90% ipsilat-eral carotid artery obstruction. In up to 50% of cases, there may be a complete ipsilateral carotid artery obstruction. The obstruction is most commonly located at the bifurcation of the common carotid into the internal and external carotids, but can be located anywhere from the aortic arch distally (Fig. 1).

Involvement is bilateral in 90% of cases, and men comprise about two-thirds of cases. The mean age is 65 years, and most patients are over the age of 50. No racial predilection has been identified. The exact incidence is unknown, but is probably at least in the range of 7–8 per million patients per year.

Symptoms

Approximately 90% of patients relate a history of visual loss that is typically gradual, occurring over a period of weeks or longer, but is abrupt in about 12% of cases. In this latter instance, a cherry-red spot may be seen, indicating more acute retinal ischemia. Amaurosis fugax is present in about 10% of cases.

An intermittent, dull aching pain is found in about 40% of cases. Patients generally localize it to the orbital area of the affected eye. The pain has been called "ocular angina" and may occur secondary to ischemia to the globe, increased intraocular pressure from neovascular glaucoma, ipsilateral dural ischemia, or a combination of these mechanisms.

Prolonged visual recovery following exposure to bright light is also a symptom frequently experienced by patients with the ocular ischemic syndrome.

Signs

Collateral vessels on the forehead can sometimes be seen in patients with the ocular ischemic syndrome, and these vessels most often shift blood from the external carotid system

G. C. Brown, M.D.: Department of Ophthalmology, Thomas Jefferson University; and Retina Vascular Unit, Wills Eye Hospital, Philadelphia, PA 19107

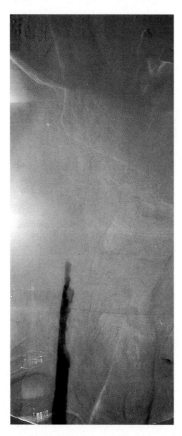

FIG. 1. Carotid arteriogram in a patient with an ipsilateral ocular ischemic syndrome. There is a 100% common carotid artery obstruction.

on one side to that on the side with severe carotid artery obstruction (Fig. 2).

The visual acuity in ocular ischemic syndrome eyes is highly variable. About 35% of affected eyes have 20/20 to 20/40 vision at the time of discovery, although at the end of a year over 70% of eyes have counting-fingers vision or

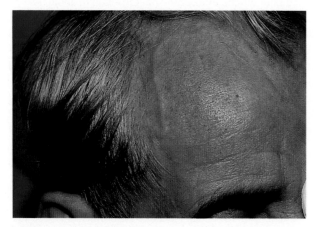

FIG. 2. Collateral vessels traversing from the right external carotid system to the left external carotid arterial system in an eye with a left internal carotid artery obstruction and the ocular ischemic syndrome.

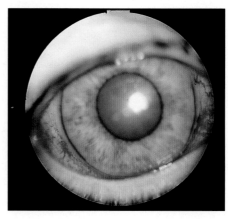

FIG. 3. Rubeosis iridis (iris neovascularization) is an eye with the ocular ischemic syndrome. The eye is injected and the new vessels are most pronounced nasally and temporally in region of the anterior chamber angle.

worse. About 30% initially have 20/50 to 20/400 vision, and 35% have counting-fingers vision or worse.

Anterior segment: Rubeosis iridis is seen in about two-thirds of eyes at the time of presentation of the ocular ischemic syndrome (Fig. 3). Accompanying ciliary injection is often seen when the intraocular pressure is elevated. Despite the prevalence of iris neovascularization, only one-half of these eyes (one-third of all patients) have an increase in intraocular pressure. In some cases, the anterior chamber angle can actually be closed by fibrovascular tissue, and the intraocular pressure is normal or low because of impaired ciliary body perfusion and decreased aqueous production. It should be remembered that after carotid endarterectomy the ciliary body perfusion can improve, but the anterior chamber angle still remains closed. In these instances, the intraocular pressure can rise acutely, with severe accompanying pain.

Flare is present in the majority of eyes with iris neovascularization, but there is also an anterior chamber cellular response in 20% of ocular ischemic syndrome eyes that is usually mild and rarely accompanied by large keratic precip-

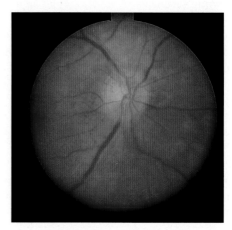

FIG. 4. Ocular ischemic syndrome fundus reveals dilated, but not tortuous, retinal veins.

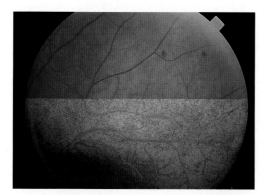

FIG. 5. Retinal hemorrhages in the midperiphery of an ocular ischemic syndrome eye.

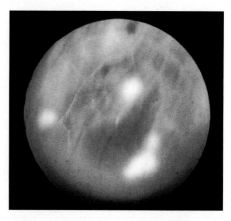

FIG. 7. A: Hyperfluorescence occurring secondary to neovascularization of the retina in an ocular ischemic syndrome. Retinal capillary nonperfusion can be seen inferiorly, peripheral to the retinal neovascularization.

itates. Cataracts can occur in eyes with the advanced ocular ischemic syndrome, but are not usually a prominent feature of the earlier stages.

Posterior segment: Retinal arterial narrowing is commonly present in ocular ischemic syndrome eyes. The retinal veins are usually dilated (Fig. 4) and may be beaded. Retinal tortuosity is typically *not* a feature of the ocular ischemic syndrome and is more commonly seen with central retinal vein obstruction, in which there is an outflow obstruction.

Retinal hemorrhages, which are found in about 80% of affected eyes, are usually dot and blot and are most commonly located on the midperiphery (Fig. 5).

Neovascularization of the optic disc (Fig. 6) is encountered in about 35% of eyes, and neovascularization elsewhere in the retina (Fig. 7) is seen in about 8% of eyes. Rarely, the neovascularization can become sufficiently severe to cause traction retinal detachment. Retinal capillary nonperfusion can be seen with fluorescein angiography (Fig. 7).

Microaneurysms are often present, most commonly in the retinal periphery. In the posterior pole, they can leak and contribute to macular edema. The macular edema is often more pronounced with fluorescein angiography (Fig. 8) than clinically, and marked cystic changes are usually absent. Telangiectatic vascular changes may also be present.

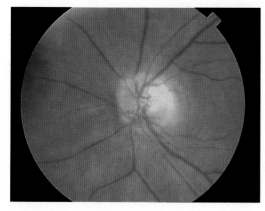

FIG. 6. Neovascularization of the optic disc in an ocular ischemic syndrome eye.

Cotton-wool spots are occasionally found, as are spontaneous retinal arterial pulsations. The latter are most pronounced over the optic disc and extend to 1–2 disc diameters from the edge of the disc. Although spontaneous retinal arterial pulsations are also seen with cardiac disease and increased intraocular pressure, their presence in a person over the age of 50 should strongly arouse suspicion of the ocular ischemic syndrome.

If spontaneous retinal arterial pulsations are not present, light digital pressure on the lid will often induce them. This is not usually the case with central retinal vein obstruction and can be a helpful differentiating feature between the two diseases.

Ischemic optic neuropathy, characterized by acute visual loss and optic disc swelling, can rarely be seen. Retinal pigment epithelial disturbance is not typically a feature of the ocular ischemic syndrome.

Ancillary Tests

Fluorescein angiography reveals delayed filling of the choroid in approximately 60% of ocular ischemic syndrome eyes (Fig. 9). Normally, the choroid is completely filled within 5 seconds of the first appearance of dye within it. Delayed retinal arteriovenous transit time (the time from the first appearance of dye within the temporal retinal arteries until the corresponding retinal veins are completely filled; normally less than 11 seconds) is found in 95% of affected eyes, but is not as specific for the ocular ischemic syndrome as is delayed choroidal filling. It can also be seen with central retinal artery obstruction or central retinal vein obstruction. Staining of the retinal vessels (Fig. 10), often more so the arteries than the veins, is seen in about 85% of ocular ischemic syndrome eyes, probably due to endothelial cell ischemia.

Electroretinography often reveals diminution of the amplitudes of the a and b waves (Fig. 11), corresponding to the

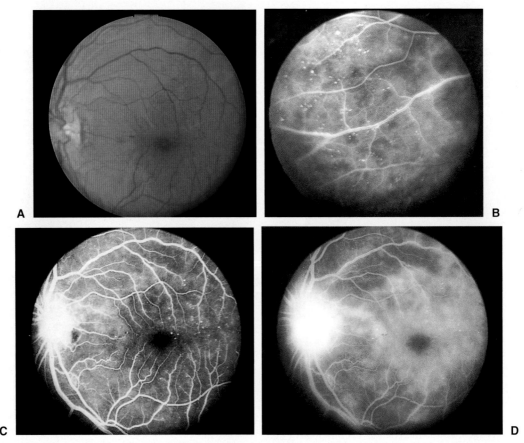

FIG. 8. A: Macular cyst in an ocular ischemic syndrome eye of a patient with an ipsilateral 100% internal carotid artery obstruction. The visual acuity was 20/40. **B:** Fluorescein angiogram of the eye shown in A at 70 seconds after injection reveals hyperfluorescence due to numerous retinal microaneurysms. **C:** Microaneurysms can be seen in the macula at 78 seconds after injection. **D:** At 446 seconds after injection, there is marked intraretinal leakage of dye, as well as hyperfluorescence of the optic disc.

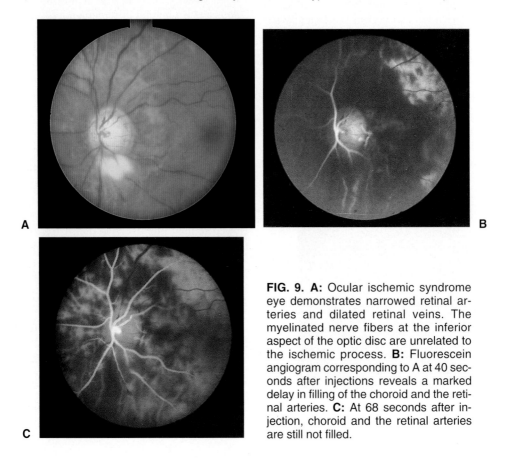

FIG. 9. A: Ocular ischemic syndrome eye demonstrates narrowed retinal arteries and dilated retinal veins. The myelinated nerve fibers at the inferior aspect of the optic disc are unrelated to the ischemic process. **B:** Fluorescein angiogram corresponding to A at 40 seconds after injections reveals a marked delay in filling of the choroid and the retinal arteries. **C:** At 68 seconds after injection, choroid and the retinal arteries are still not filled.

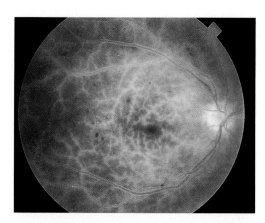

FIG. 10. Late fluorescein angiogram of an eye with the ocular ischemic syndrome reveals staining of the retinal vessels.

outer and inner retinal ischemia, respectively. Histopathologic evaluation reveals damage to both the inner and outer retinal layers (Fig. 12).

Carotid noninvasive tests (ultrasonography and Doppler testing) are approximately 90% accurate in detecting a carotid artery stenosis of 50% or greater and can be used for screening in suspected cases. Digital subtraction angiography and magnetic resonance angiography can be employed as confirmatory tests. In instances where the carotid arteries appear normal with noninvasive testing, color Doppler ultrasonography of the eye and orbital vessels can be helpful in detecting an underlying ophthalmic artery obstruction.

Associated Systemic Diseases

As might be expected, there is a high prevalence of diseases associated with systemic atherosclerosis in patients with the ocular ischemic syndrome. Over half have diabetes mellitus, and nearly half have ischemic cardiac disease. Approximately one-quarter of patients have had a previous cerebrovascular accident, and almost one-fifth have required peripheral bypass surgery prior to the discovery of the ocular ischemic syndrome.

The 5-year mortality rate in patients with the ocular ischemic syndrome is 40%. Despite a stroke rate of 4% per year, the leading cause of death is cardiac disease.

Treatment

Local therapy for the ocular ischemic syndrome is usually temporizing. Eyes with iris neovascularization and an open anterior chamber angle can be considered for laser panretinal photocoagulation, which is successful in eradicating the new vessels in about 35% of cases.

Although no clinical trials have evaluated surgical therapy for vision in the ocular ischemic syndrome, carotid endarterectomy appears to be beneficial for maintaining an improving vision in some cases. Unfortunately, once rubeosis iridis is present, over 90% of eyes are legally blind at the end of 1 year, with or without surgery.

Overall, carotid endarterectomy has been proven to be of benefit in preventing disabling stroke in symptomatic patients (those with amaurosis fugax, hemispheric transient ischemic attack, or nondisabling stroke) with 70%–99% carotid artery stenosis. As compared with a control group using aspirin, the North American Symptomatic Carotid Endarterectomy Trial Collaborators found that the stroke rate among endarterectomy patients at 2 years was 9%, whereas the stroke rate was 26% in the control group. For symptomatic patients with an associated 0–29% carotid artery stenosis, carotid endarterectomy has not been shown to be beneficial for preventing stroke, when compared with treatment with aspirin. In asymptomatic patients with a carotid artery stenosis of 60% or greater, the stroke rate at 5 years is approximately 10% in patients treated with aspirin, versus 5% in those treated with endarterectomy.

When a 100% carotid artery stenosis is present, a thrombus usually propagates distally, usually precluding successful endarterectomy. In such instances, extracranial to in-

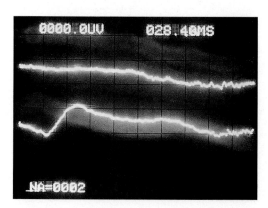

FIG. 11. Electroretinogram of an ocular ischemic syndrome eye in the *top tracing* discloses diminution of the amplitudes of both the a and b waves. The normal *bottom tracing* was taken in the unaffected contralateral eye.

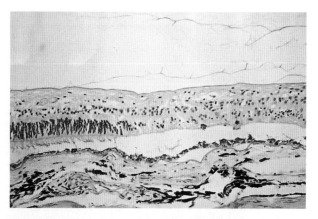

FIG. 12. Light-microscopic section of the retina from an ocular ischemic syndrome eye reveals loss of cellularity of the ganglion cell layer (inner retinal ischemia), as well as photoreceptor loss (outer layer ischemia). The retinal pigment epithelium is intact. Hematoxylin–eosin, ×40. (Courtesy of Dr. W. Richard Green, Wilmer Eye Institute.)

tracranial bypass (for example, superficial temporal artery to middle cerebral artery) has been attempted. While it may transiently help the vision, at 1 year there appears to be no advantage over observation. Additionally, this procedure has been shown in a clinical trial not to be more beneficial than aspirin in preventing stroke.

ACUTE OPHTHALMIC ARTERY OBSTRUCTION

Approximately 5%–10% of cases of acute central retinal artery obstruction are probably, in reality, acute ophthalmic artery obstruction, which is characterized by sudden severe visual loss. Light perception is often lost, and there is marked opacification of the retina in the macular region and more peripherally (Fig. 13). In some eyes, the whitening is so severe that there is ischemic opacification of the retinal pigment epithelium and choroid. Approximately 30% of cases lack a cherry-red spot, in 40% it is questionable, and in the remaining 30% it is present.

Fluorescein angiography often reveals choroidal perfusion defects in addition to delayed arteriovenous transit time. In the later phases, there may be focal or generalized staining of the retinal pigment epithelium (Fig. 14).

Because of the choroidal ischemia, often long-term retinal pigment epithelium changes can occur in both the posterior pole and the peripheral fundus.

The etiologies are similar to those for acute central retinal artery obstruction. In particular, giant cell arteritis should be considered in patients over the age of 55.

Treatment is generally unsatisfactory.

CENTRAL RETINAL ARTERY OBSTRUCTION

In 1859, von Graefe reported the case of a patient with endocarditis who experienced an acute central retinal artery obstruction. By the beginning of the 20th century, over two dozen cases of retinal arterial obstruction had appeared in the

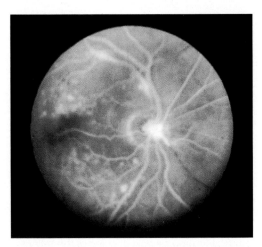

FIG. 14. Areas of focal staining at the level of the retinal pigment epithelium in an eye with an acute ophthalmic artery obstruction.

literature. Some of the mechanisms responsible for central retinal artery obstruction include embolization, thrombus (including under atherosclerotic plaque), dissecting aneurysm, hypertensive arterial necrosis, spasm, and inflammation.

Clinical Features

Patients with acute central artery obstruction typically relate a history of abrupt, painless, unilateral visual loss occurring over a period of seconds. Some may have a previous history of amaurosis prior to the episode of several visual loss.

The visual acuity in eyes with central retinal artery obstruction is usually in the counting-fingers to hand-motions range unless a patent cilioretinal artery supplies the foveola. In most instances, at least a temporal island of vision remains. An afferent pupillary defect can appear within seconds after the development of the obstruction.

Fundus examination discloses superficial whitening of the

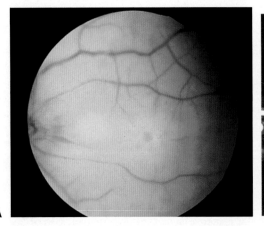
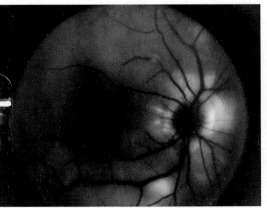

FIG. 13. A: Acute ophthalmic artery obstruction. Marked retinal opacification, due to inner and outer retinal layer ischemia, is present and no cherry-red spot can be seen. **B:** Fluorescein angiogram corresponding to A reveals lack of dye in the retinal arteries and only peripapillary filling in the choroid.

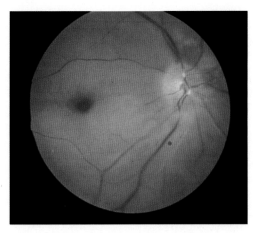

FIG. 15. Acute central retinal artery obstruction. Superficial retinal opacification is present and a cherry-red spot can be seen in the foveola. Larger retinal emboli, suggestive of the calcific variant, can be seen on the optic disc.

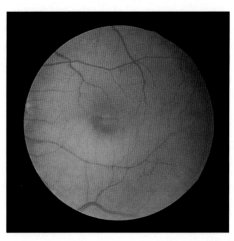

FIG. 17. Cholesterol embolus (Hollenhorst plaque) in a retinal branch artery in the temporal macula.

retina that is most pronounced in the macular region (Fig. 15). The whitening typically develops within hours, although in the primate model it can develop within minutes with complete obstruction. In the foveola, where the retina is only 0.1 mm thick, a cherry-red spot can be seen. Segmentation of the blood column, or "boxcarring," is present in severe obstructions in both the retinal arteries and the retinal veins. In approximately 10% of eyes, a patent cilioretinal artery supplies the foveola (Fig. 16). In these instances, the visual acuity improves to 20/50 or better in 80% of eyes over a period of weeks.

Emboli (Figs. 15 and 17) are seen within the retinal arterial system in approximately 20%–40% of eyes with central retinal artery obstruction. Calcific emboli, from the cardiac valves, are usually large and white and have a greater tendency to cause obstruction than do smaller, yellow, glistening cholesterol emboli (Hollenhorst plaques). Some other forms of emboli reported include platelet-fibrin thrombi,

corticosteroids, and white blood cell aggregates (leukoemboli).

An evaluation should be undertaken to ascertain the cause of the central artery obstruction. Among the more common underlying associated abnormalities are carotid artery obstructive disease, cardiac valvular disease, collagen vascular disease, and coagulopathy. A more complete list of abnormalities associated with central retinal artery obstruction is presented in Table 1. A similar workup should be considered for patients with acute ophthalmic artery obstruction, for those with branch retinal artery obstruction, and in cases of cotton-wool spots in which no underlying cause is obvious.

Treatment

No treatment has been shown to be consistently effective for improving vision in eyes with acute central retinal artery obstruction. Ocular massage, anterior chamber paracentesis, inhalation treatment with a combination of oxygen and carbon dioxide, antithrombolytic agents via the carotid system and intravenously, and oral vasodilators have all been tried without convincing success.

The upper time limit for any treatment modality is uncertain. Animal studies have suggested that the window of opportunity is less than 2 hours. Nevertheless, in the clinical situation, in which there is often some limited flow through the obstructed artery, visual improvement has been seen clinically as late as 3 days after obstruction. In the Retina Vascular Unit at Wills Eye Hospital, ocular massage and anterior chamber paracentesis are still generally performed if the obstruction is less than 24 hours in duration..

Approximately 18% of eyes with central retinal artery obstruction will progress to develop iris neovascularization, usually at 1–3 months after the obstruction, with a mean time of 6 weeks after the obstruction. Thus, for the first 1–3 months, these eyes should be followed relatively frequently. If iris neovascularization develops, laser panretinal photoco-

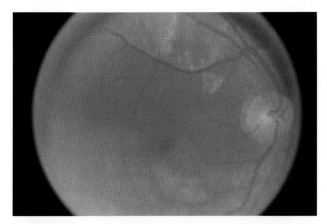

FIG. 16. Central retinal artery obstruction with cilioretinal arterial sparing of the foveola. The visual acuity improved to 20/20.

TABLE 1. *Disease entities associated with central retinal artery obstruction*

Abnormalities contributing to embolus formation
    Systemic arterial hypertension (via atherosclerotic plaque formation; can also cause hypertensive necrosis)
    Carotid artery atherosclerosis
    Cardiac valvular disease
        Rheumatic
        Mitral valve prolapse
    Thrombus after myocardial infarction
    Cardiac myxoma
    Tumors
    Intravenous drug abuse
    Lipid emboli (also possible white blood cell emboli)
        Pancreatitis
        Purtscher's retinopathy
    Loiasis
    Radiologic studies
        Carotid arteriography
        Lymphangiography
        Hysterosalpingography
    Head and neck corticosteroid injection
    Retrobulbar corticosteroids
    Deep vein thrombobis (via paradoxical embolus)

Trauma
    Retrobulbar injection
    Orbital fracture repair
    Anesthesia
    Penetrating injury
    Drug-induced and/or alcohol-induced stupor
    Nasal surgery

Coagulopathies
    Sickle hemoglobinopathies
    Homocystinuria
    Oral contraceptives

    Pregnancy
    Platelet and/or factor abnormalities
    Lupus anticoagulants
    Protein S deficiency
    Protein C deficiency
    Antithrombin III deficiency

Ocular conditions associated with retinal arterial obstruction
    Prepapillary arterial loops
    Optic disc drusen
    Increased intraocular pressure (with sickling hemoglobinopathy)
    Toxoplasmosis
    Optic neuritis

Collagen vascular diseases
    Systemic lupus erythematosus
    Polyarteritis nodosa
    Giant cell arteritis
    Wegener's granulomatosis
    Liebow's lymphoid granulomatosis

Other vasculitides
    Orbital mucormycosis
    Radiation retinopathy
    Behçet's disease

Miscellaneous associations
    Ventriculography
    Fabry's disease
    Sydenham's chorea
    Migraine
    Hypotension
    Fibromuscular hyperplasia
    Nasal oxymethazalone use
    Lyme disease

Modified from Brown GC. Retinal arterial obstructive disease. In: Ryan SJ, ed. *Retina.* Baltimore: CV Mosby, 1994: 1361–1377, with permission.

agulation successfully achieves regression in about 65% of cases and will likely reduce progression to neovascular glaucoma. If iris neovascularization is present at the time of the acute central retinal artery obstruction, carotid artery obstructive disease and the ocular ischemic syndrome should be suspected. In these instances, severe carotid artery obstruction can lead to neovascular glaucoma and an intraocular pressure that exceeds the perfusion pressure in the central retinal artery.

Giant cell arteritis accounts for approximately 1% of cases of acute central retinal artery obstruction. If the disease is suspected, evaluating the erythrocyte sedimentation rate should be considered, since the second eye can develop a central retinal artery obstruction within hours of the first. Prompt administration of high-dose corticosteroids should be considered when giant cell arteritis is suspected, probably more so to protect the second eye than to help the first.

CENTRAL RETINAL ARTERY–VEIN OBSTRUCTION

Patients with combined central retinal artery–vein obstruction typically relate a history of abrupt visual loss and present with the clinical features of both entities. The visual acuity is usually in the counting-fingers to hand-motions range, and the fundus examination findings are characterized by superficial retinal whitening, a cherry-red spot, dilated and tortuous retinal veins, retinal hemorrhage, and retinal edema (Fig. 18). The prognosis for visual recovery is poor,

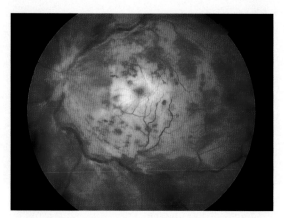

FIG. 18. Central retinal artery–vein obstruction in the eye of a 20-year-old woman with systemic lupus erythematosus.

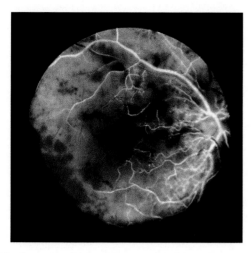

FIG. 19. Severe retinal capillary nonperfusion in an eye with a central retinal artery–vein obstruction.

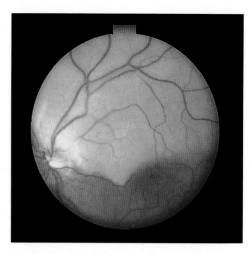

FIG. 20. Branch retinal artery obstruction.

and effective treatment for the improvement of visual acuity is lacking.

The pathophysiologic mechanisms that lead to this entity are unclear. One acute case has been reported in which there was histopathologic obstruction in both the central retinal artery and vein. The artery obstruction can occur prior to obstruction in the vein, the vein obstruction can occur prior to the artery obstruction, or both can present simultaneously to clinicians.

Systemic associations encountered with acute central retinal artery–vein obstruction are similar to those seen with acute central retinal artery obstruction. Nonetheless, almost one-quarter of reported cases occur secondary to complications from retrobulbar injection at the time of ocular surgery.

Fluorescein angiography most often reveals severe retinal capillary nonperfusion (Fig. 19). The macular retina is often markedly thickened clinically, although in many instances there does not appear to be substantial leakage of dye, probably because of shutdown of much of the retinal vascular bed.

BRANCH RETINAL ARTERY OBSTRUCTION

Branch retinal artery obstruction causes acute visual field loss in distribution corresponding to the impaired retina. Although the central visual acuity may be decreased, it often improves to 20/20 as the zone of hypoxia at the border of the obstruction improves.

Fundus examination in eyes with acute branch retinal artery obstruction reveals superficial retinal opacification in the affected area (Fig. 20). The systemic workup is essentially similar to that for eyes with central retinal artery obstruction.

One variant of branch retinal artery obstruction is cilioretinal artery obstruction. Cilioretinal arteries are derived from the short posterior ciliary arteries, either directly or via the choroid. Most commonly, a cilioretinal artery enters the fundus on the optic disc separately from the central retinal

artery or its branches. Three variants of cilioretinal artery obstruction have been described:

1. Isolated cilioretinal artery obstruction.
2. Cilioretinal artery obstruction in conjunction with central retinal vein obstruction.
3. Cilioretinal artery obstruction in association with anterior ischemic optic neuropathy.

Eyes with isolated cilioretinal artery obstruction demonstrate superficial retinal opacification in the distribution of the obstructed vessel (Fig. 21). The visual acuity returns to 20/40 or better in 9% of cases.

In eyes with cilioretinal obstruction and central retinal vein obstruction, there is superficial retinal opacification in the distribution of the obstructed artery and features of central retinal vein obstruction, including retinal hemorrhage, dilated retinal veins, and retinal edema. Approximately 70% of these eyes will improve to a vision of 20/40 or better.

It is not surprising that anterior ischemic optic neuropathy can be associated with cilioretinal artery obstruction since both abnormalities occur secondary to obstruction of vessels derived from the posterior ciliary circulation. Ophthalmoscopically, there is superficial retinal opacification in associ-

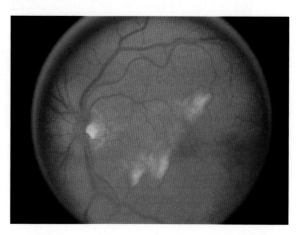

FIG. 21. Isolated cilioretinal artery obstruction.

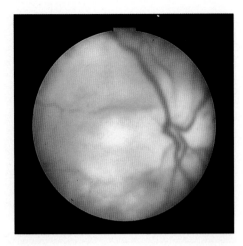

FIG. 22. Cilioretinal artery obstruction associated with anterior ischemic optic neuropathy in a patient with giant cell arteritis.

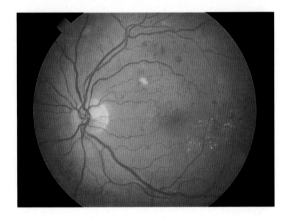

FIG. 23. Cotton-wool spot superotemporal to the optic disc in the eye of a patient with diabetic retinopathy.

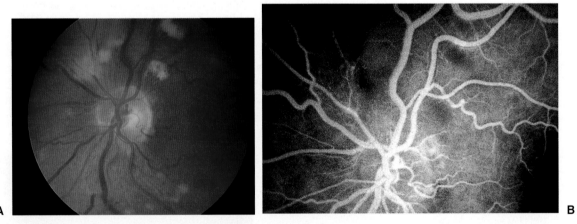

FIG. 24. A: Multiple cotton-wool spots in the eye of a patient with metastatic carcinoma. A superonasal branch retinal artery obstruction is also present. **B:** Fluorescein angiogram of A reveals areas of hypofluorescence corresponding to the cotton-wool spots.

ation with optic disc swelling (Fig. 22). The visual acuity in these eyes typically remains in the 20/400 range of worse. In these instances, the possibility of giant cell arteritis should be considered as an underlying cause.

Cotton-wool Spots

A cotton-wool spot appears clinically as an area of superficial retinal whitening less than one-quarter disc area in size (Fig. 23). Cotton-wool spots are typically located in the peripapillary region or along the retinal vascular arcades. Often they are multiple (Fig. 24).

Diabetic retinopathy is the leading cause of cotton-wool spots, and approximately 32%–44% of patients with diabetic retinopathy have them. When known diabetics are excluded, eyes with a fundus appearance characterized by the presence of at least one cotton-wool spot, or a predominance of cotton-wool spots, will have an associated systemic disease in about 95% of cases. In theses cases, undiagnosed diabetes mellitus accounts for about 20% of cases, and systemic arterial hypertension accounts for another 20%, as does collagen vascular disease. With cases of systemic arterial hypertension, the diastolic blood pressure in adults is usually at least in the range of 110–115 mm Hg.

Other causes of cotton-wool spots include AIDS retinopathy, cardiac valvular disease, and carotid artery obstructive disease. A more complete list of entities causing cotton-wool spots is presented in Table 2. Theoretically, any etiologic abnormality associated with retinal arterial obstruction can also be encountered with cotton-wool spots.

TABLE 2. *Disease entities associated with cotton-wool spots*

Diabetes mellitus
Systemic arterial hypertension
Collagen vascular diseases
   Systemic lupus erythematosus
   Dermatomyositis
   Polyarteritis nodosa
   Scleroderma
   Giant cell arteritis
Cardiac valvular disease
   Mitral valve prolapse
   Rheumatic heart disease
   Endocarditis
Acquired immunodeficiency syndrome
Leukemia
Trauma
Radiation retinopathy
Central retinal artery obstruction (partial)
Retinal venous obstruction
Metastatic carcinoma
Leptospirosis
Rocky Mountain spotted fever
High-altitude retinopathy
Severe anemia
Acute blood loss
Papilledema
Papillitis
Carotid artery obstruction
Dysproteinemias
Septicemia
Aortic arch syndrome (pulseless disease)
Intravenous drug abuse
Acute pancreatitis
Onchocerciasis

From Brown GC, et al. Cotton-wool spots. *Retina* 1985;5:206–214, with permission.

BIBLIOGRAPHY

Atebara NH, Brown GC, Cater J. Efficacy of anterior chamber paracentesis and carbogen in treating acute nonarteritic central retinal artery obstruction. *Ophthalmology* 1995;102:2029–2034.

Brown GC. Retinal arterial obstructive disease. In: Ryan S, ed. *Retina.* Baltimore: CV Mosby, 1994:1361–1377.

Brown GC, Magargal LE. Central retinal artery obstruction and visual acuity. *Ophthalmology* 1982;89:14–19.

Brown GC, Shields JA. Cilioretinal arteries and retinal arterial occlusion. *Arch Ophthalmol* 1979;97:84–92.

Brown GC, Magargal LE. The ocular ischemic syndrome: clinical, fluorescein angiographic and carotid angiographic features. *Int Ophthalmol.*

Brown GC, Magargal LE, Shields JA, Goldberg RE, Walsh PN. Retinal arterial obstruction in children and young adults. *Ophthalmology* 1981;88:18–25.

Brown GC, Moffat K, Cruess A, Magargal LE, Goldberg RE. Cilioretinal artery obstruction. *Retina* 1983;3:182–187.

Brown GC, Brown MM, Hiller T, Fischer D, Benson WE. Cotton-wool spots. *Retina* 1985;5:206–214.

Brown GC, Magargal LE, Sergott R. Acute obstruction of the retinal and choroidal circulations. *Ophthalmology* 1986;93:1371–1382.

European Carotid Surgery Trialists' Collaborative Group. European carotid surgery trial interim results for symptomatic patients with severe (70–99%) or with mild (0–29%) carotid stenosis. *Lancet* 1991;337:1235–1243.

Karjalainen K. Occlusion of the central retinal artery and retinal branch arterioles. *Acta Ophthalmol Suppl* 1971;109:5–96.

Kearns TP, Hollenhorst RW. Venous-stasis retinopathy of occlusive disease of the carotid artery. *Mayo Clin Proc* 1963;38:304–312.

North American Symptomatic Carotid Endarterectomy Trial Collaborators. Beneficial effect of carotid endarterectomy in symptomatic patients with high-grade carotid stenosis. *N Engl J Med* 1991;325:445–453.

Sivalingam A, Brown GC, Magargal LE. The ocular ischemic syndrome. II. Mortality and systemic morbidity. *Int Ophthalmol* 1990;13:187–191.

Sivalingam A, Brown GC, Magargal LE. The ocular ischemic syndrome. III. Visual prognosis and the effect of treatment. *Int Ophthalmol* 1991;15:15–20.

Practical Atlas of Retinal Disease and Therapy, Second Edition
edited by William R. Freeman,
Lippincott–Raven Publishers, Philadelphia © 1997.

· 20 ·

Submacular Surgery

Antonio Capone, Jr., and Paul Sternberg, Jr.

Laser photocoagulation is the treatment of choice for most eyes harboring choroidal neovascularization (CNV) located juxtafoveally (close to the fovea) or extrafoveally (outside of the fovea proper). Retina overlying CNV is destroyed along with the CNV. In many eyes, CNV is subfoveal. Submacular surgery evolved as an alternative method for treating subfoveal CNV (and submacular hemorrhage) with the hope of preserving the fovea.

Patients with CNV caused by age-related macular degeneration (ARMD) and ocular histoplasmosis (OH) comprise the vast majority of submacular surgical candidates. Additional conditions that may benefit from submacular surgery include idiopathic CNV, and CNV complicating multifocal choroiditis, punctate inner choroidopathy (PIC), toxoplasmic chorioretinitis, and traumatic macular choroidal rupture. To date, all published reports on submacular surgery—both evacuation of subretinal hemorrhage and excision of choroidal neovascular membranes—are of uncontrolled studies, neither prospective nor randomized, with limited data regarding long-term visual outcome. A prospective, randomized, and controlled multicenter clinical trial of submacular surgery (the Submacular Surgery Trial) is currently in progress.

Most conditions amenable to submacular surgery are commonly encountered. This chapter provides an overview of submacular surgical techniques, relevant anatomic considerations, recent advances, and future horizons.

TECHNIQUE

Subfoveal Choroidal Neovascularization

A pars plana vitrectomy is performed, and the posterior hyaloid is detached if a posterior vitreous separation is not already present (Fig. 1). Usually the retina is separated from the underlying CNV due to fluid exuded by the neovascular complex (that is, neurosensory detachment). When there is little or no neurosensory detachment, fluid is injected beneath the retina to separate the retina from the CNV and to establish a "working space" between the photoreceptors and retinal pigment epithelium (RPE). The CNV is then gently separated from the surrounding retina and RPE with a subretinal spatula, grasped with a forceps, and extracted through the retinotomy. The infusion bottles are elevated during removal of the neovascular complex and for several minutes thereafter for hemostasis. A limited air–fluid exchange is performed at the conclusion of the procedure to assist in retinal reattachment.

Submacular Hemorrhage

In eyes with subretinal hemorrhage, tissue plasminogen activator (tPA) is injected beneath the retina (6 μg/0.1 ml, using up to approximately 50 μg), and 20 minutes or more are allowed to pass. Liquefied subretinal blood is aspirated. The neovascular complex is usually not visible, and thus not removed, in such cases.

CLINICAL AND ANATOMIC CONSIDERATIONS

Choroidal Neovascularization

Visual acuity often improves following excision of CNV caused by OH, PIC, or multifocal choroiditis. Conversely, experience to date suggests that eyes with exudative ARMD experiencing an initial improvement in vision generally go on to lose vision, even in the absence of recurrent neovascularization. Several investigators observed preservation of RPE following subfoveal CNV excision in eyes with histoplasmosis. However, excision of subfoveal CNV caused by ARMD almost invariably results in concomitant excision of a broad carpet of RPE (1). With loss of subfoveal RPE, there is loss of photoreceptor viability and atrophy of the choriocapillaris, analogous to atrophic ARMD.

A. Capone, Jr., M.D., and P. Sternberg, Jr., M.D., Department of Ophthalmology, Emory University, Atlanta, GA 30322.

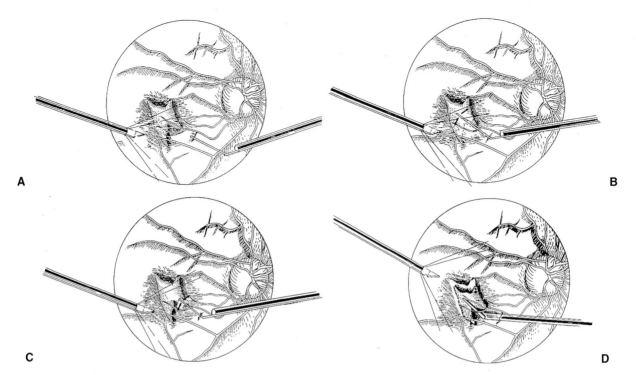

FIG. 1. Vitrectomy is performed and the posterior hyaloid elevated. **A:** Creation of retinotomy with microsurgical pick. **B:** Fluid dissection of the CNV from the overlying retinal photoreceptors. **C:** Separation of the CNV from surrounding RPE–Bruchs' membrane. **D:** The CNV is grasped with forceps and removed from beneath the macula.

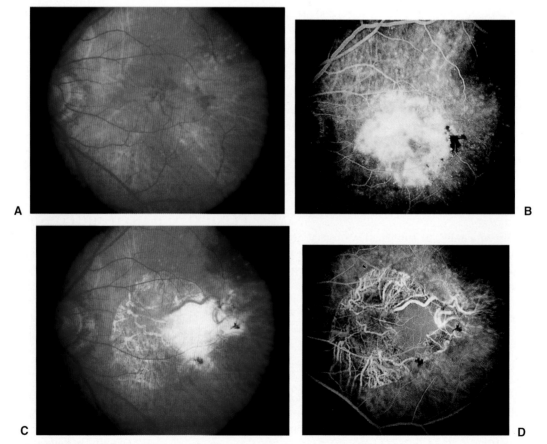

FIG. 2. Type 1 CNV-ARMD. **A:** Subfoveal CNV resulting in vision of 20/300. **B:** Fluorescein angiogram demonstrates a broad area of flat, ill-defined choroidal neovascularization. **C:** Visual acuity 1 month postoperatively was 20/100. By 18 months postoperatively (this figure), vision had dropped to 3/200. Note the broad area of loss of RPE. **D:** Choriocapillaris loss is angiographically apparent, with relative preservation of medium-caliber choroidal vessels outside the retinotomy site.

358

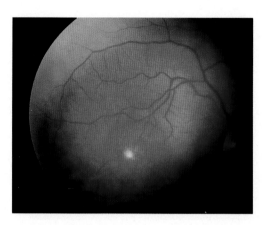

FIG. 3. Postoperative image of an eye after excision of histoplasmic type 2 CNV. Note the postoperative preservation of subfoveal retinal pigment epithelium outside of the hypopigmented CNV ingrowth site. Vision at 8 months postoperatively was 20/25.

Gass (2) provided histopathologic evidence gleaned from autopsy eyes to propose a classification scheme for CNV based on its position relative to the RPE. In type 1 CNV, typical of eyes with diffusely abnormal Bruchs' membrane and RPE (that is, ARMD), a flat plate of CNV insinuates itself between native RPE and Bruchs' membrane. In type 2 CNV, typical of eyes with a focal defect in the Bruchs' membrane–RPE complex but otherwise healthy RPE (that is, OH), a focus of CNV grows out through the focal defect from a stalk to lie on top of the native RPE, surrounded over time by "reactive" RPE. This theoretical construct reconciles the clinical experience of excision of a geographic area of native RPE overlying type 1 CNV (Fig. 2), with poor visual outcome, versus relative preservation of native RPE following excision of type 2 CNV (Fig. 3), often with favorable

outcome. Exceptions, of course, do occur (Fig. 4: type 2 CNV in ARMD).

The decision as to whether submacular surgery will provide a result superior to the natural history of the disorder can be perplexing. Eyes with well-defined type 2 CNV occasionally fare well without surgery (Fig. 5). As with photocoagulation, fluorescein angiography is useful in determining whether submacular surgery is feasible for a given eye—particularly in ARMD. At least some component of the CNV must be angiographically well defined in order for the surgeon to have an identifiable edge of the CNV. Eyes with ill-defined CNV (Fig. 6) or disciform features (Fig. 7) are not considered for submacular surgery. Long-standing cystoid macular edema associated with disciform-phase CNV precludes visual improvement, even after CNV removal and flattening of neurosensory detachment.

Submacular Hemorrhage

Ideal surgical candidates for evacuation of submacular hemorrhage have blood restricted to the space between the RPE and the outer retina (Fig. 8). Blood located beneath the RPE is not effectively liquefied by tPA, and removal of sub-RPE blood results in removal of overlying RPE. Visual outcome is best among eyes with hemorrhage restricted to within the arcades (3). Eyes with subretinal blood extending to the equator and beyond have little chance of attaining a visual acuity better than 9/200.

The timing of surgical evacuation of subretinal blood is an important determinant of visual outcome (4). Irreversible degenerative change occurs in the overlying retina in animal models within 24 hours, with moderate-to-severe outer retinal destruction at 3–7 days progressing to full-thickness retinal degeneration by day 14 (5,6). Prompt evacuation of sub-

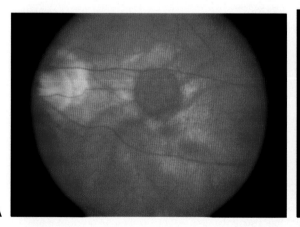
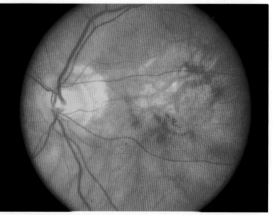

A   **B**

FIG. 4. Type 2 CNV in ARMD. **A:** Vision had dropped to 1/400 in the eye of this 74-year-old man with fine drusen, type 2 CNV, and a broad neurosensory detachment. **B:** One month following CNV excision, vision was 20/400. There was a small amount of residual subsensory blood. Finely stippled retinal pigment epithelium remains where the CNV had lain.

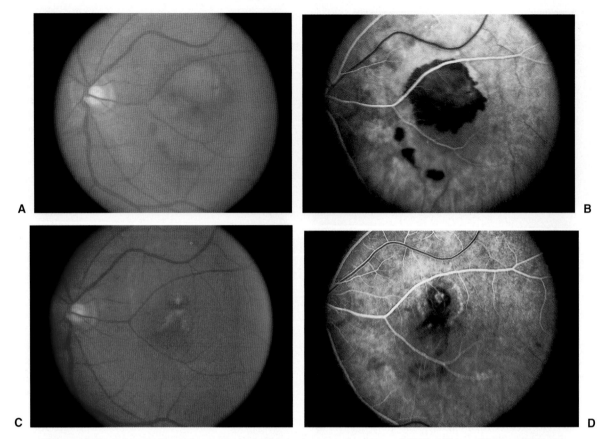

FIG. 5. A,B: Color photograph and fluorescein angiogram of an eye with idiopathic subfoveal CNV. Vision is 20/200. **C,D:** Several months later, the CNV has involuted and retracted to its extrafoveal ingrowth site. (Photographs are courtesy of Patrick Rubsamen, M.D., Bascom Palmer Eye Institute, Miami, FL.)

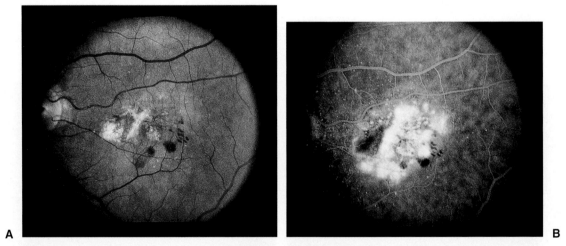

FIG. 6. A: Ill-defined choroidal neovascularization (CNV) caused by age-related macular degeneration, ineligible for submacular surgery. A prior photocoagulation scar is seen nasal to the fovea. White fibrotic features are present in the subfoveal component, with subsensory blood temporally. **B:** The photocoagulation scar at the nasal aspect of the lesion is hypofluorescent in this venous recirculation-phase angiographic frame, demonstrating diffuse ill-defined CNV-related hyperfluorescence.

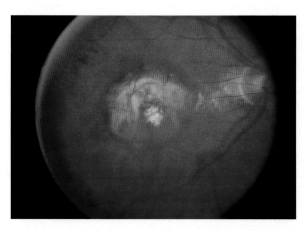

FIG. 7. Cicatricial-phase (disciform) choroidal neovascularization caused by age-related macular degeneration, ineligible for submacular surgery. A prior photocoagulation scar is seen centrally, with subsensory blood temporally.

macular hemorrhage is ideal, as intervention after seven days will likely offer only modest benefit.

COMPLICATIONS

Two changes in the macular milieu that occur in the setting of CNV have a practical impact on surgical technique and visual prognosis: cystoid macular edema and fibrin-related and/or photocoagulation-related retinal adhesion to CNV. Cystoid degenerative changes render the fovea vulnerable to iatrogenic macular hole (*blowout*) due to the increase in subretinal pressure, which occurs either during fluid-assisted separation (hydrodissection) of the retina from the subjacent neovascular complex or during irrigation of subretinal blood with a fibrinolytic agent. Incomplete separation of the overlying retina from underlying CNV or prior photocoagulation scar places the fovea at risk of avulsion (*pull through*) during subretinal CNV removal.

As with vitrectomy in general, development of nuclear sclerotic cataract is commonly accelerated postoperatively. Though dramatic, foveal blowout and pull through are rare surgical complications. Subretinal hemorrhage generally occurs intraoperatively, either due to iatrogenic choroidal trauma or when antiplatelet agents have not been discontinued prior to surgery. In most cases, raising the infusion bottles will prevent bleeding during CNV excision. In the event that bleeding does occur, fresh subretinal blood will often clot and may be removed manually after 5 minutes. Retinal detachment is usually seen postoperatively, typically as a consequence of tears close to the sclerotomy sites. The risk of vitreous incarceration and retinal tears related to a sclerotomy is increased when intraocular pressure (elevated for hemostasis) is not lowered prior to removal of intraocular instruments, as well as with attempted removal of a large subretinal clot or CNV via the sclerotomy.

As with photocoagulation, recurrent CNV plagues those who have undergone otherwise successful submacular surgery. The Submacular Surgery Trial will provide prospective data on this topic. It has been the experience of most surgeons active in this area that 1-year recurrence rates are on the order of 40%.

RECENT ADVANCES

The last several years have witnessed a decline in ocular morbidity in submacular surgical cases, due in part to advances in technique. The trend in anterior segment surgery in the last decade has been to reduce surgical incision size. Submacular surgery has evolved along similar lines, with design of subretinal surgical tools as fine as 36 gauge (7–9). The last several years have also witnessed a growing literature on the clot-specific fibrinolytic agent tPA. With new instruments and adjuncts, subretinal blood and choroidal neovascular membranes may be removed through incisions measured in fractions of a millimeter.

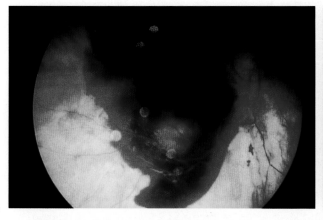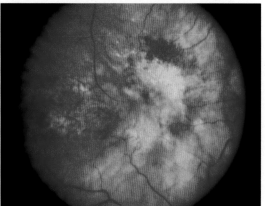

FIG. 8. A: Submacular hemorrhage caused by exudative age-related macular degeneration. **B:** One month after removal of the subretinal blood.

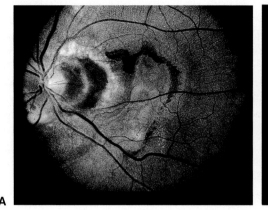
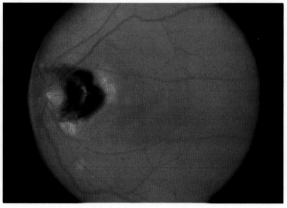

A   B

FIG. 9. A: Red-free photograph of histoplasmic CNV (at 5 o'clock relative to a hyperpigmented previously photocoagulated peripapillary CNV) extending beneath the fovea, with an associated neurosensory detachment and subsensory blood. Preoperative visual acuity was 3/400. Clinically, the CNV was well defined and plaquelike with a sharp, elevated edge. **B:** Visual acuity had improved to 20/40 by the time of this 3-week postoperative photograph. Note preservation of retinal pigment epithelium throughout the prior CNV bed.

OTHER CONDITIONS

Experience with other forms of CNV is limited. Peripapillary histoplasmic CNV extending beneath the fovea may fare well surgically, as CNV growth often occurs on the RPE surface, and RPE is often preserved following excision (Fig. 9). With the caveat that the numbers are small, eyes with idiopathic membranes behave similarly to eyes with exudative histoplasmic eyes with regard to both outcome and recurrence rate. The same appears to be true of eyes with CNV in association with inflammatory conditions such as toxoplasmosis (Fig. 10) and multifocal choroiditis/PIC. Little is known regarding recurrence rates for such conditions, because the number of cases to date is small. Outcome following excision of CNV complicating myopia and angioid streaks has been disappointing: visual results are poor and recurrences are common.

SUMMARY

Submacular surgery is vitreoretinal surgery's most exciting and controversial new frontier. Conditions amenable to surgical intervention are either focal (histoplasmosis, idiopathic CNV, and multifocal choroiditis/PIC) or diffuse (ARMD and pathologic myopia) with regard to pathologic changes of the RPE–Bruchs' membrane complex. Submacular surgery, though, is still in its infancy. The merits of such surgery are currently under study in the prospective, randomized, and controlled multicenter Submacular Surgery Trial.

ACKNOWLEDGMENTS

This work has been supported in part by a departmental grant from Research to Prevent Blindness, Inc., and a depart-

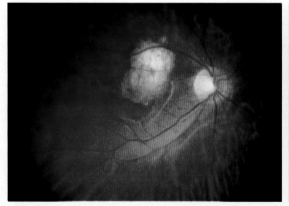
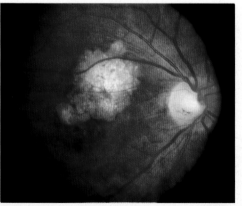

A   B

FIG. 10. A: This patient had bilateral toxoplasmic involvement of the macula. Surgery was performed on the better right eye when fixation was compromised by CNV with associated subsensory fluid and blood. Note the dense CNV pigmentation. **B:** One-year follow-up vision is 20/60 without recurrence. Again, RPE persists in the prior CNV bed.

mental core grant from the National Institutes of Health (P30 EY06360).

REFERENCES

1. Grossniklaus HE, Hutchinson AK, Capone A, Woolfson J, Lambert HM. Clinicopathologic features of surgically excised choroidal neovascular membranes. *Ophthalmology* 1994;101:1099–111.
2. Gass JMD. Biomicroscopic and histopathologic considerations regarding the feasibility of surgical excision of subfoveal neovascular membranes. *Am J Ophthalmol* 1994;118:285–298.
3. Lewis H. Intraoperative fibrinolysis of submacular hemorrhage with tissue plasminogen activator and surgical drainage. *Am J Ophthalmol* 1994;118:559–568.
4. Toth CA, Morse LS, Hjelmeland LM, Landers MB. Fibrin directs early retinal drainage after experimental subretinal hemorrhage. *Arch Ophthalmol* 1991;109:723–729.
5. Lewis H, Resnick SC, Flannery JG, Straatsma BR. Tissue plasminogen activator treatment of experimental subretinal hemorrhage. *Am J Ophthalmol* 1991;11:197–204.
6. Glatt H, Machemer R. Experimental subretinal hemorrhage in rabbits. *Am J Ophthalmol* 1982;94:762–773.
7. Thomas MA, Ibanez HE. Instruments for submacular surgery. *Retina* 1994;14:84–87.
8. Thomas MA, Lee CM, Pesin S, Lowe M. New instruments for submacular surgery. *Am J Ophthalmol* 1991;112:733–734.
9. Peyman GA, Lee KJ. A new subretinal forceps. *Retina* 1994;114:88–89.

Practical Atlas of Retinal Disease and Therapy, Second Edition
edited by William R. Freeman,
Lippincott–Raven Publishers, Philadelphia © 1997.

· 21 ·

Macular Holes and Other Surgical Macular Disorders

Serge de Bustros

This chapter reviews macular holes and other surgical macular disorders of the vitreoretinal interface. The emphasis is on macular holes in view of the exciting developments in the field; macular puckers and the vitreomacular traction syndrome are also discussed. Each of these three disorders is a distinct and separate clinical entity that is linked in some way to age-related vitreous syneresis.

MACULAR HOLES

Macular holes are circular full-thickness retinal defects affecting the central macula and causing significant visual loss. They can occur following blunt trauma, but most macular holes are idiopathic with no associated ocular pathology. Idiopathic macular holes appear to be more prevalent than previously thought. The highest incidence is in individuals in their seventh decade of life, with women being affected twice as often as men, although the sex difference diminishes with advancing age. The disease is bilateral in at least 10% of cases. When the first eye is affected, individuals with normal good vision in the fellow eye may not detect the visual loss right away and often discover the decreased vision upon covering the fellow eye. When the fellow eye develops a hole, patients will usually describe a sudden visual loss.

Our understanding of the pathogenesis of idiopathic macular holes is evolving. The current thinking is that most idiopathic macular holes start as a central dehiscence that gradually enlarges over a period of months until it reaches the size of approximately 500 μm or one-third of a disc diameter. As the hole enlarges, the visual acuity drops. Age-related vitreous syneresis and vitreous traction, primarily tangential vitreous traction exerted by a layer of cortical vitreous, appear to play an important role in the occurrence of the central de-

hiscence and its subsequent enlargement. Condensation of vitreous along with some cellular elements may form an opacity overlying the dehiscence termed pseudo-operculum.

Tangential vitreous traction initially results in foveal detachment, seen clinically as a yellow spot or yellow ring (Fig. 1); the yellow color may be due to alterations in the distribution of xanthophyll pigment. This stage is transient and may easily go unnoticed. Persistent tangential vitreous traction will usually result in dehiscence and full-thickness defect. Vitreous traction may be released spontaneously at the early stage, resulting in subsidence of signs and symptoms.

The diagnosis of fully developed macular holes is usually straightforward: there is a full-thickness circular retinal defect in the central macula with a surrounding cuff of subretinal fluid (Fig. 2). There usually is a variable amount of surrounding retinal detachment that extends beyond the cuff. There often are yellow deposits at the base of the macular hole. The hole usually measures a few hundred micrometers in diameter, and the visual acuity usually drops to 20/80 to 20/400. Patients will usually see an interruption in a thin slit beam of light focused on the macular hole corresponding to the retinal defect (positive Watzke–Allen sign). Fluorescein angiography shows an early bright hyperfluorescence (Fig. 3B), except in darkly pigmented individuals where it may be absent.

The diagnosis may be more difficult in early (smaller) macular holes when the visual acuity loss may be minimal (Fig. 3). In such cases, the slit-beam test is done with a very thin slit beam focused over the lesion. Fluorescein angiography will usually reveal a bright pinpoint hyperfluorescence. More sophisticated diagnostic methods, including ultrasonography and optical coherence tomography, may be useful when the diagnosis is in doubt.

The only possible treatment for macular holes is vitreous

S. de Bustros, M.D.: Department of Ophthalmology, Rush Medical College, Chicago, IL 60612; and Retina Center, Munster, IN 46321; and Illinois Retina Associates, Harvey, IL 60426.

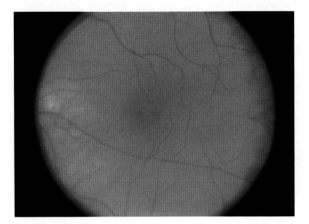

FIG. 1. Premacular hole with a yellow halo or ring. Visual acuity is 20/30.

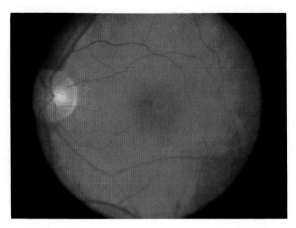

FIG. 3. Small macular hole. Visual acuity is 20/80.

surgery. Vitreous surgery for macular holes is still in its infancy, and the technique is still evolving at the time of this writing. The goals of the surgery are to relieve vitreous traction and perform a complete fluid–gas exchange followed by prone postoperative positioning of patients for a period ranging from 1 to several weeks. The ultimate goal of the surgery is to make the hole smaller, flatten the surrounding retina, and seal the edges of the hole. The benefit of surgery has been confirmed by a prospective randomized clinical trial.

A core vitrectomy is first done, followed by identification and removal of a layer of cortical vitreous from over the posterior pole. This layer is present in most cases unless the macular hole has been present for some time and spontaneous posterior vitreous detachment has occurred. The safest and most effective way to identify and remove the cortical vitreous is to use a suction method that can be combined with incision of the cortical vitreous by a sharp instrument. Various methods and instruments have been developed for this purpose, including a blunt cannula, a cannula with a soft flexible tip that can bend upon engaging the cortical vitreous

(fish-strike sign), or the vitrectomy probe itself placed on the suction mode. At present, the latter appears to be the most commonly used method probably because it is readily available, fast, and effective. The probe is placed in the peripapillary area and suction is applied (usually 150 mm Hg is sufficient, although a higher suction can be used). Striations from the instrument port engaging cortical vitreous will be visible (Fig. 4), or the Weiss ring will suddenly come off. The separation of the cortical vitreous is extended over the posterior pole and then excised with the vitrectomy probe. Every attempt is made to avoid direct suction over the macular hole for fear of damage, and no attempt is made to extend the peeling of the cortical vitreous to the anterior retina for fear of creating peripheral retinal breaks. The peripheral retina is then examined with the indirect ophthalmoscope and scleral indentation to look for iatrogenic peripheral tears, paying particular attention to the inferior retina. Retinal tears are treated with transconjunctival cryopexy or laser photocoagulation by using the indirect laser ophthalmoscope.

A complete fluid–gas exchange is then performed. As it

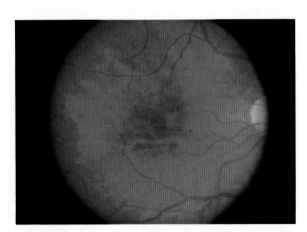

FIG. 2. Macular hole with a surrounding cuff of subretinal fluid. Notice the yellow deposits at the base of the hole. Visual acuity is 20/200.

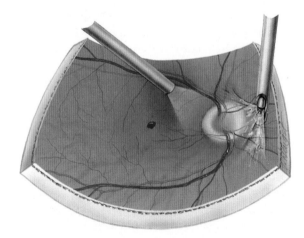

FIG. 4. Peeling of the cortical vitreous. The vitrectomy probe is placed on the suction mode and is positioned near the optic nerve; vitreous strands are drawn into the vitrectomy probe.

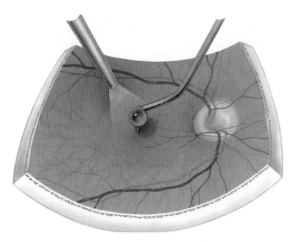

FIG. 5. Addition of pharmacologic agents. A drop of plasma is applied over the macular hole; this will be followed by a drop of thrombin. This is done after fluid–air exchange. Notice that the hole is usually smaller at this stage of the procedure.

turns out, after a complete fluid–gas exchange is done, waiting a few minutes will invariably lead to reaccumulation of fluid over the posterior pole, probably fluid originating at the vitreous base and trickling posteriorly. We therefore wait approximately 15 minutes and then go back inside the eye and aspirate more fluid. At this point, some surgeons will add adjuvants or cytokines over the macular hole to increase the likelihood of sealing the edges of the hole. I personally have been using a drop or two from the patient's plasma, followed by a drop or two of thrombin at a concentration of 100 units/ml (Fig. 5). We developed this concentration for control of intraocular bleeding in an animal model. In the presence of plasma, the thrombin forms a sticky fibrin plug that may aid in sealing of the hole. This method, which was first described by Dr. Mark Blumenkranz, is cheap and readily available, although its value remains unproven. An air–gas exchange is then performed by using a long-acting gas. I use a nonexpansile concentration of perfluoropropane gas

(C_3F_8). The surgery is then completed with closure of the incisions. The patient is then placed face down as soon as possible after surgery. I ask the patient to keep the face down most of the time for 2 weeks.

The anatomic and visual results of vitreous surgery for macular holes have steadily improved over the past few years probably because of case selection, improvement in surgical techniques, and patient compliance with postoperative prone positioning, and I now find the surgery to be quite rewarding in most instances.

Better preoperative visual acuity, smaller holes, and a shorter duration of macular holes appear to be good prognostic factors for good results. In successful cases, the visual acuity improves within 2 or 3 months, usually by three or more lines on the Snellen visual acuity chart, and the hole edges are sealed and hard to visualize; there might be some mild pigmentary changes in the fovea, and the rim of subretinal fluid subsides (Figs. 6 and 7). Interestingly, the preoperative central hyperfluorescence seen on angiography often disappears (Figs. 6 and 7). The importance of and techniques for postoperative prone positioning are discussed extensively with the patient and family preoperatively. The patient is urged to practice prone positioning at home in preparation for the difficult postoperative period.

A side effect of the surgery is the occurrence or progression of nuclear sclerotic cataracts. The pathogenesis of increased nuclear sclerosis remains undetermined. The risk factors for its occurrence appear to be similar to the risk factors of nuclear sclerosis following vitreous surgery for macular puckers (namely, older age and longer follow-up), although nuclear sclerosis following macular hole surgery appears earlier and seems to progress faster than after macular pucker surgery. Therefore, patients are counseled preoperatively about the need for cataract surgery and are counseled about lens implantation approximately 1 year after the macular hole surgery. I have seen macular holes reopen in conjunction with cystoid macular edema following cataract surgery, and therefore I ask the cataract surgeon to prescribe

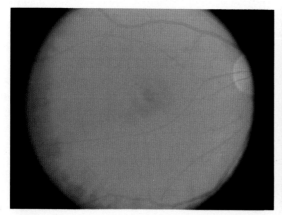
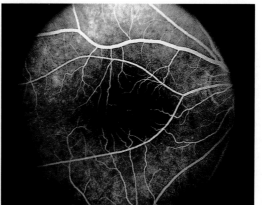

FIG. 6. A: Preoperative fundus photograph showing macular hole; visual acuity is 20/200. **B:** Preoperative fluorescein angiogram showing central hyperfluorescence corresponding to the macular hole.

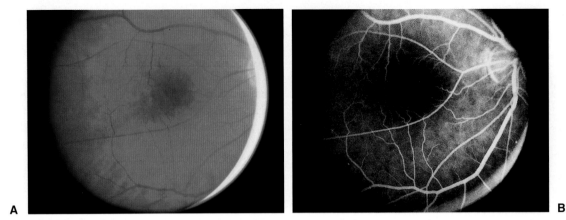

FIG. 7. A: Postoperative fundus appearance following successful macular hole surgery and cataract surgery with lens implantation. The macular hole edges are sealed. This patient had an unusually good visual result (visual acuity is 20/20). **B:** Postoperative fluorescein angiogram showing subsidence of central hyperfluorescence.

topical antiprostaglandins to decrease the incidence of postoperative cystoid macular edema.

Rhegmatogenous retinal detachment can complicate otherwise successful macular hole surgery. Unlike retinal tears following vitrectomy for other vitreoretinal disorders, the tears in this situation are usually in the inferior quadrants and are probably related to forceful separation of the cortical vitreous and extension of the separation anteriorly. These retinal detachments respond well to additional surgery, and interestingly they often do not seem to jeopardize closure of the macular hole. This complication can be lessened by avoiding anterior extension of the separation of the cortical vitreous and by careful intraoperative examination of the peripheral retina with scleral indentation, after separation of the cortical vitreous and before fluid–gas exchange.

As mentioned earlier, macular hole surgery is still in its infancy, and the list of complications will probably grow over time. For example, a recently described postoperative complication is loss of temporal peripheral visual field in some patients. The mechanism for this complication is unclear; it appears to be due to surgical trauma, possibly during forceful peeling of posterior cortical vitreous from the peripapillary area. Other complications include retinal pigment epithelium damage under the hole, phototoxicity, and enlargement of the macular hole causing further visual loss; the latter may occur intraoperatively and underscores the need to minimize manipulation of the hole itself. Microbial endophthalmitis and intraocular hemorrhage are complications common to all intraocular procedures.

There remain unanswered questions in macular hole surgery, including the need for removal of associated epiretinal membranes or internal limiting membrane, the duration of postoperative prone positioning, the use of pharmacologic agents to help seal the macular hole, the need to develop gentler methods to separate the posterior cortical vitreous, and so on. Some of these questions may remain unanswered, or there may be more than one way to achieve a good result, just as there are many different ways to repair a rhegmatogenous

retinal detachment. Future research should also focus on simplifying and shortening the patient's postoperative course.

All in all, the developments in macular hole surgery over the past few years are remarkable considering that this blinding disease was declared untreatable for so long; the next few years will undoubtedly reveal further refinement in surgical techniques and further progress in visual outcome. Macular hole surgery has improved our ability to identify and remove the cortical vitreous in other vitreoretinal diseases; it has also improved our ability to perform a more complete fluid–gas exchange.

MACULAR PUCKER

Macular pucker is a fairly common macular disorder characterized by the migration and proliferation of cells over the posterior pole; these cells secrete collagen and other extracellular material, resulting in an epiretinal membrane. The cells, which can be retinal pigment epithelial, fibrous astrocytes or myofibroblasts, often contract, resulting in retinal distortion: hence the term macular "pucker" (Fig. 8).

Epiretinal membranes can be secondary to a peripheral retinal disease such as retinal tear or retinal detachment, a retinal vascular disease such as branch retinal vein occlusion, inflammation, or trauma, or they can occur for no apparent reason (idiopathic). Idiopathic epiretinal membranes are often thin and translucent and can create an abnormal glistening sheen over the macula: hence the term "cellophane" maculopathy or "surface wrinkling" retinopathy (Fig. 9). Most idiopathic epiretinal membranes are mild and nonprogressive. In case of significant progression causing significant distortion and visual loss, surgical removal is considered. Epiretinal membranes occurring after retinal tear or retinal detachment repair are usually more prominent than idiopathic epiretinal membranes (Fig. 10); they can be pigmented and can obscure visualization of retinal vessels. In

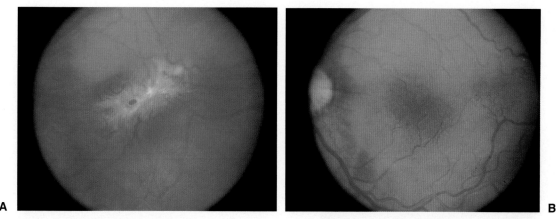

FIG. 8. A: Preoperative appearance of a macular pucker. Visual acuity is 20/100. Notice the presence of retinal striae and a small oval pseudomacular hole. **B:** Postoperative appearance following vitrectomy and removal of the macular pucker. Visual acuity is 20/50. The macula has regained a normal appearance.

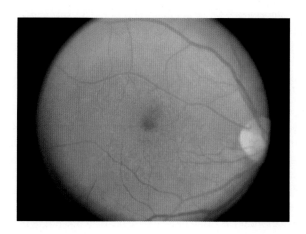

FIG. 9. Idiopathic epiretinal membrane (cellophane maculopathy). Visual acuity is 20/40 and has remained unchanged for five years.

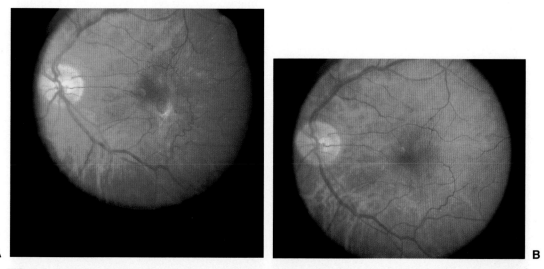

FIG. 10. A: Preoperative appearance of macular pucker secondary to successful retinal detachment surgery. Notice the retinal striae. Visual acuity is 20/40. The patient's has significant visual distortion. **B:** Postoperative appearance following vitrectomy and peeling of the macular pucker. Visual acuity is 20/20. The visual distortion has subsided.

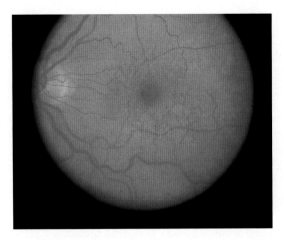

FIG. 11. Epiretinal membrane with a pseudomacular hole. Visual acuity is 20/30.

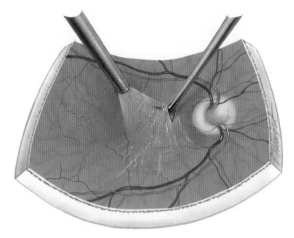

FIG. 13. A sharp vitreoretinal pick is used to create an edge that will be used to dissect and peel the thin epiretinal membrane.

this clinical setting, they can be described as a limited form of proliferative vitreoretinopathy.

The diagnosis of epiretinal membrane is made by ophthalmoscopy. A posterior vitreous separation is present in most cases. The fluorescein angiogram usually highlights the vascular distortion and may reveal some nonspecific leakage in the macula. The angiogram might also reveal an underlying disorder such as retinal vascular abnormalities secondary to a previous branch retinal vein occlusion.

An interesting variant of macular puckers is epiretinal membrane with pseudomacular holes, where a hole develops within the epiretinal membrane, giving the appearance of a macular hole (Fig. 11). Unlike macular holes, there is no surrounding halo or rim of subretinal fluid and the visual acuity is relatively good. The central defect may be oval (Fig. 12A). Fluorescein angiography often shows mild spotty hyperfluorescence but no bright transmission defect, which is seen in most patients with macular holes (Fig. 12B). Patients do not usually see an interruption in the slit-beam test, although there can be some bending or variation in the thickness of the beam.

Vitreous surgery can be considered in patients with significant visual loss or metamorphopsia. The surgical technique involves a core vitrectomy followed by peeling of epiretinal membrane. As mentioned earlier, most of these eyes have a posterior vitreous detachment. The peeling of the epiretinal membrane is usually done in two steps: creation of a good edge followed by grasping of the membrane with forceps to peel it from over the macula and remove it from the eye (Figs. 13 and 14). Sometimes there can be some difficulty in finding or creating an edge, and sometimes the membrane shreds in several pieces. Creation of an edge might require a sharp instrument such as a sharp micropick that the surgeon can slide over the retinal surface until an edge is engaged (Fig. 13). Thicker membranes are often easier to peel. The membrane is often more extensive than one might think. Immature membranes tend to be more friable and, whenever possible, it is helpful to wait 6–8 weeks before surgery is performed. This applies mainly to epiretinal membranes developing after treated retinal tears or retinal detachment surgery, where such membranes can be considered a limited form of proliferative vitreoretinopathy. Small retinal hemor-

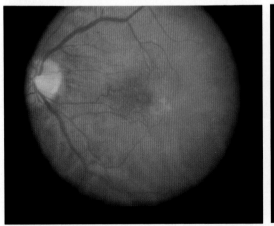
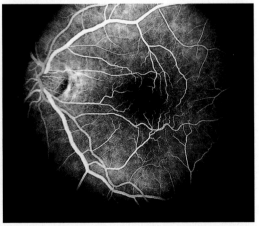

A   B

FIG. 12. A: Epiretinal membrane with a pseudomacular hole. The hole is oval. Visual acuity is 20/30. **B:** Fluorescein angiogram showing a faint transmission defect corresponding to the pseudomacular hole.

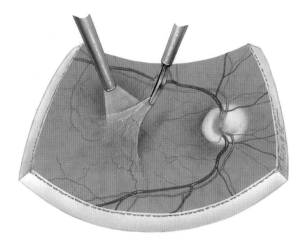

FIG. 14. A positive-action forceps is used to grasp the partially dissected epiretinal membrane and remove it from the eye. The membrane is often more extensive than is apparent.

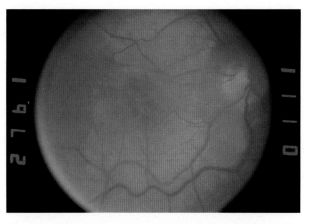

FIG. 15. Vitreomacular traction syndrome. Notice the traction in the superior peripapillary area and across the superior macula, creating a retinal fold. Visual acuity is 20/100.

rhages often occur during peeling of the membrane, and these usually clear within a few days without any adverse effect. There sometimes are white intraretinal deposits in the macula that may become apparent intraoperatively after peeling of the membrane; these presumably represent deposits from impaired axoplasmic flow, and they clear spontaneously within a few days of the surgery.

Most patients will experience a moderate visual improvement after surgery and a significant improvement in the metamorphopsia. The final visual acuity is often halfway between initial visual acuity and normal vision (Figs. 8 and 10). Good prognostic factors for visual recovery include better preoperative visual acuity and shorter duration of the macular pucker.

A side effect or complication of the surgery is the development or progression of nuclear sclerotic cataracts. The cause of this complication is unknown, and risk factors include older age and increased duration of follow-up. By 3 years after surgery, the majority of phakic eyes will develop significant nuclear sclerosis. Cataract surgery and lens implantation result in significant visual improvement in most cases. Recurrence of epiretinal membranes after surgery is rare, even though some fragments often remain after peeling.

In summary, epiretinal membranes causing macular pucker are a common disorder of the vitreomacular interface. Most of the time, the visual loss is mild and nonprogressive. In patients with significant visual loss or distortion, vitreous surgery can be used to peel the epiretinal membrane. Surgery usually results in modest visual improvement and significant improvement in the metamorphopsia.

VITREOMACULAR TRACTION SYNDROME

The vitreomacular traction syndrome is an uncommon disorder of the vitreoretinal interface characterized by incomplete posterior vitreous separation and vitreoretinal trac-

tion over the posterior pole, causing visual loss. The area of posterior vitreous attachment is thickened because of some cellular proliferation; it varies in shape and extent, and it often involves the peripapillary retina, sometimes resulting in a dumbbell configuration. Traction at the optic nerve may cause some elevation sometimes referred to as the "fleshy doughnut" sign (Fig. 15).

Examination of the fundus usually reveals a thin epiretinal membrane in the posterior pole. The mild-appearing pathology is often deceiving. Diagnosis is made with biomicroscopy and the use of a fundus lens such as a 78-diopter Volk lens; this will reveal partial posterior vitreous separation with visible vitreoretinal traction over the posterior pole. Fluorescein angiography often reveals mild nonspecific

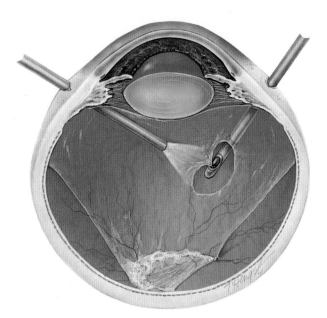

FIG. 16. A vitrectomy is done to relieve anteroposterior vitreous traction. Notice the thickened posterior cortical vitreous over the posterior pole.

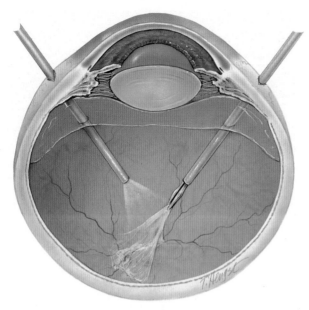

FIG. 17. The thickened posterior cortical vitreous is grasped with positive-action forceps and gently peeled over the macula.

leakage. Ultrasonography may be helpful in defining the configuration of the posterior vitreous.

Vitreous surgery should be considered in patients with significant visual impairment. The surgery involves relief of anteroposterior vitreous traction and peeling of the thickened posterior cortical vitreous (Fig. 16). A dissection plane is readily developed, and the thickened posterior cortical vitreous is then grasped with forceps and peeled over the macula (Fig. 17). Occasionally one encounters a strong attachment at the optic nerve head that is severed with the vitrectomy probe. Sometimes a thin epiretinal membrane is present under the thickened posterior cortical vitreous, and it should be peeled to maximize the visual improvement. Traction at the vitreous base should be minimized to avoid creation of peripheral retinal tears. Most patients will experience some visual improvement following surgery. Development or progression of nuclear sclerotic cataracts occurs at a rate similar to nuclear sclerosis following vitrectomy for macular pucker.

BIBLIOGRAPHY

Bluemenkranz MS. Adjuvant therapy for treating macular holes. *Vitreoretinal Surgery and Technology* 1995;7:5–8.

de Bustros S, and the Vitrectomy for Prevention of Macular Hole Study Group. Vitrectomy for prevention of macular holes: results of a randomized multi-center clinical trial. *Ophthalmology* 1994;101:1055–1060.

de Bustros S, Thompson JT, Michels RG, Enger C, Rice TA, Glaser BM. Nuclear sclerosis after vitrectomy for idiopathic epiretinal membranes. *Am J Ophthalmol* 1988;105:160–164.

de Bustros S, Rice TA, Michels RG, Thompson JT, Marcus S, Glaser BM. Vitrectomy for macular pucker after treatment of retinal tears or retinal detachment. *Arch Ophthalmol* 1988;106:758–760.

Fisher YL, Slakter JS, Yannuzzi LA, Guyer DR. A prospective natural history study and kinetic ultrasound evaluation of idiopathic macular holes. *Ophthalmology* 1994;101:5–11.

Freeman WR, Kim JW, Azen SP, El-Haig W, Mishell D, Bailey I, and the Vitrectomy for Macular Hole Study Group. Vitrectomy for the treatment of full-thickness stage III or IV macular holes. *Arch Ophthalmol* 1997;115:11–21.

Gass JDM. (1988) Reappraisal of biomicroscopic classification of stages of development of a macular hole. *Am J Ophthalmol* 1995;119:752–759.

Glaser BM, Michels RG, Kuppermann BD, Sjaarda RN, Pena RA. Transforming growth factor-B2 for the treatment of full-thickness macular holes. *Ophthalmology* 1992;99:1162–1173.

Hikichi T, Yoshida A, Trempe CL. Course of vitreomacular traction syndrome. *Am J Ophthalmol* 1995;119:55–61.

Klein BR, Hiner CJ, Glaser BM, Murphy RP, Sjaarda RN, Thompson JT. Fundus photographic and fluorescein angiographic characteristics of pseudoholes of the macula in eyes with epiretinal membranes. *Ophthalmology* 1995;102:768–774.

Kokame GT. Clinical correlation of ultrasonographic findings in macular holes. *Am J Ophthalmol* 1994;119:441–451.

Madreperla SA, McCuen BW II, Hickingbotham D, Green WR. Clinicopathologic correlation of surgically removed macular hole opercula. *Am J Ophthalmol* 1995;120:197–207.

Margherio RR, Cox MS Jr, Trese MT, Murphy PL, Johnson J, Minor LA. Removal of epimacular membranes. *Ophthalmology* 1985;92:1075–1083.

McDonald HR, Johnson RN, Schatz H. Surgical results in the vitreomacular traction syndrome. *Ophthalmology* 1994;101:1397–1403.

Melberg NS, Thomas MA. Visual field loss after pars plana vitrectomy with air/fluid exchange. *Am J Ophthalmol* 1995;120:386–388.

Park SS, Marcus DM, Duker JS, et al. Posterior segment complications after vitrectomy for macular hole. *Ophthalmology* 1995;102:775–781.

Poliner LS, Olk RJ, Grand MG, Escoffery RF, Okun E, Boniuk I. The surgical management of premacular fibroplasia. *Arch Ophthalmol* 1988;106:761–764.

Ruby AJ, Williams DF, Grand MG, et al. Pars plana vitrectomy for treatment of stage 2 macular holes. *Arch Ophthalmol* 1994;112:359–364.

Ryan EH Jr, Gilbert HD. Results of surgical treatment of recent-onset full-thickness idiopathic macular holes. *Arch Ophthalmol* 1994;112:1545–1553.

Smiddy WE, Michels RG, Glaser BM, de Bustros S. Vitrectomy for macular traction caused by incomplete vitreous separation. *Arch Ophthalmol* 1988;106:624–628.

Wendel RT, Patel AC, Kelly NE, Salzano TC, Wells JW, Novack GD. (1991) Vitreous surgery for macular holes. *Ophthalmology* 1993;100:1671–1976.

Practical Atlas of Retinal Disease and Therapy, Second Edition
edited by William R. Freeman,
Lippincott–Raven Publishers, Philadelphia © 1997.

· 22 ·

Endophthalmitis

Dennis P. Han

Endophthalmitis is a serious intraocular inflammatory disorder resulting from infection of the vitreous cavity. *Exogenous* endophthalmitis occurs when infecting organisms gain entry into the eye by direct inoculation, such as from intraocular surgery, penetrating trauma, or contiguous spread from adjacent tissues. *Endogenous* endophthalmitis occurs when infectious agents are hematogenously disseminated into the eye from a distant focus of infection or during transient bacteremia or fungemia. Treatment strategies differ between these two main forms of endophthalmitis. In exogenous endophthalmitis, the infection is initially localized to the vitreous cavity and adjacent ocular structures, and antimicrobial therapy administered directly at the site of infection constitutes the mainstay of treatment. In contrast, treatment of endogenous endophthalmitis must address systemic, as well as local, sites of infection.

Progressive vitritis is a hallmark of any form of endophthalmitis. Histologically, there is massive infiltration of the vitreous cavity with inflammatory cells, primarily neutrophils (Fig. 1). In most instances, vitreous infiltration is accompanied by progressive intraocular inflammation associated with loss of vision, pain, and hypopyon. Further progression may lead to panophthalmitis, corneal infiltration and perforation, orbital cellulitis, and phthisis bulbi. Common forms of endophthalmitis and their management strategies are described below.

ACUTE POSTOPERATIVE BACTERIAL ENDOPHTHALMITIS

Acute postoperative endophthalmitis, which is one of the most feared complications following ocular surgery, may occur after any type of intraocular surgery or as a complication of inadvertent globe penetration during extraocular procedures. Procedures that have been associated with endophthalmitis include cataract extraction, glaucoma surgery, penetrating keratoplasty, strabismus surgery, radial keratotomy, drainage of subretinal fluid, pars plana vitrectomy, and postoperative suture removal.

Cataract surgery is the most common intraocular procedure performed in the United States, resulting in more than 1,000 cases of endophthalmitis per year (1). The incidence of endophthalmitis after cataract extraction is approximately 0.1%. Bacteria are the most common infecting agents, although fungal infection may also occur, particularly in association with the use of contaminated ocular irrigation fluids (2). Table 1 shows the various agents responsible for acute postoperative endophthalmitis occurring within 6 weeks of cataract or secondary lens implantation surgery in the Endophthalmitis Vitrectomy Study (EVS) (3). Numerous studies suggest that the patients' own flora are the source of the infection and that introduction of organisms into the eye occurs at the time of surgery (4,5).

Most patients present with postoperative endophthalmitis within 1–2 weeks of surgery, often within a few days. However, patients may present several weeks or more after surgery as a result of infection with organisms of relatively low virulence such as *Propionibacterium acnes*, *Staphylococcus epidermidis*, or fungi. Other causes of delayed presentation include wound dehiscence, inadvertent filtering bleb, suture abscess or postoperative suture removal (Fig. 2), and the vitreous wick syndrome (Fig. 3). Erosion through overlying conjunctiva by scleral sutures fixating posterior chamber intraocular lenses may also be associated with endophthalmitis.

Symptoms of acute postoperative bacterial endophthalmitis include blurred vision, pain, ocular redness, and lid swelling. Any patient who develops unexplained visual loss or pain soon after cataract surgery should be suspected of having endophthalmitis. The absence of pain does not exclude the possibility of endophthalmitis; one-fourth of patients in the EVS did not experience ocular discomfort.

Clinical signs of endophthalmitis include decreased visual acuity, vitreous opacification, hypopyon (Fig. 2A), chemo-

D.P. Han, M.D.: Department of Ophthalmology, Medical College of Wisconsin, Milwaukee, WI 53226.

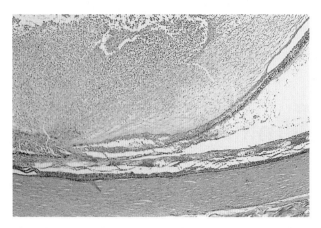

FIG. 1. Histopathology of an enucleated eye with advanced acute bacterial endophthalmitis demonstrates severe infiltration of the retina, choroid, subretinal space, and vitreous cavity with inflammatory cells (primarily neutrophils). (Courtesy of Kenneth B. Simons, M.D., Medical College of Wisconsin, Milwaukee, WI.)

TABLE 1. *Microbiologic spectrum of bacterial isolates in the Endophthalmitis Vitrectomy Study (3)*

Organism type	Percent[a]
Gram-positive, coagulase-negative micrococci	70.0
Other gram-positive organisms	24.2
Staphylococcus aureus	9.9
Streptococcus spp.	
Viridans streptococci	3.7
S. pneumoniae	2.2
Other streptococci	3.1
Enterococcus spp.	2.2
Miscellaneous	3.1
Gram-negative organisms	5.9

[a] Figures represent number of isolates as a proportion of 323 isolates with confirmed growth obtained from 291 of the 420 enrolled patients.

sis, lid edema, and corneal edema or infiltration (Fig. 4). Retinal periphlebitis may be the earliest sign (Fig. 5) (6). However, any eye with inflammation greater than the usual clinical course should be suspected of having endophthalmitis. Such cases should be referred to a vitreoretinal specialist for evaluation or, in questionable cases, be observed at frequent intervals until the clinical course can be determined. In some cases, a follow-up examination later in the same day may be appropriate. The differential diagnosis of infectious endophthalmitis includes inflammation from a retained lens nucleus, hypopyon uveitis (for example, Behçet's disease or rifabutin toxicity), corneal ulcer or infiltrate with secondary hypopyon, and "toxic lens syndrome" associated with residual compounds left on the intraocular lens.

When endophthalmitis is diagnosed, treatment must be initiated without delay to prevent severe, irreversible visual loss. In one study, delay of treatment for more than 24 hours was associated with a loss of light perception in 70% of cases compared with 25% when treatment was begun sooner (7). Treatment should be initiated when a clinical diagnosis of endophthalmitis is made, usually before culture results are available.

Ultrasound evaluation of the globe should be performed if significant media opacification prevents an adequate view of the fundus. Findings consistent with endophthalmitis include dispersed vitreous opacities from associated vitritis and, in advanced cases, chorioretinal thickening (Fig. 6). These may be detected with either A-scan or B-scan techniques. In cases with anterior loci of infection (for example, infected cataract wound or filtration bleb), the vitreous opacities may be concentrated more anteriorly. The ultrasound examination should also rule out associated retinal or choroidal detachment, dislocated lens material, or retained foreign bodies, which may influence management.

Management of acute postoperative endophthalmitis consists principally of (a) acquiring aqueous and vitreous specimens for culture and gram stain (Fig. 7), (b) injecting intra-

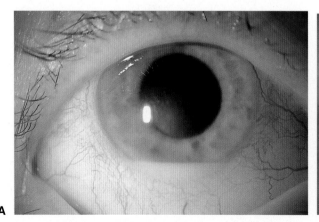

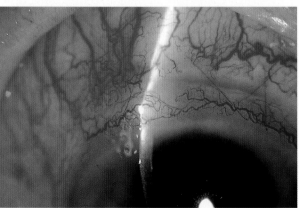

FIG. 2. A: Endophthalmitis with hypopyon formation and reduced vision following previous cataract extraction and suture fragment removal. **B:** The same eye as in A, with a suture abscess at trimmed end of the running suture. Cultures from the abscess grew *Staphylococcus aureus*.

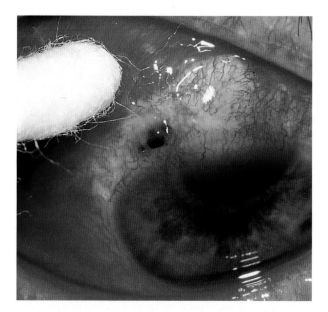

FIG. 3. Vitreous wick syndrome. Endophthalmitis is associated with a wick of vitreous and uveal tissue incarcerated in the cataract wound. Bacteria may enter the eye through the fistula at the site of incarceration.

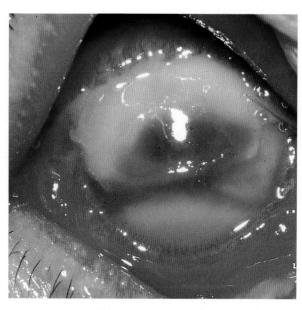

FIG. 4. Corneal infiltration and hypopyon in postoperative *Proteus* endophthalmitis. (Courtesy of Robert A. Hyndiuk, M.D., Medical College of Wisconsin, Milwaukee, WI.)

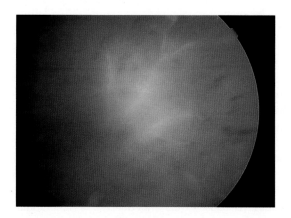

FIG. 5. Periphlebitis and vitritis in a patient with postoperative bacterial endophthalmitis. Sheathing of retinal venules and retinal hemorrhages are present.

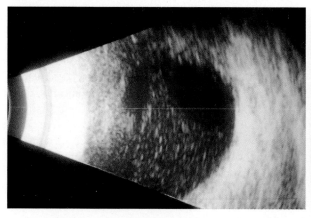
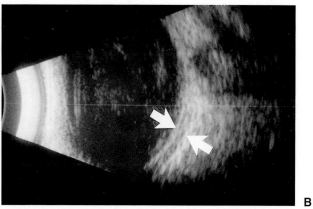

FIG. 6. A: B-scan ultrasound of an eye with endophthalmitis shows dispersed, mobile opacities in the vitreous cavity. **B:** The same eye as in A. With progression of endophthalmitis, retinochoroidal thickening has become evident posteriorly (*between the arrows*). Vitreous opacities remain but are less visible because of the lower tissue sensitivity setting.

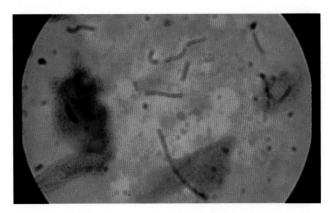

FIG. 7. Gram stain showing gram-positive cocci in chains in a patient with streptococcal endophthalmitis. (Courtesy of Robert A. Hyndiuk, M.D., Medical College of Wisconsin, Milwaukee, WI.)

vitreal and periocular antibiotics, and (c) performing therapeutic vitrectomy in selected cases. Obtaining an aqueous specimen alone for microbiologic study is not sufficient because of its lower yield relative to the vitreous. If possible, both specimens should be obtained, since each adds significantly to the overall yield. Intravitreal antibiotic injection should not be delayed until the results of cultures are available. Administration of subconjunctival or sub-Tenon's antibiotics without intravitreal injection is generally ineffective in established cases of endophthalmitis.

Aqueous and vitreous specimens may be obtained at the time of pars plana vitrectomy, in the event that it is indicated (see below). Otherwise, a limited procedure is required to obtain these specimens. Retrobulbar anesthesia may be necessary but must be administered cautiously in the presence of a recent ocular surgical wound. The eye is surgically prepped with Betadine (povidone–iodine) 5% solution and rinsed thoroughly with sterile Balanced Salt Solution or normal saline to remove residual antiseptic from the ocular surface. A surgical drape, lid speculum, and operating microscope may be used. A 30-gauge needle attached to a tuberculin syringe is inserted through the limbus into the anterior chamber, and an aqueous specimen is aspirated without collapsing the anterior chamber. A quantity of approximately 0.1 ml can usually be obtained. A vitreous specimen may be obtained either by vitreous needle tap or by vitreous biopsy with a cutting/aspirating probe. Vitreous biopsy is the author's preferred method. After conjunctival incision, a vitrectomy probe attached to a tuberculin syringe is inserted into the vitreous cavity through a sclerotomy incision placed 3 mm posterior to the limbus. Approximately 0.1–0.3 ml of vitreous is removed from the anterior vitreous cavity by using the automated cutting mechanism of the probe and slow, manual aspiration into the syringe. The alternate method, vitreous needle tap, is performed by inserting a 27- to 22-gauge needle attached to a tuberculin syringe into the vitreous cavity through the pars plana, and slowly aspirating a similar volume of fluid vitreous. If no fluid vitreous can be obtained with a needle tap, a vitreous biopsy must be performed instead to avoid aspirating formed vitreous. After the aqueous and vitreous specimens are obtained, intravitreal antibiotics are injected, and the pars plana entry sites and conjunctiva are sutured closed if necessary.

If the eye is hypotonous after these procedures, sterile Balanced Salt Solution should be injected to normalize the intraocular pressure. Subconjunctival and topical antimicrobials and corticosteroids are also initiated at this time. Topical antimicrobials are continued for at least 1 week, or longer, depending on the clinical circumstances (for example, wound infection or stitch abscess). Topical cycloplegic agents are also important to reduce the risk of posterior synechiae.

Antimicrobial therapy should be directed at both gram-negative and gram-positive bacteria. In cases of suspected fungal endophthalmitis, intravitreal antifungal agents should be administered. A list of these agents and their respective dosages and methods of delivery is presented in the Table 2, which also indicates drugs chosen by the EVS for treatment of acute bacterial endophthalmitis. Potential complications relating to intravitreal antimicrobial therapy include inadvertent overdosage from mixing error, macular infarction, corneal opacification, and loss of retinal function as measured by electroretinography.

The role of immediate pars plana vitrectomy for bacterial endophthalmitis after cataract or secondary intraocular lens implantation surgery was also evaluated by the EVS (8). Immediate pars plana vitrectomy was beneficial only for patients who presented with severe visual loss to the level of light perception only, which constituted one-fourth of patients. In contrast, there was no advantage to immediate vitrectomy over vitreous tap/biopsy in patients with hand-motions visual acuity or better. In the EVS, however, patients not doing well 36–60 hours after vitreous tap/biopsy underwent delayed vitrectomy and reinjection of intravitreal antibiotics. [Because of the importance of assessing initial visual acuity, it was recommended that the ophthalmologist be directly involved in visual acuity measurement. Hand-motions visual acuity required that the patient correctly identify four of five presentations of a moving hand at a distance of 2 feet from the patient (8).]

Intravenous antimicrobial therapy for postoperative bacterial endophthalmitis after cataract surgery was found to be of no benefit in the EVS. The role of direct injection of intraocular corticosteroids in acute bacterial endophthalmitis is controversial. A recommended intraocular dosage of dexamethasone is 400 μg [0.1 ml of Decadron (dexamethasone) 4/mg/ml solution]. Experimentally, a beneficial effect from intravitreal dexamethasone was observed in rabbit eyes infected with toxin-nonproducing organisms, but none was observed in eyes infected with cytolytic toxin-producing organisms (9). These observations suggest that measures other than corticosteroids may be needed to counter the destructive effects of elaborated toxins. In most cases of acute postoperative endophthalmitis, the intraocular lens need not be removed as part of routine treatment.

TABLE 2. *Topical, subconjunctival, and intraocular dosages of selected antibiotics used in the treatment of endophthalmitis*

	Topical	Subconjunctival	Intravitreal
Amikacin	20 mg/ml[a]	40 mg	400 μg[a]
Amphotericin B	0.15–0.5%	—	5–10 μg
Ampicillin	50 mg/ml	100 mg	5 mg
Cefamandole	50 mg/ml	75 mg	2 mg
Cefazolin	50 mg/mg	100 mg	2.25 mg
Ceftazidime	50 mg/ml	100 mg[a]	2.25 mg
Clindamycin	—	30 mg	250 μg
Gentamicin	10–20 mg/ml	20 mg	200 μg
Methicillin	1% solution	100 mg	2 mg
Miconazole	10 mg/ml	5 mg	25 μg
Tobramycin	8–15 mg/ml	20 mg	200 μg
Vancomycin	50 mg/ml[a]	25 mg[a]	1 mg[a]

[a] Drugs used in the Endophthalmitis Vitrectomy Study (8).

For postoperative endophthalmitis following cataract surgery, the prognosis is generally good, due to the predominance of infection with organisms of relatively low virulence, such as *Staphylococcus epidermidis* and other gram-positive, coagulase-negative micrococci, which constitute approximately 50% of cases. Approximately 80% of patients infected with these organisms may be expected to achieve visual acuity of 20/100 or better, and 60% may achieve visual acuity of 20/40 or better (8). Culture-negative cases have a similar prognosis. In contrast, patients infected with gram negatives, *Staphylococcus aureus*, and streptococci may be expected to achieve visual acuity of 20/100 or better in only 30%–50%. These toxin-producing organisms are more likely to cause irreversible retinal or optic nerve damage. Despite treatment, permanent visual loss may result from macular pigmentary degeneration, macular edema, macular ischemia, epiretinal membrane formation, optic nerve damage, corneal opacification, or retinal detachment.

MICROBIOLOGIC EVALUATION OF ENDOPHTHALMITIS

Aqueous and vitreous specimens should be submitted for aerobic, anaerobic, and fungal cultures. Inoculation of culture media by the surgeon within minutes of obtaining specimens is ideal to maximize recovery of organisms. Aerobes are best isolated with chocolate and blood agars incubated in air enriched with 5%–10% CO_2 or in liquid media (for example, brain–heart infusion and thioglycolate) incubated at 37°C. Anaerobes may be recovered with broths of chopped-meat glucose or thioglycolate enriched with hemin and vitamin K or by blood agar incubated anaerobically at 37°C. A spinal needle should be used to inject the specimen deeply into liquid media. Residual specimen trapped in the dead space of the needle may be flushed out by aspirating the liquid media in and out of the needle at the end of injection. Anaerobic cultures should be kept for at least 14 days to recover slow-growing species (for example, *P. acnes*). Fungi may be recovered with Sabouraud's dextrose agar incubated aerobically at room temperature and kept for several weeks.

Alternative methods of culturing organisms include injection of specimens into aerobic and anaerobic blood culture bottles and various automated techniques that continuously monitor for growth. Because ocular specimens obtained from eyes with endophthalmitis are small, the ophthalmologist must select culture media with the greatest chance of successful yield. If unusual organisms are suspected, consultation with the microbiologist is important to choose the best technique available in the laboratory.

Cultures results may determine subsequent intravitreal antimicrobial therapy in cases responding poorly to initial treatment. In such cases, reinjection of antibiotic may be required, at which time the culture results and susceptibilities from the initial specimen may help to determine appropriate therapy. However, in vitro tests alone should not be used to judge whether reinjection should be considered, since levels of antibiotics achieved with intravitreal injection may far exceed the laboratory thresholds used to judge resistance. Reinjection may also be associated with an increased risk of retinal toxicity to the injected medication.

CHRONIC POSTOPERATIVE ENDOPHTHALMITIS

Chronic postoperative endophthalmitis is a low-grade inflammation that occurs due to infection with a variety of indolent microorganisms after intraocular surgery. It may result from infection with *P. acnes*, *Corynebacterium* species, *Staphylococcus epidermidis*, other gram-positive, coagulase-negative micrococci, or fungi. A prototypic organism, *P. acnes*, is an anaerobic, gram-positive, pleomorphic *Bacillus* that has been observed to have adjuvantlike properties in enhancing lens-induced granulomatous uveitis. Such organisms may sequester in the capsular bag, where they may incite chronic inflammation, and require surgical excision to effect a cure. Because *P. acnes* has only been recently recognized as a definitive pathogen in chronic postoperative endophthalmitis (10), previously described cases of "sterile" endophthalmitis might have actually represented *P. acnes* infection.

Chronic postoperative endophthalmitis may be associated with mild or no pain and minimal or no conjunctival hyperemia and may begin within a few days or up to several months after surgery. In these cases, a low-grade inflammation or granulomatous uveitis may develop, which is initially or partially responsive to corticosteroids. Notably, *P. acnes* infection has also been associated with residual lens material or a white, indistinct plaque on the lens capsule that represents the sequestered organisms (Fig. 8). In this condition, extremely late presentations may occur if yttrium–aluminum–Garnet capsulotomy is performed, presumably freeing sequestered organisms from disrupted lens capsule that subsequently incite an inflammatory response.

In addition to the usual measures taken for postoperative endophthalmitis, adjunctive therapy may be required for chronic postoperative endophthalmitis. Management of *P. acnes* infection consists of initial pars plana vitrectomy and capsulectomy to excise involved portions of the posterior capsule, accompanied by intravitreal (possibly intracapsular) injection of vancomycin or an alternative drug. Postoperative topical corticosteroids are administered and gradually tapered. If there is no response, more aggressive intervention with repeat vitrectomy, complete capsulectomy, intraocular lens removal, and reinjection of antibiotics may be required. In some instances, low-grade inflammation may be recalcitrant and require many weeks of topical anti-inflammatory therapy. Similar measures may be needed for chronic infection from other indolent organisms.

Microbiologic evaluation of chronic postoperative endophthalmitis should involve the usual methods, plus special measures to recover anaerobes. Vitreous and capsulectomy specimens may be best cultured anaerobically by inoculating

deeply the appropriate broth media (chopped meat or thioglycolate enriched with hemin and vitamin K). If specimen size permits, sectioning of a portion of the capsular tissue for histologic evaluation may be helpful. Culture media should be incubated for at least 14 days to allow recovery of slow-growing organisms. Fungal cultures should also be obtained and kept for several weeks.

FILTERING BLEB-ASSOCIATED ENDOPHTHALMITIS

Filtering bleb-associated endophthalmitis typically occurs months to years after glaucoma filtration surgery or development of an inadvertent filtration bleb. The incidence of late-onset, posttrabeculectomy endophthalmitis is estimated at 0.2%–1.8% (11). Presumably, bacteria enter the eye through the filtering bleb rather than being introduced into the eye at the time of surgery. A conjunctivitis or contact lens wear in the presence of a filtration bleb may be risk factors for endophthalmitis.

In contrast to acute postoperative endophthalmitis after cataract surgery, in which a majority of cases involve gram-positive, coagulase-negative micrococcal infection, the predominant infecting agents in bleb-associated endophthalmitis consist of more virulent organisms. In one series (12), the infecting organisms included streptococci (57%), *Haemophilus influenzae* (23%), *Staphylococcus aureus* (7%), *Pseudomonas aeruginosa* (7%), *Moraxella nonliquefaciens* (3%), and *Fusarium* species (3%). The difference in the spectrum of infecting organisms in bleb-associated en-

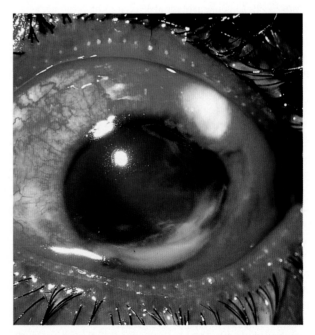

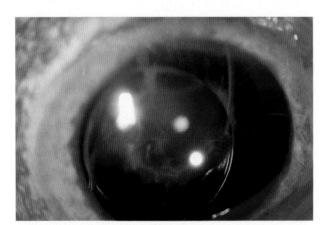

FIG. 8. Posterior capsular opacities associated with *Propionibacterium acnes* endophthalmitis in a patient presenting several weeks after cataract extraction and posterior chamber intraocular lens implantation.

FIG. 9. Inadvertent filtration bleb with development of endophthalmitis 3 years after cataract extraction. Note the severe conjunctival injection, purulent bleb, hypopyon formation, and associated meibomitis.

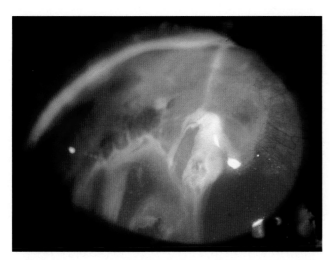

FIG. 10. Seidel's positive bleb leak associated with infected filtering bleb and endophthalmitis. (Courtesy of Jeffrey W. Kalenak, M.D.)

dophthalmitis may relate to preferential infection by bacteria that are more effective in penetrating intact conjunctiva.

The visual prognosis in bleb-associated endophthalmitis is much poorer than in endophthalmitis after cataract surgery, due to the virulent nature of the infecting organisms. In one series, only 32% obtained 20/400 or better visual acuity, and 41% lost light perception (12).

Patients with bleb-associated endophthalmitis may present with ocular irritation, redness, discharge, pain, and loss of vision. Early in its course, clinical examination often demonstrates conjunctival injection and purulent material within the bleb (Fig. 9). The conjunctiva overlying the bleb is usually intact but may be Seidel positive (Fig. 10). In the absence of intraocular infection, the term "blebitis" has been coined for inflammation involving the bleb (Fig. 11). However, with subsequent progression to anterior chamber and vitreous inflammation, an established endophthalmitis should be strongly suspected.

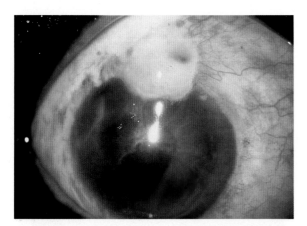

FIG. 11. Blebitis. Infected filtering bleb is present with minimal associated intraocular inflammation. (Courtesy of Jeffrey W. Kalenak, M.D.)

Treatment of an eye with an infected bleb depends on the degree of suspicion for endophthalmitis. A blebitis without significant intraocular inflammation may respond to conservative treatment with intravenous and topical fortified antibiotic therapy (13). Rarely, such cases may develop a hypopyon and be difficult to differentiate from endophthalmitis. Eyes with intraocular inflammation severe enough to cause vitritis or acute hypopyon formation should be suspected as having endophthalmitis. In this instance, vitreous and aqueous specimens should be obtained for culture and gram stain, and intraocular injection of antibiotics administered. Needle aspiration of the conjunctival bleb is not advised, since it is usually not effective in yielding a specimen and may compromise occasional late retention of a functioning filtration site. It has been recommended that vancomycin and an aminoglycoside be injected intravitreally because of their potential synergism against *Enterococcus faecalis*. Immediate pars plana vitrectomy has also been advocated to facilitate clearing of both virulent organisms and their toxins, which may cause subsequent retinal damage (13). As in acute postoperative endophthalmitis, subconjunctival antibiotics and corticosteroids, and intensive topical cycloplegia, antibiotics, and corticosteroids, are administered. Intraocular and systemic corticosteroids may also be considered.

ENDOGENOUS ENDOPHTHALMITIS

Host factors play an important role in determining the risk for endogenous endophthalmitis. Predisposing factors include intravenous drug use, indwelling catheters, total parenteral nutrition, diabetes mellitus, recent surgery or trauma, cardiac abnormalities, the newborn state and prematurity, leukemia or lymphoma, and immunosuppressed states. Endogenous endophthalmitis may be bacterial or fungal and may rarely be due to parasites (for example, *Toxocara canis* or toxoplasmosis). Treatment depends on the source of infection and the infecting agent.

Endogenous bacterial endophthalmitis may result from seeding of bacteria from any remote focus of bacterial infection, such as meningitis, endocarditis, urinary tract infection, gastrointestinal/abdominal infection, and pneumonia (Fig. 12A). It may also be associated with bacteremia without an identifiable focus of infection. Because infection involves the eye hematogenously, uveal or retinal involvement usually precedes infection of the vitreous cavity.

The spectrum of organisms reflects those of the systemic bacteremia or infection. Common gram-positive bacterial agents include streptococci, *Staphylococcus aureus*, and *Bacillus cereus*. Streptococcal infection is particularly common. Group B streptococci are observed in newborns with meningitis, and group G streptococci are found in elderly patients with skin wounds or malignant neoplasms (14). *Bacillus cereus* is typically associated with intravenous injections, usually in the setting of intravenous drug abuse. Gram-negative organisms include *Neisseria meningitides* and *H. in-*

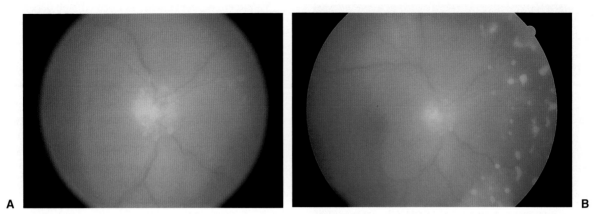

FIG. 12. A: Focal periphlebitic exudates on the optic disc remaining after systemic treatment of endogenous endophthalmitis in a patient with pneumonia caused by gram-positive cocci. **B:** The same eye as in A. Preretinal exudates remaining after systemic therapy for endogenous endophthalmitis.

fluenzae, often associated with meningitis. However, many other gram-negative species may cause endophthalmitis, typically as a result of dissemination from the urinary or gastrointestinal tract. In immunosuppressed patients or patients with AIDS, a variety of opportunistic organisms, such as *Nocardia*, an acid-fast filamentous bacteria (Fig. 13), may infect the choroid and eventually cause endophthalmitis. *Staphylococcus epidermidis* rarely causes endogenous endophthalmitis, in contradistinction to its prominent role in postoperative endophthalmitis.

Fungi are a common cause of endogenous endophthalmitis, particularly *Candida albicans*, which commonly infects the immunosuppressed, high-risk patient. Other common organisms include *Aspergillus*, *Cryptococcus*, and *Fusarium*. Intravenous drug abusers, premature infants, and patients who have undergone recent abdominal surgery are at particular risk of developing fungal endophthalmitis. Infection may begin as a focal chorioretinitis (Fig. 14), followed by vitritis and endophthalmitis. In early stages, little inflammation may be seen, and white–gray infiltrates may be visible in the fundi. Patients with multiple episodes of candidemia,

infection with *C. albicans* (versus non-*C. albicans species*), or who are immunosuppressed are at particular risk of developing intraocular candidiasis (15).

Patients with endogenous endophthalmitis of any cause often present with symptoms and signs of systemic infection, associated with floaters, visual loss, ocular redness, or pain. Endophthalmitis may develop while the patient is hospitalized for treatment of the systemic infection. Ocular findings may include lid edema, conjunctival injection, corneal haze, keratic precipitates, hypopyon, iris abscesses, chorioretinal infiltrates, vitreous opacification, choroidal abscess, and panophthalmitis. As in other forms of endophthalmitis, the diagnosis must usually be made clinically, because of the necessary wait for culture results to become positive.

Treatment of endogenous bacterial or fungal intraocular infection depends on whether there is localized chorioretinal involvement or whether the vitreous has become involved. Focal bacterial or fungal chorioretinitis or focal anterior uveal involvement (for example, iris microabscess) may respond to systemic antimicrobial therapy alone because of high levels of drug that can be obtained at the site of infec-

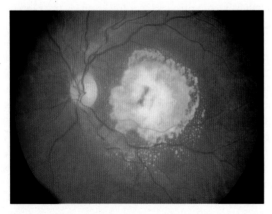

FIG. 13. *Nocardia* chorioretinal infiltrate in an immunosuppressed 9-year-old bone marrow transplant patient with acute lymphocytic leukemia.

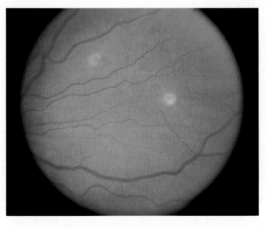

FIG. 14. *Candida* chorioretinal infiltrates in a patient with candidemia from an indwelling Hickman catheter.

tion with this method of drug delivery. Some cases with focal chorioretinitis and associated mild vitreous haze have been noted to respond to systemic therapy. If progressive or severe vitreous opacification is noted, however, endophthalmitis must be presumed, and both aqueous and vitreous specimens should be obtained for microbiologic study. In bacterial cases, direct intravitreal injection of an appropriate antimicrobial agent should be administered. Vitrectomy should be strongly considered because of the predominance of virulent organisms, such as the exotoxin-producing streptococci and *B. cereus*. In most cases, the infecting organism must initially be presumed to be that causing the systemic infection. Culture results from systemic sources may determine initial empiric antibiotic therapy directed at the eye. Intensive topical corticosteroid therapy and cycloplegia should also be administered to prevent inflammatory ocular sequelae.

In endogenous endophthalmitis caused by fungi, definitive treatment may consist of vitrectomy and either intravitreal or possibly systemic antifungal therapy (16,17). The intraocular penetration of systemic amphotericin B is poor, so intravitreal injection of this medication may be required for adequate intraocular levels to be obtained (18). However, intravenous administration may be required for treatment of systemic infection. The availability of new azole antifungal agents that penetrate the vitreous well when administered systemically (for example, fluconazole) may alter our treatment strategy of endogenous fungal endophthalmitis.

TRAUMATIC ENDOPHTHALMITIS

The visual prognosis of endophthalmitis after penetrating injury is poorer than in postoperative endophthalmitis due to ocular damage from coexisting trauma. Ocular sequelae from the injury may mask early manifestations of posttraumatic endophthalmitis, requiring a high index of suspicion for its detection (Fig. 15). Traumatic endophthalmitis may occur within a few days or up to several weeks between injury and onset, depending on the virulence of the infecting organism. Symptoms and signs include pain, loss of vision, a greater than expected degree of inflammation, hypopyon, vitritis, chemosis and lid edema, and corneal ring ulcer. Endophthalmitis may also develop from contiguous spread from an infected corneal or scleral wound.

The incidence of endophthalmitis after penetrating trauma is 2%–7% and somewhat higher, 9%–11%, for cases with retained intraocular foreign bodies (19,20). Gram-positive organisms are the predominant infecting agents in traumatic endophthalmitis. In a review of eight published series, infection was reported as being due to *Staphylococcus epidermidis* (24%), *Staphylococcus aureus* (8%), *Streptococcus* species (13%), and gram-negative organisms (11%). Infection with fungi occurred in 8% and with anaerobes in 3%. *Bacillus* species were particularly common, infecting approximately 22% of traumatic cases (20). The course of

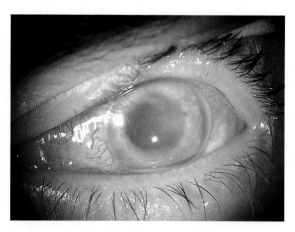

FIG. 15. Patient with corneal perforation, retained intraocular foreign body, and endophthalmitis. Severe anterior chamber inflammation and fibrin deposition are present.

Bacillus endophthalmitis is usually rapid and destructive, carrying with it a poor visual prognosis. Cases with retained foreign bodies, which are likely to be contaminated with soil, are at particular risk of infection with *Bacillus*. Tree branch injuries are notorious for causing fungal infection.

Initial evaluation of traumatic endophthalmitis must exclude the possibility of an occult, retained intraocular foreign body. If there is an inadequate view of intraocular structures by slit-lamp examination and indirect ophthalmoscopy, imaging studies of the globe must be performed. In an eye with an unclosed wound, noncontact studies such as computed tomography scanning with thin (2/mm) radiographic cuts or plain films may be appropriate. Computed tomography may be most sensitive in detecting small metallic foreign bodies. Magnetic resonance imaging is to be avoided because of the possibility that a retained foreign body may be magnetic. In an eye with a self-sealing or previously sutured wound, ultrasound evaluation may be possible. This technique is useful in determining the position of a foreign body in relation to other intraocular structures, such as the retina, and may be particularly useful in detecting nonmetallic or organic foreign bodies that have a radiographic density similar to that of ocular structures.

Management of traumatic endophthalmitis consists of obtaining aqueous and vitreous specimens for culture and gram stain, as described for postoperative endophthalmitis. In addition, Giemsa, Gomori's methenamine–silver, or periodic acid–Schiff stains may be particularly helpful if fungi are suspected. Definitive treatment consists of intravitreal injection of an appropriate antimicrobial agent. Although the exact role of vitrectomy in traumatic endophthalmitis is not clear, it should be strongly considered, especially for severe cases. Initial empiric intravitreal injection of vancomycin 1.0 mg and ceftazidime 2.25 mg may be appropriate to cover both gram-positive organisms (including *Bacillus* species) and gram-negative organisms. Like vitrectomy, the exact role of systemic antimicrobial therapy for traumatic endophthalmitis is also not clear.

Prophylactic systemic antibiotic treatment may be appropriate for prevention of endophthalmitis after penetrating trauma. Conceivably, such treatment might protect against endophthalmitis caused by an initially small inoculum of microorganisms introduced at the time of the injury. A broad-spectrum antimicrobial regimen may be appropriate in this circumstance, possibly consisting of intravenous cefazolin (1/g every 6 hours for 48–72 hours), followed by an oral agent with good vitreous penetration, such as ciprofloxacin (750 mg p.o. every 12 hours for 7–10 days). In penicillin-sensitive patients, intravenous vancomycin or oral ciprofloxacin could be substituted for cefazolin as initial therapy.

The role of prophylactic intravitreal antibiotics in penetrating trauma to prevent endophthalmitis is controversial. It may be considered for particularly dirty injuries and those with retained intraocular foreign bodies, in which the vitreous cavity has been violated. Vancomycin 1.0 mg may be an appropriate choice for prophylactic intravitreal injection because of its excellent coverage of *Bacillus* species and other gram-positive organisms. Intravitreal ceftazidim 2.25/mg may be a useful adjunct for gram-negative coverage, particularly in cases involving contamination with organic matter (21). Intravitreal aminoglycosides should probably not be used for prophylaxis in eyes without established endophthalmitis because of the reported risk of retinal toxicity.

SUMMARY

Early diagnosis and treatment with antimicrobial therapy are critical to optimize visual outcome in cases of infectious endophthalmitis. Usually, the diagnosis must be made on clinical grounds, and empiric antimicrobial therapy must be chosen based on the spectrum of microorganisms most likely to be encountered under the clinical circumstances.

Intravitreal antimicrobial therapy is the mainstay of treatment of infectious endophthalmitis. In addition, the EVS showed that pars plana vitrectomy was of benefit in patients with endophthalmitis following cataract extraction or secondary intraocular lens implantation that presented with light-perception-only visual acuity. Although the role of vitrectomy in other forms of endophthalmitis is unclear, it is currently an accepted adjunct to intravitreal antimicrobial therapy for treatment of moderate-to-severe cases of infectious endophthalmitis from other causes.

The EVS also showed that systemic antimicrobial therapy was of no benefit in endophthalmitis following cataract extraction or secondary intraocular lens implantation. Systemic antimicrobial therapy also remains controversial for other forms of exogenous endophthalmitis, for which intravitreal antibiotic therapy is strongly recommended. Systemic antimicrobial therapy may be of particular value in early cases of endogenous endophthalmitis with chorioretinal lesions and minimal vitritis, or if it is suspected that an active focus of infection is present elsewhere in the body. In most cases of endophthalmitis, adjunctive corticosteroid therapy directed at suppressing intraocular inflammation is important to reduce the risk of postinflammatory complications.

ACKNOWLEDGMENT

This work was supported in part by an unrestricted grant from Research to Prevent Blindness, Inc., New York, NY, U.S.A.

REFERENCES

1. Menikoff JA, Speaker MG, Marmor M, Raskin EM. A case control study of risk factors for postoperative endophthalmitis. *Ophthalmology* 1991;98:1761–1768.
2. McCray E, Rampell N, Solomon SL, Bond WW, Martone WJ, O'Day D. Outbreak of *Candida parapsilosis* endophthalmitis after cataract extraction and intraocular lens implantation. *J Clin Microbiol* 1986;24: 625–628.
3. Han DP, Wisniewski SR, Wilson LA, et al., and the Endophthalmitis Vitrectomy Study Group. Spectrum and susceptibilities of microbiologic isolates in the Endophthalmitis Vitrectomy Study. *Am J Ophthalmol* 1996;122:1–7.
4. Speaker MG, Milch FA, Shah MK, Eisner W, Kreiswirth BN. Role of external bacterial flora in the pathogenesis of acute postoperative endophthalmitis. *Ophthalmology* 1991;98:639–649.
5. Dickey JB, Thompson KD, Jay WM. Anterior chamber aspirate cultures after uncomplicated cataract surgery. *Am J Ophthalmol* 1991; 112:278–282.
6. Packer AJ, Weingeist TA, Abrams GW. Retinal periphlebitis as an early sign of bacterial endophthalmitis. *Am J Ophthalmol* 1983;96: 66–71.
7. Puliafito CA, Baker AS, Haaf J, Foster CS. Infectious endophthalmitis. *Ophthalmology* 1982;89:921–929.
8. Endophthalmitis Vitrectomy Study Group. Results of the Endophthalmitis Vitrectomy Study: a randomized trial of immediate vitrectomy and of intravenous antibiotics for the treatment of postoperative bacterial endophthalmitis. *Arch Ophthalmol* 1995;113:1479–1496.
9. Jett BD, Jensen HG, Atkuri RV, Gilmore MS. Evaluation of therapeutic measures for treating endophthalmitis caused by isogenic toxin-producing and toxin-nonproducing *Enterococcus faecalis* strains. *Invest Ophthalmol Vis Sci* 1995;36:9–15.
10. Meisler DM, Palestine AG, Vastine DW, et al. Chronic *Propionibacterium* endophthalmitis after extracapsular cataract extraction and intraocular lens implantation. *Am J Ophthalmol* 1986;102:733–739.
11. Katz LJ, Cantor LB, Spaeth GL. Complications of surgery in glaucoma. *Ophthalmology* 1985;92:959–963.
12. Mandelbaum S, Forster RK, Gelender H, Culbertson W. Late onset endophthalmitis associated with filtering blebs. *Ophthalmology* 1985;92: 964–972.
13. Brown RH, Yang LH, Walker SD, Lynch MG, Martinez LA, Wilson LA. Treatment of bleb infection after glaucoma surgery. *Arch Ophthalmol* 1994;112:57–61.
14. Greenwald MJ, Wohl LG, Sell CH. Metastatic bacterial endophthalmitis. *Surv Ophthalmol* 1986;31:81–99.
15. Donahue SP, Greven CM, Zuravleff JJ, et al. Intraocular candidiasis in patients with candidemia: clinical implications derived from a prospective multicenter study. *Ophthalmology* 1994;101:1302–1309.
16. Barrie T. The place of elective vitrectomy in the management of patients with *Candida* endophthalmitis. *Graefes Arch Clin Exp Ophthalmol* 1987; 225:107–113.
17. Kroll P, Emmerich K-H, Fegeler W. *Candida albicans* endophthalmitis: results of pars plana vitrectomy without intraocular antimycotic therapy. *Klin Monatsbl Augenheilkd* 1984;184:104–108.
18. Brod RD, Flynn HW Jr, Clarkson JG, Pflugfelder SC, Culbertson WW, Miller D. Endogenous *Candida* endophthalmitis. *Ophthalmology* 1990; 97:666–674.
19. Brinton GS, Topping TM, Hyndiuk RA, Aaberg TM, Reeser F, Abrams GW. Posttraumatic endophthalmitis. *Arch Ophthalmol* 1984;102: 547–550.
20. Parrish CM, O'Day DM. Traumatic endophthalmitis. *Int Ophthalmol Clin* 1987;27:112–119.
21. Boldt HC, Pulido JS, Blodi CF, Folk JC, Weingeist TA. Rural endophthalmitis. *Ophthalmology* 1989;96:1722–1726.

Subject Index

Page numbers in italic indicate illustrations. Page numbers followed by a t indicate tables.